INPATIENT PSYCHIATRY

Diagnosis
and Treatment

SECOND EDITION

INPATIENT PSYCHIATRY

Diagnosis
and Treatment

SECOND EDITION

EDITOR

Lloyd I. Sederer, M.D.

Mount Auburn Hospital
Harvard Medical School
Cambridge, Massachusetts

WILLIAMS & WILKINS

Baltimore • London • Los Angeles • Sydney

Editor: Nancy McSherry-Collins
Associate Editor: Brian K. Smith
Copy Editor: Stephen C. Siegforth
Design: JoAnne Janowiak
Illustration Planning: Wayne Hubbel
Production: Raymond E. Reter

Copyright ©, 1986
Williams & Wilkins
428 East Preston Street
Baltimore, MD 21202, U.S.A.

Printed in the United States of America

First Edition, 1983

Library of Congress Cataloging in Publication Data

Main entry under title:

Inpatient psychiatry.

Includes bibliographies and index.
1. Psychiatric hospital care. 2. Psychiatry. I. Sederer, Lloyd I. [DNLM: 1. Mental Disorders—diagnosis. 2. Mental Disorders—therapy. 3. Psychiatry—methods. WM 100 I56]
RC439.I5 1986   616.89   85-22670
ISBN 0-683-07628-0

Printed at the
Waverly Press, Inc.

86 87 88 89 90
10 9 8 7 6 5 4 3 2 1

To my son

preface

The opportunity to publish a second edition of this text, offered to me by John Gardner, now Editor-in-Chief of Williams & Wilkins, came as a source of particular satisfaction for me. The universal wish, " . . . if only I had another chance . . . ," had been granted to me. I would have another chance to work with my fellow authors and clinicians on further defining and academically organizing the subspecialty of Inpatient Psychiatry. More knowledge had accumulated. Some practices had been changed, and some had become outdated. My mistakes, and those of others, could be recognized and remedied. New ideas and treatment approaches had sprung forth like spring perennials. Legal and financial exigencies had spread mercilessly, demanding sharper clinical acumen, renovations in care, and fastidious documentation. New voices had emerged. Old voices had seasoned. A second edition would grant me the opportunity to revise and add anew, all the while enjoying the company of my colleagues. This volume is the product of that opportunity.

In the more than 15 years that I have habituated inpatient units, as resident, staff, director, supervisor, and consultant, I have never suffered from ennui. Inpatient units are beehives of emotional intensity and, when run well, of healing activities. They exhaust and excite the staff, few of whom, especially those in leadership positions, last more than 4 or 5 years. This text was in its first edition, and is in its second, an effort to provide those hearty enough to practice inpatient psychiatry with a *specific* body of knowledge to help diminish the clinical confusion and worry that is endemic to psychiatric units.

The Diagnostic and Statistical Manual of Mental Disorders, ed. 3, of the American Psychiatric Association (DSM-III) remains the established nomenclature of American psychiatry. Explicit in its criteria, reliable in its use by trained professionals, and familiar to many other countries, DSM-III, though not the bearer of Platonic truth, is the foremost diagnostic system we have available. DSM-III is employed throughout this text. Another convention that the reader will recognize is that of the pronoun *he* (or *his*) as referring to male or female. Though the he/she construction may reduce gender bias, it is awkward and violates the rule of parsimony. Until a suitable alternative arrives, I will follow standard English practice.

This edition does not depart from its original structure of examining inpatient psychiatry in two principal ways (which are represented by the two parts of the book). The first part of the text describes the principal diagnostic disorders that afflict hospitalized psychiatric patients. Matters of diagnosis, differential diagnosis, pathogenesis, course, and inpatient treatment are the substance of each chapter in this section. The second part of the text aims to be simultaneously more general and more specific. Herein lie detailed accounts of the particular treatments, populations, problems, and resources unique to the subspecialty of Inpatient Psychiatry. Throughout both parts of the text, and the different approaches they represent, lives a unifying philosophical perspective. Disease, person, and circumstance *all* converge to create human misery. If psychiatric pathogenesis is multifold, so must be its remedies. The contributors have consequently endeavored to present as their philosophy a biopsychosocial perspective for understanding and action in psychiatric practice.

I want to begin my acknowledgments with an expression of deep gratitude to the patients, trainees, staff, and leadership of the inpatient units with which I have been affiliated. It has been a privilege to come so close to the griefs and passions of these people.

To Margaret Richardson, Sara Egan, and many other support staff go my special thanks for laboring with me on this project.

I have Dr. Gregory Rochlin to thank for helping me strive toward a curious and comprehensive "cast of mind." Once again I offer Dr. Jane Thorbeck my greatest thanks for her unyielding insistence on accuracy and clarity and for her critical intellectual assistance. My final thanks go to my contributors, who have given me the pleasure of being an Editor.

L.I.S.

contributors

Janet Abeles, M.Ed., O.T.R.
Clinical Supervisor of Psychiatric Occupational Therapy, Mount Auburn Hospital, Cambridge, Massachusetts

Eugene V. Beresin, M.D.
Director, Child Psychiatry Residency Training; Associate Director, Adult Psychiatry Residency Training; and Associate Director, Continuing Education Division, Department of Psychiatry, Massachusetts General Hospital;
Instructor in Psychiatry, Harvard Medical School, Boston, Massachusetts

Gerald P. Borofsky, Ph.D.
Director of Psychology and Associate Psychologist, Massachusetts General Hospital;
Instructor in Psychology, Harvard Medical School, Boston, Massachusetts

Harold Bursztajn, M.D.
Co-Director, Program in Psychiatry and the Law, Massachusetts Mental Health Center;
Assistant Clinical Professor of Psychiatry, Harvard Medical School, Boston, Massachusetts

John F. Clarkin, Ph.D.
Chief of Psychology, Westchester Division, The New York Hospital;
Professor of Clinical Psychology in Psychiatry, Cornell University Medical College, New York, New York

Bonnie Cummins
Research Associate, Program in Psychiatry and the Law, Massachusetts Mental Health Center, Boston, Massachusetts

Joseph T. English, M.D.
Director, Department of Psychiatry, St. Vincent's Hospital and Medical Center of New York City;
Professor of Psychiatry and Associate Dean, New York Medical College, New York, New York

Irl Extein, M.D.
Medical Director, Fair Oaks Hospital, Delray Beach, Florida

Ira D. Glick, M.D.
Associate Medical Director, Payne Whitney Psychiatric Clinic at New York Hospital;
Professor of Psychiatry, Cornell University Medical College, New York, New York

Mark S. Gold, M.D.
Director of Research, Fair Oaks Hospital, Delray Beach, Florida, and Summit, New Jersey

Thomas G. Gutheil, M.D.
Co-director, Program in Psychiatry and the Law and President, Law and Psychiatry Resource Center, Massachusetts Mental Health Center;
Visiting Lecturer, Harvard Law School;
Associate Professor of Psychiatry, Harvard Medical School, Boston, Massachusetts

Gordon Harper, M.D.
Chief of Service, Psychosomatic Unit, Judge Baker Guidance Center, Children's Hospital Medical Center;
Assistant Professor of Psychiatry, Harvard Medical School, Boston, Massachusetts

Cavin P. Leeman, M.D.
Clinical Professor of Psychiatry, State University of New York, Downstate Medical Center, Brooklyn, New York

Richard G. McCarrick, M.D.
Assistant Director and Chief of Training and Education, Department of Psychiatry, St. Vincent's Hospital and Medical Center of New York City;
Assistant Professor of Psychiatry, New York Medical College, New York, New York

Dean X. Parmelee, M.D.
Director of Psychiatry, Cumberland Hospital for Children and Adolescents, New Kent, Virginia;
Clinical Assistant Professor in Child Psychiatry, Medical College of Virginia-Virginia Treatment Center for Children, Richmond, Virginia

A. L. C. Pottash, M.D.
Executive Medical Director, Fair Oaks Hospital, Delray Beach, Florida, and Summit, New Jersey

John A. Renner, Jr., M.D.
Chief, Center for Problem Drinking, Boston Veterans Administration Outpatient Clinic;
Associate Professor of Psychiatry, Boston University School of Medicine;
Clinical Instructor, Harvard Medical School, Boston, Massachusetts

Jerome Rogoff, M.D.
Associate Chief of Psychiatry and Director, Inpatient Psychiatric Unit, Faulkner Hospital, Jamaica Plain, Massachusetts;
Associate Clinical Professor of Psychiatry, Tufts University School of Medicine, Boston, Massachusetts

Irene E. Rutchick, M.S.S.S.
Director of Group Services and Unit Supervisor of Inpatient Psychiatry, Social Services Department, Massachusetts General Hospital;
Instructor, Massachusetts General Hospital Institute for Health Professions, Boston, Massachusetts

Sharan L. Schwartzberg, Ed.D., O.T.R.
Associate Professor of Occupational Therapy, Tufts University-Boston School of Occupational Therapy, Medford, Massachusetts;
Associate Staff, Department of Psychiatry, and Adjunct Occupational Therapy Staff, Mount Auburn Hospital, Cambridge, Massachusetts

Lloyd I. Sederer, M.D.
Formerly, Director of Inpatient Psychiatric Services, Massachusetts General Hospital, Boston, Massachusetts
Currently, Associate Chief of Psychiatry, Mount Auburn Hospital, Cambridge, Massachusetts
Assistant Professor of Psychiatry, Harvard Medical School, Boston, Massachusetts

Andrew E. Slaby, M.D., Ph.D., M.P.H.
Psychiatrist-in-Chief, Rhode Island Hospital/Women and Infants Hospital;
Professor of Psychiatry and Human Behavior, Brown University, Providence, Rhode Island

Jane Thorbeck, Ed.D.
Clinical Assistant in Psychology, Massachusetts General Hospital;
Instructor in Psychology, Harvard Medical School, Boston, Massachusetts

contents

part 1

inpatient diagnosis and treatment

chapter 1

depression

Lloyd I. Sederer, M.D.

DEFINITION

Depression is the most common of the major psychiatric disorders. It has been estimated that in excess of 15% of all adults will experience a depressive episode at some point in the course of their lives.[1-3] Depression is also the most common cause for psychiatric hospitalization.[4] Furthermore, depression is widely found among medically and surgically hospitalized patients.

When depression is severe, persistent, and disabling of everyday bodily and social functioning, it is easily discernible. At other times the distinction between a normal fluctuation of mood and a depression may not be very clear. Feelings of sadness, blueness, frustration, and discouragement are part of the normal range of human emotions. These fluctuations in mood, however, tend to be short-lasting, do not become overwhelming in their experience, do not impair reality testing, and do not generate suicidal thoughts or behavior. In addition, normal mood fluctuations do not produce persistent disturbances in sleep, appetite, or motoric activity.

The central feature of clinical depression generally is a subjective experience of sadness, despondency, hopelessness, or gloom. This feeling of depressed mood is accompanied by a loss of interest and pleasure in life and its activities and responsibilities. Some patients will present with anxiety as the prominent mood disturbance, whereas other patients may present with the experience of agitation as their major subjective emotional complaint. In some cases, patients will report no mood disturbance, despite the presence of a host of other symptoms and clear cause for an alteration in mood.

A feeling of lowered self-esteem is common, as are feelings of helplessness. Depressed patients show an inability to perform even the simplest of daily tasks. They are frequently preoccupied (sometimes obsessed) with work, family, money, and their own health. They approach these matters with marked pessimism and hopelessness. In some patients, hopelessness, pessimism, extremely low self-esteem, and guilt, in concert, prompt thoughts of death and suicide.

The predominance of depressed patients show a loss of appetite and consequent weight loss. Some patients, many of whom are younger and show milder depressions, present with symptoms of increased appetite with consequent weight gain.[5, 6]

Sleep disturbance is a very common symptom of depression. Disturbances of sleep are described according to whether they present as difficulty falling asleep, difficulty remaining asleep, or early morning awakening (initial, middle, and terminal insomnia).

Many patients have psychomotor disturbances. Those patients with an increase in psychomotor activity are described as having agitation. They may be unable to remain still; instead they pace about, wring their hands, bite their nails, smoke, or talk incessantly. Those patients showing decreased psychomotor activity are described as psychomotorically retarded. These patients typically complain of lethargy and fatigue. Objectively, their body movements are slowed and limited, and there is a poverty, monotony, and latency to their speech. In some severely retarded patients, a clinical syndrome approaching catatonia may occur. In these cases, the patient is virtually mute and is without spontaneous movement.[7] Self-care slips away, and the patient shows no interest in eating or taking care of his bodily needs.

Decreased libido is a common finding in depression. The loss of libido reflects a general loss of cathexis, or energy, for living. Work, play, friends, and family are all neglected.

Difficulty with concentration and memory may occur. Thinking may be slowed and indecision frequent. These cognitive disturbances can become so marked as to appear like dementia. Patients in whom the primary disturbance is depression and who demonstrate a severe, cognitive disorder that mimics dementia are said to have depressive pseudodementia.[8]

Furthermore, many depressed patients complain of bodily disturbances involving almost every organ in the body. Gastrointestinal disturbances, headache, backache, and urinary difficulties are common. Often, patients with a mild, pre-existing bodily disorder will present with an exacerbation of this symptomatology. In these cases, the patients come to the attention of their internists and primary care physicians because of their physical complaints. Upon more careful examination the diagnosis of depression aggravating their pre-existing disorder can be made.

In a small number of depressed patients, disturbances in reality functioning may occur. These are called delusional or psychotic depressions. These patients show delusions and/or hallucinations that tend to reflect the person's sense of self-reproach or pessimism. Examples include somatic delusions or auditory hallucinations that are highly critical.

In essence, depression is a syndrome characterized by a persistent, severe, and abnormal disturbance of mood, with neurovegetative symptomatology, and with or without psychosis. The syndrome of depression has varied etiologies which are discussed later in this chapter.

DIAGNOSIS

The *Diagnostic and Statistical Manual of Mental Disorders* (DSM-III) of the American Psychiatric Association[9] offers the following diagnostic criteria for a major (clinical) depression:

1. A dysphoric (depressed, blue, sad, irritable, hopeless) mood or loss of interest in most daily activities. This dysphoria does not show transient shifts from one mood to another. The mood disturbance of depression is persistent and prominent.

2. At least four of the following symptoms that have been present daily for at least 2 weeks:
   a. Decreased appetite and weight loss or increased appetite and weight gain
   b. Insomnia or hypersomnia
   c. Psychomotor agitation or retardation
   d. A loss of interest or pleasure (anhedonia); decreased libido
   e. Loss of energy and fatigue
   f. Feelings of worthlessness, self-reproach, or excessive and inappropriate guilt (which may reach delusional proportions);
   g. Subjective complaints or objective evidence of decreased ability to think or concentrate; memory difficulties and indecisiveness without the presence of loosened associations or incoherence
   h. Recurrent thoughts of death, suicidal ideation, wishes to be dead, or a history of attempted suicide

3. This symptom picture is not superimposed on schizophrenia, a schizophreniform disorder, or a paranoid disorder.

4. This disorder is not due to any organic mental disorder or uncomplicated bereavement.

In summary, the DSM-III defines depression as a particular constellation of symptoms lasting for at least 2 or more weeks. DSM-III does allow for distinctions between psychotic and nonpsychotic depressions, but it does not concern itself with specific syndromal or etiological differences between psychotic and nonpsychotic depressions.

Nosological research in psychiatry over recent years has attempted to develop valid and reliable systems for classifying affective disorders. Figure 1.1 shows a widely accepted nosology of the affective disorders and of depression in particular. This diagnostic system provides a distinction between primary and secondary affective disorders. Primary affective disorders (whether they are depressive or manic in nature) have no previous history of another psychiatric disorder and are not secondary to any systemic medical disease. Within the primary affective disorder group is the distinction between bipolar and unipolar affective disorders. Bipolar affective disorders are mood disorders in which the patient has had a history of either mania or both manic and depressive episodes. A unipolar affective disorder is diagnosed only when the patient has had a history of primary depressive illness only.

The primary-secondary diagnostic distinction grew out of efforts to enhance research of the depressive disorders.[10–12] This distinction allows the researcher to examine the depressive syndrome on the basis of etiologic differences. Questions of reactive versus endogenous depression and psychotic versus neurotic depression do not pertain to this diagnostic scheme. The unipolar and bipolar distinctions have become increasingly important as greater specificity in the treatment of the mood disorders is gained. Research in psychopharmacology indicates significant dif-

ferences between bipolar and unipolar patient response to lithium and to the antidepressant drugs.

Over a half century ago Gillespie[13] proposed a nosology of depression in which reactive and endogenous terms were applied. These are terms that remain alive, although they are less popular and do create some semantic confusion. Klerman[14] has suggested that the term endogenous depression signifies more than a lack of precipitating event or external cause. He has suggested that endogenous depressions show certain "state" characteristics (i.e., characteristic of the acute illness, as opposed to trait, or inborn and persistent), as well as an autonomy to the disorder that renders it unresponsive to environmental alterations. Furthermore, there is data to support abnormalities in neurophysiology and specific differences in response to organic treatment for the so-called endogenous depressions.[15–17] What is clear and most important is that the biological treatment of depression is symptom specific. The presence of certain neurovegetative signs (especially early morning awakening, weight loss, and psychomotor retardation) all augur a good response to antidepressant medication or electroconvulsive (shock) therapy (ECT). Furthermore, in support of this observation, patients with endogenous depression are responsive to combined treatment with

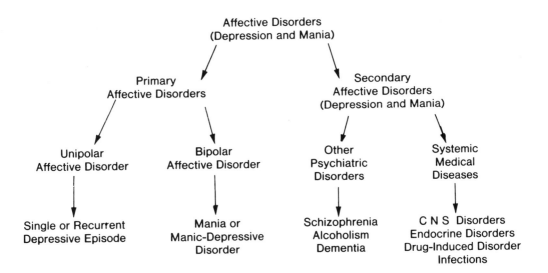

Figure 1.1. Nosology of depression.[10–12]

medication and psychotherapy but are not responsive to psychotherapy alone. On the other hand, patients with reactive (situational) depression have been shown to be responsive to either tricyclic medication or psychotherapy alone.[18]

The neurotic-psychotic distinction in the nosology of depression bears a few words. It is of crucial importance to diagnose the presence of psychotic features because this generally calls for the use of antipsychotic medications or ECT, rather than the use of antidepressants or psychotherapy alone. The term neurotic depression has fallen into disuse and appropriately so. It has come to mean so many different things to so many different people that it has lost its clinical utility.[19]

DSM-III has introduced a new term, *dysthymic disorder,* for an old condition, known previously as neurotic depression. Dysthymia means "ill-humored" and refers to an individual who is habitually gloomy, brooding, and preoccupied with his feelings. Dysthymic disorder is classified in DSM-III on Axis I (as a clinical syndrome), rather than as a personality disorder on Axis II. Clinically, dysthymic disorder presents as a low-grade depression that lasts for 2 or more years.[20, 21] Multicenter collaborative research studies have indicated that one-fourth of patients seen in clinics and university hospitals and diagnosed as having major depression demonstrate a history of dysthymic disorder. Patients who have both major depression and dysthmic disorder are said to suffer from "double depression." Furthermore, the longer the duration of the chronic, low-grade depression, the greater the probability of relapse into major depression, and consequent persistence of chronicity.[22, 23]

Akiskal's work[22-25] suggests that one-third of chronic depressions are residual symptomatic states of primary unipolar disorder; patients who develop these residual states are typically older and presumably have subaffective disorders. A second third of chronic depressions occur in early life, often the teenage years, and evidence fluctuations over time; these disorders may best be conceptualized as characterological depressions. The final third of chronic depressions are secondary to non-affective disorders, including severe anxiety disorders, somatization disorder, and disabling medical and neurological illnesses. REM (rapid eye movement) latency disturbances may aid in distinguishing characterological subtypes from antidepressant medication-responsive subaffective dysthymic disorders.

Although DSM-III did not include *involutional melancholia,* it did provide criteria for the diagnosis of melancholia. Among the indicators are excessive or inappropriate guilt; diurnal variation in mood (worse in the morning); early morning awakening; and significant anorexia and psychomotor disturbances. Significant evidence to establish this disorder as a separate entity remains to be established. However, those patients with late onset depressions do appear to be significantly different in their symptomatic profiles and more refractory to nonbiological treatments.[26]

Finally, a subgroup of affectively disordered patients appear to suffer from what has been termed *seasonal affective disorder.*[27] These patients have hypersomnia, overeating, carbohydrate craving, and recurrent depressions, with onset annually at the same time of year. Changes in climate and latitude are often remedial. Preliminary studies suggest that these patients are light sensitive and respond favorably to extending their exposure to bright artificial light.

DIFFERENTIAL DIAGNOSIS

The differential diagnosis of depression requires a thorough knowledge of organic and functional (nonorganic) disorders that can present looking like depressive syndromes. In other words, secondary depressions must be separated from primary depressions. Failure to distinguish an organic disorder will result not only in the patient's failure to respond to treatment for his ersatz depression but will also allow another disorder to progress without diagnosis and specific treatment. The failure to separate a primary depressive illness from a variety of other functional psychiatric disorders will result in lack of specificity of treatment, with a consequent effect on course and prognosis.

Organic Disorders that Can Mimic Depression

The first order of business for the inpatient psychiatrist is to rule out any organic disorder that presents mimicking a depression. It is important not to let the presence of a powerful precipitating event or a past history of depression bias the clinician against considering an organic etiology for the current depressive episode.

Table 1.1 presents an extensive differential diagnosis for the organic causes of depression. Careful history-taking with additional, collaborative information from family members, a full review of systems, a complete physical and neurological examination, as well as appropriate laboratory tests (see pages 13–15), will inform the clinician of the possibility of an organic disorder.

Psychiatric Disorders That May Be Confused with Depression

There are a variety of psychiatric disorders that may appear to be depressive illness.

Schizophrenia

Schizophrenic patients often demonstrate depressive affect or symptomatology. Further, depressed patients can have psychotic symptoms.

In psychotically depressed patients, the affective symptoms occur first. The psychotic symptoms then follow as the disorder increases in severity. In schizophrenia, the psychotic symptoms precede the mood disturbance thereby making the mood symptoms of shorter duration than the psychosis. Premorbid and family histories are very helpful in differentiating schizophrenic patients from those with an affective disorder. Furthermore, the autognostic, or subjective, experience of the clinician is one of distance and difficulty in comprehending the schizophrenic patient. In contrast, the depressed patient tends to evoke feelings of sadness and empathy. Finally, schizophrenia is a diagnosis that is made only when there are persistent thought-disordered symptoms lasting more than 6 months (see Chapter 3).

Table 1.1.
Organic Causes of Depression [a]

I. Drugs and Poisons

Amphetamine	Other sedatives
Cocaine	Bromides
Reserpine	Digitalis
Methyldopa	Steroids
Alcohol	Oral contraceptives
Antabuse	Lead poisoning
Propanolol	Other heavy metals
Opiates	Carbon disulfide
Barbiturates	

II. Metabolic Disturbances and Endocrine Disorders

Hyperthryoidism	Diabetes
Hypothyroidism	Uremia
Hyponatremia	Hypopituitarism
Hypokalemia	Porphyria
Cushing's disease	Hepatic disease
Addison's disease	Hyperparathyroidism
Pernicious anemia	Wernicke-Korsakoff
Pellagra	syndrome
Severe anemia (any	
Wilson's disease	
cause)	

III. Infectious Diseases

TB	Hepatitis
Subacute bacterial	Brucellosis
endocarditis	Encephalitis
Lues	Postencephalitic states
Mononucleosis	

IV. Degenerative Diseases

Parkinson's disease
Huntington's disease
Alzheimer's disease
Multiple sclerosis
Other CNS degenerations

V. Neoplasia

Carcinomatosis
Cancer of the pancreas
Primary cerebral tumor
Cerebral metastasis

VI. Miscellaneous Conditions

Pancreatitis
Lupus and other collagen disorders
Chronic pyelonephritis
Chronic subdural hematoma
Normal pressure hydrocephalus
Postconcussion syndrome
Postpartum syndrome
Meniere's disease

[a]Reproduced with permission from WH Anderson: Depression, in Lazare, A (ed): *Outpatient Psychiatry: Diagnosis and Treatment*, p. 259, Baltimore, Williams & Wilkins, © 1979.

Schizoaffective Disorder

This disorder may be a subset of the affective disorders, although the diagnosis has come under considerable question.[28] Family history, acute treatment with lithium and/or neuroleptics, and long-term outcome all support considering this syndrome an affective disorder. However, until greater nosological clarity is obtained, it may be best to avoid this diagnosis.

Dysthymic and Cyclothymic Disorders

The dysthymic disorder in the DSM-III is what was previously called a depressive neurosis (see Diagnosis). Though the dysthymic disorder or depressive neurosis resembles a depression, the signs and symptoms are not as severe nor as persistent as those of a depressive episode. It does happen, however, that patients with dysthymic disorders can develop a depressive episode. In these cases the diagnosis is dysthymic disorder with a unipolar depression ("double depression").[19–25]

Cyclothymic disorder is a chronic mood disorder in which the patient demonstrates repetitive episodes of depression and hypomania. Like the dysthymic disorder, the periods of depression do not meet the criteria for a clinical depression. Hypomania, by definition, is less severe than mania.

Personality Disorders

Personality disorders may present with depressive features. For example, obsessive-compulsive patients can show signs of depression when esteem is low or when a loss has occurred. In all cases of personality disorder, the basis for making the diagnosis of a full depressive syndrome is a demonstration of the presence of a constellation of depressive symptoms that have been severe and persistent.

Alcoholism and Drug Abuse

Depressive symptoms are common among patients who abuse alcohol and other drugs that depress the central nervous system. The diagnosis of primary depression can only be made after the patient has been abstinent for at least several months. Interestingly, however, depression, when present, may be associated with higher rates of relapse into addictive behaviors.[29]

Uncomplicated Bereavement

Persons who have suffered the death of an intimate demonstrate a normal human response called bereavement.[30] Bereavement may be indistinguishable in its symptomatology from a depression. Sadness and neurovegetative disturbances are common. Unlike a depression, bereavement does not tend to be associated with worthlessness and self-reproach. In addition, uncomplicated bereavement is a state that improves over the course of several months.

Bereaved patients who show persistent symptomatology for more than several months or who show severe self-reproach and persistent social disability may have developed a depression superimposed on their bereavement.

Unresolved grief is a disorder that has been recognized as a disabling syndrome. The reader is referred to Lazare,[31] for a discussion of this disorder.

EPIDEMIOLOGY

Though alcoholism and phobias are more common in the general population than is depression, primary and secondary unipolar depressions are the most common causes of psychiatric hospitalization. It has been estimated that in excess of 15% of adults are at risk to develop a clinical depression during the course of their lives.[1–3, 32, 33] Some estimates suggest that these figures are low because they are based on a research definition of depression. If dysthymic or neurotic depressions are included, the risk for depression in the course of a lifetime appears to rise as high as 20–30%.[34] Furthermore, only a portion of patients with clinical depression seek out medical or psychiatric care. As a consequence, these figures may be falsely low because of a high number of unreported cases.[35]

Incidence

The incidence of a disorder is the number of new cases in a given population in one year. Estimates for first admissions to a psychiatric facility with a diagnosis of affective disorder range from about 10–20 per 100,000. This is an incidence of 0.01–0.02%. Because approximately 10–20% of these cases are manias, the adjusted incidence for depression would be that much less.

Epidemiological findings arising out of multicenter collaborative research on depression suggests that there has been a progressive increase in rates of depression in successive birth cohorts through the 20th century. Furthermore, each birth cohort evidenced an earlier age of onset and a decrease in the magnitude of female-male ratio.[36]

Prevalence

The period prevalence of a disorder is the total cases that exist in a population in a given year.

DSM-III indicates that epidemiological figures for the United States and Europe approximate that 18–23% of adult females and 8–11% of adult males have had a depressive episode at some time in their lives. It is also estimated that the depression was severe enough to require hospitalization in 6% of the females and 3% of the males.

Age, Sex, and Race

Depression may occur at any age. Admissions to a hospital for depressive disorders peak in the age group from 40 to 60. Any major psychiatric disorder (excluding dementia and delirium) that presents for the first time in a person's life after the age of 35 is likely to be a depression.

Depressive disorders are twice as prevalent in women as they are in men.[37, 38] This appears to be true of the range of depressive disorders, with a large difference for less severe forms of depression. Weissman and Klerman[38] have demonstrated that the differences in the prevalence of depression in men and women are true findings, without methodological error or significant differences in health-seeking behavior. They begin to hypothesize that these differences are multifactorial, with biological influences (either genetic or endocrinological) and psychosocial elements (such as sex discrimination or learned helplessness) acting to render the female more vulnerable to depression.

Differences in the racial distribution of depression have not been established in studies that control sex and social class variables.

Socioeconomic and Marital Status

At one time manic-depressive illness was considered a disorder of the upper and middle classes.[39] Recent epidemiological research, however, has shown no highly valid or reliable data to indicate that depression is found in one particular socioeconomic stratum.

Several authors have hypothesized that the status disadvantage a married woman experiences is related to her vulnerability to depression.[38, 40–43] Their data indicate that married women show higher rates of depression than married men, and that unmarried women show a lower rate of psychiatric disorder than unmarried men. It will be interesting to see whether these figures sustain themselves as women continue to enter the work force, enhance their role versatility and financial and personal prestige, and decrease their time in the home.

THEORIES OF ETIOLOGY

Biochemical Hypotheses

Biochemical hypotheses of the etiology of depression have centered on disturbances of CNS neurotransmitters.[44, 45] The primary neurotransmitters implicated in depressive illness are norepinephrine, a catecholamine, and serotonin, an indoleamine. Acetylcholine has also been hypothesized in the etiology of depression.[46, 47]

Neurotransmitters are chemicals found in the brain that regulate nerve impulse transmission across synapses. The presynaptic neuron releases norepinephrine or serotonin from the neuron into the synaptic space. Once in the synaptic junction, the neurotransmitter excites the postsynaptic neuron to fire. The neurotransmitter is then inactivated by a process of reuptake in which it is taken back into storage vescicles in the presynaptic neuron. The neurotransmitter may also be destroyed within this cell by the action of a monoamine oxidase enzyme.

The amine hypothesis has been derived from clinical research with a number of centrally active medications. Experiments with reserpine have demonstrated that norepinephrine and serotonin are depleted by this drug. A monoamine oxidase inhibitor (MAOI), isoniazid, has been shown to increase CNS catecholamines. The tricyclic antidepressants (TCAs) are known to block the reuptake of neurotransmitters in the synapse, thereby delaying their inactivation. Lithium has been shown to increase the reuptake of catecholamines, thereby decreasing the availability of these transmitters. ECT has been demonstrated to result in increased norepinephrine levels.

The amine hypothesis of depression posits a deficiency of catecholamines (norepinephrine) or indoleamines (serotonin) in the neural synaptic juncture. Antidepressants were thought to alleviate depression by correcting this deficiency, which they achieve by inhibiting uptake or decreasing catabolism once uptake has occurred.[48-50] This hypothesis has undergone modification because of antidepressants that do not inhibit amine uptake or breakdown and evidence that inhibition of amine uptake does not always ameliorate depression.[51] Receptor sensitivity is now the center of research efforts as findings point to a decrease in the number of postsynaptic beta-adrenergic receptors by almost all antidepressants. The decrease in receptors has been called "down-regulation"; interestingly, drugs that increase postsynaptic receptors (e.g., reserpine, propanolol) can induce depression.[52, 53] The amine theory still applies, however, in that disturbances in norepinephrine and serotonin are etiologic and corrected by antidepressants, but by a process that involves "down-regulation" of synaptic receptors, perhaps both presynaptically as well as postsynaptically.[54, 55]

Research on metabolites of CNS neurotransmitters as well as responsiveness to different TCA's suggests that some depressions are related to catechol (norepinephrine) disturbances while others are related to serotonergic (serotonin) disturbances.[48, 49] Of these two different depressive subtypes, the group with deficient catecholamine (norepinephrine) demonstrates low urinary excretion of 3-methoxy-4-hydroxyphenylglycol (MHPG), a metabolite of norepinephrine. The serotonin-deficient depressive subgroup shows normal urinary levels of MHPG and has been shown to have low levels of 5-hydroxyindoleacetic acid (5-HIAA), a metabolite of serotonin. Though there have been claims that low-MHPG levels predict response to antidepressants that enhance norepinephrine (e.g., desipramine, imipramine) and that low 5-HIAA levels predict response to serotonergic drugs (e.g., amitriptyline), there is no consistent evidence for these claims.[48, 56-59] There is, however, evidence to suggest that patients who respond transiently to methylphenidate (a centrally active catecholamine releaser) may do better on antidepressants that enhance norepinephrine, rather than serotonin.[60, 61]

Genetic Hypotheses

Genetic hypotheses on unipolar depression have drawn their data from twin studies, family studies, and adoption studies. Concordance rates for affective disorder (unipolar and bipolar) in monozygotic twins are estimated to be 75%, whereas concordance for dizygotic twins is 20% (which approximates the morbidity risk among siblings).[62-70] Furthermore, monozygotic twins reared apart showed a concordance equal to monozygotes reared together.[71] There are no reports of one twin developing affective disorder and another schizophrenia. Data that separates unipolar from bipolar disorders among twins revealed a concordance of 41% for monozygotic twins with unipolar depression and 13% for dizygotic twins with unipolar depression.[70] The degree of difference of concordance rates is similar to that of the combined unipolar/bipolar studies, and dizygotic twins still had a morbidity risk approximating that of siblings.

Family studies of unipolar affective disorder indicate that first-degree relatives have a morbidity risk of approximately 15%. Male first-degree relatives had a risk rate of 11%, compared to 18% for females. Morbidity risk for affective disorder among parents was 13%, among siblings 15%, and among children 20%.[72-78]

Adoption studies have been developed to try to control for familial factors that are not genetic. Cadoret[79] followed the adopted-away offspring of normal and affectively disordered (unipolar and bipolar) biological parents. Adopted children of affectively disordered biological parents had a risk of 38%, and the normal controls had a risk rate of 7%.

While the mode of transmission of affective disorder remains to be established, these findings strongly support a genetic factor in the etiology of unipolar depression. The data also indicates that unipolar and bipolar disorders are genetically distinct entities and that affective disorders are genetically distinct from schizophrenia.

Psychodynamic Hypotheses

Abraham[80] was the first to psychodynamically link grief and melancholy. He stated that normal mourning, or grief, becomes melancholy, or depression, when anger and hostility accompany love for the lost object.

Freud,[81] in his famous paper on mourning and melancholia, advanced these ideas. In addition to ambivalent feelings toward the lost object, Freud considered melancholia as a "disturbance of self-regard." The melancholic, unlike the mourner, suffers a loss of self-respect. Furthermore, he described mourning as occurring only in response to a realistically lost object, whereas melancholia could occur in reaction to the unconsciously perceived or imagined loss of an object.

In melancholia, the rage experienced toward the real or imagined loss of the loved object is hypothetically turned upon the self. This "retroflexed rage"[82] is a well-known psychodynamic formulation of melancholy or depression. It helps to explain the self-reproach and loss of self-esteem seen in depression, as well as the melancholic's need for punishment. This theory argues that the aggressive wish is, however, actually meant for the lost object and not the self.

Hostility directed toward the self rather than toward the lost object has epidemiological support in the inverse relationship seen between suicide and homicide.[83, 84]

Further, one clinical study[85] demonstrated that depressed patients show less expressed anger than do normal controls.

The universality of the retroflexed rage hypothesis is, however, brought into question by the existence of a clearly identified group of "hostile depressives"[86] who show concomitant anger and depression. Furthermore, Weissman et al.[87] demonstrated coexistent hostility and depression in certain patients. Finally, the expression of hostility by depressed patients toward the lost object does not correlate with clinical improvement and may even result in a worsening of the depression.[88]

As psychoanalytic theory evolved and the ego became more the locus of study, depression was seen as a disorder of esteem.[89] Mourning was not truly for the lost object, but for the mourner's loss of self-esteem. The lost person or object would then be understood as symbolic of the individual's lost self-esteem. Kierkegaard perhaps put this best when he said, "despair is never ultimately over the external object but always over ourselves."[90]

Klein's[91] work posits that a capacity for depression exists in all of us. She postulated the "normal depressive position" as the stage of life from 6 to 12 months. In this stage the infant experiences a fall from the omnipotence of early infancy to the experience of being separate, dependent, and vulnerable. In depression there may be a regression to this former sense of helplessness with a concomitant loss of esteem.

Bibring's[92] psychoanalytic explorations focused on the ego, the lost object, and self-esteem. He regarded depression as an ego state that was independent of aggressive drives. Bibring hypothesized that the depressed person has failed to live up to his ego ideal and has suffered a narcissistic injury. In this theory, the ego's failure to attain its goals (e.g., the wish to be loved, to be strong, to be good and loving) stimulates a feeling of helplessness. It is this helplessness that injures the ego's narcissism and results in the loss of self-esteem that Bibring regarded as central to depression.

Bibring's theory is drawn from adult psychoanalytic inquiry. Efforts to apply this hypothesis to the development of depressive affect in children or to the understanding of self-esteem and narcissism in children should be regarded with caution. As the child's ego (and narcissism) is considerably different from that of an adult, so would be the experience of narcissistic injury to the ego. Bibring's theory, therefore, could not take us to the childhood genetic roots of depression.[93]

The relationship between separation in early life and depression has been considered. Bowlby[94] posited that an interruption in the normal course of development, by separation or loss, produces "anxious attachment." Spitz[95] studied normal infants, after 6 months of age who had been separated from their mothers and placed in foundling homes. He described a triphasic reaction of protest, despair and, finally, detachment which he called anaclitic depression.

Brown[96] specifically studied the incidence of childhood bereavement (parental death before the age of 15) in depressed patients. Forty-one percent of depressed patients, in contrast to 16% and 12% in control groups, had experienced parental death. The loss of mother was significant throughout the first 15 years of life, whereas the loss of father was significant between the ages of 5 and 15.

A number of studies have tried to clarify the role of separation in acute-onset adult depressive states.[97-101] The data allow us to tentatively conclude that though separation events are common precipitants in depressive disorders, separation is not a specific, nor sufficient, cause for depression.

Clinicians have been impressed, over time, that certain personality types appear prone to depression. Obsessive-compulsive personalities, for example, are frequently found in the premorbid personality evaluation of depressed patients, as are passive-dependent personalities. The obsessive's tenuous hold on self-esteem and need for the almost constant presence of external reinforcers can render him vulnerable to depression. This vulnerability is enhanced by a punitive superego which is forever ready to criticize and is unable to forgive. The passive-dependent person is always in a helpless position and, consequently, deeply sensitive to loss and self-deprecation. Empirical work has, however, brought these clinical impressions

into question. For one thing, assessment of personality cannot be accurately accomplished when the patient is in a depressed state.[102] Though there is modest evidence for obsessive and dependent character constellations in unipolar depressions, the data are strongest for the premorbid trait of introversion.[103] There is no evidence that a specific personality constellation (or pathology) exists for subjects who will develop unipolar affective disorder.

Beck's behavioral model of depression[104-107] is built on a cognition of negative expectations. Beck considered hopelessness and helplessness to be central to the experience of depression. His hypothesis is that these affects succeed, not precede, a set of cognitive processes involving a negative self-conception, negative interpretations of one's life events, and a pessimistic view of the future. Helplessness and hopelessness can only ensue in view of this cognitive set. His cognitive psychotherapy for depression, which has demonstrated efficacy, is aimed at altering cognition. Though cognitive treatment works, it remains to be established that maladaptive attitudes cause depression, rather than exist as a symptom of the disorder.[108, 109]

The clinician should be theoretically well-informed when meeting the hospitalized depressed patient. Nevertheless, as Klerman has repeatedly stated, anybody may develop a depression: there is no single psychodynamic process, personality type, stressful life event, or developmental experience that is unique to depressive states.

Family and Social Hypotheses

For certain depressed patients, the family is etiologic through the genetic pool. The nuclear family can also contribute to the etiology of depression in ways other than the cell nucleus.

In all families, models of adaptiveness or helplessness are learned. If, as behaviorists suggest, depression is a learned form of helplessness, it would be important to look for models of helplessness within the family. Further, disruptions in the family early in the individual's life, and more specifically, disturbances in the early mother-child relationship, can leave a person vulnerable to depression.

Events in a person's life or social field show a clear relationship to the development of depression.[110-115] Major losses, including death, divorce, health, and money, are frequently associated with depression. These stressful life events may, in some persons, be a necessary cause but have not been shown to be a sufficient cause for depression.

BIOPSYCHOSOCIAL EVALUATION

Biological Evaluation

A thorough biological evaluation is the first step in the evaluation of any patient who presents with depression. The clinician must feel confident that an organic cause of depression has been ruled out before proceeding with the conventional methods for treating a primary depression. Every psychiatric hospital should have access to the necessary diagnostic resources for this evaluation to occur.

The disorders to be ruled out are comprehensively listed on Table 1.1 (Organic Causes of Depression).

History

A detailed history of the patient's *chief complaint* and *present illness* must be obtained. *Past medical and psychiatric illnesses*, including any medications or treatment that the patient has undergone or is currently taking, are essential. A *family history*, with particular emphasis on inheritable medical and psychiatric disorders, is part of the comprehensive history. The person's *habits*, including drug and dietary habits, must also be included.

In taking the history, the physician must be alert to any information regarding recent prescribed or nonprescribed drug ingestion or ingestion of any toxic substance. A history of infection, abnormal neurological activity, or medical treatment of any sort must also be sought.

History-taking is done best when the patient's account is augmented by collaborative information from the family and significant others. Any person who has had occasion to witness the patient's behavior or who has pertinent knowledge about the events prior to hospitalization should be contacted.

In the *mental status examination* the clinician must search for any signs of an altered sensorium or prominent cognitive deficits. A SET test or a mini-mental status may be administered to help document cognitive impairment and to help discriminate between dementia and the pseudodementia of depression (see Table 6.3). A thorough *review of systems* must be taken. A previous history of depression only suggests that the current episode is a recurrence. It is unfair to any patient to presumptively conclude, on the basis of past history, that this episode is simply a recurrence. For sure, the odds are high that such is the case. Nevertheless, the patient warrants a thorough medical evaluation to rule out the development of an autonomous medical disorder presenting as depression.

Physical Examination

A thorough physical examination must be completed to complement the history. Careful attention must be paid to the patient's vital signs and to the neurological examination.

Laboratory Studies

Regular Studies. Complete blood cell count (CBC), urine analysis, serum test for syphilis, blood glucose, Na, K, Cl, CO_2, Ca, PO_4, creatinine, BUN, alkaline phosphatase, SGOT, bilirubin-T/D (Total/Direct), and thyroxine (T4).

Special Studies.
1. Toxic screening of the blood and/or urine for any suspected drug or toxin, including stimulants, steroids, barbiturates and opiates, bromine, lead, and other heavy metals
2. Serum B_{12} and folic acid
3. Serum ceruloplasmin
4. Thyroid-stimulating hormone (TSH), triiodothyroxine (T_3) resin uptake, thyroid antibodies[116]
5. ESR
6. Antinuclear antibody
7. Skin tests for tuberculosis and brucellosis
8. Blood cultures
9. Mono spot test
10. Serum lead level
11. Lumbar puncture with special vi-

ral studies and/or colloidal gold curve

12. Urine for uroporphyrins
13. 8 a.m. cortisol

Neuroendocrine Studies. A disturbance in hypothalamic-pituitary-adrenal functioning has been demonstrated in a significant number of patients with primary unipolar depression.[117–121] The most specific and documented measure of hypothalamic-pituitary-adrenal axis activity (HPA axis) is the *dexamethasone suppression test* (DST).

In the DST, a baseline 8 a.m. serum cortisol level is obtained. One milligram of dexamethasone is then given orally at 10 p.m. on day 1 of testing. Samples are drawn at 4 p.m. and 10 p.m. of day 2. The day 2 samples are then compared to the baseline serum cortisol studies. A cortisol level of greater than 5 µg/dl is considered diagnostic of nonsuppression.

Somewhat less than 50% of primary, unipolar depressed patients do not show the normal suppression of serum cortisol by dexamethasone. These patients show pituitary-adrenal nonsuppression or cortisol hypersecretion which cannot be accounted for by physical or emotional stress or by the presence of psychotropic medications. Hypersecretors do not show an all-or-nothing pattern. These patients show a release from suppression generally within 12–24 hours after dexamethasone administration. More severely depressed patients tend to show escape early in the day and may have a high cortisol level by 8 a.m. Less severely depressed patients may not demonstrate escape until late day or late evening, hence the 4 p.m. and 10 p.m. samples.

The initial promise of the DST has given way to a studied consideration of its utility.[122–124] Marked inconsistencies have appeared over time in the rates of DST nonsuppression in different subtypes of depression. Furthermore, rates of nonsuppression have also varied among diagnostic groups (e.g., mania, schizophrenia, personality disorders). Finally, increasing evidence of false-positive and false-negative results is accumulating. The most striking finding of a false-positive DST was in primary depressives admitted to the hospital: nonsuppression was found in the first couple of days after admission, with return to the suppressed state in the ensuing few days.[125]

Where the DST may prove useful is as a predictor of prognosis. Those patients who have nonsuppression and fail to revert to the suppressed state during treatment are more likely to relapse than those depressed patients whose DST did become normal. For those DST nonsuppressors who fail to revert, continuation on medication appears indicated.

Neuroendocrine studies are at the frontier of contemporary psychobiological research in depression. Their promise and utility will be clearer in the years to come.[126] The reader is referred to Chapter 9 for further discussion of this subject.

Radiological Studies

Regular Studies. Chest film.
Special Studies. Skull films, CT scan, brain scan, metastatic survey.

Additional Diagnostic Studies

EKG, EEG with wake and sleep tracings.

Psychological Testing

Psychological testing can be very helpful in the differential diagnosis of depression. The Bender-Gestalt and WAIS tests can be highly discriminant of organic deficits and can help rule in or out a dementia.

Psychological testing can also inform the clinician about the presence of suicidal ideation and can help assess the patient's impulsivity. A careful assessment of impulsivity gives the clinician further information as to whether the patient can be relied upon not to act on his suicidal ideas.

Psychological testing can also uncover the presence of well-guarded psychotic thought processes which, if present, may call for the addition of antipsychotic medication. Finally, psychological testing can offer a profile on the patient's personality formation, both premorbid and current. An understanding of the patient's personality is helpful in devising strategies for allying with the patient and offers prognostic information. Patients with good premorbid functioning and high level personality construction fare better prognostically.

Baseline Thyroid Studies for Lithium Therapy

Lithium can be helpful in certain cases of depression. For these patients, baseline thyroid studies done before administering lithium include TSH, T_4, T_3 resin uptake, and T_4 index (see Chapter 2).

Psychodynamic Evaluation and Formulation

Depression is not specific to any psychosocial stage of development or to any personality configuration. Anyone can develop a depression. For this reason, particularly, the psychodynamic evaluation of the hospitalized depressed patient calls for a careful assessment of the patient's underlying psychological structure.

A hierarchical model of development and psychic structure has been offered by Gedo and Goldberg.[127] They trace, hierarchize, and show the interaction among the following developmental lines: typical situations of danger; object relations; narcissism; sense of reality; and typical defenses. By examining the person from these perspectives, the clinician can assess the degree of functional organization and formulate whether there is a psychotic core, a narcissistic personality disorder, a neurotic character disorder, or mature adult functioning.

For example, does the patient typically experience danger in the form of moral (good/bad) anxiety; with self and object differentiation and the object a source of gratification; with the reality principle operant and guided by the ego ideal; and with repression the typical defense? If so, a neurotic character structure seems likely. If, however, the typical danger is separation, a grandiose self exists with magical illusions, and projection and introjection are the typical defenses, a psychotic psychic organization is apt to be operant.

It is beyond the scope of this section or chapter to fully develop and present such a model with the complexity and caveats attached to its use. It is a rich model for the psychodynamic assessment of the depressed patient who inherently fails to fit any specific psychosexual stage or developmental niche.

In addition to a developmental, hierarchical model for psychodynamic assessment of the depressed patient, there are aspects of his early life and current inner life that bear examination.

Death or early separation from a parent is a common historical event for depressed patients. As noted earlier, this is not specific, nor sufficient cause for a depressive disorder. Family influences extend beyond loss. Depressed patients often come from a family in which low self-esteem and concomitant high expectations exist and are transmitted from one generation to the next.[128] Frequently, one child is chosen to bear the parental aspirations and grows to believe that love is contingent on success. At the same time, this child, outwardly loved and protected, is asked to deny his dependent yearnings and provide a facade of adequacy and aspirations. He is urged to work hard and to not complain (deny hostility), without being provided the fundamentals of self-confidence, which entail adequate sources of early love and esteem. In time "... self-esteem depends on a combination of support from external objects, maintenance of his own adaptive capacity, and protection from unusual demands or expectations from others. The result is such a fragile balance that recurrent disruptions are inevitable, and life is series of repeated depressions."[128]

Self-esteem and depression are intimately linked. Self-esteem can be considered a self-representation or image of one's *capacity* to obtain gratification for one's needs: self-esteem is invariably compromised in depression. The ego ideal is what a person wishes himself to be like; it is an internal collection of goals and aspirations.[129] Esteem is high when a person feels close to his ego-ideal and, conversely, diminution of self-confidence and self-esteem accompany falling short of one's ego ideal (or its goals). Failure thereby can herald loss of self-esteem and depressive symptomatology.

In depression-prone people, self-esteem is overly based on continuing approval, admiration and love from important objects. A disruption or loss (real or imagined) of a sustained relationship will jeopardize sources of esteem and gratification. Depression may then ensue. In this schema, expression of hostility is dangerous, for the patient may destroy who it is he most needs. Furthermore, there is often concomitant guilt over conscious (or unconscious) hostility.

Another area that warrants exploration and understanding in the depressed patient is that of masochism. The degree to which pain is a condition for pleasure, the necessity of abuse in assuring the person that he is loved (corroborating earlier life experiences), the need for self-inflicted pain to demonstrate that one's misery is not out of one's control, and the secondary gain of masochism (compassion from others and the moral superiority of the martyr) are all aspects of masochism that can be considered in the evaluation of the depressed patient. MacKinnon and Michels[128] provide an excellent discussion of the problem of masochism in depression. They also remind us how the sufferer can torment others by the repeated presentation of his miseries.

A final and critical area for assessment is that of suicide potential. Suicidality can be assessed along two principal lines: 1) the history and mental status examination and 2) a psychodynamic exploration into the motives for suicide and the adequacy of the patient's sustaining environment.

Active inquiry into the patient's suicidality should *never* be omitted from the history and mental status examination of the depressed patient. Inquiry is *not* suggestive; the clinician should not fear introducing an idea that the patient may later act upon. Instead, careful examination of this subject tends to be reassuring to the patient for it demonstrates that the examiner is willing to hear the patient's most powerful wishes and fears. The patient is asked whether he has had thoughts about taking his life. If so, a thorough exploration of what these thoughts are, what *method* or *plan* of self-destruction he has considered, whether he has the *means* to do so (e.g., pills, gun), and whether he *intends* to act and *when*. A thorough history of self-destructive behavior and suicidal attempts should then be conducted. As much detail as possible should be obtained in order to assess whether these behaviors were high or low *risk* and

whether *rescue* possibilities were high or low.

The history and examination described above are augmented by an empathic reading of the patient's self-destructiveness. Empathy is, however, often limited in the assessment of the suicidal patient because of the patient's limited capacity to relate and to convey a sense of his despair.[130]

An understanding of the motives for suicide and their careful assessment through an accurate psychodynamic evaluation and formulation add additional depth and trustworthiness to the suicidal assessment.[131-134] The principal *motives* for suicide are murder and escape from pain. Murderous wishes must be searched for in the depressed patient. They may occur when a sustaining object (i.e., a person, job, institution) is lost, in jeopardy, or unavailable. Murderous rage can be felt towards the lost object if the self fears or experiences intense, intolerable aloneness and severe worthlessness and self-contempt. Because the sustaining object is also loved and is a part of the self (through a process of introjection), these murderous wishes may be unconsciously turned on the self to spare the loved object or to kill the object as it exists within the person. The latter case is seen particularly, but not exclusively, in psychotic patients who poorly distinguish self from other. Powerful, primitive guilt may also be stirred by this rage, thereby adding the additional suicide motive to destroy oneself for wishing another destroyed.

The suicidal motive of escape from pain must also be explored. In these instances death images can be elicited in which peace, comfort, soothing, reunion, and rebirth are envisioned.

The psychodynamic exploration into these motives will allow the clinician to understand the patient's inner life, with its wishes, drives, and feeling states. It is, however, the capacity of the patient's external world of people and events and his inner world of objects and images to provide a sufficient sense of soothing connection with others and of self-worth that are crucial. Such a capacity, or lack of it, will inform the clinician as to whether the patient may be predisposed to act upon these underlying motives. An *insufficient sustaining external and internal life* will expose the patient to unbearable aloneness and self-contempt and predispose him to suicidal action.

Sociocultural Evaluation

An assessment of the home and social environment of the depressed patient is a crucial aspect of the complete patient evaluation.

Social stressors, especially those of loss, are involved in the development of many depressive disorders. In evaluating the patient's social field, the clinician should examine for sources of stress as well as for the patient's resources. Finally, friends and work supports will be important in enabling the patient to return to prior functioning, if these supports are not invested in maintaining the patient's illness. Financial factors also play an important role in how debilitating a depressive illness can become.

HOSPITAL TREATMENT

Psychopharmacological Treatment of Depression

The psychopharmacological treatment of clinical depression is a critical aspect of caring for the hospitalized depressed patient. By the time hospitalization occurs, the depressed patient's symptoms are generally severe or life-threatening. Suicidal thoughts and behavior may be active, and environmental and psychosocial interventions will have had limited impact. Furthermore, significant morbidity and mortality are associated with untreated depression, especially in the elderly and in cases of psychotic depression.[135] As a general rule, when the depressed patient enters the hospital, he will require biological treatment.

Great advances have occurred in the somatic treatment of depression in the past 25 years. Estimates indicate that 80–90% of patients with a diagnosed major DSM-III depression will improve with a carefully chosen and administered biological therapy regimen.

Figure 1.2 is a flow sheet that provides general guidelines for the somatic treatment of nonpsychotic unipolar depression. Nonpsychotic unipolar depressions are generally first treated with a tricyclic antidepressant (TCA). The choice of whether to begin with a noradrenergic (i.e., principally enhancing norepinephrine) or a serotonergic (i.e., principally enhancing serotonin) tricyclic and which one to employ is discussed below in the section on the tricyclic medications. If a patient has had adequate dosages, evidenced by adequate serum levels for 3–6 weeks,[136] without clinical response, a variety of clinical alternatives then exist for continued treatment. Most simply, the patient may be switched to a second TCA and given an adequate trial on this second agent. Exciting alternatives, involving a briefer trial period, exist in the potentiation of TCA's by L-triiodothyronine (T_3) or lithium. Dosages of 900–1200 mg/day of lithium or 25–50 µg/day of T_3 (added to the TCA) have been effective treatments, within days, for refractory unipolar depression.[137–141]

Seventy to eighty percent of patients with nonpsychotic, unipolar depression will improve with tricyclic treatment alone or with lithium or T_3 augmentation. Of the remaining 10–30%, a small number may respond to treatment with a monoamine oxidase inhibitor (MAOI), lithium alone, or with a psychostimulant. Figure 1.2 graphically represents these treatment choices. Lithium, MAOI's, and stimulants are discussed in more detail later in this chapter. Of the 20–30% non-responders, about half, or 10–15%, will respond to ECT. These figures are the basis for the estimate that approximately 85% of patients with nonpsychotic, unipolar depression will respond to a well-planned somatic treatment program.

As Figure 1.2 also indicates, some patients may begin their hospital treatment with lithium or a MAOI or proceed directly to ECT. These are patients for whom tricyclics may be contraindicated or who already have been tricyclic failures. In some patients with an atypical depressive syndrome (see Monoamine Oxidase Inhibitors), the use of MAOI is indicated. Finally, for some patients, the immediate use of ECT will be indicated. These are

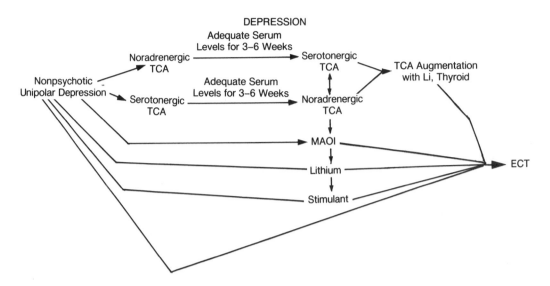

Figure 1.2. Guidelines for somatic treatment of nonpsychotic unipolar depression.

patients for whom antidepressant medication is contraindicated or who present with life-threatening behavior. This will be discussed further in the section on ECT.

Those patients who present with depression and a history of mania or hypomania have a bipolar depression. Figure 1.3 provides guidelines for the treatment of this disorder. Though lithium is less likely to provide antidepressant action than a TCA (50% improvement is reported in 1-month trials), there are several important reasons for considering this agent, if clinically feasible. First, TCA's put the patient at risk for a TCA-induced mania or rapid mood cycling. Second, if the patient does not develop mania initially, he is at greater risk (on TCA's) for developing more rapid mood cycles in the maintenance phase of treatment. Finally, if the patient responds to lithium, he will be

taking a medication that will be useful for prophylaxis as well as treatment.[142–144] Lithium and TCA can be used concurrently, as in unipolar disorders, and lithium may be combined with a MAOI. There are suggestions that bipolar patients are more responsive to MAOI's than to other antidepressants.[144] Failure to respond to pharmacological treatment, or inability to tolerate these agents, or life-threatening illness are indications for the use of ECT.

Patients with psychotic, or delusional, depressions require a different treatment protocol, which is outlined on Figure 1.4. These patients do not respond favorably to TCA alone and may, in fact, do worse.[145, 146] Antipsychotic (neuroleptic) medications in combination with tricyclic antidepressants show better results than either agent alone.[147] ECT is highly effective for psychotic depression, has a more rapid

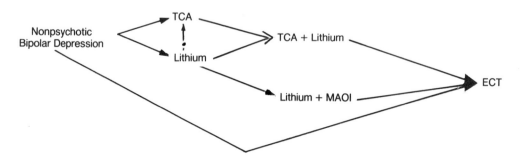

Figure 1.3. Guidelines for somatic treatment of nonpsychotic bipolar depression.

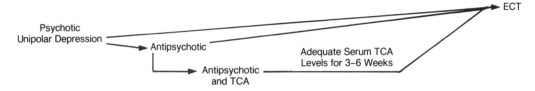

Figure 1.4. Guidelines for somatic treatment of psychotic unipolar depression.

onset of action, and, for many patients, is better tolerated than combined drug regimens.

Tricyclic Antidepressants

The tricyclic antidepressants (TCA) have been in clinical practice since the mid-1950's. They were inadvertently discovered during research on the phenothiazines. Imipramine was found to have no antipsychotic properties but did result in improvement in mood in a significant number of patients.

The tricyclics exert their biochemical effect in the synaptic space of neurons responsible for mood regulation. By inhibiting the reuptake of norepinephrine and/or serotonin, and by altering pre- and postsynaptic receptor activity, the tricyclics produce a functional increase in catecholamines and, hypothetically, an improvement in mood. Guidelines for their clinical use are as follows.

Who? Any patient admitted to the hospital who meets the criteria for nonpsychotic depression with symptoms lasting at least several weeks is a candidate for tricyclic treatment. Psychotically depressed patients tend to require antipsychotics or ECT as a first line somatic treatment. Atypically depressed patients with a symptom picture characterized by increased sleep and weight gain, irritability and sensitivity to rejection, reversed diurnal variation, anxiety, and phobic behavior may do better on a MAOI.[148-150] Elderly patients who are intolerant of tricyclic treatment or whose medical condition contraindicates the use of tricyclics may do well with a stimulant drug like methylphenidate,[151] as may older depressed patients with concomitant dementia.[152]

Contraindications. *Absolute Contraindications.*

1. Acute myocardial infarction.
2. Narrow angle glaucoma. The anticholinergic effects of the tricyclics can induce acute glaucoma.

Relative Contraindications.

1. Cardiac conduction deficits. Patients with His bundle conduction defects (e.g., bundle branch block, anterior hemiblock) are sensitive to the conduction effects of most of the tricyclics. Doxepin has had a reputation for relative cardiac safety in patients with conduction disorders, though this may not be true if doxepin is given in doses equipotent to other TCA's.[153-156]
2. Congestive heart failure. The anticholinergic effects of the tricyclics induce sinus tachycardia, which can drive a marginally compensated heart into failure. Any patient with a compensated cardiac status must be carefully reviewed before these medications are prescribed. If a tricyclic is to be used, desipramine would be the first drug of choice because it has the least anticholinergic effect. A small initial dose (e.g., 10–25 mg) of desipramine, followed by small incremental increases (10–25 mg), with regular cardiac monitoring, enhances patient safety.
3. An otherwise abnormal EKG or cardiac history. There is evidence to suggest that the tricyclics depress the myocardium in susceptible patients. In these cases, prudence dictates the collaboration of a cardiologist and the patient before tricyclics are prescribed.
4. Pregnancy and lactation. Tricyclics pass through the placenta and are found in breast milk. Collaborative consultation with the patient and an obstetrician are essential before

both mother and fetus are affected.[157, 158]

5. Seizure disorders. Tricyclics lower seizure thresholds.

6. Prostatism. The anticholinergic effects of TCA's can cause urinary retention 2° to increased sphincter tone. If a tricyclic is to be used, desipramine would be the drug of choice.

Which One? In addition to the side effects to be avoided, which are discussed above, several other factors can help the clinician determine which tricyclic to choose.[159]

1. A past history in the patient, or in a family member, of response to a specific drug strongly suggests the use of that tricyclic.

2. Side effects can be desirable as well as detrimental. Patients who show anergic or retarded depression may do better without any sedative action, but with the activating effect derived from protriptyline or imipramine. The treatment of agitated depressives may not require a minor tranquilizer or neuroleptic if adequate sedation results from treatment with amitriptyline or doxepin.

3. As previously discussed, there is conflicting research evidence as to whether different types of depression are based on differing biogenic amine alterations.[48, 49, 56–59]

    3-Methoxy-4-hydroxyphenylglycol (MHPG) is the major metabolite of CNS norepinephrine. Low levels of MHPG in the urine of depressed patients may suggest norepinephrine depletion in the brain. Furthermore,, there may be a more favorable response to treatment with imipramine and desipramine in patients with low urinary MHPG. Patients with normal or high urinary MGPG may be more likely to respond to amitriptyline, which exerts its effects on serotonin.[160, 161] More definitive research is needed before these laboratory tests become a part of clinical practice.

4. Efforts to correlate the depressed patient's response to dexamethasone (either suppression or nonsuppres-

sion) and the efficacy of noradrenergic (imipramine, desipramine) or serotonergic (amitriptyline) tricyclics have been explored and are discussed earlier in this chapter.

Predictors of Response.[60, 61, 159, 162–166]

Positive Predictors.

1. A past history of response to a tricyclic in the patient or family member.

2. Anorexia and weight loss; middle and terminal insomnia; psychomotor retardation.

3. Premorbid personality traits of obsessive compulsiveness.

4. Higher socioeconomic status.

5. A positive response (improved mood and increased activity) to a brief trial on amphetamine or methylphenidate is associated with a response to imipramine.

Negative Predictors.

1. Hypochondriasis.

2. Multiple previous episodes of depression. "Double depression."

3. Delusions. The treatment of delusional depression generally requires addition of antipsychotic medication or administration of ECT.

4. "Atypical" depression. MAOI's show considerable promise in treating this disorder, which is generally refractory to TCA's.

In addition to these negative predictors of response to the tricyclic treatment of unipolar depression, several other factors are responsible for *treatment failure*. First, and perhaps foremost, is *compliance*. An effective treatment alliance with the patient and the family and a schedule of drug administration that reduces complexity will help to enhance compliance.

A second source of treatment problems is the interaction between TCA's and other drugs. The clinician should keep in mind that a variety of prescribed drugs may lower levels of antidepressant drugs.

A third factor is the wide interindividual *differences in serum tricyclic levels* that patients achieve at the same dosage. Some patients on high dosages of TCA's may not obtain adequate plasma levels of the drug, while others, on low doses, may obtain adequate or even toxic levels. Fur-

Table 1.2.
Tricyclic Antidepressants[160, 163, 167-169]

Drug Generic (Trade Name)	Dosage Range[a]	Amine Grouping	Biogenic Amine Affected		Sedative Potency	Anti-cholinergic Potency	Desired Plasma Tricyclic Levels[b]
			Serotonin	Norepinephrine			
	mg/day						ng/ml or μg/L
Amitriptyline (Elavil and others)	150–300	3°	⊬⊬⊬	0	High	High	More than 160–200 (amitryptiline and nortriptyline)
Imipramine (Tofranil and others)	150–300	3°	⊬⊬	⊬	Low	Moderate	More than 200 (imipramine and desipramine)
Doxepin (Sinequan or Adapin)	150–400	3°	?	?	High	Moderate	More than 100 (doxepin and desmethyl-doxepin)
Trimipramine (Surmontil)	75–200	3°	?	?	High	Moderate	?
Desipramine (Norpramine or Pertofrane)	150–300	2°	0	⊬⊬⊬	Low	Low	40–160
Nortriptyline (Aventyl or Pamelor)	75–200	2°	⊬	⊬	Moderate	Moderate	50–150
Protriptyline (Vivactyl)	20–80	2°	?	?	Very low	Low	130–250

[a]Geriatric patients generally require lower dosages.
[b]Levels are of TCA and its major metabolite.

ther, the secondary amine tricyclics (see Table 1.2) (e.g., desipramine and protriptyline) show optimal clinical effect in what has been called a "therapeutic window." The therapeutic window is a plasma level below *and* above which the patient will not experience an optimal effect from the medication. The standard use of serum tricyclic levels for the hospitalized patient will help to diminish this third cause of treatment failure.

How? TCA's are available in oral and intramuscular forms. I.M. tricyclics have not been shown to be more effective and do increase the toxic effects of the drug.

There has been considerable controversy about the quality control of generically sold tricyclics. Standard brands or generics produced by major pharmaceutical firms offer the best quality control and help to ensure maximal drug absorption.

How Much and How Long? Table 1.2 describes the dosage ranges and serum levels desired for the commonly used TCA's.

Hospitalized depressed patients in otherwise good health can be started on 50 mg of desipramine or equally potent doses of another TCA, increasing the dosage 25–50 mg/day up to 150–200 mg/day or until adverse effects occur. A plasma level can be drawn and sent for analysis while the patient remains at this level or is given further increases. Adjustments in dosage then follow the clinical response and plasma level determinations. Though the routine use of serum levels in outpatient practice is debatable, the regular use of levels seem sensible in intensive, highly expensive inpatient settings.[170]

Once a patient has achieved an optimal serum level he should be allowed to remain on that dose of medication for at *least 3–6 weeks*.[136] Tricyclics are well-known to produce their antidepressant effect at least 2 weeks after adequate levels occur.

At this time the decision to continue or change medications can be made.

The problem in providing excessive dosages of secondary amine tricyclics is twofold. First, clinical response actually decreases after a certain dose, and, second, side effects increase. Excessively high doses of tertiary amines bring only the increased side effects.

When? Single daily bedtime dosage of a tricyclic increases compliance, aids in any difficulty falling asleep, and generally results in unwelcomed side effects (e.g., hypotension) occurring while the patient is asleep. No clinical efficacy is lost with once daily dosage.

Other dosage schedules may be more suitable for specific patients and may minimize some side effects. The physician is wise to include his patient in choosing the patient's medication schedule.

Barbiturates, as sleeping medications, ought to be *avoided*. They are no more efficacious than nonbarbiturate hypnotics, show tolerance, *and* increase liver microsomal activity with consequent increased TCA metabolism and decreased TCA levels.

Side Effects.
1. Cardiac toxicity.
2. Dry mouth, blurred vision, urinary retention, and constipation (anticholinergic effects that tend to improve with time).
3. Dizziness (postural hypotension), restlessness, insomnia, tremor.
4. Delirium—anticholinergic CNS toxicity that is responsive to parenteral physostigmine salicylate (Antilirium).
5. Skin rashes.
6. Allergic-obstructive jaundice.

Second Generation Antidepressants (Table 1.3)

A variety of new antidepressants have been introduced in recent years. The impetus for new agents was prompted by the multitude of undesirable side effects of the so-called first generation antidepressants. Anticholinergic side effects (dry mouth, constipation, urinary retention), orthostatic hypotension, and cardiotoxicity were among the adverse effects that led to

Table 1.3.
Second Generation Antidepressant Agents

Four Rings	Three Rings	One Ring
Amoxapine	Nomifensene	Buproprion
Maprotiline		
Trazodone		
Alprazolam		

poor tolerance and poor compliance. The principal agents that have been offered as new alternatives to the first generation drugs are amoxapine, maprotiline, trazodone, nomifensene, buproprion, and alprazolam.[171-175]

Amoxapine is a metabolite of the neuroleptic loxapine. Its mode of action is believed to be by uptake inhibition of norepinephrine and dopamine receptor blockade. The dopamine blockade, as with neuroleptics, may have antipsychotic qualities, but the efficacy of amoxapine in psychotic depression has yet to be established. Extrapyramidal problems have, however, occurred commonly and numerous reports of amoxapine-induced seizures from overdosage have resulted in limited use of this new agent.

Maprotiline has a tetracyclic structure and clinical action similar to standard tricyclics, though it is of a fully separate class of compounds. Maprotiline appears to be a norepinephrine uptake inhibitor that resembles desipramine. Maprotiline's record of seizure induction is an adverse effect that does not occur with desipramine, rendering the former as having little clinical advantage over the latter.

Trazodone is also chemically distinct from the TCAs and was introduced as an alternative to serotonergic agents like amitriptyline. It is an inhibitor of serotonin uptake and has relatively low anticholinergic properties, which adds to its value. Many patients find its sedative effects intolerable when therapeutic doses are obtained. For other patients, the sedation provides significant anxiolytic action.

Nomifensene is an isoquinolone antidepressant, differing in structure from TCAs and MAOIs. The drug exerts both norepinephrine and dopamine uptake inhibition and appears to have fewer sedative and anticholinergic side effects than imipramine and has not demonstrated epileptogenic properties. More clinical experience is needed with this promising new antidepressant.

Buproprion is a moncyclic drug that is structurally and pharmacologically different from the TCAs. Its action is as a norepinephrine uptake inhibitor and a dopamine agonist. Buproprion is a highly activating antidepressant and, while helpful for some anergic patients, is poorly tolerated by agitated patients. The drug has minimal anticholinergic and sedative effects, but has been associated with seizures.

Alprazolam is a triazolobenzodiazepine with properties quite similar to the benzodiazepine diazepam, though 5 to 10 times more potent. It has clear anxiolytic and antipanic properties. Alprazolam's capacity to "downregulate" receptor sites led to inquiry into its antidepressant potential. Though still investigational as an antidepressant, Alprazolam is demonstrating clinical efficacy. Whether this drug offers more than its predecessor, diazepam, is unclear; it does, like diazepam, have the capacity to induce tolerance and disinhibition and withdrawal states.

In *summary*, there is no evidence that the newer antidepressants demonstrate any greater efficacy than their tricyclic predecessors. Side effects accompany these new agents, though profiles may be different. There is little to suggest initiating treatment with a new agent: tricyclics should be tried first. Those patients who cannot tolerate TCAs or do not respond can then be candidates for treatment with these second generation agents.

Monoamine Oxidase Inhibitors

The monoamine oxidase inhibitors (MAOI) were discovered serendipitously about 30 years ago during research on antitubercular medications. After initial enthusiasm, clinicians virtually abandoned these drugs because of their association with hypertensive crises. In the past 10 years the MAOI's have regained clinical popularity for primarily two reasons. First, their risk has been overestimated[176, 177] and, second, research has demonstrated their specificity and efficacy in the treatment of "atypical" depressions [148–150, 178] and in some depressed patients who are refractory to tricyclic therapy. They remain, nevertheless, underutilized and hold promise for many patients.

Monoamine oxidases are enzymes found within the neuron that metabolize mood-regulating amines. Inhibition of this enzyme, by a MAOI, results in an increase in CNS biogenic amines. The two more commonly used MAOI's are phenelzine (Nardil) and tranylcypromine (Parnate). Phenelzine is a nonreversible inhibitor (a hydrazine) whose action lasts about 2 weeks after its discontinuation. Its value in the treatment of atypical depression and phobic-anxiety states has been established. Phenelzine shows a lower incidence of hypertensive reactions and is a less activating compound. Tranylcypromine is a reversible inhibitor (a nonhydrazine) whose action persists for several days after its discontinuation. This drug has a higher incidence of hypertensive reactions and is a highly activating compound that can be helpful with anergic patients.

Both phenelzine and tranylcypromine can cause hypertensive reactions when the drug interacts with exogenous tyramine and similar sympathomimetic substances. Tyramine is found in a variety of foods that have been produced by putrefaction (e.g., aged cheeses and wines, yogurt, yeast extract, chocolate) and certain medications which contain sympathetic-like compounds (e.g., ephedrine, L-dopa, amphetamine). Patients must be reliable, allied with treatment, and educated in taking their medication before the physician prescribes a MAOI. Dietary lists are available and can be distributed to patients and families.

Dosages of at least 60 mg/day of phenelzine (about 1 mg/kg) are associated with greater rates of improvement. Divided dosages with a larger portion given at bedtime seem to reduce hypotensive effects which, empirically, correlate with response to phenelzine. Tranylcypromine dosages range upward from 20 mg/day, as tolerated.

A pretreatment platelet MAO activity level is drawn by serum sample. Analysis is available at major laboratories. Clinical improvement is associated with greater than 80% inhibition of the baseline value. Samples for assessment of inhibition can be obtained after 10 days of stabilization on a given dose.

Lithium

Lithium carbonate has been reported to show antidepressant properties in patients with diagnosed bipolar affective disorder.[169, 179, 180] A family history of bipolar disorder and the presence of neurovegetative disturbances that are persistent and independent of environmental influences are also associated with an antidepressant response to lithium.

Patients who are refractory to conventional treatment and who demonstrate the historical or clinical features noted above should be considered for a trial on lithium. Furthermore, lithium carbonate can be *added* to tricyclic or MAOI-treated patients who show a minimal response to the antidepressant alone (see Figs. 1.2 and 1.3).

Stimulants

Amphetamine (Dexedrine and Benzedrine) and methylphenidate (Ritalin) may be effective in the treatment of some demented patients with secondary depressions and in other elderly patients whose medical status does not permit the use of antidepressant medications.[151, 152] Doses are administered early in the day to avoid causing insomnia. Five to ten milligrams of amphetamine b.i.d. or t.i.d. or 10 mg of methylphenidate b.i.d. or t.i.d. are prescribed as tolerated. If effective, results are apparent within several days. Tolerance does not appear to become a problem.

Combined Drug Treatment

Treatment resistant unipolar depressions, which account for about 15% of cases, have prompted clinicians to search for new methods of treatment. Chronic depression is a severely painful disorder for the patient and his intimates. Clinicians are to be encouraged to try less conventional treatments in collaboration with their patients when concerted somatic and psychosocial efforts fail.

As discussed earlier, augmentation of TCA or MAOI agents can be done with Lithium. T_3 can be added to TCA's and may be helpful with female patients.[181] A partial response to a tricyclic may be enhanced by adding a stimulant drug (methylphenidate or amphetamine).[182]

The use of a MAOI added to an established tricyclic regimen (but *not* vice versa) may be beneficial in some refractory depressions.[183] Tyrosine, an amine precursor, has been reported to show an antidepressant effect.[184]

Finally, a number of novel drug combinations and research antidepressants are being studied and employed at various university centers. Treatment resistant patients and their families can be referred to specialty psychopharmacologists when conventional methods prove unsatisfactory.

Nonpharmacological Somatic Interventions

Potentiation of antidepressant medication has been achieved by advancing the patient's sleep cycle. Simply put, patients sleep from 6:00 p.m. to 2:00 a.m. and are not permitted to nap during the day. This advance in the sleep-wake cycle holds promise because of its rapid effect and lack of biological toxicity. Patients are gradually shifted back to their normal cycle.[185]

Patients with seasonal affective disorder[27, 186] may benefit from exposure to bright fluorescent lights before dawn and after dusk. Though more work needs to be done to establish efficacy, this is a simple and nontoxic measure that can be considered for certain patients.

Electroconvulsive Therapy

Electroconvulsive therapy (ECT) is the most specific and efficacious of treatments for psychotic, unipolar depression.[146, 162, 187] Also, in excess of 50% of nonpsychotic, unipolar depressives who did not respond to tricyclic treatment will respond to ECT.[188–191] In essence, ECT offers the most breadth and the highest efficacy of all biological treatments for depression.

As a general rule, ECT is reserved for patients who have not responded to adequate trials on antidepressants or who have not been able to tolerate these often toxic drugs. Elderly and medically ill patients may be more safely treated with ECT than with TCA's and, therefore, represent possible exceptions to this rule. Severely depressed patients with active suicidal intent or catatonically or psychotically depressed patients may also bypass medications, for they may require the more rapid action that ECT provides.

ECT increases norepinephrine turnover in the CNS.[192] An increased turnover of norepinephrine increases the functional availability of this catecholamine and suggests that the mode of action of ECT is similar to that of the antidepressant medications.

ECT can be used with remarkable safety in ill, debilitated, elderly, and most tricyclic intolerant patients when measures are taken to monitor and manage any medical disorder concomitant to the patient's depression. The contraindications to ECT are an intracranial space-occupying lesion (e.g., tumor, subdural) and a history of myocardial infarction within the previous 6 weeks.

Mandel et al.[188] reported prediction of response to ECT on the basis of clinical symptomatology. A positive response to ECT is associated with delusions (somatic or paranoid), sudden onset of symptoms, guilt, mood lability, fluctuating course and, I would add, a previous history of response to ECT. Concomitant personality pathology (especially, borderline, hypochondriacal, and dependent features) augurs a poorer response to ECT.

The *work up* for ECT proceeds along two lines. First, informed consent must be obtained from the patient.[193] Informed consent is the written version of the establishment of a trusting, working alliance with the patient *and* his family. The second part of the work-up is the medical evaluation which includes:

1. Medical history and review of systems
2. Physical examination
3. CBC, urine analysis, VDRL, BUN, blood glucose, SGOT
4. EKG
5. Chest films, spine films

In addition, the patient's psychotropic medication regimen must be carefully reviewed. Barbiturates should be avoided because they affect seizure threshold. If evening or morning sedation is needed, hydroxyzine or oxazepam may be used. If the patient has been on tricyclics, they should be discontinued as far in advance of ECT as possible. Tricyclics can cause complications with blood pressure during anaesthesia and are cardiac depressants. Patients who are receiving neuroleptics should be managed on as low a dose as possible during the course of ECT.

ECT can be administered unilaterally or bilaterally. Unilateral, nondominant hemisphere treatment reduces post-ECT cognitive difficulties without increasing the number of treatments needed.[191, 194]

Generally, six treatments are given in a series, though some patients may require more to obtain relief. Patients are premedicated with I.M. atropine to reduce secretions and minimize vagal cardiac dysrhythmias. Intravenous (I.V.) methohexital (Brevital), a rapid-acting barbiturate, is used for anesthesia and I.V. succinylcholine (Anectine) is used for muscular relaxation.

The electrical stimulus is administered once medication effects are established and oxygenation achieved via an airway. Many centers try to minimize the "dose," which is measured in time and voltage. Current research on the use of ECT instruments will provide Federal standards for these devices as well as further inform clinicians about recommended duration, frequency, and waveform of the electrical stimulus.[195]

Upon completion of the seizure, oxygenation is resumed, and the patient is carefully monitored. Most patients are up and about an hour after the treatment is completed.

Considerable misinformation and mystique surrounds ECT. It is a safe and highly effective treatment for major depression. All clinicians should be familiar with this treatment and know when to prescribe it, for it holds the remedy for many patients who cannot be treated by other methods.

Milieu Management

The salient aspects of the milieu management of the hospitalized, depressed patient are safety, remoralization,[196] and education.

The great preponderance of depressed patients will get better if they do not seriously injure or kill themselves during the course of their illness. Delusionally depressed patients are at significantly higher risk for suicide than nonpsychotic depressives. Hospitalization of the depressed person often occurs when suicidal ideation or behavior has developed.[197-199]

As a consequence, the first order of business for the hospital staff is to assess the patient's suicidality and establish appropriate safety measures. The patient's possessions are checked for sharp objects or materials that could be used for suicide (e.g., drugs, belt, rope). Many patients will be able to establish a *verbal* (or written) *contract* in which the patient agrees to inform a member of the staff if he experiences a compelling impulse to hurt himself. Patients are told that in hospital (and thereafter) they can learn to talk, rather than act, on their impulses.

Those patients who are unable to form this contract may require *constant observation,* where they are always in the company of a staff member or are visible in a ward community space. Severely suicidal patients may require treatment on a closed ward to prevent elopement. Others will require one-to-one supervision to prevent suicidal behavior. The improving depressed patient may gain hope and become less suicidal *or* may acquire the energy to act on his impulses.

Remoralization is the re-experience of confidence in the self. The depressed patient has lost morale, and the hospital can serve to help restore it. The nursing and milieu staff provide the patient with empathic listeners who enable the patient to tolerate his despair. Staff, as well as other patients, offer surcease from the aloneness or guilt that can prompt self-destruction. Ventilation of affects is encouraged in patients at a rate they can tolerate.

The regular rhythm of the ward with its shelter and structure appears to help many depressed patients. Staff also begin to create expectations for dress, self-care, and meal behaviors that had waned prior to admission. Socialization is encouraged but not forced. Structured activities in the occupational therapy shop and through patient activity groups enable the depressed patient to re-experience his competence. The ward community provides an ambience of belief in each individual's capacity to improve, while gently asserting the person's responsibility to participate in his care. The depressed patient slowly emerges from his preoccupation with himself and rediscovers himself, his world, and his morale.

The milieu can also offer the patient an educational experience that can be corrective cognitively as well as emotionally. The depressed patient can learn that depression is a highly treatable disorder that affects large numbers of people. This sense of universality and treatability may be a corrective cognitive experience. Negative self-concepts, maladaptive coping patterns, and indirect or confused communicational styles all become apparent in the ward community. Constructive feedback from patients and staff can foster alternative thinking and behavior. Furthermore, the patient can rediscover that he is a person who can care about others and have others care about him.

Group therapy, two to three times weekly, during the patient's hospital stay can focus on current stresses and on ways of coping with these stresses. Interpersonal and communicational styles emerge quickly in these groups. Patients can be helped to relearn social skills and to correct relating and communicating difficulties in an atmosphere of group acceptance and support.

Individual Psychotherapy

Individual psychotherapy has a very important place in the treatment of the hospitalized depressed patient. Somatic treatments and psychotherapy complement each other in quite specific ways. Medications or ECT are efficacious in treating the neurovegetative symptoms (eating, sleeping, motor and cognitive disturbances), while psychotherapy acts as a specific and effective treatment for the interpersonal and social disturbances that accompany depression (e.g., isolation, dependence, constricted or hostile communication, rumination, and work performance).[109, 200-202]

Arieti[203] has suggested that for some treatment-refractory depressed patients psychotherapy alone is the treatment of choice. He implies that in some cases medications may interfere with the treatment process. Though Arieti's thoughts may apply in some specific cases, it is my view, and that of others,[204] that most hospitalized depressed patients require a biological treatment to enable them to form a relationship with a therapist and to have adequate energy and cognitive capacity for psychotherapy.

In-hospital psychotherapy can begin on a daily basis. Meetings may be shorter, e.g., 20–30 minutes, initially if this is all the time the patient can tolerate. As improvement occurs, the time can be increased to 30–50 minutes with the frequency of individual meetings continuing daily or decreasing to 3–4 times per week.

Conventional principles of outpatient exploratory or reconstructive psychotherapy, which entail a nondirective, interpretative therapeutic posture as well as necessary silence, should be eschewed with the hospitalized depressed patient. Nondirective, exploratory psychotherapy unduly stresses the severely depressed person and reinforces his unconscious view of unavailable, uncaring caregivers who wish to reject him.

Instead, hospital psychotherapy aims to be supportive and restitutive. The therapist should be active and persistent in his inquiry, flexible in his scheduling, friendly in his demeanor, and interested in contact with relatives.[205] Defenses are reinforced, and areas of adaptive functioning are sought and encouraged. Restitutive psychotherapy involves empathic listening, for the depressed patient wants to share his grief. The therapist must be able to bear the patient's pain with him; extra time may be needed for this affect to emerge, especially in view of the depressed patient's psychomotor retardation. The therapist needs to *not* be too warm, or too funny. The depressed patient feels unworthy of excessive warmth and tends to withdraw and feel worse when this is offered. Excessive humor on the part of the therapist denies the patient his grief and is devaluing.

The therapist wishes to convey a sense of hope to the depressed patient. This does not take the form of simple reassurance or universal optimism. The therapist must seek out and understand with his patient the underlying fears and anxieties. For example, the fear that depression is an illness that will last forever was understood in one patient to be a fear of becoming like his mother, who became depressed and remained ill for a lifetime. Only when these underlying concerns are clear can the patient be responded to, reassured, and given hope.

The hospital therapist faces the difficult dilemma of how to be supportive and even protective (in cases of self-destructive behavior) without reinforcing the depressed patient's sense of helplessness. Therapeutic directiveness and permission to be taken care of can stimulate child-like helplessness, as well as diminish the patient's self-esteem. Therapeutic efforts to foster autonomy, on the other hand, can be seen as rejection by the patient. In general, the acutely depressed patient requires dependency gratification and needs to be encouraged to accept the care he has previously refused. The therapist can indicate that the patient needs help at this time, while informing the patient that these interventions are only temporary and will change as the patient grows clearer about his needs and is more able to care for himself.

Aside from establishing clear safety measures to prevent the depressed patient from hurting himself, the clinician should avoid taking responsibility for decisions the patient must make. Most important decisions can be deferred until the patient has obtained some significant improvement in his depression. Once the depression has improved, as it generally does, the clinician can then aide his patient in carefully exploring his life dilemmas and determining his own cast of mind.

Dependent needs are pronounced and generally unacceptable to the depressed person, who also assumes that he will not get what he wants. Anger, conscious and unconscious, may develop as dependent needs are perceived as being unmet. The depressed patient often seeks nurturance through his suffering. This dynamic of deprivation, intense and forbidden dependent needs, and anger over deprivation and anticipted rejecton will live itself out in the transference (the historically determined relationship the patient will develop with the therapist). The therapist can never fully satisfy the patient's dependent needs, and anger will soon occupy the therapeutic arena, particularly if the therapist appropriately avoids taking unnecessary control of the patient's life. Anger in the transference needs to be allowed and should spontaneously lead to anger toward other important people and losses that the patient has experienced. Careful examination and working through in this area allows the clinician to promote patient autonomy and to curtail the helplessness and suffering that is aimed at securing caring. The direct expression of hostility, in therapy or with important others, has not been shown to universally result in clinical improvement.[87, 88] The technique just described regards anger as an affect that will naturally accompany (and therefore need not be provoked) the understanding and working through of dependency conflicts, learned helplessness, and the secondary gains of depression. Work of this sort can begin in the hospital, to be continued after discharge in a more explorative and reconstructive manner.

Coyne,[206] a social psychologist, studied the response of others to the depressed patient. Subjects who spoke with depressed patients felt themselves to be anxious with and hostile and rejecting to the depressed group when compared to their responses to the control population. Depressives seemed to elicit this response by persistently offering high self-disclosure statements about their suffering. Psychotherapeutic work at helping the patient limit to whom, when, and how much he shares his grief can be helpful, as is Beck's[104-107] reshaping of the depressive's negative self-image.

Countertransference feelings can become quite powerful in the treatment of depressed and suicidal patients.[128, 207] When the therapist is feeling guilt or anger he should suspect covert aggression on the part of the patient. This may occur when the patient is subtly making overwhelming or impossible demands which render the therapist first helpless, then guilty or angry. Boredom and impatience may also be felt in the countertransference, but these feelings are more difficult to work through. The patient has somehow gotten the therapist to reject him through boredom and impatience. When this is occurring, the therapist must understand that the patient is unconsciously driving away the very source of nurturance he desperately needs. Careful self-inspection, supervision, or consultation may be needed to assist the therapist in understanding his part in this process.

As this short-term, restitutive therapy progresses, the therapist and patient begin to make plans for follow-up care. Posthospital psychotherapy in conjunction with appropriate family work and psychopharmacological treatment will improve long-term prognosis. If the patient is to be transferred to another therapist upon discharge, this transfer is best done while the patient is still in the hospital. Two or three meetings for getting acquainted and planning a treatment contract with the outpatient therapist will increase posthospital compliance.

The termination phase of inpatient psychotherapy is often characterized by a looking back on the severe depression and feeling vulnerable to the stresses that did and will continue to exist outside the hospital. Loss of the hospital and the intense contact with the therapist may echo earlier losses and frustrations. Adequate time should be allotted to the termination phase of hospitalization in order to allow the patient time to work through these feelings and to say good-bye to hospital staff and fellow patients.

Family Work

Family Evaluation and Therapy

Most spouses and families of depressed patients welcome contact from the hospital psychiatric social worker or a member of the ward staff. Families often feel left out, unrecognized and uncared for, because the identified patient has generally been the focus of previous professional contact.

An effective alliance with the patient's spouse or family is critical in several ways.

First, additional collaborative history may be essential diagnostically. Second, distortions shaped by the patient's illness can be corrected in the minds of the hospital staff. Contact with the family also allows for a clearer exploration and identification of stressors. Furthermore, an effective alliance with the family will reduce the possibility of their sabotaging treatment for reasons intrinsic to the family's psychopathology or its need to maintain its current equilibrium, which may be dependent on one person being ill. Finally, there is evidence that family intervention positively influences treatment compliance, which correlates with outcome. This appears especially true of poor prehospital compliers: family intervention improves compliance and thereby improves long-term outcome.[208]

The evaluation of the family can be done with once or twice weekly meetings for as many meetings as needed. The family can be encouraged to attend any additional family groups that the hospital may offer (e.g., family orientation meetings or a multiple family support group).

Throughout the family contact and therapy the therapist needs to adopt a posture of listening, calming, and educating. Families experience the distress wrought upon them by the depressed person and are often emotionally and financially drained by the time the patient enters the hospital. Many families do not understand depression and can view some symptoms as thoroughly willful. When the family feels heard and empathically responded to, the members can then listen to the therapist educate them about depression.

On the basis of the evaluation, a recommendation for continued family contact or inhospital marital or family therapy is made, when indicated. Indications include marital distress (very common in depression)[209]; family psychopathology that rests, at least in part, on the patient occupying a sick role; or an impasse in the development of the family (e.g., children leaving home) that appears associated with the patient's depression. In brief hospital family therapy, issues and affects are identified, alliances with *all* family members fostered, and goals for change negotiated. Plans for follow-up are established, when

indicated, and concretely set in place prior to discharge to maximize compliance.

Genetic Counseling

Many family members have concerns about the genetic transmission of depression. A parent may worry what he might convey to his children, and a child may worry about his vulnerability to depression.

If family members do not spontaneously raise these concerns, the clinician ought to mention, in a family meeting, that these are frequent questions and concerns that families have and thereby encourage their expression.

Genetic factors in the etiology of depression can be candidly reviewed with family members. It is estimated that the risk of developing a depression in first degree relatives of an affected patient is 15%. A child with one parent with depressive illness is at 26% risk, and a child with both parents affected is at 43% risk. Concordance for dizogytic twins is 13% and is 41% for monozygotic twins.[62-78, 210]

As the clinician explores family concerns and educates its members about the biology of depression, he should also emphasize the psychosocial aspects of this disorder and its manageability with early diagnosis and treatment.

COURSE AND PROGNOSIS

Eighty-five percent or more of patients with unipolar depressions will improve from a specific, carefully chosen biopsychosocial treatment plan. Untreated depressions have been reported to spontaneously remit in 6–9 months.[211] Treated depressions can respond in weeks to months. Predictors of recovery from acute symptoms of depression include acute onset, severe illness in those who have no chronic history of depression, and superimposition of an acute episode on a chronic underlying depression.[212]

Ten to fifteen percent of depressed patients will have a chronic course. Statistically significant increases in rate of relapse are associated with underlying chronic depression and three or more previous episodes of affective disorder.[213] The multiaxial (biopsychosocial) perspective is helpful in understanding a chronic course.

Depression involves an interplay between biology, person, and environment. Patients with personality disorders whose ego offers less resources and poor resilience to depression are apt to have a poorer course and a worse prognosis. Similarly, those patients with limited social resources (family, money, access to medical care) are also apt to demonstrate a poorer course and prognosis.

Weissman et al.[201] have shown that patients treated with a combination of drugs and psychotherapy will have a better prognosis, perhaps because of the interplay between personality and social axes.

Fifty percent of patients who have one episode of depression will have a second, recurrent episode. Patients with two or more episodes show increased risk as the number of episodes increases.

The course and prognosis of depression is, of course, affected by suicide. Bipolar patients show a suicide rate of about 15%. Unipolar patients (including chronic cases) show higher rates.[214] In effect, in excess of 15–20% of patients with depressive disorders will take their own lives. The optimism for treating depression must be tempered by caution, concern, and careful assessment and management of suicidal behavior.

REFERENCES

1. Weissman M, Myers J: *The New Haven Community Survey 1967-1975: Depressive Symptoms and Diagnoses.* Presented to Society for Life History Research in Psychopathology, Fort Worth, Texas, October 1976.
2. Srole L, Langner TS, et al.: *Mental Health in the Metropolis,* New York, McGraw-Hill, 1962.
3. Baldessarini RJ: *Risk rates for depression (letter to the editor).* Arch Gen Psychiatry, *41:* 103–106, 1984.
4. Williams TA, et al.: *Special Report on the Depressive Illnesses.* Washington, D.C., U.S. Department of Health, Education and Welfare, November 1970.
5. Davidson JRT, Miller RD, et al.: *Atypical depression.* Arch Gen Psychiatry, *39:* 527–534, 1982.
6. Aarons SF, Frances AJ, et al.: *Atypical depression: a review of diagnosis and treatment.* Hosp Community, Pyschiatry *36:* 275–282, 1985.
7. Gelenberg AJ: The catatonic syndrome. Lancet *1:* 1339–1341, 1976.
8. McAllister, TW: *Overview: pseudodemintia.* Am J Psychiatry *140:* 528–533, 1983.
9. American Psychiatric Association. *Diagnostic and Statistical Manual of Mental Disorders,* ed. 3 (DSM-III), Washington, D.C., American Psychiatric Association, APA Task Force on Nomenclature, 1980.
10. Robins E, et al.: Primary and secondary affective disorders, in Zubin J, Freyhan FA (eds): *Disorders of Mood,* Baltimore, Johns Hopkins University Press, 1972.
11. Guze SB, et al.: "Secondary" affective disorder: A study of 95 cases. Psychol Med *1:* 426–428, 1971.
12. Akiskal HS, Rosenthal RH, et al.: Differentiation of primary affective illness from situational, somatic and secondary depressions. Arch Gen Psychiatry, *36:* 635–643, 1979.
13. Gillespie RD: The clinical differentiation of types of depression. Guy's Hosp Rep, *79:* 306–344, 1929.
14. Klerman GL: Clinical phenomenology of depression: Implications for research strategy in the psychobiology of the affective disorders, in Williams TA, et al. (eds): *Recent Advances in the Psychobiology of the Depressive Illnesses,* DHEW Publ. No. (HSM) 70-0953, Washington, D.C., U.S. Government Printing Office, 1972.
15. Rosenthal SH, Gudeman JE: The endogenous depressive pattern. Arch Gen Psychiatry, *16:* 241–249, 1967.
16. Klein DF: Endogenomorphic depression. Arch Gen Psychiatry, *31:* 447–454, 1974.
17. Nelson JC, Charney DS: Primary affective disorder criteria and the endogenous-reactive distinction. Arch Gen Psychiatry, *37:* 787-793, 1980.
18. Prusoff BA, Weissman MM, et al.: Research diagnostic criteria subtypes of depression: Their role as predictors of differential response to psychotherapy and drug treatment. Arch Gen Psychiatry, *37:* 796–801, 1980.
19. Klerman GL, et al.: Neurotic depressions: A systematic analysis of multiple criteria and meanings. Am J Psychiatry, *136:* 57–61, 1979.
20. Akiskal HS: Dysthymic disorder: Psychopathology of proposed chronic depressive subtypes. Am J Psychiatry, *140:* 11–20, 1983.
21. Akiskal HS, Webb WL: Affective disorders. I. Recent advances in clinical conceptualization. Hosp Community Psychiatry, *34:* 695–702, 1983.
22. Keller MB, Shapiro RW: "Double depression." Am J Psychiatry, *139:* 438–442, 1982.
23. Keller MB, Lavori PW, et al.: "Double depression": two year follow-up. Am J Psychiatry, *140:* 689–694, 1983.
24. Akiskal HS: Dysthymic disorder: psychopathology of proposed chronic depressive subtypes. Am J Psychiatry, *140:* 11–20, 1983.
25. Akiskal HS: Factors associated with incomplete recovery in primary depressive illness. J Clin Psychiatry, *43:* 266–271, 1982.
26. Brown RP, Sweeney JP, et al.: Involutional melancholia revisited. Am J Psychiatry, *141:* 24–28, 1984.
27. Rosenthal NE, Sack DA, et al.: Seasonal affective disorder. *41:* 72–80, 1984.

28. Pope HG, Lipinski JF, et al.: "Schizoaffective disorder": An invalid diagnosis? A comparison of schizoaffective disorder, schizophrenia and affective disorder. Am J Psychiatry, *137:* 921–927, 1980.

29. Hatsukami D, Pickens RW: Posttreatment depression in an alcohol and drug abuse population. Am J Psychiatry, *139:* 1563–1566, 1982.

30. Lindemann E: Symptomatology and management of acute grief. Am J Psychiatry, *101:* 141–148, 1944.

31. Lazare A: Unresolved grief, in Lazare A (ed): *Outpatient Psychiatry: Diagnosis and Treatment,* pp. 498–512, Baltimore, Williams & Wilkins, 1979.

32. Boyd JH, Weissman MM: Epidemiology of affective disorders: A re-examination and future directions. Arch Gen Psychiatry, *38:* 1039–1046, 1981.

33. Helgason T: Epidemiologic investigations concerning affective disorders, in Schou M, Stromgren E: Origin, Prevention, and Treatment of Affective Disorders, New York, Academic Press, 1979.

34. Essen-Moller E, Hagnell O: The frequency and risk of depression within a rural population group in Scandinavia. Acta Psychiatr Scand [Suppl 162], *37:* 28–32, 1961.

35. Klerman GL, Barrett JE: The affective disorders: Clinical and epidemiological aspects, in Gershow S, Shobsin B (eds): *Lithium: Its Role in Psychiatric Treatment and Research,* New York, Plenum Press, 1973.

36. Klerman GL, Lavori PW, et al.: Birth-cohort trends in rates of major depressive disorder among relatives of patients with affective disorder. Arch Gen Psychiatry, *42:* 689–693, 1985.

37. Silverman C: *The Epidemiology of Depression,* Baltimore, Johns Hopkins University Press, 1968.

38. Weissman MM, Klerman GL: Sex differences and the epidemiology of depression. Arch Gen Psychiatry, *34:* 98–111, 1977.

39. Faris RE, Dunham HW: *Mental Disorders in Urban Areas,* Chicago, University of Chicago Press, 1939.

40. Gove WR: The relationship between sex roles, marital status and mental illness. Soc. Forces, *51:* 34–44, 1972.

41. Gove WR: Sex, marital status and mortality. Am J Sociol, *79:* 45–67, 1973.

42. Radloff L: Sex differences in depression. The effects of occupation and marital status. Sex Roles, *1:* 249–269, 1975.

43. Weissman MM, Paykel ES: *The Depressed Woman: A Study of Social Relationships,* Chicago, University of Chicago Press, 1974.

44. Goodwin FK, Bunney WE: A psychobiological approach to affective illness. Psychiatric Ann, *3:* 19, 1973.

45. Schildkraut JT: The catecholamine hypothesis of affective disorders: A review of supporting evidence. Am J Psychiatry, *122:* 509–522, 1965.

46. Janowsky DS, El Yousef MK, et al.: A cholinergic-adrenergic hypothesis of mania and depression. Lancet, *1:* 632–635, 1972.

47. Snyder SH: Cholinergic mechanisms in affective disorders. N Engl J Med *311:* 254–255, 1984.

48. Maas JW: Biogenic amines and depression. Biochemical and pharmacological separation of two types of depression. Arch Gen Psychiatry, *32:* 1357–1361, 1975.

49. Baldessarini RJ: Biogenic amine hypotheses in affective disorders. Arch Gen Psychiatry, *32:* 1087–1093, 1975.

50. Brown RP, Mann JJ: A clinical perspective on the role of neurotransmitters in mental disorders.

51. Hewinger GR, Charney DS: The monoamine receptor sensitivity hypothesis of antidepressant drug action. *Psychopharmacol Bull, 18:* 130–135, 1982.

52. Sulser F: Mode of action of antidepressant drugs. *J Clin Psychiatry, 44(5):* 14–20, 1983.

53. Richelson E: The newer antidepressants: Structures, pharmacokinetics, pharmacodynamics, and proposed mechanisms of action. *Psychopharmacol Bull 20(2):* 213–223, 1984.

54. Charney DS, Heninger GR, Sternberg DE: The effect of mianserin on alpha-2 adrenergic receptor function in depressed patients. *Br J Psychiatry, 144:* 407–416, 1984.

55. Hyttel J: Experimental pharmacology of selective 5-HT reuptake inhibitors. *Clin Neuropharmacol 7(suppl 1):* 866–867, 1984.

56. Schildkraut JJ: *Neuropsychopharmacology and the Affective Disorders,* Boston, Little, Brown & Co., 1970.

57. Asberg N, et al.: Serotonin depression—A biochemical subgroup within the affective disorders? Science, *191:* 478–480, 1976.

58. Koslow SH, Maas JW, et al.: CSF and urinary biogenic amines and metabolites in depression and mania. Arch Gen Psychiatry, *40:* 999–1010, 1983.

59. Muscettola G, Potter WZ, et al.: Urinary MHPG and major affective disorders. Arch Gen Psychiatry, *41:* 337–342, 1984.

60. Sabelli HC, Fawcett J, et al.: The methylphenidate test. Am J Psychiatry, *140:* 212–214, 1983.

61. Brown P, Brawley P: Dexamethasone suppression test and mood response to methylphenidate in primary depression. Am J Psychiatry, *140:* 990–993, 1983.

62. Rosanoff AJ, Handy LM, Plesset IR: The etiology of manic-depressive syndromes with special reference to their occurrence to twins. Am J Psychiatry, *91:* 725–762, 1935.

63. Essen-Moller E: Psychiatrische Untersuchungen an einer Serie von Zwillingen. Copenhagen, Munksgaard, 1941.

64. Gedda L: Studio dei Gemelli. Rome, Edizioni Orizzonte Medico, 1951.

65. Slater E: Psychotic and Neurotic Illnesses in Twins. MRC Special Report Series, no 278. London, Her Majesty's Stationer's Office, 1953.

66. Kallmann FJ: Genetic principles in manic-depressive psychosis, in Hoch P, Zubin J (eds):

Depression, New York, Grune & Stratton, 1954.

67. DaFonseca AF: Analise Heredo-Clinica das Perturbacoes Afectivas. Oporto, Faculdade de Medicina, 1959.

68. Kringlen E: *Heredity and Environment in the Functional Psychoses,* Oslo, Universitets-Forlaget, 1967.

69. Allen MG, Cohen S, Pollin W, et al.: Affective illness in veteran twins: A diagnostic review. Am J Psychiatry, *131:* 1234–1239, 1974.

70. Bertelsen A, Harvald B, Hange M: A Danish twin study of manic-depressive disorders. Br J Psychiatry, *130:* 330–351, 1977.

71. Price JS: The genetics of depressive behaviour, in Coppen A, Walk A (eds): *Recent Developments in Affective Disorders: A Symposium,* Kent, England, Royal Medico-Psychological Association, 1968.

72. Angst J: Zur atiologie und nosologie endogener depressiver psychosen. Monogr Neurol Psychiatry, *112:* 1–118, 1966.

73. Perris C: A study of bipolar (manic-depressive) and unipolar recurrent depressive psychoses. Acta Psychiatr Scand Suppl, *194:* 1–189, 1966.

74. Gershon E, Mark A, Cohen N, et al.: Transmitted factors in the morbid risk of affective disorders: A controlled study. J Psychiatr Res, *12:* 283–299, 1975.

75. James NM, Chapman CJ: A genetic study of bipolar affective disorder. Br J Psychiatry, *126:* 449–456, 1975.

76. Trzebiatowska-Trzeciak O: Genetical analysis of unipolar and bipolar endogenous affective psychoses. Br J Psychiatry, *131:* 478–485, 1977.

77. Tsuang MT, Winokur G, Crowe R: Morbidity risks of schizophrenia and affective disorders among first-degree relatives of patients with schizophrenia, mania, depression, and surgical conditions. Br J Psychiatry, *137:* 497–504, 1980.

78. Winokur G, Cadoret R, Dorzab J, et al.: Depressive disease: A genetic study. Arch Gen Psychiatry, *24:* 135–144, 1971.

79. Cadoret RJ: Evidence for genetic inheritance of primary affective disorder in adoptees. Am J Psychiatry, *135:* 463–466, 1978.

80. Abraham K: Notes on the psychoanalytical investigation and treatment of manic-depressive insanity and allied conditions, in: *The Selected Papers of Karl Abraham,* London, Hogarth Press, 1927.

81. Freud S: Mourning and melancholia, in Strachey J (ed): *Standard Edition,* vol. 14, London, Hogarth Press (1917), 1958.

82. Fenichel O: Depression and mania, in: *The Psychoanalytic Theory of Neurosis,* New York, Norton, 1945.

83. Kendell R: Relationship between aggression and depression: Epidemiological implications of a hypothesis. Arch Gen Psychiatry, *22:* 308–318, 1970.

84. Henry A, Short J: *Suicide and Homicide,* Chicago, Free Press of Glencoe, Ill., 1954.

85. Friedman A: Hostility factors and clinical improvement in depressed patients. Arch Gen Psychiatry, *23:* 524–537, 1970.

86. Paykel E: Classification of depressed patients: A cluster analysis derived grouping. Br J Psychiatry, *118:*275–288, 1971.

87. Weissman M, Fox K, et al.: Hostility and depression associated with suicide attempts. Am J Psychiatry, *130:* 450–455, 1973.

88. Klerman G, Gershon, E: Imipramine effects upon hostility in depression. J Nerv Ment Dis, *150:* 127–132, 1970.

89. Bibring E: The mechanism of depression, in Greenacre P (ed): *Affective Disorders,* New York, International Universities Press, 1953.

90. Kierkegaard S: *The Sickness Unto Death,* Princeton, N.J., Princeton University Press, 1941.

91. Klein M: A contribution to the psychogenesis of manic-depressive states, in *Contributions to Psychoanalysis,* pp. 228–310, London, Hogarth Press, 1945.

92. Bibring E: The mechanism of depression, in Greenacre P (ed): *Affective Disorders,* pp. 13–48, New York, International Universities Press, 1965.

93. Rochlin G: Personal communication.

94. Bowlby J: The process of mourning. Int J Psychoanal, *42:* 317–340, 1961.

95. Spitz RA: Anaclitic depression, in: *The Psychoanalytic Study of the Child,* vol. 2, New York, International Universities Press, 1946.

96. Brown F: Depression and childhood bereavement. J Ment Sci, *107:* 754–777, 1961.

97. Leff M, Roatch J, et al.: Environmental factors preceding the onset of severe depressions. Psychiatry, *33:* 293–311, 1970.

98. Paykel E, Myers J, et al.: Life events and depression. Arch Gen Psychiatry, *21:* 753–760, 1970.

99. Clayton P, Halikas J, et al.: The depression of widowhood. Br J Psychiatry, *120:* 71–77, 1972.

100. Parkes C: Bereavement and mental illness: A clinical study of the grief of bereaved psychiatric patients. Br J Med Psychol, *38:* 1–12, 1965.

101. Schmale A: Relationship of separation and depression to disease. Psychosom Med, *20:* 259–277, 1958.

102. Hirschfeld RMA, Klerman GL, et al.: Assessing personality: Affects of the depressive state on trait measurement. Am J Psychiatry, *140:* 695–699, 1983.

103. Akiskal HS, Hirschfeld RMA, el al.: The relationship of personality to affective disorders. Arch Gen Psychiatry, *40:* 801–810, 1983.

104. Beck AT: Depressive neurosis, in Arieti S, Brody EB (eds): *American Handbook of Psychiatry,* pp. 61–90, ed. 2, vol. 3, New York, Basic Books, 1974.

105. Rush AJ, Beck AT, et al.: Comparative efficacy of cognitive therapy and pharmacotherapy in the treatment of depressed outpatients. Cognit Ther Res, *1:* 17–37, 1977.

106. Kovacs M, Beck AT: Maladaptive cognitive structures in depression. Am J Psychiatry, *135:* 525–533, 1978.

107. Seligman ME: *Helplessness: On Depression, Development, and Death.* San Francisco, W. H. Freeman, 1975.
108. Silverman JS, Silverman JA, et al.: Do maladaptive attitudes cause depression? Arch Gen Psychiatry, *41:* 28–30, 1984.
109. Simons AD, Garfield SL, et al.: The process of change in cognitive therapy and pharmacotherapy for depression. Arch Gen Psychiatry, *41:* 45–51, 1984.
110. Ilfeld FW: Current social stressors and symptoms of depression. Am J Psychiatry, *134:* 161–166, 1977.
111. Gunderson EK, Rahe RH: *Life Stress and Illness,* Springfield, Ill., Charles C Thomas, 1974.
112. Lloyd C: Life events and depressive disorder reviewed. II. Events as precipitating factors. Arch Gen Psychiatry, *37:* 541–548, 1980.
113. Paykel ES: Life stress, depression, and attempted suicide. J Hum Stress, *2:* 3–12, 1976.
114. Paykel ES, Myers JK, Dienelt MN, et al.: Life events and depression: A controlled study. Arch Gen Psychiatry, *21:* 753–760, 1969.
115. Fava GA, Munari F, Pavan L, et al.: Life events and depression: A replication. J Affect Dis *3:* 159–165, 1981.
116. Green AI: Thyroid function and affective disorders. Hosp Community Psychiatry, *35:* 1188–1189, 1984.
117. Schlesser MA, Winokur G, et al.: Hypothalamic-pituitary-adrenal axis activity in depressive illness: Its relation to classification. Arch Gen Psychiatry, *37:* 737–743, 1980.
118. Carroll BJ, Curtis GC, et al.: Neuroendocrine regulation in depression. I. Limbic system—Adrenocortical dysfunction. Arch Gen Psychiatry, *33:* 1039–1044, 1976.
119. Brown WA, Shuey I: Response to dexamethasone and subtype of depression. Arch Gen Psychiatry, *37:* 747–751, 1980.
120. Carroll BJ, Greden JF, et al.: Neuroendocrine disturbances and the diagnosis and etiology of endogenous depression. Lancet: 321–322, 1980.
121. Goldberg IK: Dexamethasone suppression test as indicator of safe withdrawal of antidepressant therapy. Lancet: 376, 1980.
122. Hirschfeld RMA, Koslow SH, Kupfer DJ: The clinical utility of the dexamethasone suppression test in psychiatry: Summary of a National Institute of Mental Health Workshop. JAMA *250:* 2172–2174, 1983.
123. Baldessarini RJ: *Biomedical Aspects of Depression and Its Treatment,* pp 59–66. Washington, D.C., American Psychiatric Press, 1983, pp. 59–66.
124. Gelenberg, AJ: The DST in even greater perspective. Biol Ther Psychiatry, *7:* 1, 1984.
125. Coccaro EF, Prudic J, et al.: Effect of hospital admission on DST results. Am J Psychiatry, *141:* 982–985, 1984.
126. Baldessarini RJ, Finklestein S, et al.: The predictive power of diagnostic tests and the effect of prevalence of illness. Arch Gen Psychiatry, *40:* 569–573, 1983.
127. Gedo JE, Goldberg A: *Models of the Mind: A Psychoanalytic Theory,* chaps. 6, 7, 11, and 12, Chicago, University of Chicago Press, 1973.
128. MacKinnon RA, Michels R: *The Psychiatric Interview in Clinical Practice,* pp. 174–229, Philadelphia, W. B. Saunders Co., 1971.
129. Sederer LI: Heiress to an empty throne: Egoideal problems in contemporary women. Contemp Psychoanal, *12:* 240–251, 1976.
130. Buie DH: Empathy: Its nature and limitations, Presented at the Annual Fall Meeting of the American Psychoanalytic Association, New York, December 1979.
131. Havens L: The anatomy of a suicide. N Engl J Med, *272:* 401–406, 1965.
132. Havens L: Recognition of suicidal risks through the psychological examination. N Engl J Med, *276:* 210–215, 1967.
133. Maltsberger JJ, Buie DH: The devices of suicide. Int Rev Psychoanal, *7:* 61–72, 1980.
134. Buie DH, Maltsberger JJ: The practical formulation of suicide risk. Cambridge, Mass., Firefly Press, 1983.
135. Avery D, Winokur G: Mortality in depressed patients treated with electroconvulsive therapy and antidepressants. Arch Gen Psychiatry, *33:* 1029–1937, 1976.
136. Quitkin FM, Rabkin JG, et al.: Duration of antidepressant drug treatment: What is an adequate trial? Arch Gen Psychiatry, *41:* 238–245, 1984.
137. Heninger GR, Charney DS, et al.: Lithium carbonate augmentation of antidepressant treatment. Arch Gen Psychiatry, *40:* 1335–1342, 1983.
138. Montigny C, Cournoyes G, et al.: Lithium carbonate addition in tricyclic antidepressant-resistant unipolar depression. Arch Gen Psychiatry, *40:* 1327–1334, 1983.
139. Montigny, CP, Elie R, et al.: Rapid response to the addition of lithium in iprindole-resistant unipolar depression. Am J Psychiatry *142:* 220–223, 1985.
140. Goodwin FK, Prange AJ: Potentiation of Antidepressant effects by L-triiodo thyronine in tricyclic nonresponders. Am J Psychiatry, *139:* 34–38, 1982.
141. Schwarcz G, Halaris A, et al.: Normal thyroid function in desipramine nonresponders converted to responders by the addition of L-triiodothyronine. Am J Psychiatry, *141:* 1614–1616, 1984.
142. Baldessarini RJ: Drugs and the treatment of psychiatric disorders, in Gilman AG, Goodman LS (eds.): *The Pharmacological Basis of Therapeutics,* ed. 6, pp. 391–447. New York, MacMillan Publishing Co., 1980.
143. Klein DF, Gittelman R, et al.: Diagnosis and drug treatment of psychiatric disorders. Baltimore, Williams & Wilkins, 1980.
144. Prieu RF, Kupfer DJ, et al.: Drug treatment in the prevention of recurrences in unipolar and bipolar affective disorders. Arch Gen Psychiatry, *41:* 1096–1104, 1984.
145. Glassman AH, Roose SP: Delusional de-

pression: A distinct clinical entity? Arch Gen Psychiatry, *38:* 424–427, 1981.

146. Minter RE, Mandel MR: The treatment of psychotic major depressive disorder with drugs and ECT. J Nerv Ment Dis, *167:* 726–733, 1979.

147. Spiker DG, Weiss JC, et al.: The pharmacological treatment of delusional depression. Am J Psychiatry, *142:* 430–436, 1985.

148. Quitkin F, Rifkin A, et al.: Monoamine oxidase inhibitors. Arch Gen Psychiatry, *35:* 749–760, 1979.

149. Robinson DS, Nies A, et al.: Clinical pharmacology of phenelzine. Arch Gen Psychiatry, *35:* 629–635, 1978.

150. Liebowitz MR, Quitkin FM, et al.: Phenelzine vs. imipramine in atypical depression. Arch Gen Psychiatry, *41:* 669–677, 1984.

151. Katon W, Raskind M: Treatment of depression in the medically ill elderly with methylphenidate. Am J Psychiatry, *137:* 963–965, 1980.

152. Kaplitz SE: Withdrawn apathetic geriatric patients responsive to methylphenidate. J Am Geriatr Soc, *23:* 271–276, 1975.

153. Carney MWP: Tricyclics and the heart. Br J Psychiatry, *134:* 637–639, 1979.

154. Burrows GD, et al.: Cardiac effects of different tricyclic antidepressant drugs. Br J Psychiatry, *129:* 335–341, 1976.

155. Luchins DJ: Review of clinical and animal studies comparing the cardiovascular effects of doxepin and other tricyclic antidepressants. *Am J Psychiatry, 140:* 1006–1009, 1983.

156. Glassman AH: Cardiovascular effects of tricyclic antidepressants. Ann Rev Med, *35:* 503–511, 1984.

157. Nurnberg HG, Prudic J: Guidelines for treatment of psychosis during pregnancy. Hosp Community Psychiatry, *35:* 67–71, 1984.

158. Calabrese JR, Gulledge AD: Psychotropics during pregnancy and lactation: A review. Psychosomatics, *26:* 413–426, 1985.

159. Stern SL, Rush AJ, et al.: Toward a rational pharmacotherapy of depression. Am J Psychiatry, *137:* 545–552, 1980.

160. Maas JW, Fawcett JA, et al.: Catecholamine metabolism, depressive illness and drug response. Arch Gen Psychiatry, *26:* 252–262, 1972.

161. Beckman H, Goodwin FK: Antidepressant response to tricyclics and urinary MHPG in unipolar patients. Arch Gen Psychiatry, *32:* 17–21, 1975.

162. Bielski RJ, Friedel RO: Prediction of tricyclic antidepressant response: A critical review. Arch Gen Psychiatry, *33:* 1479–1489, 1976.

163. Amsterdam J, Brunswick D, et al.: The clinical application of tricyclic antidepressant pharmacokinetics and plasma levels. Am J Psychiatry, *137:* 653–662, 1980.

164. Van Kammen DP, Murphy DL: Prediction of imipramine antidepressant response by a one-day-d-amphetamine trial. Am J Psychiatry, *135:* 1179–1184, 1978.

165. Fawcett J, Siomopoulos V: Dextroamphetamine response as a possible predictor of improvement with tricyclic therapy in depression. Arch Gen Psychiatry, *25:* 247–255, 1971.

166. Maas JW, Koslow, SH, et al.: Pretreatment neurotransmitter metabolite levels and response to tricyclic antidepressant drugs. Am J Psychiatry, *141:* 1159–1171, 1984.

167. Silverman JJ, Brennan P, et al.: Clinical significance of tricyclic antidepressant plasma levels. Psychosomatics, *20:* 736–746, 1979.

168. Snyder SH, Yamamura HI: Antidepressants and the muscarinic acetylcholine receptor. Arch Gen Psychiatry, *34:* 236–239, 1977.

169. U'Prichard DC, Greenberg DA, et al.: Tricyclic antidepressants: Therapeutic properties and affinity for noradrenergic receptor binding sites in the brain. Science, *199:* 197–198, 1978.

170. Task Force on the Use of Laboratory Tests in Psychiatry: Tricyclic antidepressants—blood level measurements and clinical outcome. Am J Psychiatry, *142:* 155–162, 1985.

171. Dominquez, RA: Evaluating the effectiveness of the new antidepressants. Hosp Community Psychiatry, *34:* 405–407, 1983.

172. Prien RF, Blaine JD, et al.: Antidepressant drug therapy: The role of the new antidepressants. Hosp Community Psychiatry, *36:* 513–516, 1985.

173. Dufresne RL, Weber SS, Becker RE: Bupropion hydrochloride. *Drug Intell Clin Pharmacol, 18:* 957–964, 1984.

174. Gelenberg A: Alprazolam: Is it an antidepressant? Biol Ther Psychiatry *7:* 1, 1984.

175. Stonier, PD: a review of the clinical safety and tolerability of nomifensine. J Clin Psychiatry, *45:* 89–95, 1984.

176. Davis JM: A Review of the New Antidepressant Medications, in Davis JM, Maas JW (eds): *The Affective Disorders,* Washington, D.C., Am Psychiatric Association, 1983.

177. Baldessarini RJ: *Chemotherapy in Psychiatry,* p. 115, Cambridge, Mass., Harvard University Press, 1977.

178. Sheehan DV, Ballenger J, et al.: Treatment of endogenous anxiety with phobic, hysterical and hypochondriacal symptoms. Arch Gen Psychiatry, *37:* 51–59, 1980.

179. Mendels J: Lithium in the treatment of depression. Am J Psychiatry, *133:* 373–378, 1976.

180. Doyal LE, Morton WA: The clinical usefulness of lithium as an antidepressant. Hosp. Community Psychiatry *35:* 685–691, 1984.

181. Wilson IC, Prange, AJ, et al.: Thyroid hormone enhancement of imipramine in nonretarded depressions. N Engl J Med, *282:* 1063–1067, 1970.

182. Wharton RN, Perel JM, et al.: A potential clinical use for methylphenidate with tricyclic antidepressants. Am J Psychiatry, *127:* 1619–1625, 1971.

183. White K, Pistole T, et al.: Combined MAOI-TCA treatment. Am J Psychiatry, *137:* 1422–1425, 1980.

184. Gelenberg AJ, Wojcik JD, et al.: Tyrosine for

the treatment of depression. Am J Psychiatry, *137:* 622–623, 1980.

185. Sack DA, Nurnberger J, et al.: Potentiation of antidepressant medications by phase advance of the sleep-wake cycle. Am J Psychiatry, *142:* 606–608, 1985.

186. Kripke DF, Risch SC, et al.: Lighting up depression. Psychopharmacol Bull *19:* 526–530, 1983.

187. Glassman AH, Kantor SJ, et al.: Depression, delusion and drug response. Am J Psychiatry, *132:* 716–719, 1975.

188. Mandel MR, Welch CA, et al.: Prediction of response to ECT in tricyclic-intolerant or tricyclic-resistant depressed ptients. McLean Hosp J, *2:* 203–209, 1977.

189. Medical Research Council: Clinical trial of the treatment of depressive illness. Br Med J, *5439:* 881–886, 1965.

190. Weiner RD: The psychiatric use of electrically induced seizures. Am J Psychiatry, *136:* 1507–1517, 1979.

191. Crowe RR: Electroconvulsive therapy: A current perspective. N. Engl J Med *311:* 163–167, 1984.

192. Schildkraut JJ, Draskoczy P: Effects of electroconvulsive shock on norepinephrine turnover and metabolism: Basic and clinical studies, in Fink M, Kety S, et al. (eds): *Psychobiology of Convulsive Therapy,* Washington, D.C., VH Winston & Sons, 1974.

193. Culver CM, Ferrell RB, et al.: ECT and special problems of informed consent. Am J Psychiatry, *137:* 586–591, 1980.

194. Abrams R, Fink M, et al.: Unilateral and bilateral ECT: Effects on depression, memory and the EEG. Arch Gen Psychiatry, *27:* 88–91, 1972.

195. Mandel M: Personal communication.

196. Frank J, Hoehn-Saric R, et al.: *Effective Ingredients of Successful Psychotherapy,* New York, Brunner/Mazel, 1978.

197. Roose SP, Glassman AH, et al.: Depression delusions and suicide. Am J Psychiatry, *140:* 1159–1162, 1983.

198. Cotton PG, Drake RE, et al.: Dealing with suicide on a psychiatric inpatient unit. Hosp Community Psychiatry, *34:* 55–59, 1983.

199. Schoonover, SC: Intensive Care for Suicidal patients, in Bassuk EL, Schoonover SC (eds): Lifelines: *Clinical perspectives on Suicide,* pp. 137–152, New York, Plenum, 1982.

200. Klerman GL, DiMascio A, et al.: Treatment of depression by drugs and psychotherapy. Am J Psychiatry, *131:* 186–191, 1974.

201. Weissman MM, Prusoff BA, et al.: The efficacy of drugs and psychotherapy in the treatment of acute depressive episodes. Am J Psychiatry, *136:* 555-558, 1979.

202. Weissman MM, Klerman GL, et al.: Treatment effects on the social adjustment of depressed patients. Arch Gen Psychiatry, *30:* 771–778, 1974.

203. Arieti S: Psychotherapy of severe depression. Am J Psychiatry, *134:* 864–868, 1971.

204. Rounsaville BJ, Klerman GL, et al.: Do psychotherapy and pharmacotherapy for depression conflict? Arch Gen Psychiatry, *38:* 24–29, 1981.

205. Klerman GL: Depression in the medically ill. Psychiatr Clin North Am, *4*(2): 301–317, 1981.

206. Coyne JC: Depression and the response of others. J Abnorm Psychol, *85:* 186–193, 1976.

207. Maltsberger JT, Buie DH: Countertransference hate in the treatment of suicidal patients. Arch Gen Psychiatry, *30:* 625–633, 1974.

208. Glick ID, et al.: Family therapy and affective disorders. Paper presentation at the Annual Meeting of the American Psychiatric Association, Dallas, 1985.

209. Friedman AS: Interaction of drug therapy with marital therapy in depressive patients. Arch Gen Psychiatry, *32:* 619–637, 1975.

210. Tsuang MT: Genetic counseling for psychiatric patients and their families. Am J Psychiatry, *135:* 1465–1475, 1978.

211. Robins E, Guze SB: Classification in affective disorders, in Williams TA, Katz MM, et al. (eds): *Recent Advances in the Psychobiology of the Depressive Illnesses,* Washington, D.C., U.S. Government Printing Office, 1972.

212. Keller MB, Shapiro RW, et al.: Recovery in major depressive disorder. Arch Gen Psychiatry, *39:* 905–910, 1982.

213. Keller MB, Shapiro RW, et al.: Relapse in major depressive disorder. Arch Gen Psychiatry, *39:* 911–915, 1982.

214. Miles CP: Conditions predisposing to suicide: A review. J Nerv Ment Dis, *164:* 231–246, 1977.

mania

Lloyd I. Sederer, M.D.

DEFINITION

Mania is a *syndrome* with multiple etiologies. The features of mania include a disturbance of mood, characterized by either an elated, irritable, or expansive mood; hyperactivity; pressured speech; flight of ideas; distractibility; and poor judgment.[1, 2]

In recent years an important distinction has been made in the nosology of mania.[3] Mania is now conceived of as either *primary* or *secondary*. *Primary mania* is the mania of an affective disorder (either a manic disorder or a bipolar affective disorder presenting with a manic episode). *Secondary mania* is the mania that occurs secondary to a variety of organic disorders which include drug intake, infection, neoplasm, epilepsy, and metabolic disturbances.

Case Example: Primary Mania. Mr. B., a 23-year-old college student, was transferred from a locked unit to an open voluntary general hospital psychiatry unit at the request of his family.

Though Mr. B.'s admission to the locked unit was his first psychiatric contact, he reported a psychiatric history that went back to about the age of 17. Since that time the patient reported an annual mood cycle that was characterized by periods of social withdrawal, increased sleep, weight gain, and the general feeling of sadness during the fall and winter months. This was contrasted by periods of elation, increased energy, a decreased need to sleep, and increased activity during the late spring and summer months. During the summer prior to admission the patient reported feeling very elated with little need for sleep. He began working three jobs simultaneously, one of which involved his participation in a somewhat shaky business scheme in which half-fare airline coupons were resold. In addition to this,

Mr. B. had also attempted to purchase, as an investment, the apartment house in which he lived.

As Mr. B.'s business endeavors began to fail, he became increasingly irritable and disorganized. In the week prior to admission the patient maintained that he did not sleep at all and began to believe that he was hearing special messages from the radio. Finally, he became extremely suspicious of other people and, on the night of admission, he became combative when approached by friends.

These friends were able to usher him to an emergency ward, where his thoughts were severely disorganized; he continued to be combative. He required treatment with I.M. haloperidol and the use of mechanical restraints. It was from the emergency ward that the patient was involuntarily hospitalized on a locked inpatient unit.

DIAGNOSIS AND DIFFERENTIAL DIAGNOSIS

Primary Mania

Primary mania is the manic syndrome seen in patients with an affective disorder either of the manic or bipolar type (see Fig. 1.1). The third edition of the *Diagnostic and Statistical Manual of Mental Disorders* of the American Psychiatric Association (DSM-III) offers the following diagnostic criteria for a manic episode:

1. One or more distinct periods with a predominantly elevated, expansive, or irritable mood. The elevated or irritable mood must be a prominent part of the illness and relatively persistent, although it may alternate or intermingle with depressive mood.

2. Duration of at least 1 week (or any duration if hospitalization is necessary) during which, for most of the

time, at least three of the following symptoms have persisted (four if the mood is only irritable) and have been present to a significant degree:

a. increase in activity (either socially, at work, or sexually) or physical restlessness
b. more talkative than usual or pressure to keep talking
c. flight of ideas or subjective experience that thoughts are racing
d. inflated self-esteem (grandiosity, which may be delusional)
e. decreased need for sleep
f. distractibility, i.e., attention is too easily drawn to unimportant or irrelevant external stimuli
g. excessive involvement in activities that have a high potential for painful consequences which is not recognized, e.g., buying sprees, sexual indiscretions, foolish business investments, reckless driving

3. Neither of the following dominates the clinical picture when an affective syndrome is absent (i.e., symptoms in criteria 1 and 2 above):
   a. preoccupation with a mood-incongruent delusion or hallucination
   b. bizarre behavior
4. Not superimposed on either schizophrenia, schizophreniform disorder, or a paranoid disorder.
5. Not due to any organic mental disorder, such as substance intoxication.

Stages of Mania

Carlson and Goodwin[4] have offered an analysis of the sequence of a manic episode or the stages of mania. In their study of 20 primary mania patients, they describe three stages of mania: the *initial* phase, the *intermediate* phase, and the *final* phase. All patients entered the *initial* phase, characterized by increased speech and physical activity; by a labile mood in which euphoria predominated, though patients became irritable when their demands were not met; and by cognitive features which included grandiosity and tangentiality, though thoughts remained coherent.

The *intermediary* stage was also seen in all patients in their study. In the *intermediary* stage, speech became more pressured and physical activity increased. In this stage, mood became increasingly dysphoric with euphoric and depressed aspects. Irritability had grown to general hostility and to a capacity for explosiveness and combativeness. What were racing thoughts in the initial phase were now a flight of ideas. Grandiosity reached delusional proportions.

Seventy percent of patients entered the *final* stage, which was a desperate, dysphoric panic characterized by bizarre behavior and incoherent thought processes. Delusions and hallucinations were present, and disorientation occurred in some patients.

Carlson and Goodwin noted that this sequence was consistent in all patients, though the rate of entry from the initial stage to the second and third stages varied from several hours to several days. They also noted that the sequence was also consistent in its reverse order, namely, that those patients who entered the final stage would detumesce to the intermediary stage before they would re-enter the initial stage.

These authors suggest, as do others, that cross-sectional symptom constellations are not sufficient for the final diagnosis because acute mania can mimic schizophrenia.[5] It also appears that the level of acute disorganization is not an accurate harbinger of future clinical status. In other words, the patient's prognosis bears no relationship to the severity of the mania.

Differential Diagnosis of Primary Mania

1. Organic mental disorders or secondary mania (see following section).
2. Schizophrenia. As discussed in Chapter 3, the diagnosis of schizophrenia is made longitudinally with the duration of illness in excess of 6 months. Acute manic-like episodes are never to be initially diagnosed as schizophrenia, regardless of their severity or bizarreness.[6, 7]
3. Schizoaffective disorder. Controversy

exists about the diagnosis of schizo-affective disorder. The DSM-III[1] holds to this diagnostic category but indicates the lack of consensus in its use. Furthermore, recent work[8, 9] has brought this diagnosis into serious question.

4. Personality disorders. Chronic hypomanic or cyclothymic personality disorders may present in an aggravated state that resembles mania. In these cases, a diagnosis of mania with a personality diagnosis of hypomanic or cyclothymic personality would be in order.

5. Delirium. Acute, severe mania can show the disorientation, emotional lability, and bizarre hallucinations and delusions typical of delirium. This form of mania, called acute delirious mania, can mimic delirium.[9]

6. Dementia. Manic pseudodementia is a syndrome of reversible cognitive impairment. In elderly bipolar patients this manic presentation may be mistaken for dementia.[11-13]

Secondary Mania

Secondary mania is a manic syndrome of organic etiology with clinical features indistinguishable from primary mania.[3] The *exclusionary criteria* of secondary mania are (1) the presence of a confusional state or delirium or (2) a past history of affective disorder. In the case of manic symptoms associated with delirium, the diagnosis would be delirium. In the presence of a past history of affective disorder, the diagnosis would be affective disorder induced by an organic stressor.

The clinician is wise to consider the diagnosis of secondary mania in patients who present with manic symptomatology without a past history of affective disorder or a family history of affective disorder. In addition, secondary mania typically has a later age of onset.

Differential Diagnosis of 2° Mania

1. *Drug Ingestion*
   a. Steroids
   b. Stimulants
      Amphetamine
      Methylphenidate
      Cocaine
   c. L-Dopa
2. *Toxin Ingestion*
   Bromine
3. *Metabolic Disturbances*
   Postoperative states
   Hemodialysis
4. *Infection*
   General paresis, neurosyphilis[14]
   Postencephalitic mania
   Q-fever
   Influenza
5. *Neoplasm*
   CNS tumors
6. *Epilepsy*
7. *Vascular Lesions of the CNS*

Case Example: Secondary Mania. Glaser[15] has described the case of a 41-year-old woman who developed manic symptoms following intramuscular cortisone for treatment of severe rheumatoid arthritis. As he describes it, the patient received 300 mg of cortisone on day 1, 200 mg on day 2 and day 3, and then 100 mg thereafter for 9 days. On day 2 of treament, the patient's arthritic symptoms began to improve, and on the 3rd day the patient developed a clinical picture of pressured speech, elation, and jocularity. Over the next few days the patient became increasingly elated, irritable, unable to sleep, and hostile. By the 12th day of treatment, the patient was in what would be described as the final stage of mania and was delusional and assaultive. Throughout the course of this manic symptomatology the patient had a clear sensorium.

The patient was admitted to a psychiatric unit. After receiving four electroconvulsive treatments, her manic symptomatology cleared completely. A review of the patient's past personal and psychiatric history revealed no prominent psychopathology.

EPIDEMIOLOGY

Epidemiological studies have typically been conducted for the affective disorders in general. As a consequence, it is difficult to separate out the information for manic or bipolar disorders from the larger group of affective disorders. The epidemiological information provided below is drawn from the literature available and may represent a more rough or uncertain approximation than is available for the other major psychiatric disorders described in this book. In addition, the information below pertains *only* to primary manic or bipolar disorders. Incidence and prevalence rates for secondary mania are not available.

Incidence

The incidence of a disorder is the number of new cases in a given population during the course of one year. Estimates for first admissions with the diagnosis of affective disorder to psychiatric facilities range from about 10 to 20 per 100,000, or an incidence of 0.01–0.02%.[16] It has been estimated that one-fifth of affective disorders are manic and bipolar affective disorders.[13] Thus, 0.002–0.004% is an estimate of the incidence of primary manic and bipolar affective disorders.

On the basis of epidemiological data collected in Scandinavia and the U.S., for bipolar illness exclusively, incidence is estimated to be 0.009–0.015% for men and 0.007–0.03% for women.[17]

Prevalence

The period prevalence of a disorder is total cases that exist in a population in any given year. Krauthammer and Klerman[18] estimate period prevalence for bipolar disorder to be in the range of 0.1–0.8 per thousand per year.

The DSM-III[1] reports that between 0.4 and 1.2% of adults have had bipolar affective disorder.

Age, Sex, and Race

The age of onset for manic and bipolar affective disorders is generally in the 20's. Onset after 30 suggests a less severe genotypical endowment and a better prognosis.[19] As described in Chapter 1, unipolar affective disorder is found to be about twice as prevalent in women as in men. Bipolar affective disorder appears to be more common in women than in men, but at far less than the rate of 2:1 found in unipolar disorder.

Information about the racial distribution of bipolar disorder is not available.

Socioeconomic Status

Affective disorder, in contrast to schizophrenia, has been said to be a disorder of the upper social classes.[20, 21] In support of this is a study that suggests that bipolar affective disorder is linked with superior educational and occupational achievement.[22] Other work, however, has failed to demonstrate a relationship between social class and affective disorder.[23]

In summary, then, it appears that in contrast to schizophrenia, which has a higher prevalence in the lower socioeconomic classes, affective disorders may have a higher prevalence in the higher socioeconomic groups. However, these figures do not appear to be consistent or strongly conclusive.

Families

The risk for development of bipolar affective disease among first degree relatives of afflicted patients is in the range of 10 times the magnitude of that found in the general population. The prevalence of affective illness in relatives of patients diagnosed with affective disorder of any type (unipolar or bipolar affective disorder) is estimated at 10–25% for first degree relatives of diagnosed patients. However, studies indicate the prevalence is *more pronounced* in relatives of bipolar disordered than it is in relatives of unipolar disordered patients.[16, 17, 24–27]

Twin studies support the high rate of affective disorder found in relatives of manic patients. Those twin studies that do exist show concordance rates for bipolar disorder of 68% for monozygotic twins and 23% for same sex dizygotic twins.

THEORIES OF ETIOLOGY

Biochemical Hypotheses

The biochemical understanding of affective disorders has focused primarily on the biogenic amines, a group of chemical transmitters active in certain selective sections of the CNS. The biogenic amines most frequently discussed are norepinephrine, dopamine, and serotonin.

The hypothesis that mania is characterized by an increase in biogenic amines, particularly norepinephrine has been postulated.[28, 29]

Data to support this view is derived from indirect evidence obtained from drug effects. We know that mania can be precipitated by drugs that enhance central nervous system amine transmission and that mania can be suppressed by drugs that decrease amine transmission. For example, lithium has been shown to decrease the amount of norepinephrine available at receptor sites, with consequent clinical improvement. Furthermore, dopamine-stimulating and blocking agents have been shown to respectively induce and mute mania in some patients.[30-32]

Norepinephrine has been considered the specific amine involved because its cerebrospinal fluid metabolite, 3-methoxy-4-hydroxyphenylglycol (MHPG) has been abnormal across several studies, unlike the metabolites of dopamine and serotonin. MHPG has also been shown to be the only metabolite to correlate with manic symptomatology.[33]

Should mania be associated with increased norepinephrine, we cannot conclude that a primary disturbance in norepinephrine exists. High levels of norepinephrine metabolites could be the result of a primary increase in their synthesis during mania but also could reflect a feedback-induced increase in their production secondary to a disturbance in the recognition of norepinephrine at its receptor sites.

Finally, the clinical states associated with biogenic amine changes may reflect a disturbance in the balance that exists between the different brain transmitters. Physostigmine (an acetylcholine precursor) has been shown to suppress manic symptoms in some patients with clinical mania.[34] These findings may be the result of the effect of a direct increase in brain cholinergic activity or, perhaps more likely, the result of altering the balance between brain neurotransmitter systems.[35, 36]

In *summary,* research in the areas of biochemical neurotransmitters and their excreted metabolites as well as the action of lithium all point to the importance of biogenic amines, especially norepinephrine, in clinical states of mania. It remains uncertain whether amines are the primary etiologic factors or whether mania reflects a disturbed balance of general neurotransmitter activity.

Genetic Hypotheses

As noted earlier, the risk for first degree relatives of affective disordered patients ranges from 10–25%.[16, 24-27] This is in contrast to a risk of only 1–2% in the general population. A greater than 10-fold magnitude of risk for morbidity among first degree relatives as opposed to the general population supports a dominant gene theory of genetic transmission.

As also noted, the concordance rates for bipolar affective disorders are 68% for monozygotic twins and 23% for same sex dizygotic twins. These figures also support a significant genetic contribution and represent a pattern that is consistent with an autosomal dominant gene with incomplete penetrance.

It has been suggested that bipolar disorder may be X-linked, though evidence is conflicting for this theory.[37-40] Furthermore, polygenic inheritance has also been suggested. This theory also remains inconclusive.

In *summary,* genetic factors in bipolar affective disorder are indisputable. Morbidity risk in first degree relatives as well as twin studies strongly support a genetic contribution to bipolar affective disorder. The mode of genetic transmission remains uncertain, with evidence pointing to a dominant gene with incomplete penetrance.

Psychodynamic Hypotheses

Early in this century Karl Abraham[41] hypothesized that in mania the superego merges with the ego, thereby endowing the ego with excess libidinous energy and narcissism. This merger would appear clinically as grandiosity, excess energy, and hedonistic pursuit. This psychodynamic construction is in contrast to Abraham's notion of depression, in which the superego is excessively punitive and critical of the ego.

Psychoanalytic literature since Abraham's time has generally described mania as a defense against melancholia.[42] The importance of denial as the basic defense mechanism in mania and hypomania has been repeatedly described.[43]

Rado[44] described the personality of bipolar patients as particularly sensitive to and dependent upon approval and affection from others. He saw self-esteem in bipolars as thereby fluctuating on the basis of the attitudes of others. Gibson et al.[45] and Cohen et al.[46] later confirmed these observations.

Rochlin[47] studied the "disorder of depression and elation" from a psychoanalytic perspective. He posited mood lability based on shifts between an intense but denied identification with a seductive, masochistic mother who is devalued and aggressive, and sadistic masculine wishes which serve to strengthen the denial of the identification with mother and to repress passive and masochistic longings. In Rochlin's clinical description, depression is associated with identification with the devalued, weak mother, and elation is associated with a denial of this hated identification through aggressive and sadistic impulses and wishes.

Cohen et al.[46] provided a classic paper in which the character of patients with manic-depressive disorder was examined from the perspective of having 12 such patients involved in intensive psychoanalytic psychotherapy. As a group these patients demonstrated dependent character features and were highly dependent upon the approval of others as a means of managing their self-esteem. In addition, and correlated with this, were findings that these patients held the most conventional of values. Presumably, their dependency on universal approval for the management of their esteem resulted in their tendency to be conventional and conformist and not to risk the disapproval of the objects upon whom they were dependent. Furthermore, as a group, they were remarkably competitive and employed denial as a major defense. This study's findings on the family will be discussed below.

The psychodynamic factors described by Cohen et al. have been disputed by MacVane et al.[48] His group studied the psychological functioning of bipolar affective disordered patients in remission and did not find the presence of dependent character features and conventional, conformist behaviors. This work casts doubt on Cohen's psychodynamic view of bipolar patients. What is central to MacVane's work is that all patients studied were well stabilized on lithium. The effect of stabilization of a mood disorder on the psychological functioning of bipolar patients in remission is an important area that will require further study.

In *summary,* psychodynamic contributions to mania have been reported but have been called into question by lithium treatment. More research in this area is needed.

Family Hypotheses

The family may contribute to mania through its genetic pool and through socioeconomic factors, both of which have been discussed.

Cohen's work[46] has demonstrated, in her sample of 12 cases, how these families were socially different in a significant way from their surrounding milieu. In all cases, the family of a bipolar patient felt a keen social difference. Furthermore, these families reacted to this felt difference by attempting to improve their acceptability in the community and to win social prestige through economic fortune, honor, or achievement. Frequently, the bipolar patient became the trailblazer for the family and assumed the duty of bringing success to the family. Cohen's data, if still valid, suggests the type of environment in which the bipolar patient may be raised as well as the extent to which the patient may have become employed as a means for the family to reach its desired ends.

THE BIOPSYCHOSOCIAL EVALUATION

The Biological Evaluation

The inpatient unit must have ready access to diagnostic facilities for the biological assessment of mania. The clinician's first task is to separate out 2° mania from 1° mania.

History

Mania in a patient 40 years or older with a negative psychiatric and family history should be considered 2° mania until proven otherwise.

In taking the history, the physician must be alert to any information regarding recent prescribed or nonprescribed drug ingestion or ingestion of any toxic substance. A history of infection, abnormal neurological activity, or medical treatment of any sort must also be sought.

In the *mental status examination* the clinician should search for any signs of an altered sensorium.

In addition, a detailed history of the present illness, of past medical and psychiatric illnesses, including any medications or treatment that the patient has undergone or is currently taking; the family history, with particular emphasis on inheritable disorders and psychiatric syndromes in the family; habits, including drug and dietary habits; and a thorough *review of systems* are all to be included in taking a comprehensive history.

History-taking is done best when the patient's account is augmented with collaborative information from the family, significant others, and any person who has had occasion to witness the patient's behavior or have pertinent knowledge about the events prior to hospitalization.

Physical Examination

Particular attention must be paid to the patient's vital signs and to the neurological examination, with careful inspection for any focal signs.

Laboratory Studies

1. **Regular Studies.** Complete blood cell count (CBC), urine analysis, serum test for syphilis, blood glucose, Na, K, Cl, CO_2, Ca, PO_4, creatine, BUN, alkaline phosphatase, SGOT, bilirubin-T/D, and thyroxine (T_4).

2. **Special Studies.** Toxic screening of the urine and/or blood for any suspected drug or toxin (including stimulants, steroids, L-dopa, and bromine), ESR, blood culture, lumbar puncture, pregnancy test.

Radiological Studies

1. **Regular Studies.** Chest film.

2. **Special Studies.** Skull series, CT scan, brain scan.

Additional Diagnostic Studies

EEG (with wake and sleep tracings); EKG; urine osmolality and specific gravity following a 12-hour fast for baseline urine concentrating ability.

The thyrotropin-releasing hormone (TRH) test, in which the magnitude of the release of thyroid-stimulating hormone (TSH) after infusion of TRH is measured, has been reported as a biological marker in distinguishing mania from schizophrenia.[49-51]

Psychological testing can be particularly helpful, especially once the mania has subsided. Psychological testing ought to examine for the persistence of any thought disorder as well as for any evidence of organic impairment.

Baseline Thyroid Studies for Lithium Therapy

T_4, TSH, T_3 resin uptake, FT_4 index.

Psychodynamic Evaluation

A careful developmental history, including prenatal, infancy, toddler, preschool, latency, and adolescent information, is the foundation for beginning the psychodynamic evaluation. A work, military, play, marital, and sexual history can be obtained as an elaboration of the developmental history.

An examination of the patient's ego functioning, including past and present functioning, defensive style, object relations, and capacity for adaptation and pleasure, follows the developmental assessment. Particular attention needs to be paid to how the patient's early history helped shape his ego functioning.

With this information, the clinician should be able to develop an hypothesis as to why the patient's ego has decompensated at this time.

Sociocultural and Family Evaluation

The sociocultural evaluation focuses on obtaining information on the patient's social class as well as ethnic and religious background. How home, community, and work have shaped the patient's belief system should emerge from this evaluation.

Particular attention should be paid to the current life events that are identifiable precipitants in the patient's disorder. The response of the patient's family, friends, and colleagues to these stressors and to the patient should be carefully sought.

The patient's value system about medical care and his mode of entry into the care giving system will often be critical to the clinician's knowing how to develop a working alliance with the patient.

Mania is a destructive process for both the patient and his family. In mania, intimate relations with family members, friends, and professional associates are often severely disturbed. In addition, errors in judgment during the manic illness can create financial difficulties and even catastrophy. Employment may be jeopardized or lost.

A sensitive exploration of the impact of the manic episode on the patient's family, professional, and social world is a critical part of the inpatient assessment. Such a discussion may provide the opportunity to begin the process of rebuilding a world that was severely disrupted by the patient's illness.

HOSPITAL TREATMENT

Hospital Treatment of Primary Mania

Psychopharmacological Management

Psychopharmacological management is the mainstay of treating the acutely manic patient. Although lithium is the most specific antimanic agent, its onset of action is generally 7–10 days after initiation of treatment.

Most patients with suspected mania, therefore, will be started on antipsychotic medications. Lithium may then be started if the diagnosis of mania is confirmed. As therapeutic levels of lithium begin to develop, the need for antipsychotic medications will diminish, and the clinician can then lower the dose of antipsychotic medications accordingly. Many patients will be able to come off antipsychotic medications completely and be treated with lithium alone for the latter part of their hospitalization and for their post-hospital psychopharmacological treatment.

Combined lithium and neuroleptic treatment is common and often necessary. This combination is generally safe, though reports of toxicity and persistent organic dysfunction call for judicious use and careful monitoring of this combined drug regimen. The hospitalized manic patient is especially prone to severe side effects and toxicity a week or two after lithium has been initiated. This is a time when the patient is generally on high doses of neuroleptic, which then interacts with the then substantial action of lithium. Many patients can tolerate a decrease in neuroleptic as adequate lithium levels are obtained, thus sparing them undue side effects.[54-56]

1. Antipsychotics. The antipsychotic medications are highly effective in the treatment of target symptoms of hyperactivity, anxiety, hostility, delusions, hallucinations, insomnia, and negativism. Antipsychotic medications are the first line treatment of the acute manic state. The patient can be started on a protocol for antipsychotic medications outlined in Chapter 3.

Though the antipsychotics will be effective in reducing many of the symptoms of mania, they are *not specifically antimanic*.

If the clinician decides to begin the patient on lithium, he will notice that after 5–10 days of treatment the patient will begin to show a reduced need for antipsychotic medication. An early sign of excess antipsychotic medication is sedation, particularly in the morning. As the patient begins to obtain the therapeutic effect of lithium, the antipsychotic medication may then be reduced slowly, observing for breakthrough of manic symptomatology. If there is no breakthrough of manic symptomatology, the antipsychotic medication can be slowly decreased and discontinued over the course of 1–3 weeks, leaving the patient only on lithium.

Some patients, however, will require combined treatment throughout hospitalization with both antipsychotic medications and lithium. For these patients every effort must be made to place them on the lowest amount of antipsychotic medication necessary to contain their symptomatology. The patient may be discharged on an antipsychotic medication with follow-up aimed at having the patient on the lowest dose of medication needed for effective treatment. A clear discussion with the patient (and family, when indicated) as to the risks and benefits of neuroleptic treatment should be held once the patient has stabilized on medications.

2. Lithium Carbonate. This drug is the lithium salt commonly used in clinical practice. The use of lithium has expanded considerably in the past 20 years. It offers a unique chemical agent for the treatment of acute mania as well as for the prophylactic treatment of bipolar affective disorders.[57-59]

a. Indications. Lithium is a *specific antimanic agent.* Though slow in its action, it is highly specific for the mood disorder of mania, as well as for the associated features of hyperactivity, pressured speech, flight of ideas, distractibility, and grandiosity.

Lithium is also indicated in the prophylactic treatment of bipolar affective disorder. It is beyond the scope of this chapter to discuss maintenance treatment. The reader is referred elsewhere for a review of lithium maintenance and prophylaxis.[59-61]

Barring specific contraindications to its usage, lithium is the *drug of choice* for the treatment of 1° mania.

b. Preliminary Evaluation Studies and Contraindications to Lithium Treatment. The patient's *thyroid, renal, electrolyte,* and *cardiac* status are essential aspects of the preliminary evaluation. Any abnormality in any of these systems is a possible contraindication to the use of lithium. Medical consultation must be obtained if lithium is to be considered in the presence of any abnormality.

Lithium should be avoided, if possible, with pregnancy, especially during the first trimester. Teratogenic effects are primarily on the heart. A serum test for pregnancy should be considered before administering lithium to a woman of child-bearing capacity.[61, 62]

In addition, the patient's *general physical status* must also be examined and a *personality assessment* made. Because of the nature of lithium treatment, which calls for daily administration as well as careful blood monitoring, the patient needs to be judged reliable to take medications as prescribed and not impulsively liable to take large amounts of medications that could result in severe toxicity or death.

c. Administration. Lithium carbonate is administered as a 300 mg oral capsule or tablet. It is also available as lithium citrate, a liquid that can be dispensed in smaller dosages. Lithium is never administered parenterally. Lithium is absorbed readily in the gut and is metabolized almost completely by the kidney.

The half-life of lithium ranges from about 18 to 36 hours, according to the person's renal function. As a rule, younger people excrete lithium more quickly and, therefore, show a lower half-life and tend to require higher doses.

Lithium is administered in divided doses, three to four times per day. Administering the drug with or after meals appears to diminish gastrointestinal irritation. Sustained action lithium preparations may also be helpful in reducing gastrointestinal and other side effects.

In acute mania, the clinician is seeking to obtain a serum lithium level of around 1.0 meq/L. Blood levels are drawn in the morning, approximately 12 hours after the previous evening's dose. *No* morning dose of medication is provided until blood is drawn. In the 1st week of hospitalization blood levels may be drawn every other day in order to most closely monitor the effects of the medication and to observe for entrance into the therapeutic range. Once the patient has entered this range, blood levels may be drawn several times per week. Thereafter, blood levels may be drawn once or twice a week according to clinical needs. After several weeks the patients may go to a less frequent schedule of blood levels, e.g., once a week, then to every other week, then to once a month.

Generally, a *slow induction* process is adequate. With slow induction, the patient is generally begun on 900 mg/day of lithium, or one tablet t.i.d. The dose is then increased every several days with guidelines drawn from the serum lithium levels.

In some patients, a *rapid induction* may be indicated in order to provide the agent as quickly as possible. This situation may arise particularly in an open unit of a general hospital, where manic symptomatology may not be tolerated. The aim would be to bring the manic symptomatology under control quickly in order to avoid transfer to a closed unit in another hospital. In the rapid induction protocol, patients may be started on 600 mg of lithium t.i.d., with blood levels monitored every day and dosages adjusted upwards or downwards according to the serum lithium level. Acutely manic patients will generally require daily doses between 1200 and 3600 mg of lithium carbonate. As the mania subsides and the patient enters the subacute phase of mania, the dose will need to be decreased.

Furthermore, once the mania has subsided, the clinician seeks to obtain a lithium level in the range of 0.8 meq/L. This maintenance level of lithium is indicated for the postmanic phase in hospital and for posthospital prophylaxis. Some patients will do well at a lower blood level, while some will require higher levels. It is always the patient's clinical status, not his blood level, that determines the proper dose of lithium.

d. Side Effects. Intoxication from lithium generally occurs when the dose is in excess of clinical needs. Some patients, however, will demonstrate lithium toxicity at normal dosages. This appears to be more common in elderly patients. The *signs and symptoms* of lithium toxicity are *nausea and vomiting, diarrhea, tremor, muscular weakness, ataxia, and drowsiness.* If intoxication becomes more severe, the patient may demonstrate muscle hyperirritability with increased deep tendon reflexes, twitching, fasciculation, and nystagmus. The patient's mental status changes with increasing intoxication, with the patient initially showing confusion which may progress to stupor and then coma. Seizures may occur with severe intoxication.

The management of lithium toxicity begins with discontinuing the administration of lithium. Frequently, if intoxication is discovered early, this alone will be adequate. In more severe cases, medical consultation is indicated, and the use of gastric lavage, fluid loading, and careful electrolyte balance will be needed.

Cardiovascular side effects of lithium include EKG changes (T-wave flattening or inversion), hypotension, and arrhythmias.

Renal side effects of lithium include a diabetes insipidus with polyuria and polydipsia. Lithium-induced diabetes insipidus is generally responsive to a reduction in the lithium dose or the administration of a thiazide diuretic. Amiloride, a potassium-sparing diuretic that acts on the collecting tubule, has also been effective in ameliorating lithium-induced polyuria.[64, 65]

Recent reports[66–69] have demonstrated an *interstitial fibrotic process* found in patients on long-term lithium therapy. If lithium does cause structural changes in the kidney with subsequent renal compromise, the risk of long-term maintenance therapy with lithium must be considered and discussed with the patient. The possibility of structural renal damage calls for even *more careful selection* of patients needing lithium treatment, *baseline and regular follow-up renal functioning testing,* and *maintenance of the patient at blood levels as low as possible for clinical control.* Lithium is also implicated in the development of *goiter.* This goiter is benign and diffuse and generally patients are euthyroid or mildly hypothyroid.

Hematologic side effects are generally infrequent. They include leucocytosis and thrombocytosis; both effects reverse promptly if lithium is discontinued.[70]

Tremor is a common and often troublesome side effect of lithium treatment. Though lowering the dose of lithium may sometimes alleviate the tremor, it often persists. Beta-adrenergic blockers, such as propanolol, are often very helpful. Metoprolol, a cardioselective blocker, may be used for patients who can not take propanolol because of bronchospasm.[71, 72] *Skin* changes with lithium treatment include dry skin, folliculitis, and ulcerations.

Lithium has been demonstrated to be *teratogenic.*[62, 63, 73] The clinician must keep this in mind in prescribing lithium to women who are of childbearing age. The use of lithium during pregnancy is contraindicated except under the most special of circumstances.

e. Caveats. Keep in mind that toxicity from antipsychotic agents and from lithium is enhanced by the combined action of the two drugs.[54, 55] A clinician needs to be acutely aware of the effects of this drug combination several days to 1 week into treatment when the patient is approaching the therapeutic range of lithium while still on high doses of antipsychotic medications.

Some patients may show lithium intoxication in the normal range. The serum lithium level is a guide; it is not a commandment. The patient's clinical state is the primary determinant in adjusting dosage.

A number of medications can alter the kinetics of lithium and thereby change the serum concentration. Lithium levels should be monitored carefully when a patient is taking other medications, or if another drug is prescribed for a patient on lithium.[74, 75] All older patients, especially those with impaired renal functioning, excrete lithium more slowly, rendering them more susceptible to lithium toxicity.

A significant number of manic patients engage in self-medication prior to admission. Alcohol and sedatives appear to be frequent drugs used by these patients in their effort to modulate their dysphoric mood. Clinicians should be alert to signs of nonprescribed drug use on admission and be alert to the possibility of any withdrawal syndrome from CNS depressants while the patient is in the hospital.

3. Barbiturates. Barbiturates may be helpful adjunctively in the treatment of acute mania. Highly agitated patients who are on high doses of antipsychotic medication, as well as beginning on lithium, may benefit from an h.s. dose of 120–180 mg p.o. of sodium amytal.

4. Novel Treatment Approaches to Mania. Carbamazepine (Tegretol), an anticonvulsant, has shown some early success in the treatment of mania,[76-79] and should be considered for patients unable to take or refractory to lithium. Lecithin, the dietary precursor of choline, may hold some promise for the treatment of manic states.[80, 81]

A variety of other agents, including clonidine, clonazepam, verapamil, clorgyline, and L-tryptophan, have been reported to be effective for mania and should be considered when other efforts have failed.[82-87]

ECT

Electroconvulsive therapy (ECT) has long been recognized as a clinically effective treatment for mania.[88, 89]

Patients who are intolerant of antipsychotics or lithium should be considered for ECT. Further, for patients with severe excitement that borders on frenzy, with associated combativeness and difficulty administering adequate doses of medication, ECT can be considered as a first line of treatment for mania. In these severely manic patients, some of whom are known to run fatal courses, ECT may be the most sensible treatment because of its rapid action and high efficacy and safety.

Milieu Management

The manic patient's poor judgment, severe denial, grandiosity, euphoria, and hyperactivity frequently preclude his voluntary admission. Many manic patients, therefore, refuse voluntary treatment and are hospitalized involuntarily, particularly if their symptoms include danger to self or others.

Some manic patients, however, will seek voluntary admission, especially when pressured by friends, family, and work associates. For these patients a clear understanding of what *limits they must exercise on their behavior* is a critical part of the initial milieu management. Threatening or combative behaviors, abusing alcohol or nonprescribed drugs while on the ward, and being sexually provocative are behaviors that must be limited for the benefit of the individual patient as well as for the rest of the patient community. The manic patient must be told that these are behaviors that will not be tolerated on an open ward and represent grounds for transfer to a closed ward. Absolutely firm and consistent limit setting is essential to clinical management and to precluding dangerous acting out.[90]

Decreasing stimulation by restricting visitors and providing periods of time alone are part of the milieu treatment of the manic patient. Many of the milieu management techniques for the acutely psychotic patient apply to the acutely manic patient. The reader is referred to Chapter 3, where these are outlined.

Janowsky et al.[91, 92] have described what they call the interpersonal maneuvers of the manic patient, or the manic game. They hypothesize that the manic patient's central dynamic is his need to be taken care of. Dependent needs, however, are regarded by the manic as unacceptable and dangerous. The manic's activities are thereby seen as his way of being cared for without having to admit it.

Manic maneuvers include: (1) manipulating the self-esteem of others; (2) making individual and group conflict overt; (3) projecting responsibility; (4) progressive testing of limits; and (5) alienating family members.

An understanding of this interpersonal game enables a ward staff to expect the manic to attack or flatter their self-esteem, to divide staff, to deny and project personal responsibility, to constantly test limits, and to damage family relations. This understanding can help control staff anger and is critical in not allowing the manic to manipulate them by flattery or by assault on their self-esteem.

A manic patient generally has great impact on the rest of the ward community. Agitation and irritability in any patient tends to raise the general level of anxiety in the community. In addition, the manic patient may threaten legal action against the ward as well as attempt to call a variety of authorities in an attempt to support his manic denial.

The *community meeting* is an important forum for the ward community to understand the nature of the manic patient's symptomatology. Staff can attempt to allay some of the ward anxiety and try to enlist other patients in the treatment plan for the manic patient.

Individual Psychotherapy

Alliance Building in the Manic Phase

Explorative psychotherapy with the acutely manic patient is an exercise in futility. All the clinician can expect during this phase is to obtain a comprehensive history and to begin to develop an alliance with the patient through a combination of empathic support, firm limit setting, and effective chemotherapy.

The Postmanic Phase

Manic patients appear most amenable to psychiatric treatment when they are in a depressive phase of their illness. When bipolar patients are manic or euthymic, they tend to deny their illness and show little affinity for treatment.

For many bipolar patients dysphoric affect is anathema and is poorly tolerated. Sadness, shame, and guilt about their illness and anxiety about their future may typically be defended against by denial and flight. As a consequence, as the mania subsides and painful reality issues emerge, the patient may minimize his illness, reject medication, wish to flee the hospital, and not participate in plans for outpatient follow-up.

It is, therefore, at the moment when the mania is abating and the dysphoric affect emerging that the clinician may be most successful in establishing a psychotherapeutic relationship. If the clinician can, at that time, assist the patient in not resorting to manic denial or flight and aid him in bearing dysphoric affect, psychotherapy can begin.

The initial psychotherapeutic work should be aimed at *identifying* stressful events and feelings that were instrumental to the manic decompensation.

In addition, the clinician can help the patient begin to *bear feelings* without psychotic denial, grandiosity, or flight. More adaptive modes of coping with painful feelings are explored and supported in the psychotherapeutic hour.

As psychotherapy progresses, the patient can be helped in his work of repairing and re-establishing personal and professional *relationships*. As the patient's history will detail, many important relationships were inevitably damaged in the manic episode.

Finally, the patient can be *counseled* on the nature and course of bipolar illness. The clinician needs to work constantly on developing an alliance with the patient by emphasizing the treatability of his disorder with medication and psychotherapy.[93]

Family Work

Family Counseling

Single or recurrent episodes of mania are highly disruptive to the patient's family. It is highly important to help the family see mania as a treatable illness and thereby alter an often angry and limited perspective in which the patient's symptomatic behavior is interpreted as fully willful, hostile, irresponsible, or weak.

Marital instability is characteristic for bipolar patients. Fifty-seven percent of bipolars' marriages ended in divorce while only 8% of unipolar patients' marriages suffered a similar fate.[94] Spouses of unipolar patients tended to feel sympathy for their suffering, anger toward their dependency, and guilt for perhaps contributing to the depression; there was, however, little doubt that the marriage would continue. In contrast, spouses of bipolars were frequently motivated for divorce.

Spouses of bipolars are generally the principal object of the patients' anger and are seen as villains, opponents, and "bad parents." Furthermore, the spouse may be deeply wounded by the manic's infidelity. Spouses also generally find themselves answering to the complaints of the manic patients' social and professional community.[91]

Supportive, empathic meetings by a social worker or unit staff member with family members can begin without the patient. An alliance with the family can be established around treatment for the manic patient. In these meetings, the family worker can invite a discussion of the impact of the manic episode on the family as well as begin to make personality assessments of individual members of the family. Spouses of manic patients have been noted to have personality problems, including excessive rigidity and difficulties with alcoholism and gambling.[95]

Once the manic patient's symptomatology is under control, the family meetings can then be broadened to include the patient. During these metings general

family evaluation can begin. The clinician should pay particular attention to the way the family manages affective and power issues.

As the patient improves and his hospitalization is ending, the family can be involved in a short-term family therapy in which issues of mental illness and well-being, dependence and independence, mood fluctuations, and caretaking roles can be addressed. It is only after a period of sustained mood stability that family work, if indicated, can be directed at examining and correcting long-established maladaptive patterns and behaviors.[96]

Genetic Counseling

Genetic counseling for psychiatric patients and their families is a relatively new and highly valuable service that we can provide.

Tsuang[97] has provided an overview of this subject as well as an excellent description of what he calls the stages of counseling. As noted earlier, the risk for first degree relatives of patients with bipolar disorder is nearly 20-fold higher than normal. Furthermore, it has been estimated that siblings of the patient with bipolar disorder have a risk of 26% of becoming ill when one parent was also ill with affective disorder and a risk of 43% when both parents had a history of affective illness.[98]

Because these risk statistics are so high, they will need to be carefully shared with the family with follow-up discussion generally advisable. An understanding of the patient as well as family members is essential in order to provide information at a level that they can understand and at a pace they can accept.

Hospital Treatment of Secondary Mania

When manic symptomatology is secondary in nature, the clinician's task is to make a diagnosis of the underlying cause and to correct that organic disturbance. Frequently, however, the correction of the underlying cause may take considerable time or may be impossible. Furthermore, it may be essential to correct the manic symptomatology in order to proceed with diagnostic procedures.

When 2° manic symptomatology needs

to be corrected by psychopharmacological management, the same form of treatment used for 1° mania is applicable.[3, 15, 99-109] If the patient's medical state permits, and the exceptions are rare, the patient may be started on a neuroleptic medication and lithium added if the response to the neuroleptic is less than satisfactory. ECT can and has been used effectively in cases of 2° mania.

COURSE AND PROGNOSIS OF 1° MANIA

The *course* of a manic episode is generally 3–12 months, with a mean duration of 6 months.[110, 111] This time period may be truncated by effective antimanic treatment. The duration of manic episodes appears longer in those patients with recurrent manic episodes and advancing age.[16]

Prognostically, there is a high tendency for manic episodes to recur. It is estimated that 50–75% of manic patients go on to suffer one or more manic episodes.[110-113] In addition, most patients with mania also develop depressive episodes. For those patients who show recurrent manic episodes, the interval between episodes appears to grow shorter as the patient grows older.[16]

There is controversy about the interepisodic behavior and functioning of the bipolar patient. As discussed earlier, there is evidence that bipolar patients can show high functioning interepisodically, especially if they are receiving adequate treatment.[48]

REFERENCES

1. American Psychiatric Association. *Diagnostic and Statistical Manual of Mental Disorders,* ed. 3 (DSM-III). Washington, D.C., American Psychiatric Association, APA Task Force on Nomenclature, 1980.
2. Winokur G, et al.: *Manic Depressive Illness,* St. Louis, C.V. Mosby, 1969.
3. Krauthammer C, Klerman GL: Secondary mania. Arch Gen Psychiatry, *35:* 1333–1339, 1978.
4. Carlson GA, Goodwin FK: The stages of mania. Arch Gen Psychiatry, *28:* 221–228, 1973.
5. Abrams R, Taylor MA: Importance of schizophrenic symptoms in the diagnosis of mania. Am J Psychiatry, *138:* 658–661, 1981.
6. Pope HG, Lipinski JF: Diagnosis in schizo-
phrenia and manic-depressive illness. Arch Gen Psychiatry, *35:* 811–828, 1978.
7. Pope HG: Distinguishing bipolar disorder from schizophrenia in clinical practice: guidelines and case reports. Hosp Community Psychiatry, *34:* 322–325, 1983.
8. Pope HG, Lipinski JF, et al: Schizoaffective disorder: An invalid diagnosis? Am J Psychiatry, *137:* 921–927, 1980.
9. Brockington IF, Hillier VF, et al.: Definitions of mania: Concordance and prediction of outcome. Am J Psychiatry: 435–439, 1983.
10. Bond TC: Recognition of acute delirious mania. Arch Gen Psychiatry, *37:* 553–554, 1980.
11. Chiles JA, Cohen DP: Pseudodementia and mania. J Nerv Ment Dis, *167:* 357–358, 1979.
12. Cowdry RW, Goodwin FK: Dementia of bipolar illness: Diagnosis and response to lithium. Am J Psychiatry, *138:* 1118–1119, 1981.
13. Thase ME, Reynold CF: Manic pseudodementia. Psychosomatics, *25:* 256–260, 1984.
14. Mapelli G, Bellelli TP: Secondary mania (letter to the editor). Arch Gen Psychiatry, *39:* 743, 1982.
15. Glaser GH: Psychotic reactions induced by corticotropin (ACTH) and cortisone. Psychosom Med, *15:* 280–291, 1953.
16. Klerman GL, Barrett JE: The affective disorders: Clinical and epidemiological aspects, in Gershon S, Shopsin G (eds.): *Lithium: Its Role in Psychiatric Treatment and Research,* New York, Plenum Press, 1973.
17. Boyd JH, Weissman MM: Epidemiology of affective disorders. Arch Gen Psychiatry, *38:* 1039–1046, 1981.
18. Krauthammer C, Klerman GL: The epidemiology of mania. In Shopsin B (ed), *Manic Illness,* pp. 11–28, New York, Raven Press, 1979.
19. Taylor MA, Abrams R: Early and late onset bipolar illness. Arch Gen Psychiatry, *38:* 58–61, 1981.
20. Faris REL, Dunham HW: *Mental Disorders in Urban Areas: An Ecological Study of Schizophrenia and Other Psychoses,* Chicago, University of Chicago Press, 1939.
21. Maltzberg B: Mental disease in relation to economic status. J Nerv Ment Dis, *123:* 256, 1956.
22. Woodruff RA, et al: Manic depressive illness and social achievement. Acta Psychiatr Scand, *47:* 237–249, 1971.
23. Hare EH, Price JS, et al.: Parental social class in psychiatric patients. Br J Psychiatry, *121:* 515, 1972.
24. Reich T, et al.: Family history studies: V. The genetics of mania. Am J Psychiatry, *125:* 1358–1369, 1969.
25. Johnson GFS, Leeman MM: Analysis of familial factors in bipolar affective illness. Arch Gen Psychiatry, *34:* 1074–1083, 1977.
26. Weissman MM, Gershon ES, et al.: Psychiatric disorders in the relatives of probands with affective disorders. Arch Gen Psychiatry, *41:* 13–21, 1984.
27. Gershon ES, Hamovit J, et al.: A family study

of schizoaffective, bipolar I, bipolar II, unipolar, and normal control probands. Arch Gen Psychiatry, *39:* 1157–1167, 1982.

28. Annitto W, Shopsin B: Neuropharmacology, in Shopsin B (ed): *Manic Illness,* pp. 128–149, New York, Raven Press, 1979.

29. Schildkraut JJ: The catecholamine hypothesis of affective disorders. Am J Psychiatry, *122:* 509–522, 1965.

30. Schildkraut JJ: The effects of lithium on biogenic amines, in Gershon S, Shopsin B (eds): *Lithium: Its Role in Psychiatric Research and Treatment,* New York, Plenum Press, 1973.

31. Gerner RH, et al.: A dopaminergic mechanism in mania. Am J Psychiatry, *133:* 1177–1180, 1976.

32. Jouvent R, Lecrubier Y, et al.: Antimanic effect of clonidine. Am J Psychiatry, *137:* 1275–1276, 1980.

33. Swann AC, Secunda S, et al.: CSF monoamine metabolites in mania. Am J Psychiatry, *140:* 396–400, 1983.

34. Davis KL, et al.: Physostigmine in mania. Arch Gen Psychiatry, *35:* 119–122, 1978.

35. Nadi NS, Nurnberger JI, et al.: Muscarinic cholinergic receptors in skin fibroblasts in familial affective disorder. N Engl J Med, *311:* 225–230, 1984.

36. Snyder SS: Cholinergic mechanisms in affective disorders. N Engl J Med, *311:* 254–255, 1984.

37. Mendlewicz J, et al.: Color blindness linkage to bipolar manic depressive illness. Arch Gen Psychiatry, *36:* 1442–1447, 1979.

38. Gershon CS, et al.: Color blindness not closely linked to bipolar illness. Arch Gen Psychiatry, *36:* 1423–1430, 1979.

39. Leckman JF, et al.: New data do not suggest linkage between th Xg blood group and bipolar illness. Arch Gen Psychiatry, *36:* 1435–1441, 1979.

40. Mendlewicz J: X-Chromosome markers in bipolar illness (letter). Arch Gen Psychiatry, *38:* 719, 1981.

41. Abraham K: *Selected Papers on Psycho-Analysis,* London, Hogarth Press, 1950.

42. Lewin B: *The Psychoanalysis of Elation,* New York, WW Norton, 1950.

43. Deutsch H: The psychology of manic-depressive states, with particular reference to chronic hypomania, in *Neurosis and Character Types,* pp. 203–217, New York, International University Press, 1965.

44. Rado S: The problem of melancholia. Int J Psychoanal, *9:* 420–438, 1928.

45. Gibson RW, Cohen MB, et al.: On the dynamics of the manic-depressive personality. Am J Psychiatry, *115:* 1101⅛107, 1959.

46. Cohen MB, Baker G, Cohen RA, et al.: An intensive study of 12 cases of manic-depressive psychosis. Psychiatry, *17:* 103–137, 1954.

47. Rochlin G: Disorder of depression and elations. J Am Psychoanal Assoc, *1:* 438–457, 1953.

48. MacVane JR, et al.: Psychological functioning of bipolar manic-depressives in remission. Arch Gen Psychiatry, *35:* 1351–1354, 1978.

49. Extein I, Pottash ALC, et al.: Differentiating mania from schizophrenia by the TRH test. Am J Psychiatry, *137:* 981–982, 1980.

50. Extein I, Pottash ALC, et al.: Using the protirelin test to distinguish mania from schizophrenia. Arch Gen Psychiatry, *39:* 77–81, 1982.

51. Amsterdam JD, Winokur A, et al.: A neuroendocrine test battery in bipolar patients and healthy subjects. Arch Gen Psychiatry, *40:* 515–521, 1983.

52. Gelenberg A (ed): *Biological Therapies in Psychiatry Newsletter,* Massachusetts General Hospital, vol. 1, no. 2, 1978.

53. Gelenberg A (ed): *Biological Therapies in Psychiatry Newsletter,* Massachusetts General Hospital, vol. 7, no. 11, 1984.

54. Coffey EC, Ross DR: Treatment of lithium neuroleptic neurotoxicity during lithium maintenance. Am J Psychiatry, *137:* 736–737, 1980.

55. Spring G, Frankel M: New data on lithium and haldol incompatibility. Am J Psychiatry, *138:* 818–821, 1981.

56. Gelenberg A (ed): *Biological Therapies in Psychiatry Newsletter,* Massachusetts General Hospital, vol. 7, no. 6, 1984.

57. Baldessarini RJ: *Chemotherapy in Psychiatry,* pp. 57–75, Cambridge, Harvard University Press, 1977.

58. Gershon S, Shopsin B: *Lithium: Its Role in Psychiatric Research and Treatment,* New York, Plenum Press, 1973.

59. Davis JM: Overview: Maintenance therapy in psychiatry, II. Affective disorders. Am J Psychiatry, *133:* 1–13, 1976.

60. Prien RF, Kupfer DJ, et al.: Drug therapy in the prevention of recurrences in unipolar and bipolar affective disorders. Arch Gen Psychiatry, *41:* 1096–1104, 1984.

61. Prien RF: NIMH Report: Five center study clarifies use of lithium, imipramine for recurrent affective disorders. Hosp Community Psychiatry, *35:* 1097–1098, 1984.

62. Gelenberg A (ed): Lithium during pregnancy: Risks of cardiovascular malformations, in: *Biological Therapies in Psychiatry Newsletter,* Massachusetts General Hospital, vol. 4, No. 1, 1981.

63. Nurnberg HG, Prudic J: Guidelines for treatment of psychosis during pregnancy. Hosp Community Psychiatry, *35:* 67–71, 1984.

64. Ramsey TA, Cox M: Lithium and the kidney: A review. Am J Psychiatry, *139:* 443–449, 1982.

65. Battle DC, von Riotte AB, et al.: Amelioration of polyuria by amiloride in patients receiving long-term lithium therapy. N Engl J Med, *312:* 408–414, 1985.

66. Hestbech H, et al.: Chronic renal lesions following long-term treatment with lithium. Kidney Int, *12:* 205–213, 1977.

67. Burrows GD, et al.: Unique tubular lesion after lithium. Lancet, *7:* 1310, 1978.

68. Bucht G, Wahlin A: Impairment of renal concentrating capacity by lithium. Lancet, *1:* 778–779, 1978.

69. Hestbech J, Aurell M: Lithium induced uremia. Lancet, *1:* 491, 1979.
70. Prakash R: A review of the hematologic side effects of lithium. Hosp Community Psychiatry, *36:* 127–128, 1985.
71. Ebadi M: Management of tremor by beta adrenergic blocking agents. Gen Pharmacol, *11:* 257–260, 1980.
72. Gaby NS, Lefkowitz DS, et al.: Treatment of lithium tremor with metoprolol. Am J Psychiatry, *140:* 593–595, 1983.
73. Goldberg HG, DiMascio A: Psychotropic drugs in pregnancy In Lipton, MA, et al. (eds): *Psychopharmacology: A Generation of Progress,* pp. 1047–1055, New York, Raven Press, 1978.
74. Jefferson JW, Greist JH: *Primer of Lithium Therapy,* Baltimore, Williams & Wilkins, 1977, pp. 109–118.
75. Perry PJ, Calloway RA, et al.: Theophylline-precipitated alterations of lithium clearance. Acta Psychiatr Scand, *69:* 528–537, 1984.
76. Ballenger JC, Post RM: Carbamazepine in manic-depressive illness: A new treatment. Am J Psychiatry, *137:* 782–790, 1980.
77. Okuma T, Kishimoto A: Anti-manic and prophylactic effects of carbamazepine on manic-depressive psychosis. Folia Psychiatr Neurol Jpn, *27:* 283–297, 1973.
78. Klein E, Bental E, et al.: Carbamazepine and haloperidol vs. placebo and haloperidol in excited psychoses. Arch Gen Psychiatry, *41:* 165–170, 1984.
79. Nelson HB: Cost effectiveness of carbamazepine in refractory bipolar illness. Am J Psychiatry, *141:* 465, 1984.
80. Cohen BM, Miller AL, et al.: Lecithin in mania: A preliminary report. Am J Psychiatry, *137:* 242–243, 1980.
81. Cohen BM, Lipinski JF, et al. Lecithin in the treatment of mania. Am J Psychiatry, *139:* 1162–1164, 1982.
82. Giannini AJ, Extein I, et al.: Clonidine in mania. Drug Dev Res, *3:* 101–103, 1983.
83. Znbenko GS, Cohen BM, et al.: Clonidine in the treatment of mania and mixed bipolar disorder. Am J Psychiatry, *141:* 1617–1618, 1984.
84. Chouinard G, Young SN, et al.: Antimanic effect of clonazepam. Biol Psychiatry, *18:* 451–466, 1983.
85. Giannini AJ, Houser WL, et al.: Antimanic effects of verapamil. Am J Psychiatry, *141:* 1602–1603, 1984.
86. Potter WZ, Murphy DL, et al.: Clorgyline. Arch Gen Psychiatry, *39:* 505–510, 1982.
87. Beitman BD, Dunner DL: L-tryptophan in the maintenance treatment of bipolar II manic-depressive illness. Am J Psychiatry, 1498–1499, 1982.
88. McCabe MS: ECT in the treatment of mania: A controlled study. Am J Psychiatry, *133:* 688–691, 1976.
89. Weiner RD: The psychiatric use of electrically induced seizures. Am J Psychiatry, *136:* 1507–1517, 1979.
90. Gunderson JG: Management of manic states:
91. Janowsky DS, Leff M, et al.: Playing the manic game. Arch Gen Psychiatry, *22:* 252–261, 1970.
92. Janowsky DS, El-Yousef MK, et al.: Interpersonal maneuvers of manic patients. Am J Psychiatry, *131:* 250–255, 1974.
93. Jamison KR, Goodwin FK: Psychotherapeutic issues in bipolar illness. In Grinspoon L (ed): *Psychiatry Update: Volume II*, pp. 319–337, Washington D.C., 1983.
94. De-Nour AK: Psychosocial aspects of the management of mania, in Belmaker RH, Van Praag HM (eds): *Mania: An Evolving Concept,* pp. 349–365, New York, Spectrum Publications, 1980.
95. Dunner DL, Fleiss JL, et al.: Assortative mating in primary affective disorder. Biol Psychiatry, *11:* 43–51, 1976.
96. Mayo JA, O'Connell RA, et al.: Families of manic-depressive patients: Effect of treatment. Am J Psychiatry, *136:* 1535–1539, 1979.
97. Tsuang MT: Genetic counseling for psychiatric patients and their families. Am J Psychiatry, *135:* 1465–1475, 1978.
98. Winokur G, Clayton P: Family history studies: Two types of affective disorders separated according to genetic and clinical factors, in Wortis J (ed); *Recent Advances in Biological Psychiatry,* Vol. 9, New York, Plenum Publishing Corp., 1967.
99. Rosenbaum AH, Barry MJ: Positive therapeutic response to lithium in hypomania secondary to organic brain syndrome. Am J Psychiatry, *132:* 1072–1073, 1975.
100. Goolker P, Schein J: Psychic effects of ACTH and cortisone. Psychosom Med, *15:* 589–597, 1953.
101. Carney MW: Five cases of bromism. Lancet, *2:* 523–524, 1971.
102. Jefferson JW: Questioning a diagnosis. Am J Psychiatry, *133:* 1208–1209, 1976.
103. Weisert KN, Hendrie HC: Secondary mania? A case report. Am J Psychiatry, *134:* 929–930, 1977.
104. Oppler W: Manic psychosis in a case of parasagittal meningioma. Arch Neurol Psychiatry, *64:* 417–430, 1950.
105. Steinberg D, Hirsch SR, et al.: Influenza infection causing manic psychosis. Br J Psychiatry, *124:* 140–143, 1974.
106. Kane CS, Taylor TW: Mania associated with the use of INH and cocaine. Am J Psychiatry, *119:* 1098–1099, 1963.
107. Ryback RS, Schwab RS: Manic response to levodopa therapy: Report of a case. N Engl J Med, *285:* 788–789, 1971.
108. France RD, Krishnan KR: Alprazolam-induced manic reaction (letter to the editor). Am J Psychiatry, *141:* 1127–1128, 1984.
109. Price LH, Charney DS, et al.: Three cases of manic symptoms following yohimbine administration. Am J Psychiatry, *141:* 1267–1268, 1984.
110. Lundquist G: Prognosis and course in manic

The problem of fire setting. Psychiatry, *37:* 137–146, 1974.

depressive psychosis: A follow-up study of 319 first admissions. Acta Psychiatr Neurol, Suppl. 35, 1945.

111. Mayer-Gross W, et al.: *Clinical Psychiatry,* 3rd ed, London, Balliere, Tindall and Cassell, 1969.

112. Pollock HM: Recurrence of attacks in manic-depressive psychoses. Am J Psychiatry, *11:* 567, 1931.

113. Rennie TAC: Prognosis in manic-depressive psychoses. Am J Psychiatry, *98:* 801, 1942.

chapter 3

schizophrenic disorders

Lloyd I. Sederer, M.D.

DEFINITION

Schizophrenia is not a unitary disorder. Varied clinical presentations, natural histories, family histories, and responses to treatment have led to the opinion that there exists a spectrum of pathology which we can term Schizophrenic Disorders.[1]

Though there is considerable controversy in the field about the essential features of the schizophrenic disorders, the third edition of the *Diagnostic and Statistical Manual of Mental Disorders* (DSM-III)[1] details the current state of thinking in this area. The features that distinguish schizophrenia* include the absence of any organic or affective disorder that may have existed prior to or concurrent with the schizophrenic disorder; a characteristic acute symptom complex and a deterioration in functioning over time (see Diagnosis); and a tendency toward onset early in adult life and a proclivity towards chronicity.

Case Example: This was the first psychiatric hospitalization for Ms. A., a 23-year-old, unemployed, white, single female admitted to the hospital with the chief complaint of "nervousness."

The patient maintained that she had been "sick all of my life." On more specific questioning she was able to indicate that her problems dated back to the ninth grade. At that time she began to feel that she was not normal; she became suspicious of other people, withdrew from friends and family, and began to develop a "dream world" in which she imagined be-

*In this chapter schizophrenia and schizophrenic disorders will be used interchangeably, with the understanding that both terms convey a spectrum of disorders.

coming an actress. She increasingly preoccupied herself in her fantasy world, while listening to music and spending hours grooming herself in front of a mirror.

She did poorly for the remainder of high school, but did graduate and began to work in a factory doing simple assembly work. She continued to live at home. Her work was considered marginal and her isolation continued.

At age 20, Ms. A. was laid off from work. Thereafter, she became more isolated and withdrawn and began to think that she was really two people—someone who was attractive, social, and active and someone who was "deranged." She became obsessed with the idea that someone else existed who was either identical to her or that such a person could be created by surgery. She fantasized that eggs found in her menses could be recycled in such a way that clones of herself could be produced. Her suspiciousness increased and she began to experience the words "no children" inserted into her thoughts.

In the course of the next year, Ms. A. continued her isolation at home, doing little and relying heavily on her family. She developed an additional preoccupation that her face had changed its appearance. She began to worry that her nose would begin to grow if she touched it.

Several weeks prior to admission the patient became particularly despondent about her life and planned suicide by mixing bleach and toilet bowl cleaner together, thinking that this would create a gas that would poison her. Her mother discovered this plan and arranged for psychiatric consultation.

DIAGNOSIS

The diagnosis of schizophrenia remains as controversial today as it was almost a century ago. In that era, Kraepelin[2] proposed the diagnosis of dementia praecox, or an early mental deterioration leading to a chronic deteriorating course, while Bleuler[3] argued that the disorder, though specific in its symptomatology (see below), had a more variable course.

This debate continues today. The current consensus, as offered by the DSM-III of the American Psychiatric Association, is Kraepelinian in its tone. DSM-III describes schizophrenic disorders as generally occurring in adolescence or early adulthood and resulting in chronic deterioration in multiple areas of life functioning.

Patients whose psychotic presentations and course vary from this picture may represent atypical affective disorders. This hypothesis is being tested by more stringent diagnostic evaluations with longitudinal follow-up as well as by response to treatment with lithium.[4-9]

In addition to diagnostic uncertainty there are other reasons to demand care and circumspection before making the diagnosis of schizophrenia. First, this diagnosis may limit treatment considerations and potentially preclude trials on a variety of pharmacological agents used in the affective disorders. Second, the diagnosis suggests decline and chronicity, which can hamper hope in patients, families, employers, and caregivers.

Because multiple diagnostic schemes are still in use, I will briefly note the work of Bleuler and Schneider after detailing the DSM-III material.

DSM-III Diagnostic Criteria for Schizophrenic Disorders[1]

1. At least one of the following during a phase of the illness:
   a. Bizarre delusions (content is patently absurd and has no possible basis in fact), such as delusions of being controlled, thought broadcasting, thought insertion, or thought withdrawal.
   b. Somatic, grandiose, religious, nihilistic, or other delusions without persecutory or jealous content.
   c. Delusions with persecutory or jealous content if accompanied by hallucinations of any type.
   d. Auditory hallucinations in which either a voice keeps up a running commentary on the individual's behavior or thoughts, or two or more voices conversing with each other.
   e. Auditory hallucinations on several occasions with content of more than one or two words, having no apparent relation to depression or elation.
   f. Incoherence, marked loosening of associations, markedly illogical thinking, or marked poverty of content of speech if associated with at least one of the following:
      i. Blunted, flat, or inappropriate affect
      ii. Delusions or hallucinations
      iii. Catatonic or other grossly disorganized behavior
2. Deterioration from a previous level of functioning in such areas as work, social relations, and self-care.
3. Duration. Continuous signs of the illness for at least 6 months at some time during the person's life, with some signs of the illness at present. The 6-month period must include an active phase during which there were symptoms from 1, with or without a prodromal or residual phase, as defined below.
   a. Prodromal phase. A clear deterioration in functioning before the active phase of the illness not due to a disturbance in mood or to a substance use disorder and involving at least two of the symptoms noted below.
   b. Residual phase. Persistence, following the active phase of the illness, of at least two of the symptoms noted below, not due to a disturbance in mood or to a substance use disorder.

Prodromal or Residual Symptoms

a. Social isolation or withdrawal
b. Marked impairment in role functioning as wage earner, student, or homemaker
c. Markedly peculiar behavior (e.g., collecting garbage, talk-

ing to self in public, or hoarding food)

d. Marked impairment in personal hygiene and grooming

e. Blunted, flat, or inappropriate affect

f. Digressive, vague, overelaborate, circumstantial, or metaphorical speech

g. Odd or bizarre ideation or magical thinking, e.g., superstitiousness, clairvoyance, telepathy, "sixth sense," "others can feel my feelings," overvalued ideas, ideas of reference

h. Unusual perceptual experiences, e.g., recurrent illusions, sensing the presence of a force or person not actually present

Examples: Six months of prodromal symptoms with 1 week of symptoms from *1;* no prodromal symptoms with 6 months of symptoms from *1;* no prodromal symptoms with 2 weeks of symptoms from *1* and 6 months of residual symptoms; 6 months of symptoms from *1,* apparently followed by several years of complete remission, with 1 week of symptoms in *1* in current episode.

4. The full depressive or manic syndrome, if present, developed after any psychotic symptoms, or was brief in duration relative to the duration of the psychotic symptoms in *1.*

5. Onset of prodromal or active phase of the illness before age 45.

6. Not due to any organic mental disorder or mental retardation.

Bleulerian Criteria

Eugene Bleuler[3] introduced the term schizophrenia in the early 1900's in an effort to reshape the Kraepelinian[2] thinking of the generation that preceded him.[10] Kraepelin had argued for two disorders—dementia praecox (an adolescent intellectual deterioration with a chronic downhill course), and manic-depressive insanity (a disorder of remissions and exacerbations without deterioration). Bleuler's systematic work revealed that not all cases of dementia praecox resulted in such a pernicious course. His term, schizophrenia, described a soul divided against itself without suggesting the early dementing process that Kraepelin had proposed.

Bleuler's diagnostic criteria have been characterized as the four A's. His work continues to have conceptual utility.

1. *Autism:* A tendency to withdraw from reality into idiosyncratic fantasy.

2. *Association:* A loosening of thoughts or associations.

3. *Affect:* Affects or feelings tend to be split off or inappropriate to the situation at hand.

4. *Ambivalence:* Profoundly mixed or contradictory feelings or attitudes tend to preoccupy the patient, sometimes to the point of immobility.

For Bleuler, symptoms of hallucinations, delusions, catatonic stupor, and negativism were of secondary importance.

Schneiderian Criteria

Kurt Schneider hypothesized central or "first rank" symptoms of schizophrenia.[10–12] Schneider argued that the presence of any of these first rank symptoms was pathognomonic of schizophrenia, though there is evidence to strongly argue against this claim.[4, 13–15] Schneider's descriptions of schizophrenic symptoms nevertheless remain very valuable and bear noting.

1. Audible Thoughts

The patient experiences hallucinatory voices that echo or speak his thoughts aloud.

2. Voices Debating or Disagreeing

The patient experiences hallucinatory voices engaged in debate or argument, frequently about himself.

3. Voices Commentating

The patient experiences hallucinatory voices that comment on his actions.

4. Somatic Passivity

The patient believes that sensations are being imposed upon his body by an outside force.

5. Thought Withdrawal

The patient experiences his thoughts being withdrawn or taken out of his mind by an outside force.

6. Thought Insertion

The patient experiences thoughts being put into his mind by an outside force.

7. Thought Broadcasting

The patient experiences his thoughts being disseminated to the world around him.

8. "Made" Feelings

The patient has the experience that his feelings are not his own, that they have been imposed upon him.

9. "Made" Impulses

The patient experiences, and generally acts upon, a compelling impulse which he believes is not his own.

10. "Made" Acts

The patient experiences his actions and his will to be under the control of an outside force.

11. Delusional Perception

The patient takes a percept in his environment (e.g., a person or event) and ascribes idiosyncratic value to it. The perception is then developed into a delusion.

DIFFERENTIAL DIAGNOSIS

Organic Disorders

Table 3.1 outlines the organic differential diagnosis of schizophrenia. If any of these conditions is suspected, further evaluation is of course indicated. The reader is referred to Anderson[16] as well as to appropriate texts in medicine and neurology for a detailed explication of these disorders and their diagnosis.

Functional Disorders

Affective Disorders

1. Mania (see Chapter 2).
2. Delusional (psychotic) depression.

In an affective disorder the patient's symptoms meet the criteria for an affective disorder and either precede or are concurrent with the psychotic symptomatology.

Because there appear to be no pathognomonic signs of schizophrenia, the patient must be assessed longitudinally. The diagnosis of schizophrenia should be deferred until symptomatology is present for 6 months.

Schizoaffective Disorder

There has been controversy about the validity of this diagnosis.[5] Until nosological clarity is improved it is probably best to avoid this diagnosis. If affective symptomatology is present, the patient should be considered for trials on the variety of biological treatments known to be effective in affective disorders (e.g., a combined tricyclic and neuroleptic regimen, lithium, or ECT).

Paranoia

Paranoia is a disorder in which persecutory delusions or delusional jealousy is central and persistent. The syndrome occurs without evidence of an affective disorder, an organic brain syndrome, and without the characteristic acute symptoms of schizophrenia (e.g., hallucinations, bizarre delusions, loose or incoherent thought processes, disorganized behavior).[18]

Schizophreniform Psychosis

Schizophreniform psychoses are *brief* psychotic episodes in which the symptoms are indistinguishable from the symptoms of schizophrenia. When the syndrome is of less than 6 months duration, it is considered a schizophreniform psychosis.[19, 20]

Personality Disorders

Paranoid Personality. The paranoid person is unusually mistrustful and suspicious, emotionally constricted, and hypersensitive. He does not, however, evidence psychotic symptomatology.

Schizotypal Personality. This new diagnostic term was introduced in the DSM-III, though the concept it refers to is not new. The schizotypal person shows a variety of oddities in his thinking, behavior, perceptions, and speech. He is peculiar in demeanor and often shows social

Table 3.1.
Organic Differential Diagnosis of Schizophrenia

Toxins—Exogenous	Infections	Nutritional Deficiencies
Amphetamines	Viral encephalitis: Herpes	Niacine: pellagra
Cocaine	meningitis; viral or bacterial	Thiamine: Wernicke-Korsakoff's
Psychomimetics	meningitis; lues	syndrome
LSD	SBE	Vascular Abnormalities
PCP[17]	Metabolic—Endocrine	Collagen disorders
Mescaline	Thyroid	Aneurysm
Alcohol	Hyperthyroidism	Intracranial hemorrhage
Alcoholic hallucinosis	Hypothyroidism	Cerebral Hypoxia
Alcohol withdrawal states,	Adrenal disease	Secondary to severe anemia
including DT's	Addison's disease	Secondary to decreased
Barbiturates	Cushing's disease	cardiac output
Barbiturate intoxication	Porphyria	Miscellaneous
Barbiturate withdrawal	Electrolyte imbalances	Complex partial seizures:
Steroids	Space-Occupying Lesions	temporal lobe epilepsy
Anticholinergics	Tumors	Wilson's disease
	Primary tumors	Huntington's chorea
	Metastases, e.g., lung, breast	Normal pressure hydrocephalus
	Subdural hematoma	
	Brain abscess	

anxiety and isolation as well as a limited capacity for relatedness. Thinking may be magical, and ideas of reference may occur.

Though many of these features suggest schizophrenia, the schizotypal patient does not meet the criteria for schizophrenia. He falls short of showing the severe and persistent symptoms of schizophrenia. Previously, such a patient may have been called a latent, borderline, or ambulatory schizophrenic.[21]

Borderline Personality with Psychosis. Borderline patients may show transient disturbances in reality testing and may have brief psychotic episodes. The presence of other symptomatology (see Chapter 4) as well as the transiency of the psychotic process easily distinguishes these patients over time.

EPIDEMIOLOGY

Incidence

The incidence of a disorder is the number of new cases in a given population during the course of 1 year. Incidence of schizophrenia is roughly 0.05% in the United States, thereby resulting in excess of 100,000 new cases of schizophrenia each year.[22]

Lifetime Prevalence

The lifetime prevalence is the percentage of those people living who have had or are likely to develop schizophrenia. The lifetime prevalence of schizophrenia in the United States is approximately 1%, or 2 million people.[22]

Age, Sex, Race

The onset of schizophrenia is typically in adolescence or young adulthood. Schizophrenia is most prevalent in persons age 15–50 and is equally common in males and females. Schizophrenic disorders are more common in nonwhites than in whites.[22]

Socioeconomic Status

The prevalence of schizophrenia is highest in lower socioeconomic levels of society. There is controversy as to whether this is related to "social causation" or to "drift." In the former, the increased stresses of lower socioeconomic living are attributed to fostering schizophrenia. The latter hypothesis argues that social factors do not pertain etiologically but that, instead, schizophrenics "drift" toward the lower echelons of society.[23–25]

Families

In families in which there is one schizophrenic parent, 12% of the children are likely to develop schizophrenia. In families where there are two schizophrenic parents, 35–45% of the children are likely to develop schizophrenia.[22]

THEORIES OF ETIOLOGY

Genetic

The incidence of schizophrenia in the general population is approximately 0.05%, whereas the incidence in parents of schizophrenics is 5% and in the siblings and children of schizophrenics about 10%.[22, 26] Furthermore, studies of concordance in twins reveal a higher concordance of schizophrenia in monozygotic twins than in dizygotic twins. The concordance is in the range of 40–50% in the monozygotic twins in contrast to 9–10% concordance in the dizygotic twins.[27, 28]

Kety et al.,[29] in a joint project between Danish and American investigators, studied the relatives of schizophrenic patients who had been adopted. More specifically, he studied the prevalence and types of mental illness in the biological and adoptive relatives of adoptees who became schizophrenic. His findings demonstrated that 13.9% of those genetically related to the schizophrenic index cases received a diagnosis in the schizophrenic spectrum. This finding is compared to 2.7% of the adoptive relatives of the schizophrenic index cases who were found to have schizophrenic spectrum disorders. These differences, if accurate,[30–34] are highly significant statistically and strongly support the operation of genetic factors in schizophrenia.

Kety's findings support genetic transmission in schizophrenia, though they are not finally conclusive. In utero influences, trauma at birth, and very early mothering influences might account for the same findings. However, a significant percentage of schizophrenic disorders was found in the paternal half siblings of schizophrenics with whom they shared no prenatal or postnatal environment.

In summary, incidence studies in the general population, twin studies, and prevalence studies in adoptive relatives all support the hypothesis that genetic factors are operant in the transmission of schizophrenia. However, the evidence is not adequate to support a conclusion that a genetic etiology is a sufficient cause of schizophrenia. A polygenic model appears likely in which biologic liability to illness increases as the individual approaches the upper end of a bell-shaped curve that represents genetic loading. Risk to relatives of an affected proband would, therefore, be highest in first degree relatives and decrease as relatives became more distant.[8] The polygenic model would also conform to evidence that risk of schizophrenia also confers risk for schizophrenic spectrum disorders (e.g., schizoaffective disorder and schizotypal personality).[34] Such a model also, by inference, points to the importance of environmental factors in the development of schizophrenia.

Biochemical Hypotheses

Transmethylation Hypothesis

Studies on transmethylation and schizophrenia are controversial. The transmethylation hypothesis posits that low levels of the enzyme monoamine oxidase are found in schizophrenia. Because monoamine oxidase detoxifies methylated amines with hallucinogenic properties, low levels of this enzyme might account for accumulations of these hallucinogenic amines in the CNS. The accumulated hallucinogens, hypothetically, result in schizophrenic symptomatology.[35–37] Increased levels of these proposed endogenous psychomimetics have yet to be demonstrated, and there is no consistent evidence of an abnormal methylating pathway.

Dopamine Hypothesis

The dopamine hypothesis grows out of psychopharmacological findings on the action of drugs that improve schizophrenia and the action of drugs that mimic the disorder. The antipsychotic agents with their dopamine blockade, the paranoid psychosis of amphetamine toxicity, and the fact that amphetamine,[38] methylphenidate, and L-dopa can all induce psychotic episodes in schizophrenic patients all support the hypothesis that schizophrenia is a hyperdopaminergic condition that principally affects the mesolimbic and mesocortical regions of the brain.[37-40]

Endorphins

Endorphins are endogenous, morphine-like substances found in certain specific sections of the brain. Their high density presence in the periaqueductal gray matter of the brain stem, in the locus coeruleus of the midbrain, and in the limbic system suggests their role in analgesia, addiction, mood disorders, and schizophrenia.

Efforts to employ the endorphins to ameliorate psychotic symptomatology have shown mixed results. At this time the role of endorphins in schizophrenia is at best controversial. However, the role of these polypeptide chains in neurobiological functioning seems probable. Future study of the endorphins may result in greater basic science understanding of schizophrenia.[41-43]

Summary

The transmethylation hypothesis, the dopamine hypothesis, the new findings on the endorphins, as well as other studies on serotonin, acetylcholine, histamine, and GABA all strongly support biochemical factors in schizophrenia. No single factor has been identified, though treatment is empirically aimed at muting dopamine activity, especially in the mesolimbic pathways of the CNS.

Neuropathological Hypotheses

Computerized axial tomography (CAT Scanning) prompted a renaissance of interest in neuropathological and neuroanatomic theories of schizophrenia. Subsequent technical advancement has enabled researchers to monitor cerebral blood flow and to disclose brain physiology and chemistry. Accumulating evidence now supports the view that some patients with schizophrenia have larger cerebral ventricles and/or evidence of cortical atrophy when compared to same-age normal controls and the siblings of affected individuals. Poor premorbid history, cognitive impairment, negative symptoms, and poor

response to treatment have been correlated with abnormal neuroanatomical findings.[44]

Cerebral blood flow studies report deficits in frontal lobe perfusion in schizophrenic patients, especially when engaged in a task requiring frontal lobe activity. Positron emission tomography (PET), which can assay and visualize neuronal metabolism, further supports frontal deficits in schizophrenia.[45, 46]

Brain electrical activity mapping (BEAM) has been done with schizophrenic patients and has shown increased frontal and left parietal frequencies. Nuclear magnetic resonance (NMR), a technique that allows for mapping specific brain nuclides, will undoubtedly increase our knowledge in the years to come.[47]

Perceptual-Cognitive Hypotheses

Consistent with abnormal neuroanatomic and neuropathological findings are reports of cognitive impairment in schizophrenia. Though more work needs to accumulate, important data are suggestive of a dementing process as causing schizophrenic cognition.[48-50]

Perceptual theorists suggest that schizophrenic withdrawal and apathy is a defensive maneuver against being flooded by perceptions that the schizophrenic cannot receive and adequately assimilate.[51] The posited state of hyperarousal is said to result in impaired attention. It is this attentional impairment that is regarded as central to the cognitive disturbance of schizophrenia.[52]

Lidz[53] regards the schizophrenic's deficiencies in category formation as instrumental to cognitive dysfunction. Category formation, he hypothesizes, is the cognitive process by which extraneous precepts and associations are filtered out. The schizophrenic's limited (and egocentric) capacity to form categories and to filter properly thereby render him vulnerable to perceptual overload and cognitive dysfunction.

Psychodynamic Hypotheses

Ego Disturbances

Ego disturbances in schizophrenics are generally atrributed to a disturbance in the mother-infant relationship. Klein[54] hypothesized that a constitutional (biological) defect in very early ego functions (which include the capacity to regulate and control drives, to relate to objects in the environment, to understand and respond to the external reality, and for cognitive functioning) renders the child vulnerable to disturbances in the relationship with mother. A disturbance in any of these ego functions, particularly a drive disturbance with consequent intense hostility and aggression in the infant, may produce distortions in the mother-infant relationship and promote the development of a personality which will be highly vulnerable to disorganization.

Less constitutionally predisposed theorists also attribute schizophrenia to disturbances in the mother-infant relationship. Margaret Mahler[55, 56] has postulated the importance of the separation-individuation phase of childhood development as crucial in the pathogenesis of schizophrenia. The psychological task for the child at this developmental stage is the achievement of a sense of self, separate from mother, with clear self-boundaries and a capacity to appreciate the separateness and constancy of other persons in his environment. Mahler suggested that the schizophrenic person never achieves a sense of object constancy. In essence, ego disturbances and ego vulnerability leave the schizophrenic adult especially sensitive to stress, particularly loss. When stressed, the schizophrenic person undergoes a regression in ego functions. More specifically, the schizophrenic, when stressed, no longer can employ higher ego defenses which maintain boundaries and reality as well as integrate feelings and drives. Stress induces a regression, and more primitive, reality compromising defenses are employed. The typical defenses in schizophrenic psychosis are delusional denial, projection, and severe distortion.

Interpersonal Disturbances

Harry Stack Sullivan's[57, 58] theoretical writings and clinical practice perhaps stand at the heart of the interpersonal schools. Sullivan helped extricate psychoanalytic thinking from its intrapsychic

locus and relocate it to the interpersonal sphere. Sullivan believed that mental illness arises from a failure in interpersonal relationships. He maintained that psychiatric illness or well-being was the product of continuous interaction from birth onward between the individual and important others in the environment.

Sullivan considered the schizophrenic patient as a human being who had been robbed, early in life, of crucial opportunities for interpersonal learning and gratification. Built into this conception is the premise that the development of a real and corrective human relationship with the schizophrenic patient could improve the schizophrenic patient's attempts at establishing a more secure and gratifying interpersonal world.

Family Hypotheses

The families of schizophrenic patients have been examined for their communicational patterns, their psychopathology, and their relationship structures.[59-62]

Though it seems unlikely that disturbed and disordered *communication* in a family is sufficient cause for schizophrenia, it seems probable that a child will not become schizophrenic unless intrafamilial communication is severely disordered.[63-65] Communication in schizophrenic families often includes the presence of "double binds."[61] In a double bind, contradictory messages are given without the recipient's being able to escape from the transaction. For example, the mother of a schizophrenic patient arrived on the ward to visit. Upon her arrival, the patient warmly put his arms around his mother. She visibly stiffened, and he withdrew his embrace. Mother then inquired "Don't you love me anymore?" The patient appeared ashamed, and mother then said "Don't be so embarrassed about showing your feelings."

Double bind theory is based on observing a pattern of behavior or interaction. It does not aim to portray mothers as villain or as schizophrenogenic. Once this pattern has been established within the family, the entire sequence of the double bind may not be needed to induce an experience of confusion and panic in the schizophrenic patient.

Lidz[59, 66] has emphasized that the parents of schizophrenics employ defective language and categories which, in turn, transmit irrationality to the child. He believes that the parents sacrifice language and categorization in order to maintain their distorted and egocentric view of the family and the world. These parents are said to be in tenuous emotional balance and must, therefore, distort their perceptions in a profoundly egocentric manner in order to avoid deeper distress and disorganization. The child thus inhabits a family in which he must distort or invalidate his perceptions (to conform to those of his parents) or be rejected. Lidz emphasized that the severe parental egocentricity precludes their capacity to separate and appreciate their feelings and perceptions from those of the child (and others). Examples include parental intrusiveness into the child's life without consideration for his needs or feelings, a belief that the child cannot function in any way without the parent(s), and the use of the child to provide meaning and purpose for the parent(s). Lidz hypothesized that the boundary disturbances that follow are central to the origin and nature of the schizophrenic thought disorder.

A thought disorder in which distortion, diffusion, and confusion prevail in families has been described by Wynne and Singer.[62, 67, 68] Their work offers important examples of the *psychopathological signs and symptoms* seen in schizophrenic families. Schizophrenic families, they maintained, are "pseudomutual," that is, characterized by a compelling need to believe that all the members share the same needs and expectations. Unclear messages, contradictions, denial of what has been said or is perfectly obvious, and fragmented and amorphous communications making focus difficult are all examples of how the pseudomutual family disturbs thought and communication. These maneuvers serve to maintain the illusion that divergence or individuality do not exist within the family.

Cognitive disturbances in schizophrenic families also include difficulties in family members sharing the focus of attention and in bringing closure to subjects. There is a tendency toward disruptive and unusual verbal behavior that does not allow communication to proceed in a rational, goal-directed fashion. Families of schizophrenic patients may also show many other symptoms of schizophrenia, namely, loose associations, idiosyncratic thinking, paranoia, and ambivalence.

Family *structure* is the way the family organizes and hierarchizes its relationships. Schizophrenic families tend to show markedly rigid, chaotic, or disturbed structures and relationships. The parents of female schizophrenic patients have been described by Lidz[59] as "schismatic." In this marriage, overt strife exists between the parents who clearly exhibit "emotional (albeit not actual) divorce." Such parents may invite the child to join as an ally in this battle of mutual derogation. The mother's pre-existing low self-esteem and doubt about her mothering is repeatedly undermined by the father, who regards women with contempt. Mother conveys a sense of meaninglessness about her life and cannot feel gratified by a daughter because of mother's unhappiness in being a woman. The fathers, though perhaps well functioning out of the home because of their rigid organization, are as disturbed as the mothers. The father is generally deeply insecure in his masculinity and needs his wife to passively comply with whatever is needed to maintain his self-esteem. Disagreement or difference on the wife's part is seen as hostility and insubordination. Since father's needs for unwavering and unrealistic admiration are not met by mother, he turns to daughter in a manner that approximates an incestuous relationship. The girl child is torn between both parents and compromises her needs and development as she repeatedly changes alliances and constantly fends off rejection from both parents.

The families of male schizophrenics tend to show "marital skew." The mother is highly intrusive in her son's life without regard for him as a separate person with separate feelings and needs. Empty and unfulfilled as a woman, the mother conveys that life would be meaningless without her son. The boy comes to believe that mother cannot live without him and, because he has developed so rudimentary a belief in himself, that he is unable to live without her. This is true symbiosis. The father in these families is passive, inept, and subject to constant derision. The boy cannot turn to father to escape the identification from and symbiosis with mother. Severe boundary and gender disturbances then ensue.

THE BIOPSYCHOSOCIAL EVALUATION

The biopsychosocial evaluation is modern psychiatry's effort to integrate biological, psychodynamic, and social factors into the understanding, evaluation, and treatment of psychiatric disorders.

In general, schizophrenia presents to the inpatient clinician as acute psychosis. The workup for the acutely psychotic patient will be described below in its biological, psychodynamic, and social and family aspects.

The Biological Evaluation

The inpatient unit in the general hospital is particularly suited for the biological evaluation of schizophrenia because of the necessity of ruling out an organic etiology for the patient's psychotic state.

The organic differential diagnosis for schizophrenia has been detailed in Differential Diagnosis. A thorough in hospital assessment includes the following.

History

A detailed history of the present illness; of past medical and psychiatric illnesses, including any medications or treatments that the patient has undergone or is currently taking; the family history, with particular emphasis on inheritable disorders and psychiatric syndromes in the family; habits, including drug and dietary habits; a thorough review of systems, with particular attention to a history of trauma or any recent changes in any of the organ systems; and a thorough *mental status examination*.

History-taking is best done from the patient with collaborative information obtained from family and significant others who have had occasion to witness the patient's behavior.

The Physical Examination

Particular attention must be paid to the patient's vital signs and pupils; to the presence of nuchal pain and rigidity; to the presence of diaphoresis; and to the neurological examination.[16]

Laboratory Studies

Regular Studies. Complete blood cell count (CBC), urine analysis, serum test for syphilis, blood glucose, NA, K, Cl, CO_2, Ca, PO_4, creatinine, BUN, alkaline phosphatase, SGOT, bilirubin-total/direct (T/D), thyroxine (T_4), free thyroxine (FT_4).

Special Studies. Blood culture, zinc, magnesium, toxic screen (with a specific group requested according to the hypothesized exogenous toxin), bromine, ceruloplasm, NH_3, ESR, B_{12}, folic acid, arterial blood gases.

Radiologic Studies

Regular Studies. Chest film.

Special Studies. Skull series, CT scan, brain scan, metastatic survey. In addition to ruling out specific space-differentiate chronic or process schizophrenia.[44, 49, 69-72] (See Neuropathological Hypotheses.)

Special Studies

EEG with wake and sleep tracings when complex partial seizures are suspected; EKG; and lumbar puncture.

Treatment Tests

1. I.V. glucose for hypoglycemia
2. I.V. physostigmine salicylate for anticholinergic delerium
3. I.V. thiamine for Wernicke's encephalopathy

Psychodynamic Evaluation and Formulation

Cognition and Affect

Whether the clinician chooses to adhere to DSM-III, Bleuler, or Schneider is debatable. What is not debatable is the importance of a careful evaluation of the patient's cognitive, perceptual, and affective symptomatology.

The *cognitive* disorder of schizophrenia may present with disturbances in the *flow* of thought; by the experience of *thought control or possession;* with disturbances in the *content of thought*; and by a *formal thought disorder.*[73] Thought *flow* may show rate disturbances in which thinking is slowed or rapid, with the latter more characteristic of excited psychotic states. Thought flow can also be disordered by disturbances of the train (or continuity) of thinking. Common examples of discontinuity found in schizophrenia are thought blocking, tangentiality, and perseveration.

Schizophrenic patients frequently exhibit *thought control or possession.* They report that their thoughts (or mind) are controlled by alien forces, that thoughts are put into or taken out of their mind, and that they are "made to" do a variety of behaviors. These are all examples of thought control. Delusions are the characteristic disturbance in the *content of thought* found in schizophrenia. Delusions, or fixed idiosyncratic beliefs that conform to the schizophrenic's reality (and to no one else's), may be persecutory, grandiose, or somatic.

Formal disturbances of thought include logical errors, impaired abstracting ability, and incoherence. Logical errors frequently arise from egocentricity or idiosyncratic premises. Concrete interpretations of reality (e.g., How is it that you came to the hospital?—by car.) reflect impaired abstraction and are quite common to schizophrenia. Incoherence is often the result of disordered *associations,* which Bleuler described.

Perceptual disturbances in schizophrenia occur in the form of hallucinations. Auditory hallucinations include voices conversing about oneself, hearing one's thoughts aloud, or hearing an ongoing commentary about one's actions. Visual hallucinations may also occur; their presence in the absence of auditory hallucinations should prompt the clinician to search for an organic etiology. Tactile, olfactory, and gustatory hallucinations should arouse questions of organicity, though they may be found in schizophrenia.

Affective disturbances in schizophrenia are characteristically a blunted, flat, or inappropriate affect. Inappropriate affect is the presence of an affect that is not appropriate to the social situation or topic of discussion. Examples include giggling when discussing the death of a family member or smiling during an intensely hostile family meeting. As a rule these inappropriate affects become understandable as the patient's inner life becomes apparent. The affect that was so inappropriate to the immediate external context may be quite appropriate to the patient's inner thoughts, hallucinations, or delusions. *Anhedonia,* or the absence of pleasure, frequently inhabits all aspects of the schizophrenic's life.

Core Conflicts

Problems with psychological separateness and identity are central to the schizophrenic's dilemma. A defective sense of self and disturbed boundaries make it difficult for the schizophrenic to *differentiate* himself from others. He views himself as either potentially merged with another or as distinct but helpless, terrified, and abandoned. As the clinician attempts to form a therapeutic relationship he will arouse the patient's fear of fusion; yet if he is too distant the patient will continue to feel estranged and terrified. This same dilemma existed prior to admission, and if this delicate balance were disturbed (e.g., with a family member(s), therapist, friend, or lover), the precipitant for hospital admission may be revealed.

The schizophrenic's limited ego capacities and disturbed boundary and communicational skills render him vulnerable and *dependent.* Though clearly dependent, the schizophrenic fears the intimacy of a relationship that can provide for his needs. He also tends to deny this helplessness to maintain an already compromised sense of self-esteem. This dilemma may have characterized the prodrome to hospitalization and needs to be carefully understood, particularly since this situation will so powerfully obtain in the hospital.

Anger and *aggression* are particularly difficult for the schizophrenic because of boundary disturbances and weak repressive capacities. Anger may therefore threaten both inside and outside, self, other, and world, and threaten to explode into unrestrained rage. Healthy assertion and aggression may be sacrificed with consequent passivity and apathy.[74]

History and Formulation

The psychosocial history of the schizophrenic patient is no different from that of any psychiatric patient, though additional collaborative information may be needed. Early development must be understood with particular emphasis on the patient's place in the family and his relationships with family members and peers. Separations and other important stresses should be noted. The patient's educational, social, and occupational efforts are very important and are central to understanding the patient's strengths, weaknesses, and prognosis. Sexual and marital history will need to be explored tactfully, as tolerated by the patient. Past psychiatric treatment, with special attention to the patient's relationship with his therapist, also needs careful exploration.

Premorbid functioning (the patient's adaptive capacities prior to the onset of illness) can be assessed by an examination of (1) the patient's functioning in relationships, work, and play and (2) the patient's personality style and characteristic defenses employed. The clinician seeks to understand the patient's highest level of functioning and to understand whether deterioration was sudden or insidious. Furthermore, the history seeks to clarify whether the patient was schizoid, obsessional, depressed, or hysterical, or showed some other personality style premorbidly. Closely linked to this is information regarding the patient's principal defensive operations (e.g., withdrawal, reaction formation, intellectualization, denial, repression, somatization, acting-out).[75]

The case formulation lends meaning to the patient's decompensation. The clinician aims toward a formulation which will depict the stresses in the patient's life that were related to the onset of the psychosis. Detail is sought in order to carefully understand what happened to the patient, with whom, when, and where. These stressors should be understood and explained in terms of the core conflicts and dilemmas of the schizophrenic and his limited capacities to respond. The formulation should also demonstrate the regression from premorbid functioning to acute (or chronic symptomatology). This regression can be described in terms of behavior, symptomatology, and ego defenses (e.g., from work to unemployment, from withdrawal to delusional preoccupation, from intellectualization to denial, distortion, and projection).

Social and Family Evaluation

An assessment of the home and social environment of the schizophrenic patient is a crucial aspect of the complete patient evaluation.

Family studies[65, 66, 76–80] have demonstrated that schizophrenics who return to home environments that include a relative who is critical, hostile, or emotionally overinvolved tend to have a very high relapse rate. This is in contrast to those schizophrenics who can return to a more accepting and emotionally neutral environment. On the other hand, a social environment that will allow for marked isolation and absence of stimulation will also foster regression and social withdrawal and promote relapse.

In addition to evaluating the emotional tone and degree of environmental stimulation of the family, the clinician should examine the structure of the family. The family needs to be seen in order to assess whether the family has a pathological need for an ill person for the homeostasis (or balance) of the family. More precisely, the examiner should look for secondary, or conscious, gain from illness for the patient *and* other members of the family. A careful examination of the schizophrenic's relationship to mother and father and a scrutiny of the mother-father relationship are additional aspects of the family evaluation. These relationships are examined for enmeshment (overinvolvement) of the schizophrenic with one parent, for this is one mode that the family can employ to detour conflict away from the parents or to avoid intimacy problems in the couple. In order for the schizophrenic patient to develop appropriate autonomy, he must be willing to differentiate and separate from his family, *and* his family must be willing to let this happen.

HOSPITAL TREATMENT

Psychopharmacological Management and ECT

Carpenter et al.[81] explored the possibility of treatment of acute schizophrenia without drugs. They argue that in a research setting with ample staff and commitment to nondrug management, the acute psychosis of schizophrenia can be well managed without drugs. Though it may be feasible to treat acute schizophrenic episodes without medication, this approach can generally occur only under special circumstances. It has, therefore, become standard hospital practice to treat the acute psychosis of schizophrenia with medications, which in most cases are antipsychotic agents.[82]

Antipsychotic Agents

All commercially available antipsychotic agents are clinically effective. The neuroleptic medications have been unquestionably proven to be the most effective treatment in remedying the symptoms of the acute psychosis of schizophrenia.[83] Furthermore, the antipsychotic medications have been shown to be highly effective in the treatment of *particular target symptoms*. These include hallucinations, acute delusions, combativeness, anxiety, hostility, hyperactivity, negativism, insomnia, and poor general self-care.

Choice of Agent. All neuroleptic agents are effective when given in adequate dosages. The physician needs to acquaint himself with several neuroleptic medications in different classes in order to have a variety of agents with which he can treat. In choosing a medication, the following *guidelines* apply:

1. Polypharmacy must be avoided. There is no evidence that the use of two neuroleptics at the same time is more effective than the use of one agent. Polypharmacy interferes with the clinician's understanding of which agent may be working and leaves the clinician in a quandary as to which drug may be causing difficulty if problems arise.
2. The patient's history may be helpful. If a patient has responded favorably in the past, this would support the use of that drug once again. If the patient has been allergic to or responded adversely to a drug in the past, this would be a relative or absolute contraindication to the re-use of that drug.
3. Physicians choose medications with which they feel familiar. In the course of training or clinical practice, a physician ought to become familiar with the phenothiazines (chlorpromazine, thioridazine, trifluoperazine, perphenazine, fluphenazine); a butyrophenone (haloperidol); a thioxanthene (thiothixene); a dibenzoxapine (loxapine); and a dihydroindolone (molindone). A familiarity with four or five drugs spanning several classes is a solid foundation for the general practitioner in psychiatry.
4. A particular neuroleptic may be chosen for its specific side effects. When sedation is preferable, one of the more sedating agents, like chlorpromazine, may be selected. When anticholinergic side effects need to be avoided, an agent with very low anticholinergic properties, like haloperidol, would be indicated. High† potency neuroleptics (e.g., haloperidol, fluphenazine, trifluoperazine, thiothixene) are generally minimally hypotensive, sedating, and anticholinergic; they are, however, highly extrapyramidal. Low† potency neuroleptics (chlorpromazine, thioridazine) tend to have fewer extrapyrimidal problems, but often induce hypotension, sedation, and anticholinergic symptomatology. Perphenazine, loxapine, and molindone fall somewhere in between the high and low potency agents.

Route of Administration. Neuroleptic medications can be given orally or intramuscularly. Oral medications are available in elixir and tablets. Elixir is more

---

†High and low potency refer to the number of milligrams needed for clinical effect. All agents are potent; these terms refer to whether the dose required will be in the range of 2–60 (high potency) or 400–3000 mg (low potency).

rapidly absorbed than tablets, and there is less possibility of "cheeking." I.M. administration can be employed when symptoms must be rapidly treated, as in the case of a combative patient. Parental administration would also be indicated when there is some doubt about gastrointestinal absorption.

Caffeine, found in coffee, tea, and caffeinated beverages, can bind or precipitate out neuroleptic medications as well as stimulate microsomal activity in the liver (thereby increasing the catabolism of antipsychotic agents).[83-86] As a consequence, the ingestion of caffeine in combination with a neuroleptic medication may significantly interfere with the absorption and half-life of the drug and potentially limit clinical improvement. Though there is some debate as to whether the interference stems from caffeine or tannic acid,[87] clinicians may want to eliminate caffeinated beverages from the kitchen area of the hospital unit and inform patients about this interaction.

Dosage. At least 300 mg of chlorpromazine, or its equivalent in another neuroleptic, are generally necessary for antipsychotic effect. One hundred milligrams of chlorpromazine is roughly equal to 100 mg of thioridazine and to 5 mg of trifluoperazine, haloperidol, thiothixene, and fluphenazine. Table 3.2 provides a list of the commonly used antipsychotics and their equivalent dosages.

It is advisable to document a *dose-response curve* in the neuroleptic treatment of an acute psychotic episode. The effect on the target symptoms and the side effects experienced by the patient are monitored at varying doses of the medication in order to choose the most effective dose of medication for the patient. An example of a dose response curve is provided in Figure 3.1.

Neuroleptic Blood Levels. Unlike lithium and tricyclic antidepressant levels, neuroleptic levels are in the infancy of their development. A need clearly exists in order to provide the lowest possible therapeutic dose (and thereby limit exposure and consequent risk of tardive dyskinesia) as well as to minimize side effects. Difficulties in developing valid and accurate measurements are related to the presence of metabolites and cross-reactivity between metabolites, the parent compound, and any other psychoactive agent the patient may be taking. Emerging studies show that plasma levels of neuroleptics vary enormously among patients and that there probably is a therapeutic window for haloperidol. If upper and lower limits of efficacy exist (i.e., a therapeutic window) for haloperidol, clinicians will want to keep in mind that a dosage decrease may be helpful for some patients.[88-90]

Schedule of Administration. Upon admission to an inpatient unit, acutely psychotic patients have often, in recent years, been managed by a medication regimen of *rapid neuroleptization,* in which doses of antipsychotic medication are administered every half hour or hour until there is evidence of "lysing" of a psychotic episode, or until sedation sets in. Recent studies, however, have demonstrated that patients receiving rapid, and higher, dosage schedules did no better clinically than those patients who received standard doses and routine administration (e.g., t.i.d.). Furthermore, there was no evidence that those receiving rapid neuroleptization had briefer hospital stays.[91-93] Patients receiving rapid neuroleptization did show a higher incidence of extrapyramidal disorders, thereby requiring greater amounts of antiparkinson agents, and were exposed to higher doses of antipsychotic medication during the course of hospitalization.

Table 3.2.
Equivalent Oral Dosages of Antipsychotic Medications Compared to 100 mg of Chlorpromazine (Thorazine)

Drug (Trade Name)		Dose
		mg
Haloperidol	(Haldol)	2–5
Trifluoperazine	(Stelazine)	5
Perphenazine	(Trilafon)	10
Thioridazine	(Mellaril)	100
Fluphenazine	(Prolixin)	2–5
Thiothixene	(Navane)	5
Loxapine	(Loxitane)	15
Molindone	(Moban)	10

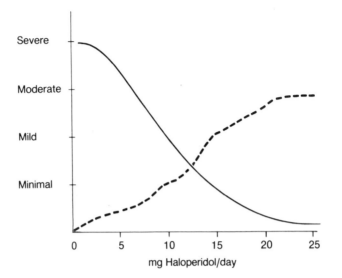

Figure 3.1.   Dose-response curve. *Dashed line,* side effects; *solid line,* degree of symptomatology.

These studies support, when clinically feasible, the judicious use of neuroleptics. Recompensation from psychosis is a process that cannot be condensed into hours: acutely psychotic patients will restitute over days to weeks to a nonpsychotic state on conservative neuroleptic regiments. And can thereby be spared excessive exposure to neuroleptics and their adverse effects.

In general, 300–600 mg/day of chlorpromazine, or its equivalent (see Table 3.2) in other neuroleptics like trifluoperazine, haloperidol, or perphenazine, will be effective for the antipsychotic treatment of acute psychosis. The use of adjunctive benzodiazepines has become increasingly employed as a method of providing additional tranquilization, without increasing the patient's exposure to neuroleptics. Lorazepam (1–2 mg p.o.) or oxazepam (10–20 mg p.o.) can be written as p.r.n. or maintenance orders and administered up to several times per day, especially in the first few days of hospitalization. Hypnotics may also be provided initially if the patient's psychosis has disrupted his sleep cycle.

Adverse Effects. *Extrapyramidal Syndromes. 1. Acute Dystonia.* This generally occurs within the first few days of treatment. It is more common in younger patients, especially males. Acute dystonic reactions are characterized by sudden, marked, and often subjectively frightening tonic contractions of the muscles of the tongue, neck, back (opisthotonus), mouth, or eyes (oculogyric crisis).

Acute dystonic reactions can be treated effectively with I.M. benztropine (Cogentin), 1 or 2 mg, or diphenhydramine (Benadryl), 25 or 50 mg, I.M. or I.V. The patient should then be placed on a maintenance dose of the agent chosen (e.g., benztropine, 1 mg b.i.d.).

2. Drug-Induced Parkinsonism. This is a common side effect from antipsychotic medication. It tends to appear within the first few weeks of treatment. The features of drug-induced parkinsonism include bradykinesia (slowed movements), rigidity, and tremor. Masked (expressionless) facies, stooped posture, drooling, and gait disturbances are also common. So called "postpsychotic depressions" are often bradykinesic parkinsonian states, which are highly treatable if accurately diagnosed.

Treatment is with oral antiparkinson agents, e.g. benztropine (Cogentin), 1–4 mg/day; diphenhydramine (Benadryl), 25–100 mg/day; or amantadine (Symmetrel), 100–300 mg/day, all in divided dosages. Antiparkinson agents often can be reduced or discontinued after several weeks. The patient is then observed to see if parkinsonism returns.

3. *Akathisia.* Akathisia is a neuroleptic-induced syndrome of motor restlessness and subjective inability to sit still or, in more severe cases, a feeling of marked anxiety and dysphoria.[94, 95] Akathisia is easily confused with worsening psychosis and mistakenly prompts the use of additional neuroleptic medication, thereby escalating the problem. Furthermore, a variety of impulsive and bizarre behaviors have been associated with the dysphoria of akathisia, including suicide attempts.[96-100]

Psychotic patients with somatic preoccupations or delusions are especially vulnerable to interpreting akathisia as a form of external influence. Patients (especially young men) who rely on the experience of body well-being and activity as a defensive style are apt to have these adaptations undermined by the akathisic experience.[101, 102] Finally, "the consumer has a point."[103]: schizophrenic patients who have a dysphoric response to a neuroleptic do poorly with further medication treatment and frequently are noncompliant. These dysphoric responses were highly correlated with the diagnosis of akathisia.

Treatment of akathisia begins with considering a decrease in the dose or changing of the neuroleptic. Antiparkinson agents provide little relief from akathisia. Benzodiazepines (diazepam, 2–5 mg p.o. b.i.d.-t.i.d., or lorazepam, 1 mg p.o. b.i.d.-t.i.d.) can be helpful and, as noted earlier, can reduce the need for antipsychotic medication. Propanolol has proven to be quite beneficial, working within days in a dosage range of 20–80 mg/day, given in divided doses.[104] Caution about the interaction between propanolol and neuroleptics is indicated, in view of one clear instance of hypotension and cardiopulmonary arrest when this betablocker was administered concurrently with haloperidol.[105] Nadolol, another betablocker, has shown efficacy, as has clonidine, a central noradrenergic blocker.[106, 107]

4. *Neuroleptic-Induced Catatonia.* A gradual development of catatonia in patients on high potency neuroleptic drugs may be a result of the drug itself.[108] Neuroleptic-induced catatonia must be diagnosed, if present, in order not to be mistaken for a worsening of the patient's psychotic symptomatology. Treatment involves changing the neuroleptic medication or adding amantadine (Symmetrel) 100 mg p.o., t.i.d.

5. *Tardive Dyskinesia.* Tardive dyskinesia is a late onset, abnormal movement disorder that appears to occur at an increasingly alarming rate in patients treated with neuroleptic medications.[109-111] The syndrome of tardive dyskinesia is often heralded by fasciculations of the tongue. Later manifestations include involuntary, persistent movements of the tongue, lips, and facial muscles (lingual-buccal-facial dyskinesia). More severe cases can demonstrate choreoathetoid (spasmodic and/or writhing) movements of any or all portions of the upper and lower extremities as well as truncal and diaphragmatic dyskinesias.

Tardive dyskinesia must be looked for in all patients on neuroleptic medication and carefully reviewed as a possible side effect with the patient when he is in a nonpsychotic state. The reader is referred elsewhere[109, 112, 113] for treatment and prognostic information on this common and complex disorder.

Other Adverse Effects. *Neuroleptic Malignant Syndrome.* The neuroleptic malignant syndrome is a quartet of muscular rigidity, fever, autonomic dysfunction, and disturbances of mental status.[114, 115] Incidence has been estimated at approximately 1%, with the disorder generally associated with high potency neuroleptics. Young men and patients with organic brain disease are reported to be at higher risk. The pathophysiology of this disorder is unknown. What is known is that this syndrome can come on rather explosively (1–2 days) and can cause death. Early recognition is therefore essential.

Treatment of the neuroleptic malignant syndrome involves immediately stopping the neuroleptic. A differential diagnosis of other possible explanations for the patient's symptoms must be explored while respiratory, renal, and cardiovascular functioning are monitored and treated accordingly. Though some patients with this disorder may respond to drug discontinuation and supportive measures,[116] the use of dantrolene sodium and bromocriptine, each alone or in combination, may be vital in refractory cases.[117–119]

Anticholinergic Effects. These include dry mouth, blurry vision, urinary retention, and slowing of the bowel. Patients with "narrow angle" glaucoma should not be prescribed neuroleptic agents without ophthalmological consultation.

Cardiovascular Side Effects. Orthostatic hypotension is commonly found with the low potency agents (e.g., chlorpromazine and thioridazine).

Hypothalamic Effects. Changes in appetite, libido, breast enlargement, and galactorrhea are the more common hypothalamic effects.

Jaundice. Jaundice is generally an allergic, cholestatic jaundice that is benign and responsive to withdrawal of medication.

Agranulocytosis. Agranulocytosis is a rare, potentially fatal side effect from neuroleptic medication. It is an allergic, nondose-related phenomenon for which the clinician must always be on the alert. Patients who show fever, sore throat, or signs of some infectious process should have an immediate white blood count to rule out agranulocytosis.

Mental Status Changes. Very little has been said or written about adverse *psychological* effects of neuroleptics on schizophrenic patients. Nevertheless, patients frequently note disagreeable changes in their mental state which add to their psychic discomfort and may cause them to discontinue medication.

Nevins[120] observes that changes may occur in ego defensive activities, in object relations, in needed psychotic restitutive symptoms, and in body image. For example, defensive denial or motor activity may be altered by medication allowing for the emergence of painful inner feelings of grief and passivity; autistic and psychotically driven autoerotic activities may cease and allow expression of repressed sexual and dependent wishes and fears; psychotic omniscience may give way to severe depression and self-derogation; and the peripheral and central effects of neuroleptics (e.g., dry mouth, sedation, rigidity) may be interpreted psychotically as brain damage or punishment from God.

Neuroleptics and Pregnancy and Lactation. Neuroleptic agents pass through the placenta and have been detected in breast milk. Every effort must be made not to expose the fetus or newborn to medication of any sort, including antipsychotic agents. When neuroleptics appear essential, risk/benefit concerns must be addressed with the patient and family and informed consent obtained.[121, 122]

Barbiturates

Barbiturates were routinely used before the era of neuroleptic medication. They are still helpful as sedating agents for highly agitated patients. A dose of 120–180 mg of sodium amytal prescribed at bedtime can be a helpful adjunct in the treatment of the acutely psychotic patient who has already received adequate antipsychotic medication.

Anxiolytic Agents

Anxiolytics (antianxiety agents or minor tranquilizers) are growing in value in the treatment of acute psychosis. Anxiolytics (e.g., lorazepam, diazepam, oxazepam) are useful in the treatment of akathisia and can be used concurrently with neuroleptics for the symptoms of acute psychosis (see Antipsychotic Agents).

Lithium

Lithium is known to be effective in the acute and maintenance treatment of affective disorders. Neuroleptic medications remain the drugs of choice for the treatment of the acute psychosis of schizophrenia. However, in cases where a considerable affective component may be suspected, or where excitement seems a primary target symptom, the use of lithium as a single agent or as an adjunct to neuroleptic medication should be considered.[123]

Propanolol

Propanolol (Inderal) is a beta-adrenergic blocker that is commonly used in the treatment of cardiovascular disorders.[124–126] Recent clinical trials have shown propanolol to be helpful as an *adjunct* to antipsychotic medications in treatment-resistant, chronically psychotic, schizophrenic patients. This may be the result of increasing plasma concentrations of the neuroleptic the patient is receiving, rather than by the direct action of propanolol.[127] Propanolol, and nadolol, are also effective in the management of akathisia (see Adverse Effects).

Electroconvulsive Therapy (ECT)

ECT is never the first line treatment for the acute psychosis of schizophrenia unless there is a catatonia that is life-threatening or the patient is intolerant to any neuroleptic medication. In general, a lack of response to a variety of medications should lead to a search for toxic psychosocial factors rather than to the immediate prescription of a course of ECT. In patients where this search proves unsuccessful, ECT may prove to be beneficial if adequate medication trials have been completed. Catatonic and affective symptoms are more responsive than apathy, autism, and delusional preoccupation.[128, 129]

Milieu Management

The question not of how, but rather, *whether* milieu treatment of schizophrenia has any benefit has been argued for at least the past decade. This debate bears summarizing, for it reveals the diversity of patients, milieu environments, and therapeutic ideologies involved.

Van Putten and May's[130–132] work, as well as that of Grinspoon et al.,[133] is seminal in questioning the therapeutic value of the milieu. The evidence from this work, which includes reviews of other work, indicates that ". . . current methods of milieu therapy . . . add little to the treatment of the ordinary schizophrenic patient once gross neglect is corrected and adequate chemotherapy is used"[131] Gunderson[134, 135] has taken exception to these findings, with evidence obtained by segregating chronic from nonchronic patients and nonintensive from intensive milieus. Drawing upon the work of Carpenter et al.,[81] Mosher and Menn,[136] and Rappaport et al.[137], Gunderson argues that the pessimism surrounding milieu therapy is premature and far too global. In his examination of successful milieus, four characteristics emerged: (1) High patient/

staff ratios on small units; (2) Distribution of responsibility among patients and staff; (3) A unit conception that psychosis has meaning, not to be abbreviated, but rather, to be understood and lived through; (4) A shared value in the unique, even counterculture, quality of what the staff are doing.

It appears likely that milieu therapy may be alternately helpful or harmful, thereby making *specificity of which milieu for which patient* the central clinical question.[138, 139]

What is most unbearable to schizophrenic patients is an overstimulating environment.[140–143] Explanations of why such a milieu may be toxic vary: overload in schizophrenics who have a basic defect in processing input[144]; the essential need for separateness, distance, privacy, and even isolation, in psychotic patients[145–147]; and the organism's need to protect itself from overwhelming external stimulation.[148] For many patients, not only will a less intense milieu prevent negative reactions, but also it may be valuable in permitting the recompensation process to occur.

Overstimulation can occur through a highly peopled or activity-filled environment. Multiple meetings, groups, lively and provocative discussions, affective exploration, and high value on interaction are the ingredients of modern milieu treatment; they are also what can be deleterious to the patient who requires privacy, quiet, and isolation. Similarly, milieus that invite self-disclosure, that place particular emphasis on "here-and-now" communication, and that encourage open expression of anger and aggression can be toxic to the psychotic patient.[149–151] Confrontation may be the most deleterious form of overstimulation, for it can simultaneously excite the patient and unravel needed defenses.

Milieus that persist in advocating principles of democracy, egalitarianism, role blurring, and absent hierarchies are apt to be quite confusing to psychotic patients who require structure, clarity, accountability, and firm authority.[138, 149–150, 152–155] Especially problematic are units in which the therapeutic milieu, in attending to "stylish" ideologies that enhance the working milieu of the staff, may conflict with the needs of these especially vulnerable patients.[156-158]

The difficulties schizophrenic patients experience in group therapy parallel those of the milieu. Interestingly, group therapy for schizophrenic patients began in a format that was responsive to the special needs of psychotic patients. Lazell, over 60 years ago, met with schizophrenics in groups which provided information through lectures.[159] His approach avoided what subsequently has been discovered to be especially toxic to schizophrenic patients, namely, excessive uncovering, insight-oriented exploration, and self disclosure.[160-163] Group therapy for schizophrenic patients can be beneficial if the group experience avoids these pitfalls and, instead, attends to what we have come to understand about these patients. Therapists must be active, must provide structure whenever needed, and must offer support and practical advice liberally. Reality testing must be done whenever needed, social skills must be enhanced, and specific problems (and solutions) must be identified. Above all, self-esteem must be protected. Homogeneous, or "level," groups appear to be more effective, in that expectations are then similar for the members, and success can be achieved by all.[164, 165]

Individual Psychotherapy

The effective psychotherapy of schizophrenic psychoses is deeply dependent on the quality of the therapist. Genuineness, accurate empathy, and warmth are the human qualities associated with successful outcome in the psychotherapy of schizophrenia.[166-168]

Schwartz[167] has likened the psychotherapy of schizophrenia to an heroic endeavor for therapist and patient alike. The schizophrenic's inner disorganization, turmoil, and profound psychic deprivation make constriction, withdrawal, and autistic preoccupation a powerfully seductive alternative to the pain and risks of psychotherapeutic engagement. The growth of a separate self for the schizophrenic, the essential task of psychotherapy, requires facing the bleakness and anguish of his past, the emptiness of his present, and the grief of being a separate person. The therapist, in turn, must provide inscrutable honesty, unwavering will, and unusual capacity to bear difficult and frightening feelings in order to allow and invite the patient onto the rigorous and awesome path of evolving a separate self. Schwartz urges the therapist not to be put off by the patient's wish to see him as special, endowed, even immortal. Immortal, heroic images of the therapist will permit and guide the genesis of the patient's personal, unique, and valued images of himself as a separate person who can stand on his own without fear of dissolution of self or other.

Paradoxically, while engaged in this heroic pursuit, the therapist is asked to maintain an attitude that his patient is simply another human being in pain with whom he is about to enter a relationship.[57-58] Furthermore, Fromm-Reichmann[169, 170] cautions the therapist against trying to cure the schizophrenic patient. Such heroism, humanity, and humility are indeed a remarkable combination when found in the same person.

The psychotherapy of schizophrenia must be *antiregressive*.[171, 172] The patient's decompensation and regression in ego functioning was in response to events, feelings, and thoughts which he could not bear. Short of death, psychosis is the ultimate form of withdrawal. The therapy process cannot condone avoidance, for it sacrifices reality, relatedness, and self-esteem. The therapist wishes to ally with the patient's frail ego in examining the life events and inner realities that prompted the flight into psychosis. Explorations into the precipitants of the decompensation and the nature of the patient's current relationships should occur only in the framework of an active, supportive, antiregressive stance on the part of the therapist.

In the most-developed empirical study to date, moderately ill, young, hospitalized schizophrenic patients were randomly assigned to intensive or supportive psychotherapy.[173, 174] Intensive psychotherapy focused on the treatment relationship, the transference, and the past. Supportive treatment focused on adjustment in the present. Those in intensive treatment were seen at least three times per week by experienced analysts. Those in supportive psychotherapy were seen weekly. Both groups received state of the art psychopharmacology. The results of this study support the central importance of providing reality-based, antiregressive, and adaptation-oriented psychotherapy for schizophrenic patients. Those schizophrenic patients seen in intensive psychotherapy remained in the hospital longer and were less likely to return to functioning at home or at a job. Furthermore, intensively treated patients showed a very high dropout rate (greater than 50% within 6 months), despite the use of senior clinicians. It appears likely that this dropout group suffered serious, negative outcomes.[175]

In an antiregressive psychotherapy, primary process (unconscious) productions and transference distortions about the therapist are met with reality explanations and a return to the therapeutic task of understanding why the patient finds his life so intolerable. All the patient's efforts, however rudimentary, to be adaptive and reality bound should be respected and encouraged.

As the therapy proceeds, the therapist can strive to understand his patient in a manner that lends coherence to the patient's psychotic productions. As the therapist comes to understand the unconscious avoidance aims and methods of the psychotic productions, he can enable the patient to begin to experience his thoughts and feelings as belonging to him rather than to others in the form of delusional and hallucinatory projections. Delusions and hallucinations should never be confronted. They will soften as the underlying need for them is attenuated.

Schizophrenic patients are particularly frightened by psychotherapy.[176, 177] Their terror of close contact with others makes them remarkably limited in their capacity to articulate feelings and ideas. Furthermore, the patient is frequently afraid of the power of his feelings, which he may imagine as having the capacity to destroy him or the therapist. These fears must be addressed as they emerge, without negating them. The therapist can state that he realizes that the patient has these fears and that the therapy will help the patient understand them and be less afraid. Lidz[178]

has emphasized that the absence of options for action, the absence of exits, finalizes the patient's entrance into a schizophrenic regression. As a consequence, the therapist must always allow the patient choice and an exit. For some patients this may entail an open door while for others it may be permission to forestall treatment until they are ready. Flexibility in meeting time (e.g., 15 minutes) and place (e.g., day room or patio) is critical to effective working with the psychotic patient, whose mental state permits only limited attention and calls for a subjectively safe milieu.

As the therapy proceeds to examine aspects of the patient's life and family relations, themes of loss and grief will emerge.[179] This may be seen most poignantly in the patient's desperate, persistent attachments to parents (or others) who provide so little and who demand so much. The patient's rage or sexual fantasies may emerge in the psychotherapy. If those areas of conversation are initiated by the patient, they can be gently explored. As a rule, however, these matters generally can wait until the ego has recompensated and can better manage the attendant affect. Concurrent work with the family is often essential during therapy in order to enlist their alliance, to preclude their sabotage of treatment, and to help enable them to grow and thereby allow for growth in the patient.

As the patient improves and his ego recompensates, he begins to see why he has considered his life intolerable. Grief and conflict can be borne, at least for brief moments, without psychotic defensive disorganization. A reality-based perspective allows the patient the opportunity to see what he can do for himself and to recognize that he is not as isolated and helpless as he has come to believe. This is the foundation for the patient's renewed self-esteem and for his efforts at modest, but realizable, life goals.

The transition out of the hospital is particularly difficult for the schizophrenic patient. The therapist should, whenever possible, continue with his patient after discharge. Continuity of psychotherapeutic care is a vital handhold for a person whose inner world is deeply fragmented and whose real and imagined losses are already staggering in their magnitude.

The Family

Family Evaluation and Therapy

The critical importance and power of the family in the schizophrenic patient's life cannot be overemphasized. For this reason, all families of hospitalized schizophrenic patients must be evaluated by a member of the inpatient staff. This evaluation will provide a better understanding of the schizophrenic patient's experience in his world, for his family has been the template from which the patient has come to comprehend and relate to his environment.

Furthermore, unless an effective alliance is established with the family, all therapeutic efforts with the patient can become abortive. Inpatient staff commonly see schizophrenic patients suddenly regress upon family visits, or see long labored treatment plans abruptly dissolve when the family voices opposition. With some schizophrenic families, it may be necessary to insist upon, or contract for, the family's involvement in therapy as a part of the requirements for the patient's admission.

The current direction of family treatment for schizophrenia began more than 20 years ago in Britain. Social psychiatry researchers discovered that hospitalized patients who returned to their families had higher rates of readmission than those patients who were discharged to hostels and boarding homes. In the sample of patients who returned to family living, the highest risk for recurrence of psychosis was found in excessively emotionally involved families.[180] Subsequent work refined the family factors involved in poor outcome: families high in "expressed emotion" (EE), that is, overinvolved, critical, and overtly hostile interactions, were those that evidenced the poorest outcome for schizophrenic patients. Patients from high-EE families relapsed at a rate of 56%, compared to 21% of patients from low-EE families. More than 35 hours per week of contact by schizophrenic patients with high-EE family members appeared to be especially harmful. The role of antipsychotic medications was also studied, and the results are quite striking. Patients who had high contact with high-EE families and no medication had a relapse rate of 92%; this rate dropped to 53% when these patients received neuroleptic medication. Patients who had low contact with high-EE families evidenced a 42% relapse rate when on no medication, which dropped to 15% when on antipsychotic agents. For schizophrenic patients of high-EE families, reducing contact with their families and prescribing antipsychotic medication was critical in averting relapse.[181-184]

The British work has been replicated in the United States, thereby ending any debate about validity of these findings in English-speaking countries.[64, 65, 185, 186] The impact of the family on the course of schizophrenia and the implications for treatment have been established for British and American patients, at the very least.

On the basis of this data, family treatment approaches have evolved which substantiate that decreasing family contact in high-EE families or teaching patients and families better methods of coping and changing negative attitudes of key family members will result in improved post-hospital functioning for schizophrenic patients.[187-190]

For families of hospitalized schizophrenic patients, education of the family and important others about the nature, course, and management of schizophrenia is essential. Family work can also involve training in effective problem-solving, particularly around stressful life events. Family training may also include shifting overinvolvement and criticism in the direction of concern and specific dissatisfactions.[65, 189, 191, 192] Family intervention can not cure schizophrenia. However, careful pharmacotherapy, family therapy, social skills training, occupational rehabilitation, alternative housing, and practical, reality-based psychotherapy can alter the course of the disorder dramatically. Families need to understand this and need to be engaged as allies in such a lifelong endeavor. Only when there is absence of response or resistance to the treatment approaches outlined above should more intensive interventions be employed (e.g., strategic and systemic family therapies).[193]

Informative and supportive texts for the families and friends of schizophrenic patients have been written.[194, 195] These books can serve as adjuncts to the direct care provided to families of schizophrenic patients.

Genetic Counseling

As noted earlier, family, twin studies, and adoption studies all point to the presence of environmental as well as genetic factors in the transmission of schizophrenia. Children of schizophrenics who have been adopted and raised in a separate environment show a high prevalence of schizophrenia as well as other psychiatric disorders, including personality disorders and mental retardation. In addition, adoptees from families without a history of schizophrenia who were raised by schizophrenic parents showed only a 4.8% rate of schizophrenia compared with a rate of 19.7% among adopted-away offspring of schizophrenic biological parents. These findings support a genetic predisposition to schizophrenia. They also suggest that schizophrenia in a parent does not promote the development of schizophrenia in a child if that child is not genetically predisposed.[196]

The risk for schizophrenia in the general population is roughly 1%. The risk rate for schizophrenia in first degree relatives of schizophrenics is approximately 10%, whereas the risk for more distant relatives is only about 3%. These risk figures are estimates for the more severe form of schizophrenia that we have been discussing in this chapter, with features of early onset, history of recurrence, and tendency toward chronicity.

COURSE AND PROGNOSIS

Schizophrenia typically begins insidiously in early adult life. Most schizophrenic patients show premorbid features of shyness, social withdrawal, awkwardness, and an inability to form close relationships. The onset of schizophrenia is highly uncommon after age 40; the clinician should suspect another diagnosis when presented with a first psychosis in a patient over 40.

Positive prognostic signs in schizophrenia include the presence of a supportive family, particularly a spouse; a family history of an affective disorder; and a premorbid history of good social relations and school performance. Poor prognosis is suggested by an insidious onset; a family history of schizophrenia; and a restricted or "blunted" affect. Schizophrenic patients are at high risk for suicide. Care must be taken to identify those patients who are at risk and to provide early intervention and protective hospital care.[197, 198]

Hogarty et al.[199, 200] examined relapse in schizophrenic patients for a 2-year period following hospitalization. They found that patients treated with placebo had 80% relapse rates, compared with 48% of those treated with neuroleptic medication. Those patients who were treated with a problem-solving, interpersonal, and rehabilitative form of psychotherapy in addition to neuroleptics showed a further decrease in the rate of relapse, though this was only apparent after 6 months of treatment. Glick and Hargreave's 2-year follow-up studies on hospitalized schizophrenic patients demonstrated that longer term hospital stays (90–120 days) resulted in a better course than shorter stays (21–28 days) for patients with good prehospital functioning. This finding was more pronounced for female patients. Their opinion is that longer term hospitalization resulted in greater compliance with long-term, posthospital treatment (medications and psychotherapy) and, consequently, reduced psychiatric morbidity.[201]

Longitudinal studies on the course of schizophrenia demonstrate varied findings. Whereas some studies disclose poor levels of adjustment in the great majority of cases,[202, 203] other work suggests a more sanguine outcome. Evidence is accumulating that schizophrenic patients can show improvement in psychosis, even after years of psychotic symptomatology, and that many schizophrenics can lead a relatively full and symptom-free existence.[204, 205]

REFERENCES

1. American Psychiatric Association: *Diagnostic and Statistical Manual*, ed. 3, (DSM-III),

Washington, D.C., American Psychiatric Association, APA Task Force on Nomenclature, 1980.

2. Kraepelin E: *Dementia Praecox,* London, Livingston, 1918.

3. Bleuler E: Dementia Praecox oder die gruppe der Schizophrenien, in Aschoffenburg (ed): *Handbuch der Psychiatrie,* Leipzig, 1911 (Trans. J Zinkin, 1960, New York).

4. Pope HG, Lipinski JF: Diagnosis in schizophrenia and manic-depressive illness. Arch Gen Psychiatry, *35:* 811–823, 1978.

5. Pope HG, Lipinski JF, et al.: Schizoaffective disorder: An invalid diagnosis? Am J Psychiatry, *137:* 921–927, 1980.

6. Hirschowitz J, Carter R, et al.: Lithium response in good prognosis schizophrenia. Am J Psychiatry, *137:* 916–920, 1980.

7. Extein I, Pottash ALC, et al.: Differentiating mania from schizophrenia by the TRH test. Am J Psychiatry, *137:* 981–982, 1980.

8. Deutsch SI, Davis KL: Schizophrenia: A review of diagnostic and biological issues. Hosp Community Psychiatry *34:* 313–322, 1983.

9. Pope HG: Distinguishing bipolar disorder from schizophrenia in clinical practice. Hosp Community Psychiatry, *34:* 322–326, 1983.

10. Fish F: The concept of schizophrenia. Br J Med Psychol, *39:* 269–273, 1966.

11. Mellor CS: First rank symptoms of schizophrenia. Br J Psychiatry, *117:* 15–23, 1970.

12. Schneider K: *Clinical Psychopathology* (Trans. M. W. Hamilton), New York, Grune & Stratton, 1959.

13. Silverstein ML, Harron M: First-rank symptoms in the post-acute schizophrenic: A followup study. Am J Psychiatry, *135:* 1481–1486, 1978.

14. Harron M, Quinlan D: Is disordered thinking unique to schizophrenia? Arch Gen Psychiatry, *34:* 15–21, 1977.

15. Koehler K: First rank symptoms of schizophrenia: questions concerning clinical boundaries. Br J Psychiatry, 134: 236–248, 1979.

16. Anderson WH: The physical examination in office practice. Am J Psychiatry, *137:* 1188–1192, 1980.

17. Allen RM, Young SJ: Phencyclidine-induced psychosis. Am J Psychiatry, *135:* 1081–1084, 1978.

18. Kendler KS: Demography of paranoid psychosis. Arch Gen Psychiatry, *39:* 890–902, 1982.

19. Fogelson DL, Cohen BM, et al.: A study of DSM-III schizophreniform disorder. Am J Psychiatry, *139:* 1281–1285, 1982.

20. Coryell W, Tsuang, MT: DSM III Schizophreniform disorder. Arch Gen Psychiatry, *39:* 66–69, 1982.

21. Zilboorg G: The problem of ambulatory schizophrenias. Am J Psychiatry, *113:* 519– 525, 1956.

22. Babigian HN: Schizophrenia: Epidemiology, in Kaplan HI, Sadock BJ (eds): *Comprehensive Textbook of Psychiatry,* ed. 4, Baltimore, Williams & Wilkins, 1985, p. 643.

23. Kohn ML. Social class and schizophrenia: A critical review, in Rosenthal D, Kety SS (eds):

The Transmission of Schizophrenia. Oxford, Pergamon Press, 1968.

24. Faris REL, Dunham HW: *Mental Disorders in Urban Areas,* Chicago, University of Chicago Press, 1939.

25. Goodman AB, Siegel C, et al.: The relationship between socioeconomic class and prevalence of schizophrenia, alcoholism, and affective disorders treated by inpatient care in a suburban area. Am J Psychiatry, *140:* 166– 170, 1983.

26. Slater E, Conie VA: *The Genetics of Mental Disorders,* London, Oxford University Press, 1971.

27. Kety SS: Genetic and biochemical aspects of schizophrenia, in Nicholi A (ed): *Harvard Guide to Modern Psychiatry,* Cambridge, Mass., Belknap Press, 1978.

28. Gottesman II, Shields J: *Schizophrenia and Genetics: A Twin Study Vantage Point,* New York, Academic Press, 1972.

29. Kety SS, et al.: Mental illness in the biological and adoptive families of adopted individuals who have become schizophrenic, in Fieve R, et al. (eds): *Genetic Research in Psychiatry,* Baltimore, Johns Hopkins University Press, 1975.

30. Lidz T, Blatt S, et al.: Critique of the Danish-American studies of the adopted-away offspring of schizophrenic parents. Am J Psychiatry, *138:* 1063–1068, 1981.

31. Lidz T, Blatt S: Critique of the Danish-American studies of the biological and adoptive relatives of adoptees who became schizophrenic. Am J Psychiatry, *140:* 426–434, 1983.

32. Baron M, Gruen R, et al.: Modern research criteria and the genetics of schizophrenia. Am J Psychiatry, *142:* 697–701, 1985.

33. Abrams R, Taylor MA: The genetics of schizophrenia: a reassessment using modern criteria. Am J Psychiatry *140:* 171–175, 1983.

34. Kendler KS, Gruenberg AM: An independent analysis of the Danish adoption study of schizophrenia. Arch Gen Psychiatry, *41:* 555–564, 1984.

35. Wyatt RJ, et al.: Reduced monoamine oxidase activity in platelets: A possible genetic marker for vulnerability to schizophrenia. Science, 179: 916–918, 1973.

36. Claridge G: Animal models of schizophrenia: The case for LSD-25. Schizophr Bull, *4:* 186–209, 1978.

37. Bowers MB: Biochemical processes in schizophrenia: an update. Schizophr Bull, *6:* 393–403, 1980.

38. Snyder SH: Amephetamine psychosis: A "model" schizophrenia mediated by catecholamines. Am J Psychiatry, *130:* 61–67, 1973.

39. Garver DL, Schlemmer RF, et al.: A schizophreniform behavioral psychosis mediated by dopamine. Am J Psychiatry, *132:* 33–38, 1975.

40. Meltzer HY, Stahl SM: The dopamine hypothesis of schizophrenia: A review. Schizophr Bull, *2:* 19–76, 1976.

41. Watson SJ, et al.: Some observations on the opiate peptides and schizophrenia. Arch Gen Psychiatry, *36:* 35–41, 1979.

42. Pickar D, Vartanian F, et al.: Short-term na-

loxone administration in schizophrenic and manic patients: A WHO collaborative study. Arch Gen Psychiatry, *39:* 313–319, 1982.

43. Berger PA, Watson SJ, et al.: Beta-endorphin and schizophrenia. Arch Gen Psychiatry, *37:* 635–640, 1980.

44. Weinberger DL, Wagner RL, et al.: Neuropathological studies in schizophrenia: A selective review. Schizophr Bull, *9:* 193–212, 1983.

45. Buchsbaum MS, Ingrar DH, et al.: Cerebral glucography and positron tomography. Arch Gen Psychiatry, *39:* 251–259, 1982.

46. Wolkin A, Jaeger J, et al.: Persistence of cerebral metabolic abnormalities in chronic schizophrenics as determined by positron emission tomography. Am J Psychiatry, *142:* 564–571, 1985.

47. Morhisa JM, Duffy FH, et al.: Brain electrical activity mapping in schizophrenic patients. Arch Gen Psychiatry, *40:* 719–728, 1983.

48. Taylor MA, Abrams R: Cognitive impairment in schizophrenia. Am J Psychiatry, *141:* 196–201, 1984.

49. Andreasen NC, Smith MR, et al.: Ventricular enlargement in schizophrenia: definition and prevalence. Am J Psychiatry, *139:* 292–296, 1982.

50. Grove, WM, Andreasen NC: Language and thinking in psychosis: Is there an input abnormality? Arch Gen Psychiatry, *42:* 26–32, 1985.

51. McReynonds P: Anxiety, perception and schizophrenia, in Jackson DD (ed): *The Etiology of Schizophrenia,* New York, Basic Books, 1960.

52. Kornetsky C, Markowitz R: Animal models of schizophrenia, in Lipton MA, Di Mascio A, Killam KF (eds): *Psychopharmacology: A Generation of Progress,* New York, Raven Press, 1978.

53. Lidz T: The family, language, and the transmission of schizophrenia, in Rosenthal D, Kety S (eds): *The Transmission of Schizophrenia,* Oxford, Pergamon Press, 1968.

54. Klein M: The significance of early anxiety situations in the development of the ego, in *The Psychoanalysis of Children,* ed. 3 (Trans A Strachey), London, Hogarth Press, 1948.

55. Mahler MS, Furer M: Observations in research regarding the symbiotic syndrome of infantile psychosis. Psychoanal Q, *29:* 317, 1960.

56. Mahler MS: *On Human Symbiosis and the Vicissitudes of Individuation,* New York, International Universities Press, 1978.

57. Sullivan HS: *The Interpersonal Theory of Psychiatry,* New York, Norton, 1953.

58. Sullivan HS: *Conceptions of Modern Psychiatry,* New York, Norton, 1953.

59. Lidz T: The intrafamilial environment of schizophrenic patients, II. Marital schism and marital skew. Am J Psychiatry, *114:* 241–248, 1957.

60. Lidz T: *The Origins and Treatment of Schizophrenic Disorders,* New York, Basic Books, 1973.

61. Bateson G, et al.: Towards a theory of schizophrenia. Behav Sci, *1:* 251–264, 1956.

62. Wynne LC, et al.: Pseudomutuality in the family relations of schizophrenics. Psychiatry, *21:* 205–220, 1958.

63. Wynne LC, Singer M, et al.: Communications of the adoptive parents of schizophrenics, in Jorstad J, Ugelstad G (eds): *Schizophrenia 75,* Oslo, Universitatforlaget, 1976.

64. Doane JA, West KL, et al: Parental communicational deviance and affective style. Arch Gen Psychiatry, *38:* 679–685, 1981.

65. Doane JA, Falloon, IRH, et al.: Parental affective style and the treatment of schizophrenia. Arch Gen Psychiatry, *42:* 34–42, 1985.

66. Lidz T: A developmental theory, in Shershow JC (ed): *Schizophrenia: Science and Practice,* pp. 69–95, Cambridge, Mass., Harvard University Press, 1978.

67. Wynne LC, Singer M: Thought disorder and family relations of schizophrenics: A research strategy. Arch Gen Psychiatry, *9:* 191–198, 1963.

68. Wynne LC, Singer M: Thought disorder and family relations of schizophrenics. A classification of forms of thinking. Arch Gen Psychiatry, *9:* 159–206, 1963.

69. Weinberger DR, Bigelow LB, et al.: Cerebral ventricular enlargement in chronic schizophrenia. Arch Gen Psychiatry, *37:* 11–13, 1980.

70. Golden CJ, Moses JA: Cerebral ventricular size and neuropsychological impairment in young chronic schizophrenics. Arch Gen Psychiatry, *37:* 619–623, 1980.

71. Golden CJ, Graber B, et al.: Structural brain deficits in schizophrenia. Arch Gen Psychiatry, *38:* 1014–1017, 1981.

72. Weinberger DR: Brain disease and psychiatric illness: When should a psychiatrist order a CAT scan? Am J Psychiatry, *141:* 1521–1527, 1984.

73. Manschreck TC, Keller MB: Disturbances of thinking, in Lazare A (ed): *Outpatient Psychiatry: Diagnosis and Treatment,* pp. 265–270, Baltimore, Williams & Wilkins, 1979.

74. MacKinnon RA, Michels R: The psychiatric interview, in *Clinical Practice,* pp. 230–258, Philadelphia, W.B. Saunders Co., 1971.

75. Vaillant G: *Adaptation to Life,* pp. 75–90, Little, Brown & Co., Boston, 1977.

76. Brown GW, et al.: Influence of family life on the course of schizophrenic disorders: A replication. Br J Psychiatry, *121:* 241–258, 1972.

77. Vaughn CE, Leff JP: The influence of family and social factors on the course of psychiatric illness. Br J Psychiatry, *129:* 125–137, 1976.

78. Falloon IRH, Boyd JL, et al.: Family management in the prevention of exacerbations of schizophrenia: A controlled study. N Engl J Med, *306:* 1437–1440, 1982.

79. Vaughn CE, Snyder KS, et al.: Family factors in schizophrenic relapse. Arch Gen Psychiatry, *41:* 1169–1177, 1984.

80. Platman SR: Family caretaking and expressed emotion: An evaluation. Hosp Community

Psychiatry, *34:* 921–925, 1983.

81. Carpenter WT, et al.: The treatment of acute schizophrenia without drugs: An investigation of some current assumptions. Am J Psychiatry, *134:* 14–20, 1977.
82. Stone AA: The new paradox of psychiatric malpractice. N Engl J Med, *311:* 1384–1387, 1984.
83. May PRA: *Treatment of Schizophrenia,* New York, Science House, 1968.
84. Kalhanek F, Linde OK, et al.: Precipitation of antipsychotic drugs in interaction with coffee or tea (letter to the editor). Lancet, *2:* 1130, 1979.
85. Hirsch SR: Precipitation of antipsychotic drugs in interaction with coffee or tea (letter to the editor). Lancet, *2:* 1130, 1979.
86. Bowen S, Taylor KM, et al.: Effect of coffee and tea on blood vessels and efficacy of antipsychotic drugs (Letter to the editor). Lancet, *1:* 1217–1218, 1981.
87. Kulhanek F, Linde OK: Coffee and tea influence pharmacokinetics of antipsychotic drugs (letter to the editor). Lancet, *2:* 359–360, 1981.
88. Van Patten T: Guidelines to the use of plasma levels: A clinical perspective. J Clin Psychiatry, *2:* 28–32, 1984.
89. Gelenberg A: Haloperidol levels: A therapeutic window? Biol Ther Psychiatry *7:* 36, 1984.
90. Simpson GM, Yadalam K: Blood levels of neuroleptics: State of the art. J Clin Psychiatry, *46* (5, sec. 2): 22–28, 1985.
91. Escobar JI, Barron A, et al.: A controlled study of "neuroleptization" with fluphenazine hydrochloride injections. J Clin Psychopharmacol (in press).
92. Smith RE, Dunner FJ, et al.: Rapid neuroleptization: A failure to find benefit. Paper presentation, Annual Meeting of the American Psychiatric Association, Toronto, 1982.
93. Neborsky R, Janowsky D, et al.: Rapid treatment of acute psychotic symptoms with high and low-dose haloperidol. Arch Gen Psychiatry, *38:* 195–199, 1981.
94. Van Putten T: The many faces of akathisia. Compr Psychiatry, *16:* 43–47, 1975.
95. Ratey JJ, Salzman C: Recognizing and managing akathisia. Hosp Community Psychiatry, *35:* 975–977, 1984.
96. Van Putten T, Mutalipassi LR, et al.: Phenothiazine-induced decompensation. Arch Gen Psychiatry, *30:* 102–105, 1974.
97. Raskin DE: Akathisia: A side effect to be remembered. Am J Psychiatry, *129:* 345–347, 1972.
98. Keckich WA: Neuroleptics: Violence as a manifestation of akathisia. JAMA, *240:* 2185, 1978.
99. Shear MK, Frances A, et al.: Suicide associated with akathisia and depot fluphenazine treatment. J Clin Psychopharmacol, *3:* 235–236, 1983.
100. Drake RE, Ehrlich J: Suicide attempts associated with akathisia. Am J Psychiatry, *142:* 499–501, 1985.
101. Anderson BG, Reker D, et al.: Prolonged adverse effects of haloperidol in normal subjects. N Engl J Med, *305:* 643–644, 1981.
102. Kendler KS: A medical student's experience with akathisia. Am J Psychiatry, *133:* 454–455, 1976.
103. Van Putten T, May PR, et al.: Response to antipsychotic medication: The doctor's and the consumer's view. Am J Psychiatry, *141:* 16–19, 1984.
104. Lipinski JF, Zubenko GS, et al.: Propanolol in the treatment of neuroleptic-induced akathisia. Am J Psychiatry, *141:* 412–415, 1984.
105. Alexander HE Jr, McCarty K, et al.: Hypotension and cardiopulmonary arrest associated with concurrent haloperidol and propanolol therapy. JAMA, *252:* 87–88, 1984.
106. Ratey JJ, Sorgi P, et al.: Nadolol as a treatment for akathisia. Am J Psychiatry, *142:* 640–642, 1985.
107. Zubenko GS, Cohen BM, et al.: Use of clonidine in treating neuroleptic-induced akathisia. Psychiatry Res, *13:* 253–259, 1985.
108. Gelenberg AJ, Mandel MR: Catatonic reactions to high potency neuroleptic drugs. Arch Gen Psychiatry, *34:* 947–950, 1977.
109. Klawans HL, Goetz CG, et al.: Tardive dyskinesia: Review and update. Am J Psychiatry, *137:* 900–908, 1980.
110. Granacher RP: Differential diagnosis of tardive dyskinesia: An overview. Am J Psychiatry, *138:* 1288–1297, 1981.
111. Yassa R, Jones BD: Complications of tardive dyskinesia: A review. Psychosomatics, *26:* 305–313, 1985.
112. Jeste DV, Wyatt RJ: Prevention and management of tardive dyskinesia. J Clin Psychiatry, *46:* 14–18, 1985.
113. Kane JM (ed): *Drug maintenance strategies in schizophrenia.* Washington, DC, American Psychiatric Association, 1984.
114. Caroff SN: The neuroleptic malignant syndrome. J Clin Psychiatry, *41:* 79–83, 1980.
115. Morris HH, McCormick WF, et al.: Neuroleptic malignant syndrome. Arch Neurol, *37:* 462–463, 1980.
116. Misiaszek JJ, Potter RL: Atypical neuroleptic malignant syndrome responsive to conservative management. Psychosomatics, *26:* 62–66, 1985.
117. Coons DJ, Hillman FJ, et al.: Treatment of neuroleptic malignant syndrome with dantrolene sodium: A case report. Am J Psychiatry, *139:* 944–945, 1982.
118. Zubenko G, Pope HG: Management of a case of neuroleptic malignant syndrome with bromocriptine. Am J Psychiatry, *140:* 1619–20, 1983.
119. Lazakus A: Treating neuroleptic malignant syndrome (letter to the editor). Am J Psychiatry, *141:* 1014–1015, 1984.
120. Nevins DP: Adverse response to neuroleptics in schizophrenia. Int J Psychoanal Psychother, *6:* 227–241, 1977.
121. Nurnberg HG, Prudic J: Guidelines for treat-

ment of psychosis during pregnancy. Hosp Community Psychiatry, 35: 67–71, 1984.

122. Calabrese JR, Gulledge AD: Psychotropics during pregnancy and lactation: A review. Psychosomatics, 26: 413–426, 1985.

123. Alexander PE: Antipsychotic effects of lithium in schizophrenia. Am J Psychiatry, 136: 283–287, 1979.

124. Hanssen T, Heyden T, et al.: Propanolol in schizophrenia. Arch Gen Psychiatry, 37: 685–690, 1980.

125. Yorkston NJ, Gruzelier JH, et al.: Propanolol as an adjunct to the treatment of schizophrenia. Lancet, 2: 575–578, 1977.

126. Gelenberg A, et al.: More on propanolol in schizophrenia, in Biological Therapies in Psychiatry Newsletter, Massachusetts General Hospital, vol. 4, no. 2, February 1981, pp. 7–8.

127. Peet M, Bethell MS, et al.: Propanolol in schizophrenia: I. Comparison of propanolol, chlorpromazine and placebo. Br J Psychiatry, 139: 105–111, 1981.

128. Greenblatt M: Efficacy of ECT in affective and schizophrenic illness. Am J Psychiatry, 134: 1001–1005, 1977.

129. Salzman C: The use of ECT in the treatment of schizophrenia. Am J Psychiatry, 137: 1032–1041, 1980.

130. May PR: Treatment of schizophrenia: A comparative study of five treatment methods, New York, Science House, 1968.

131. Van Putten T, May PR: Milieu therapies of the schizophrenias, in West LJ, Fluin ED (eds): Treatment of Schizophrenia: Progress and Prospects, p. 239, New York, Grune & Stratton, 1976.

132. May PR, Tuma HA, et al.: Schizophrenia: A follow-up study of the results of five forms of treatment. Arch Gen Psychiatry, 38: 776–784, 1981.

133. Grinspoon L, Ewalt JR, et al.: Psychotherapy and pharmacotherapy in chronic schizophrenia. Am J Psychiatry, 124: 1948–52, 1968.

134. Gunderson JG: A reevaluation of milieu therapy for non-chronic schizophrenic patients. Schizophr Bull, 6: 64–69, 1980.

135. Gunderson JG: If and when milieu therapy is therapeutic for schizophrenics, in Gunderson JG, Will O, Mosher EL (eds): Principles and Practice of Milieu Therapy, New York, Jason Aronson, 1983.

136. Mosher LR, Menn AZ: Community residential treatment for schizophrenia: Two year follow-up. Hosp Community Psychiatry, 29: 715–723, 1978.

137. Rappaport M, Hopkins HK, et al.: Are there schizophrenics for whom drugs may be unnecessary or contraindicated? Int Pharmacopsychiatry 13: 100–111, 1978.

138. Sederer LI: Inpatient psychiatry: What place the milieu? (editorial). Am J Psychiatry, 141: 673–674, 1984.

139. Goldberg A, Rubin B: Recovery of patients during periods of supposed neglect. Br J Med Psychol, 37: 265–72, 1964.

140. Van Putten T: Milieu therapy: Contraindications? Arch Gen Psychiatry, 29: 640–43, 1973.

141. Eissler KR: Psychiatric ward management of the acute schizophrenic patient. J Nerv Ment Dis, 105: 397–402, 1947.

142. McReynolds P: Anxiety perception and schizophrenia, in Jackson DD (ed): The Etiology of Schizophrenia, pp. 248–292, New York, Basic Books, 1960.

143. Spotnitz H: The need for insulation in the schizophrenic personality. Psychoanal 49: 3–25, 1962.

144. McGhie A: Psychological studies of schizophrenia. Br J Med Psychol, 39: 281–288, 1966.

145. Stierlin H: Individual therapy of schizophrenics and hospital structure, in Burton A (ed): Psychotherapy of the Psychoses, pp. 329–348. New York, Basic Books, 1961.

146. Will OA: Human relatedness and the schizophrenic reaction. Psychiatry, 22: 205–23, 1959.

147. Bouvet M: Technical variation and the concept of distance. Int J Psycho-Anal, 39: 211–221, 1958.

148. Freud S: Beyond the Pleasure Principle, standard ed., vol. 18, London, Hogarth Press, 1920.

149. Johnson JM, Parker KE: Some antitherapeutic effects of a therapeutic community. Hosp Community Psychiatry, 34: 70–71, 1983.

150. Spadoni AJ, Jackson JA: Milieu therapy in schizophrenia: A negative result. Arch Gen Psychiatry, 20: 547–551, 1969.

151. Klass DB, Grune GA, et al.: Ward treatment milieu and posthospital functioning. Arch Gen Psychiatry, 34: 1047–1052, 1977.

152. Kernberg OF: The therapeutic community: A re-evaluation. J Natl Assoc Private Psychiatr Hosp, 12: 46–55, 1981.

153. Raskin DE: Problems in the therapeutic community. Am J Psychiatry, 128: 492–493, 1971.

154. Klein RH: The patient-staff community meeting: A tea party with the mad hatter. Int J Group Psychother 31: 205–222, 1981.

155. Gersten D: Psychiatry residents in a milieu participatory democracy: A resident's view. Am J Psychiatry, 135: 1392–1395, 1978.

156. Fischer A, Weinstein MR: Mental hospitals, prestige, and the image of enlightenment. Arch Gen Psychiatry, 25: 41–48, 1971.

157. Shershow JC: Disestablishing a therapeutic community. Curr Concepts Psychiatry, 3: 8–11, 1977.

158. Islam A, Turner DL: The therapeutic community: A critical reappraisal. Hosp Community Psychiatry, 33: 651–653, 1982.

159. Lazell EW: The group treatment of dementia praecox. Psychoanal. Rev., 8: 168–179, 1921.

160. Kanas N, Rogers M, et al.: The effectiveness of group psychotherapy during the first three weeks of hospitalization: A controlled study. J Nerv Ment Dis, 168: 487–492, 1980.

161. Pattison EM, Brissenden E, et al.: Assessing special effects of inpatient group psychotherapy. Int J Group Psychother, 17: 283–297, 1967.

162. Strassberg DS, Roback HB, et al.: Self-disclosure in group therapy with schizophrenics. Arch Gen Psychiatry, *32:* 1259–1261, 1975.

163. Weiner MF: Outcome of psychoanalytically oriented group psychotherapy. Group, *8:* 3–12, 1984.

164. Yalom ID: *Inpatient Group Psychotherapy.* New York, Basic Books, 1983.

165. Maves PA, Schulz JW: Inpatient group treatment on short-term acute care units. Hosp Community Psychiatry, *36:* 69–73, 1985.

166. Rogers CR: *The Therapeutic Relationship and Its Impact,* Madison, University of Wisconsin Press, 1967.

167. Schwartz DP: Psychotherapy, in Shershow JC (ed): *Schizophrenia,* Cambridge, Mass., Harvard University Press, 1978.

168. McGlashan TH: Intensive individual psychotherapy of schizophrenia: A review of techniques. Arch Gen Psychiatry, *40:* 909–920, 1983.

169. Fromm-Reichmann F: *Principles of Intensive Psychotherapy,* Chicago, University of Chicago Press, 1950.

170. Fromm-Reichmann F: Notes on the development of treatment of schizophrenics by psychoanalytic psychotherapy. Psychiatry, *11:* 263–273, 1948.

171. Engle RP, Semrad EV: Brief hospitalization, the recompensation process, in Abroms GM, Greenfield NS (eds): *The New Hospital Psychiatry,* New York, Academic Press, 1971.

172. Drake RE, Sederer LI: Inpatient psychotherapy of chronic schizophrenia: Avoiding regression. Paper presentation, Annual Meeting of the American Psychiatric Association, Dallas, Texas, 1985.

173. Stanton AH, Gunderson JG, Knapp PH, et al.: Effects of psychotherapy in schizophrenia: I. Design and implementation of a controlled study. Schizophr Bull, *10:* 520–563, 1984.

174. Gunderson JG, Frank AF, Katz HM, et al.: Effects of psychotherapy in schizophrenia: II. Comparative outcome of two forms of treatment. Schizophr Bull *10:* 564–598, 1984.

175. Katz HM, Frank A, Gunderson JG, et al.: Psychotherapy of schizophrenia: What happens to treatment dropouts? J Nerv Ment Dis, *172:* 326–331, 1984.

176. Will AO: Psychotherapeutics and the schizophrenic reaction. J Nerv Ment Dis, *126:* 109–140, 1958.

177. Havens L: Explorations in the uses of language in psychotherapy: Counterprojective statements. Contemp Psychoanal, *16:* 53–67, 1980.

178. Lidz TS, Fleck S, et al.: *Schizophrenia and the Family,* New York, International Universities Press, 1965.

179. Semrad EV: *Teaching Psychotherapy of Psychotic Patients,* New York, Grune & Stratton, 1969.

180. Brown GW, Monck EM, Carstairs GM, et al.: Influence of family life on the course of schizophrenic illness. Br J Prev Soc Med, *16:* 55–68, 1962.

181. Brown GW, Rutter ML: The measurement of family activities and relationships. Hum Relations, *19:* 241–263, 1966.

182. Brown GW, Birley JLT, Wing JK: Influence of family life on the course of schizophrenic disorders: a replication. Br J Psychiatry, *121:* 241–258, 1972.

183. Vaughn CE, Leff JP: The influence of family and social factors on the course of psychiatric illness: A comparison of schizophrenic and depressed neurotic patients. Br J Psychiatry, *129:* 125–137, 1976.

184. Leff JP, Vaughn CE: The role of maintenance therapy and relative expressed emotion in relapse of schizophrenia: A two-year followup. Br J Psychiatry, *139:* 102–104, 1981.

185. Vaughn CE, Snyder KS, Freeman W, et al.: Family factors in schizophrenic relapse: A replication. Schizophr Bull, *8:* 425–426, 1982.

186. Vaughn CE, Snyder KS, et al.: Family factors in schizophrenic relapse: Replication in California of British Research on expressed emotion. Arch Gen Psychiatry, *41:* 1169–1177, 1984.

187. Snyder KS, Liberman RP: Family assessment and intervention with schizophrenics at risk for relapse, in *New Directions for Mental Health Services,* No. 12, *New Developments in Interventions with Families of Schizophrenics,* pp. 49–59, 1981.

188. Falloon IRH, Boyd JL, McGill CW, et al.: Family management training in the community care of schizophrenics. *New Directions for Mental Health Services,* No. 12, *New Developments in Interventions with Families of Schizophrenics:* 61–77, 1981.

189. Falloon IRH, Boyd JL, McGill CW, et al.: Family management in the prevention of exacerbations of schizophrenia: a controlled study. N Engl J Med, *306:* 1437–1440, 1982.

190. Boyd JL, McGill CW, Falloon IRH: Family participation in the community rehabilitation of schizophrenics. Hosp Community Psychiatry, *32:* 629–632, 1981.

191. Platman SR: Family caretaking and expressed emotion: An evaluation. Hosp Community Psychiatry, *34:* 921–925, 1983.

192. McGill CW, Falloon IRH, et al.: Family education intervention in the treatment of schizophrenia. Hosp Community Psychiatry, *34:* 934–938, 1983.

193. McFarlane WR, Beels CC: A decision-free model for integrating family therapies for schizophrenia, in McFarlane WR (ed): *Family Therapy in Schizophrenia,* pp. 325–335, New York, Guilford Press, 1983.

194. Arieti S: *Understanding and Helping the Schizophrenic: A Guide for Family and Friends,* New York, Basic Books, 1979.

195. Torrey EF: Surviving schizophrenia: A family manual, New York, Harper & Row, 1983.

196. Tsuang MT: Genetic counseling for psychiatric patients and their families. Am J Psychiatry, *135:* 1465–1475, 1978.

197. Drake RE, Gates C, et al.: Suicide among

schizophrenics: Who is at risk? J Nerv Ment Dis, *172:* 613–617, 1984.

198. Herz, MI: Recognizing and preventing relapse in patients with schizophrenia. Hosp Community Psychiatry, *35:* 344–349, 1984.

199. Hogarty GE, Goldberg SC, et al.: Drug and sociotherapy in the aftercare of schizophrenic patients, II. Arch Gen Psychiatry, *31:* 603–608, 1974.

200. Hogarty GE, Goldberg SC, et al.: Drug and sociotherapy in the aftercare of schizophrenic patients, III. Arch Gen Psychiatry, *31:* 609–618, 1974.

201. Glick ID, Hargreaves WA: *Psychiatric Hospital Treatment for the 1980's: A Controlled Study of Short vs. Long Hospitalization,* Lexington, Mass., Lexington Books, D.C. Heath & Co., 1979.

202. Harron M, et al.: Is modern-day schizophrenic outcome still negative? Am J Psychiatry, *135:* 1156–1162, 1978.

203. McGlashan TH: The Chestnut-Lodge follow-up study. Arch Gen Psychiatry, *41:* 586–601, 1984.

204. Harrow M, Carone BJ, et al.: The course of psychosis in early phases of schizophrenia. Am J Psychiatry, *142:* 702–707, 1985.

205. Harding CM, et al.: Vermont Longitudinal Research Project. Paper presentation, Annual Meeting of the American Psychiatric Association, Dallas, Texas, 1985.

chapter 4

borderline character disorder

Lloyd I. Sederer, M.D., and Jane Thorbeck, Ed.D.

DEFINITION

Character disordered patients of all types (including borderline characters) show disturbed, inflexible patterns of relating to themselves and others that are established by adolescence or earlier. These patients manifest impaired functioning in their relationships, work, and play, and they experience personal distress.[1, 2]

The terms borderline character disorder and borderline personality organization represent efforts to describe a type of patient who presents with a specific pathological personality organization. The character of these patients shows *specific traits* and is *not* merely a transitory state between neurosis and psychosis.[3] In fact, because *persistent instability* is characteristic of borderline patients, they have been described as being "stably unstable."[4]

Under highly structured, supportive conditions borderline characters may appear to be asymptomatic and functioning at a neurotic level. However, when stressed, they *regress* and demonstrate clear disturbances in their capacity to contain and manage feelings and impulses. This may happen in response to disappointment, loss, or absence of routine and structure, or under the influence of drugs or alcohol, or during a transference storm. This basic tendency for regression renders the borderline patient unstable. Mood, behavior, self-image, cognition, and interpersonal relationships are all subject to this instability, and symptoms may appear in any or all of these areas.

Mood disturbances are common. They include intense, labile affect with feelings of anger, emptiness, and bored depression. Borderline *behavior* is frequently impulsive and self-destructive, and the patient's *self-image* is inchoate. *Cognitively,* borderline patients can show transient reality disturbances and brief psychotic episodes. *Interpersonal relationships* show little stability over time. Intense dependent attachments, marred by manipulation, idealization, devaluation, and masochism, leave the patient repetitively disappointed, enraged, and helpless.[1, 5, 6]

Case Example. Ms. O. was a 19-year-old college freshman who presented for her first psychiatric admission with the chief complaint of "I've been depressed since Thursday."

A more careful history revealed that the patient complained of feeling "all speeded up" with difficulty falling asleep and some early morning awakening in the 2–3 weeks prior to admission. The patient reported that "it might be fun to die" and had intermittent suicidal ideation with thoughts of jumping out of a window of a moving train. Further, during this period the patient had two transient experiences where she thought a person on the television was talking to her.

These symptoms began rather precipitously following a breakup with a boyfriend whom she had known only briefly. This relationship ended after the patient had posed in the nude for a film that was being made by a male friend of her boyfriend.

The patient reported feeling depressed for much of her lifetime with intermittent feelings of being "dead inside." She had an extensive history throughout her adolescence of heterosexual relationships characterized by superficiality and promiscuity. She reported having difficulty maintaining relationships because, as she put it, "when you get to know someone you find out they are as screwed up as you are." The patient had a history of amyl nitrate, Percodan, and marijuana abuse.

On admission, the patient was surrounded by several family members, all of whom appeared anxious and exasperated. In the interview, the patient showed labile affect with periods of crying, anger, and thinly veiled seductiveness. She was not psychotic at the time of interview, nor did she show a prominent neurovegetative depression. Suicidal ideation was as described, and the patient requested hospitalization in order to "work on my self-image."

In view of the patient's suicidal ideation and precipitous decompensation, she was admitted for crisis intervention, diagnostic evaluation, and short-term hospital treatment.

ETIOLOGICAL CONSIDERATIONS

Biological Hypotheses

Evidence is accumulating for a biological (genetic) component to the etiology of the borderline personality disorder. Andrulonis et al.,[7-9] studying a long-term inpatient population of patients with marked functional impairment and past treatment failures, have identified three subcategories of borderline disorders, distinct from one another and from a schizophrenic control group. One group had no history of past or current symptoms of major or minimal brain dysfunction. This group had a history of acting-out behaviors, drug and alcohol abuse, depression, and a family history of affective disorder; these patients were predominantly female with the onset of their disorder occurring in adolescence. A second group had a past history of significant head trauma, epilepsy, or encephalitis. A third group had a history of past or current documented severe hyperactivity, distractibility, and/or learning disabilities. The second and third groups were often males, with early developmental problems and symptoms of episodic dyscontrol, adult minimal brain disorder, or limbic abnormalities; these latter two groups were considered organically brain disordered. From these findings, Andrulonis et al. posit a nonorganic borderline group who require a relationship-based, insight-oriented psychotherapy, a stable and structured living environment, and perhaps the adjunctive use of neuroleptics, antidepressants, or lithium. The

authors also posit, on the basis of the second and third groups, an organically dysfunctional dimension to some borderline patients, often men, who require structure and consistency in their relationships and environment, special education and vocational training, directive family therapy, and perhaps stimulants or anticonvulsants.

An affectively disordered component to borderline pathology has been hypothesized by numerous authors.[10-18] Evidence of an affective disorder playing an etiological role in borderline pathology is supported by the presence of depressive symptomatology, significant increases in the prevalence of affect disorders in relatives of borderline patients, epidemological lifetime prevalence rates of depression in borderline patients, similarities in EEG sleep between borderline and affectively disordered patients, and response to medications that target dysthymic symptoms. Gunderson and Elliot[15] propose that instead of primary depressive illness generating borderline pathology or depression resulting from the borderline syndrome, the observed concurrence of borderline and affective disorders occurs despite their heterogeneity. They hypothesize that individuals who develop either disorder start with a biophysiological limitation or vulnerability that increases their risk of psychological impairment in early development. The observed overlap is especially due to the convergence of innate and early environmental factors that combine to produce depression, chronic dysphoria, and borderline behavior.

Perhaps the most developed model to explain the genetic diathesis in borderline pathology has been advanced by Meissner.[19] He organizes borderline character types in a manner that clusters cases into a spectrum on the basis of whether there is the presence or absence of psychosis or mood disorder. For example, latent schizophrenia would represent the psychotic border of the borderline spectrum; hysteroid dysphoria would represent the affectively disordered border of the spectrum; and the as-if personality would represent a borderline patient without features of psychosis or mood disorder. In this model, he demonstrates the interplay between genetics and environment. Schizophrenic biological factors would play a role in the more psychotically disabled characters, and an affective diathesis would play a role in the more mood-disordered characters. Treatment planning, including choice of medication, as well as course and prognosis, would derive from accurate diagnosis along this character spectrum.

Psychodynamic and Developmental Hypotheses

Many theorists have constructed their ideas on the basis of work with adult patients, which they then inferentially relate to childhood.[20] In fact, these theories remain most accurate in describing the subjective experience of the adults we treat. Other theorists have gathered more objective data from child observation. A knowledge of both the adult borderline patient's experience in treatment and early childhood development are essential to understanding the pathology and the core dilemmas of the borderline patient.

In work based on child observation, Margaret Mahler[21] has described the 2nd to the 5th months in the infant's life as the *Symbiotic Phase* of development. In this phase the infant's dependence is absolute, and the child requires near total empathic understanding from the mother.[22] Successful completion of the symbiotic phase results in what has been termed self-object differentiation. Self-object differentiation refers to the child's ability to differentiate or separate his own experience of himself from his experience of his mother. Children who do not complete self-object differentiation are hypothetically vulnerable to psychosis later in life. Borderline patients are thought to have mastered self-object differentiation and to encounter their difficulties in the next phase of development.

The next developmental period, as described by Mahler et al.,[23] is entitled the *Separation-Individuation Phase*. This phase spans from 5 months to 3 years in the child's life. It is the time when the child begins to develop muscular and psychological autonomy. Successful maturation through the developmental tasks of separation and individuation requires what

Winnicott has called a "good enough mother."[22, 24, 25] This mother is able to contain the prominent pregenital, aggressive impulses of a child at this age by nonpunitive, nonanxious, and firm limit setting. She does this without curtailing her love and understanding. According to Adler,[26] this mother has a basic confidence in her own goodness. Believing in herself, she is able to frustrate the child (when this is appropriate) without fearing the child's anger. Her empathic qualities enable her to complement this frustration with understanding.

Theoretically, mastery of this developmental period leaves the child with the capacity to regard himself as both loving and hating (i.e., with the capacity for ambivalence) in response to an image of a mother who was both gratifying and frustrating. The child is thereby able to tolerate separation or loss by having the ability to maintain a comforting image of mother (a constant object image) despite her frustrating the child with her absence or her limit setting.

In summary, the "good enough mother" provides a "holding environment"[22, 27] in which she empathically, reliably, and firmly contains the child through the separation-individuation process. Successful mastery of this period establishes the child's capacity for ambivalence, object constancy, and tolerance of separation without serious regression.

Mahler et al.[28] have reported that failure of separation and individuation may occur when the mother has inadequately resolved her own conflicts about dependency and autonomy. In this study, mothers with difficulty with their own dependency responded with anger and hurt to the child's clinging (e.g., "A minute ago you didn't want me, now I don't want you ... "). Mothers with conflict about their autonomy responded to the child's autonomy with threats of abandonment (e.g., "You think you can manage on your own, well go ahead ... "). The former group stirs anxiety in the child about his wishes for care and comfort; the latter group threatens abandonment should the child begin to exhibit self-sufficiency. In both groups the mothers' defensive inability to distinguish their needs from those of the child (empathic failure) created the conditions for developmental failure.

Masterson[29-31] has posited that the mother of the borderline patient shows borderline features herself. He notes that the mother markedly interferes with the child's separation-individuation process by rewarding regressive clinging in the child and by withdrawing support from the child when he shows autonomous behavior.

Kernberg[5, 32] provides a different perspective on early development. He suggested that borderline patients demonstrate excessive aggression early in childhood as an outgrowth of either constitutional predisposition or persistent frustration of the child. The child's early experience with his mother does not allow him to develop an image of a mother who can tolerate powerful, negative feelings toward her. As a consequence, the ability to integrate positive and negative aspects of mother, and in turn the self, does not develop. In the absence of this integration, known as ambivalence, the child must dissociate good and bad, for they cannot be tolerated simultaneously in regard to the self or others. This dissociation is called splitting (see Psychodynamic Concepts and Character Diagnosis). Splitting weakens the ego, for it must compromise reality. This weakened ego poorly tolerates anxiety and frustration and shows a vulnerability to further regression. In addition, this limited ego has a diminished capacity for object constancy and therefore cannot sustain a stable, trusting relationship with another which would mitigate the desperate fear of aloneness.[33]

In summary, the borderline patient theoretically has suffered a failure in the separation-individuation phase of childhood development. In the absence of "good enough mothering" or because of constitutional effects (or both), the child does not develop object constancy, the capacity for ambivalence, and a tolerance for separation. These limitations, hypothetically, are the substrate for borderline pathology.

Family Hypotheses

Edward Shapiro and John Zinner[34-36] have studied adolescent borderline pa-

tients and their families. They apply the developmental perspectives and object-relations theories of Winnicott, Mahler, and Kernberg, as well as taking a *systems view of the family as a group that is collectively functioning in a regressed manner.*[37, 38] Shapiro and Zinner differ from Masterson in that they argue that neither of the parents need be borderline. Instead, they postulate that the family system as a whole functions in a regressed manner under the pressure of a shared unconscious fantasy that angry or hostile feelings can destroy a loved object. Believing in this fantasy, the family then employs the defense of splitting in order to protect their attachment to the loved object.

Shapiro and Zinner maintain that the parents of the borderline suffer from marked conflict in regard to autonomy and dependency issues. When a specific, unconsciously chosen child reaches adolescence, that child reactivates critical separation issues that were never mastered by the child or by his parents. This specific child's *dependent* wishes and needs are experienced by the rest of the family as *devouring demands* from which they withdraw. Dependent wishes are seen as so devouring, theoretically, because they represent the denied and otherwise unrecognized dependent needs of the parents, needs which they never had met.

The specific adolescent's efforts at *autonomy* are experienced by the family as a form of *hateful abandonment.* This adolescent is viewed by the family as wanting to separate because he hates and wishes to reject the family. Regressive splitting of "good and bad" feelings occurs because the family cannot function at a mature level of ambivalence. In this regressed state, the family tries to limit the adolescent's strivings for autonomy.

Masterson[29-31, 39] has also studied the borderline adolescent. He hypothesizes that the essence of the borderline dilemma is the conflict between natural autonomous growth and fear of parental abandonment. Masterson maintains that the mother (and father) suffers from a borderline syndrome. His observations suggest that mother rewards the child's regressive clinging and withdraws libidinal support in response to the child's independent efforts. In effect, according to Masterson, the borderline parents of the borderline adolescent are still tied to their respective mothers from whom they were unable to separate. The parents' developmental failure renders them incapable of facilitating the child's mastery of the separation-individuation phase of development. When separation issues are intensified by an adolescent child, these parents experience a renascence of internal conflict which they then act out with this child.

Gunderson et al.[40] provided a systematic study of the families of borderlines. Their sample is limited (12) and is comprised of white, middle class, intact families. However, their findings are supported by Walsh's work with a different sample.[41] Gunderson found marked *parental neglect* consistently in the families of borderline patients. The parents of borderline patients bonded powerfully to each other, without overt conflict. This rigidly tight bond between the parents excluded the children and did not provide warmth, empathy, and limit setting. Rule enforcement by the parents was poor, and there was a paucity of nurturance. The mothers and fathers, however, were not all borderline patients, as Masterson suggested. In these families the child enters adolescence with limited internal resources. The additional libidinal and aggressive drives of adolescence do not meet with parental understanding, support, or limits, and symptomatology predictably erupts.

In another small sample (n = 16) of families with borderline children from a wide socioeconomic spectrum and identified patients in an age range from 6 to 28 years of age, Feldman and Guttman[42] reported interactional patterns that have therapeutic implications. In these families, they observed two principal family constellations. In one family type, one of the parents was markedly literal-minded and unable to mobilize affects that would allow for empathy with a child. (These literal-minded parents were much like alexithymic patients who are unable to appreciate their inner world of feelings and fantasies.[43, 44]) In the second family type, one parent exhibited a borderline personality disorder, with the identified child-patient as the object of the parent's projections and distortions. The authors concluded that the presence of one parent (in either family type) who exercised a protective role vis-á-vis the child distinguished which children of these two pathological family constellations became borderline, and which did not. Protective factors included direct blocking of projections and distortions, reality testing, and empathic responsiveness. In both of these family types, parental protectiveness shielded the child from the development of a personality disorder, whereas lack of protection was correlated with personality disorder in the child. The therapeutic implications of these findings are several. First, exploratory, affect-oriented psychotherapy may not be useful in families with literal-minded members. Second, in both family constellations, family therapy should aim to mobilize the protective functions (noted above) of the healthier parent. Third, and this is reminiscent of family work with schizophrenic patients (see Chapter 3), in families where the milieu is emotionally disturbing and cannot be corrected by working with the family, the child may benefit from increased contacts out of the home, with other family members, school, and community programs wherein a more supportive, empathetic, and realistic environment is provided.

Family theory of borderline disorders has gained in size and substance but remains relatively new. Biological contributions and the role of temperament need further development. Families of schizophrenic patients suffered for too long under the concept of the "schizophrenogenic mother/family," adding to the family's burden and impairing our capacity to ally with, educate, and support adaptive efforts by a family. Until more is known about the etiology of borderline disorders, we must take care not to repeat this mistake with families of borderline patients, thereby fostering guilt and defensiveness, and alienating those closest to our patients.

DIAGNOSIS AND DIFFERENTIAL DIAGNOSIS

The diagnosis and differential diagnosis of the borderline patient can be approached from two major perspectives. The first is a *symptomatic* perspective in which constellations of symptoms provide a basis for nosology. The second perspective is *developmental and psychodynamic* and builds a nosology based on maturational processes and a psychology of the mind. Neither perspective need exclude the other.

Symptomatic Diagnosis and Differential Diagnosis

Symptomatic Diagnosis

Borderline characters typically show features of the following symptomatic picture[1, 3, 6, 45-47]:

1. Affective instability with rapid mood shifts to anxiety, irritability, or depression.
2. Unstable and intense interpersonal relationships.
3. Difficulty in being alone and chronic feelings of boredom and emptiness. Social contact may become compulsive.
4. Impulse disorders and addictions with the chronic, repetitive emergence of impulses in the service of gratifying an instinctual need. These include alcoholism, drug addictions, certain forms of psychogenic obesity, and kleptomania; sexual deviations that are episodic; and suicidal or self-mutilatory acts. Patients experience these behaviors as ego-dystonic or alien when they are not engaged in them. However, these behaviors are reported to be ego-syntonic and highly pleasurable during their enactment.
5. Transient psychotic experiences.
6. Polysymptomatic clinical presentation. This refers to those patients who present with multiple psychiatric symptomatology. Included are phobias, obsessive-compulsive symptoms, conversion symptoms, dissociative reactions, hypochondriasis, paranoia, and hypochondriacal trends.
7. Polymorphous perverse sexual

trends. This term refers to patients who demonstrate several coexisting perverse sexual deviations, e.g., exhibitionism with homosexual and heterosexual promiscuity with sadistic features. Patients who manifest no behavior that is perverse but whose fantasies are polymorphous and perverse are to be included under this symptom category. Patients whose genital life centers on a stable sexual deviation (for example, homosexuality) and who combine this deviation with constant object relationships are not included in this category.

The *Diagnostic and Statistical Manual of Mental Disorders* (Third Edition) of the American Psychiatric Association[1] (DSM-III) offers the following diagnostic criteria for Borderline Personality Disorder.

The following are characteristic of the individual's current and longterm functioning, are not limited to episodes of illness, and cause either significant impairment in social or occupational functioning or subjective distress.

At least five of the following are required:

1. Impulsivity or unpredictability in at least two areas that are potentially self-damaging, e.g., spending, sex, gambling, substance use, shoplifting, overeating, physically self-damaging acts
2. A pattern of unstable and intense interpersonal relationships, e.g., marked shifts of attitude, idealization, devaluation, manipulation (consistently using others for one's own ends)
3. Inappropriate, intense anger or lack of control of anger, e.g., frequent displays of temper, constant anger
4. Identity disturbances manifested by uncertainty about several issues relating to identity, such as self-image, gender identity, long-term goals or career choice, friendship patterns, values, and loyalties, e.g., "Who am I?", "I feel like I am my sister when I am good"
5. Affective instability: marked shifts from normal mood to depression, irritability, or anxiety, usually lasting a few hours and only rarely more than a few days, with a return to normal mood
6. Intolerance of being alone, e.g., frantic efforts to avoid being alone, depressed when alone
7. Physically self-damaging acts, e.g., suicidal gestures, self-mutilation, recurrent accidents or physical fights
8. Chronic feelings of emptiness or boredom

If under 18, does not meet the criteria for Identity Disorder.

Symptomatic Differential Diagnosis

The symptomatic differential diagnosis[1, 6, 19, 48–52] of the borderline patient includes the following.

Schizophrenia. As noted in Chapter 3, schizophrenia is a longitudinal diagnosis that requires greater than 6 months of thought, volitional, and affective disturbances. Borderline patients may show thought and volitional disturbances but only transiently. Affect in schizophrenia tends to be flat, while borderline affect is unstable, intense, and often angry. Schizophrenics tend to be socially isolated, unlike the compulsive and intense social contacts of the borderline patient.

Schizotypal Personality. This DSM-III term was formerly Latent or Borderline Schizophrenia. The schizotypal patient presents with various oddities of thinking, perception, communication, and behavior, but never severe enough to meet the criteria for schizophrenia.

Major Depressive Episode. A major depressive episode is marked by neurovegetative signs (appetite, sleep, and psychomotor disturbances) that have persisted for at least several weeks. The mood disturbance of a depressive episode is one of sadness, guilt, and self-reproach, whereas borderline patients complain of emptiness, boredom, and inability to be alone. A depressive picture with a history of transient psychotic experiences, drug abuse, and sexual deviance as well as poor academic and vocational achievement would suggest a diagnosis of borderline character.

It is possible for borderline patients to develop depressive episodes, and those that do would be diagnosed by DSM-III as Axis I, Depressive Episode, and Axis II, Borderline Personality.

Histrionic Personality Disorder. Histrionic patients show exaggerated expressiveness and are given to impulsive behavior. These symptoms, however, are more marked in conflicted areas (e.g., sexuality) in the histrionic person, whereas the borderline patient shows more generalized and diffuse affective and impulsive dyscontrol. Further, histrionic patients are typically dependent but not as desperately so as the borderline. Sexuality may be provocative in both but tends to be inhibited in the histrionic and promiscuous and polymorphous in the borderline. Cognitively, histrionics may be diffuse and impressionistic but without the reality disturbances that the borderline individual may evidence.

Narcissistic Character Disorder. Narcissistic characters[1, 53–55] suffer from a disturbance in self-regard. They are grandiose in their sense of self-importance and are preoccupied with fantasies of greatness, power, and privilege. In their interpersonal relationships they are exploitative, idealizing or devaluing, and entitled. Unlike the borderline, they generally do not regress to transient psychotic states or severe panic.

Drug and Alcohol Use and Abuse. Frequently, borderline patients have a history of continuous use or regular abuse of alcohol and drugs. Very often these substances were a part of the admission drama, in which the patient overdosed or in an intoxicated state acted in an impulsive and self-destructive way. Diagnostic controversy often centers on the following questions:

- "What if the patient's drug-taking is not the primary problem, but rather symptomatic of the underlying character pathology?"
- "What if the patient really has a concurrent affective disorder and is using drugs/alcohol to treat his depression?"

Each question invites a problematic response. By the very way the questions are posed, even a "perhaps," certainly an affirmative answer, would suggest that the patient should be treated for, in the first case, his character pathology and in the second case, his affective disorder. The questions regarding character pathology and concurrent affective disorder in the presence of a clear history of substance abuse are misleading, for they overlook several important clinical considerations:

1. Alcohol and drug use and abuse obscure an accurate diagnosis of a mood disorder. Mood disturbance from substance abuse can be quite similar to a depressive disorder, es-

pecially as it may occur in a borderline patient. This is particularly true of the continuous use of central nervous system depressants like alcohol, sedatives, and hypnotics.

2. Alcoholism, as Vaillant[56] has shown us, induces personality disturbances which can be mistaken for underlying character pathology, including borderline disorders. Vaillant has demonstrated that the premorbid personalities of most alcoholics do not differ substantively from those of nonalcoholics. He has also demonstrated that during periods of sobriety, alcoholics were as well-adapted, that is, non-characterologically disordered, as nonalcoholics. It is likely that these same findings would apply to other substance addictions.

3. Alcohol and drug abuse impede recovery. Patients cannot adequately proceed, biologically or psychologically, on a path of character development or remission from depression if they continue to regularly use psychoactive drugs of abuse. Biologically, drugs of abuse have a direct and deleterious effect on the brain (especially the limbic system). They also interfere with the pharmacokinetics of any prescribed mood-altering drug. Psychologically, regular use of drugs impairs ego function, represents denial of illness, and may result in life-endangering behaviors.[57]

These clinical considerations surpass differential diagnosis and stress the importance of recommending full abstinence as the first step in diagnosis and treatment, as well as for ensuring patient safety. Importantly, abstinence may or may not require specific drug treatment. (Vaillant[56] has also shown that some alcoholics can stop drinking without treatment.) If the patient cannot realize an abstinent state, because of denial and the compulsive drive of addiction, then referral for treatment of substance abuse would be in order. This can begin in the hospital and continue on an outpatient basis. A period of at least a few months is generally needed for biology and psychology to re-

constitute to a nondependent state, at which time an accurate assessment of mood disorder and character pathology can be made.

Psychodynamic Concepts and Character Diagnosis

Developmental Considerations

As discussed earlier (see Etiological Considerations), the infant and young child is confronted with specific developmental tasks which he attempts to master through a set of adaptive mechanisms collectively conceptualized as the ego. Successful mastery of the first, or symbiotic, phase of development is evidenced by the capacity to differentiate self from other. Children who fail to achieve this differentiation are severely wanting in their ego development and consequently suffer from the lack of boundaries between self and other, inside and outside, known as psychosis. Borderline patients have successfully mastered self-object differentiation but encounter their difficulties in the next phase of childhood development.

From 6 months to about 3 years of age the child confronts the task of progressive autonomy from the mother. Importantly, for this discussion, the ego must integrate or synthesize contradictory (e.g., frustrating and comforting, loving and hating) self and object-images. The ability to do so provides the child with what is termed *object constancy,* or the capacity to sustain a constant and whole relationship in which he cares for (and feels cared for by) a loved object, despite separations and frustrations. Borderline patients fail to achieve this integration and remain at a level at which self and others are limited to feeling partial and transient. Relationships at this level cannot encompass the warmth and the anger of intimacy, nor can they offer the inner security of an intimate relationship. Without an inner sense of permanence and security about others, separation and frustration evoke feelings of panic, emptiness, and anomie in the borderline patient.

The Defensive Operations of the Ego

A borderline patient is driven by powerful pregenital aggressive impulses and possesses an internal world of all good and all bad object images. His chaotic, intense, and ever-changing life behaviorally represents his ego's adaptive efforts to master these impulses and to comply with these images through the defenses of splitting, projective identification, idealization, and devaluation.

The borderline patient's inability to simultaneously maintain loving and hating aspects of his self-image or his image of another is the core dilemma for the borderline ego. The need to preserve a sense of the good and the loving in the presence of feelings of the bad and the hating is managed by the defense of splitting.

Splitting is the defense of keeping consciously separate from each other feelings and perceptions that are opposite or contradictory. In other words, positive and negative feelings and percepts are alternately, but never concomitantly, in consciousness. Splitting is different from *denial,* in which whole percepts are disavowed or denied and generally substituted by fantasies that are wish-fulfilling. Denial severely compromises reality and is seen in the psychotic disorders. Splitting is also different from *repression,* in which an intolerable affect or idea is temporarily expelled from consciousness. Repression underlies the neurotic defensive operations. Splitting is the defense that characterizes the borderline's efforts to preserve a relationship that is characterized by marked neglect, abuse, or manipulation, yet which is needed for emotional survival. Splitting also underlies the borderline defenses of projective identification, primitive idealization, omnipotence, and devaluation.

Through the defense of *projective identification,* an unacceptable part of the patient's self (e.g., an impulse or a judgment about the self) is dissociated (split) from consciousness and attributed to someone else. An identification with the other then occurs, for that person now has the projected qualities of the self, and the patient then behaves in response to this projection. If, for example, an aggressive impulse is projected, it is then easily recognized (unconsciously identified with) and responded to with distrust or retaliation. Projective identification is a primitive de-fense since the impulse or percept is not effectively mastered. The ego is weakened by the processes of splitting and projective identification, and the patient is left to respond to or control the recipient of his projections. Nevertheless, projective identification must also be understood as the borderline's *effort at a relationship,* however flawed and disturbing. Through the process of projective identification the borderline evokes feelings in the recipient that are like his own: he has made someone else feel like he does. For a therapist, projective identification allows for empathy because the therapist can experience how it is his patient is feeling.

Primitive idealization is the tendency to see someone else as totally good. Bad aspects of that person are dissociated and may be taken on by the self or attributed to others. *Omnipotence* is the conviction that the self is all powerful (through a process of identification with a magically idealized other). *Devaluation* is the tendency to see someone else as totally bad. It is the complementary defense of idealization.

Character Diagnosis

Character diagnosis, unlike descriptive diagnosis, is rooted in the developmental and ego-defensive considerations outlined in the preceding sections. It is beyond the scope of this chapter to present a thorough discussion of a theoretical organization of character pathology. For this, the reader is referred to Kernberg, who has written extensively in the area of character pathology and differential diagnosis.[3, 4, 58, 59] We will attempt to summarize some of his work here, though the reader is urged to read the primary source material. Our aim is to provide a theoretical framework on which the clinician can begin to anchor his observations about patients. In establishing a diagnosis, this framework becomes an important way of understanding patients along a *continuum of psychopathology.* It provides a tool for differentiating borderline patients from other character-disordered patients and for understanding individual patient regressions and progressions as they occur over the course of time and in psychotherapy.

Kernberg approaches the classification of character pathology from the perspectives of the *defensive operations of the ego,* from *superego* development,* from *instinctual development,* and from the nature of the person's *internalized object relationships.*† He has offered a classification of levels (higher, intermediate, and lower) of organization of character pathology. This continuum confines itself to character pathology. In doing so it omits psychosis, which would occur before the more disturbed end of the spectrum, and normality, which would represent the next and final step of development after higher level character pathology. Obsessives and hysterics are good examples of higher level characters, while borderline patients, in particular, exemplify the lower end of the character continuum. *Table 4.1* summarizes this classification, which is further detailed below.

The *defensive operations of the ego* form a continuum in which higher level characters employ repression as the major defense with the related defenses of intellectualization, rationalization, undoing, and higher levels of projection. Instinctive wishes are sublimated and do not appear in their original and primitive form in higher level characters. Intermediate level characters also employ repression but the defensive barrier is weak, and the instinct is partially expressed in behavior (e.g., passive-aggressiveness). Intermediate level characters also show traces of lower level defense mechanisms. Lower level characters use splitting as the predominant defense with the related mechanisms of projective identification, omnipotence, idealization, and devaluation. Instincts and impulses (e.g., aggression, sexuality) frequently break through these limited defenses.

The *superego development* of lower level characters is severely limited by a weak, impaired ego and its use of defensive split-

ting. Idealized notions of the self and others create unreachable expectations of power and greatness while a punitive superego insists on fearful obedience. Higher level characters have developed a stable ego identity with a capable repressive barrier which excludes unacceptable instincts and impulses from consciousness. Furthermore, the punitive superego is modified by its integration with more realistic and caring parental introjects in the form of the ego ideal.

The *instinctual development* of higher level characters reveals genital primacy and oedipal level conflicts. Intermediate level characters have reached a genital level of organization but regress repeatedly to pregenital levels, particularly to oral (or dependent) fixation points. Lower level characters evidence marked pregenital aggressiveness, which is said to pervade all their functioning.

The *internalized object relationships* of lower level characters (such as borderline and schizoid personalities) are severely disturbed. In the absence of object constancy and with splitting as a primary defense, their internal images are alternately all good and all bad. As a consequence, neither self nor others can be perceived as whole or constant. Intermediate level characters have developed a stable, integrated sense of self and others, but in a highly conflicted manner. Higher level characters possess a stable sense of self and experience a relatively limited degree of conflict.

EPIDEMIOLOGY

No accurate incidence, prevalence, and socioeconomic figures are available on borderline character disorder, particularly since diagnostic validity and reliability are still being established. Clinically, cases appear to abound. The disorder appears to be more common in women.

HOSPITAL TREATMENT

The effective hospital treatment of the borderline patient is one of the major challenges in contemporary hospital psychiatry. Borderline patients require special management strategies in order to *minimize the difficulties* they experience

---

*The superego is a theoretical construct which describes the mental functions of morality, conscience, and guilt. The superego can be punitive and critical and evoke guilt. It may also be loving and rewarding, through a component known as the ego ideal.

†Internalized object relationships are the introjections and identifications of the emotionally valued people in the person's life that form the basis of the ego's identity.

Table 4.1
Continuum of Character Pathology[5, 58]

Higher	Intermediate	Lower
Superego—well-integrated but severe.	*Superego*—punitive, rigid, and less integrated; decreased capacity for guilt; paranoid trends.	*Superego*—minimally integrated; tendency to project aspects of primitive, punitive superego; severely impaired capacity for guilt and concern.
Ego—well-integrated; ego identity with stable self-concept and stable representational world.	*Ego*—subject to contradictory demands of superego, i.e., be great, powerful, and attractive and morally perfect.	*Ego*—synthetic function seriously impaired; identity diffusion results from lack of stable self-concept and experience of stable external world; ego weakness with poor anxiety tolerance and impulse dyscontrol.
Defensive operations—repression primary; little or no instinctual infiltration into defensive character traits, which are primarily inhibitory and sublimatory.	*Defensive operations*—repression still primary but some dissociation and defensive splitting occurs in limited areas; character traits are partially infiltrated by instinctual strivings (e.g., structured impulsivity).	*Defensive operations*—splitting is primary with related projective identification, omnipotence, and devaluation; character defenses are typically impulsive and instinctually infiltrated.
Adaptation—somewhat constricted due to neurotic defenses but *not* seriously impaired.	*Adaptation*—variable; subject to mood swings, distrust.	*Adaptation*—generally paranoid secondary to projected superego aspects and projective identification; severely limited conflict-free ego and adaptive capacities; repetitive failures in work, play, and relationships.
Object relationships—deep and capable of experiencing guilt, mourning, and wide range of affects.	*Object relationships*—capacity for involvements with others is possible, but characterized by conflict.	*Object relationships*—object constancy not fully reached; relationships tend to be intensely dependent or threatening; unintegrated good and bad internal images and past object relationships.
Instincts—sexual and aggressive drives are partially inhibited; genital phase and oedipal conflicts predominate; no pathological condensation of genital level strivings with pregenital aggressiveness.	*Instincts*—genital level reached but pregenital (especially oral) conflicts emerge as major regressive trend; aggressive nature of pregenital conflicts is muted.	*Instincts*—excessive pregenital aggression fosters a condensation of pregenital and genital conflicts; polymorphous perverse drives infiltrate all relationships.
Examples—obsessive-compulsive characters; most hysterical characters; depressive-masochistic characters.	*Examples*—many narcissistic characters; passive-aggressive characters; sadomasochistic characters; hysteroid characters (lower level hysterics).	*Examples*—borderline characters; antisocial characters; many narcissistic characters; prepsychotic characters (schizoid and paranoid).

in the hospital. Primary among these difficulties is a negative response to treatment with pronounced, rapid *regression* and *acting out* of deviant and dangerous behavior.

Indications for hospitalization of the borderline patient include a life-threatening crisis; a transient psychotic episode; persistent depressive symptomatology; or an impasse or severe transference reaction in outpatient psychotherapy. Diagnostic uncertainty as to whether the patient has a concomitant affective or psychotic disorder would also be an indication for hospitalization.

The following hospital treatment guidelines are based on an understanding of the vicissitudes of the borderline patient's early life and the vulnerabilities that grow out of this period. These guidelines have also been fashioned on the education anvil of empirical experience and treatment failures.[60–63]

Preadmission Contact

As a general rule, it is advisable for the Unit's Admitting Officer (often a physician) and a member of the Unit Staff (often a nurse) to meet and develop a treatment plan with the borderline patient prior to admission. From the start, doctor and nurse, admissions officer, and ward staff present themselves to the patient in a unified manner. The *splitting and distortion* that tend to occur if the patient meets one clinician for admission evaluation and another upon arrival on the Unit are thereby minimized.

Furthermore, the preadmission meeting is designed to limit the borderline patient's defensive use of *primitive idealization*. The defensive use of primitive idealization creates, in the borderline patient, a mythic vision of the hospital and its staff as an all good, an all caring, and an all correcting experience. Unless primitive idealization is identified and defused from the start, the patient is likely to experience a major disappointment, with regression and probable acting out soon after admission.

At the preadmission meeting the following issues may be negotiated with the patient.

Goals for Hospitalization

Typically, borderline patients present with diffuse or global goals for hospitalization which, of course, can never be achieved. Discrete goals set during the preadmission meeting help prevent an interminable and directionless hospitalization.

Examples of hospital goals include the extinction of life-threatening suicidal or homicidal ideation; evaluation for and commencement of individual, outpatient psychotherapy; evaluation and treatment of transient, psychotic states or persistent, depressive symptomatology; evaluation for alternate living arrangements, including a halfway house or a new home; and consultation with a patient and ther-

apist who are experiencing a prolonged outpatient therapeutic impasse or a crisis in therapy.

Time Frame of Hospitalization

Borderline patients tend to regress in the hospital, especially after several weeks on a Unit. The preadmission meeting negotiates a time frame for hospitalization, generally *10–21 days,* within which the patient is expected to realize the goals of hospitalization. A time frame for hospitalization helps to preclude an experience of the hospital as timeless (like the unconscious). It also gives the patient a reasonable opportunity to achieve certain goals without encountering the dependency problems that an extended hospitalization fosters.

Behavioral Limits (Ward Rules)

The ward rules, which are basically behavioral limits, are explained to the patient in the preadmission meeting. A verbal contract is negotiated with the patient, in which he agrees to try to follow these rules. The sanctions for rule breaking (which include restriction of privileges, warning, transfer, and discharge) are mentioned to the patient, *emphasizing the need to maintain the patient's physical safety.* The ward rules should address the following.

1. **Violence toward the Self or Others.** Violence toward the self or others will not be condoned. Prior to admission, the patient must be able to form a *verbal contract* in which he agrees to verbally inform staff of, rather than act upon, any impulse to hurt himself or another. If the patient cannot form this verbal contract then admission to an open unit is generally not possible.

2. **Drugs.** The presence and/or use of nonprescribed drugs (legal or illegal) is strictly forbidden.

3. **Sexual Activity with Others.** Sexual activity with patients or visitors is not permitted.

4. **Ward Treatment Program.** In the preadmission meeting the nature of the Unit and the treatments it provides are explained to the patient. At this meeting the patient is asked to make a com-

mitment to hospital treatment. He is asked to agree to participate in the hospital treatment program of individual evaluation, group therapy, milieu therapy, medications when indicated, case conferences and consultations that relate to his care, and family meetings as indicated. It is often helpful to tell the patient that he is *entitled to* a full treatment program. The preadmission contact is designed to inform the patient of the nature of the treatment he will be receiving and to enlist his participation in the care he deserves.

The preadmission meeting and treatment plan can do more than minimize defensive splitting, primitive idealization, regression, and acting out. It is also an opportunity for *alliance building* with a borderline patient. The meeting is an opportunity to ally with the healthy part of the patient's ego and to create a sense of hopeful expectation. When regressions occur, as they almost inevitably do, the working alliance can then be resurrected around the preadmission plan with its goals, time frame, and agreement about permissible and nonpermissible behaviors on the Unit.

Frequently, *family work* will be integral to the patient's recompensation. In some cases the families of borderline patients will only agree to evaluation when there is a crisis. Insisting on family participation prior to admission while the crisis is alive may, in some cases, be the only time to effectively establish family participation in the patient's hospital treatment.

Psychopharmacological Management

Managing a Drug Withdrawal State

Drug abuse and drug addiction are not uncommon in borderline patients. CNS sedatives (alcohol and hypnotics) and tranquilizers are the common drugs of abuse that can produce withdrawal states. If the history, as obtained from the patient, friends, or family, is positive for drug abuse, *or* if the patient shows signs and symptoms of a withdrawal state, the clinician must establish a treatment protocol for withdrawal. The reader is referred elsewhere for the diagnosis and

treatment of alcohol, barbiturate, and hypnotic withdrawal states.[64, 65]

Antianxiety Agents

Borderline patients frequently present with marked anxiety. As a general rule, it is prudent to try to treat these patients without the use of antianxiety agents. Antianxiety agents have abusive potential which is increased by the borderline patient's addictive proclivity.

Tricyclic Antidepressants

Tricyclic antidepressants (TCA's) may be used adjunctively in a borderline patient who shows criteria for a depressive episode that has lasted for at least several weeks (see Chapter 1). Though distinct depressive episodes with a constellation of neurovegetative signs that last for several weeks are possible in borderline patients, what the clinician generally encounters is the mood lability of the borderline patient. Tricyclic antidepressants have a role in the treatment of depressive disorders and are highly effective in the management of the neurovegetative target symptoms of depression. Tricyclic antidepressants generally are not helpful in the management of characterological mood lability.[17]

Neuroleptic Medications

Borderline patients who experience episodic psychotic states; who evidence affective lability with a prominence of anger, anxiety, and/or depression; or who have a history of self-destructive behavior (including suicidal efforts, drug abuse, and sexual promiscuity) have been responsive to treatment with low dose, high potency neuroleptic medications.[66] High potency, rather than low potency, neuroleptics are preferable because they are not sedating, which appears to help considerably with compliance.

Trifluoperazine (Stelazine), fluphenazine (Prolixin), haloperidol (Haldol), and perphenazine (Trilafon) are the drugs of choice. *Titrating the correct dosage* appears to be a critical aspect of the effective neuroleptic treatment of these patients. *Small doses* of these *high potency* neuroleptics are all that are necessary. The patient may be started on 1 or 2 mg of any of these medications and built up to the range of 2–10 mg per day. The clinician should document a dose-response curve in which diminution of symptomatology is measured against the dosage and adverse effects of the neuroleptic. Once the proper dose is established, the medication may be provided on a once daily dosage schedule.

Monoamine Oxidase Inhibitors

Klein and Davis have noted the value of monoamine oxidase inhibitors (MAOI) in patients they regard as having "hysteroid dysphoria."[17, 67] These patients are characterized by repeated dysphoric states, rejection sensitivity, impulse dyscontrol, and a tendency toward substance abuse. Phenelzine (Nardil) has been used effectively in these patients. Dosages of 45 mg or more per day appear to reduce their emotional lability and, consequently, the disordered impulsive behaviors that occur during dysphoric states. Prolonged maintenance treatment appears necessary since discontinuation of medication is reported to result in a recurrence of symptomatology.

Lithium Carbonate

Rifkin et al. have recommended the use of lithium in those patients they term "emotionally unstable character disorders."[18] Rifkin bases this recommendation on the hypothesis that this disorder is an affective illness characterized by depressive and hypomanic swings that last no longer than a few days at a time.

The clinical features of the "emotionally unstable character disorder" are found in some borderline patients. Lithium carbonate could, therefore, be considered as an alternate treatment for this disorder. However, as noted in Chapter 2, lithium must be used cautiously because of its possible long-term renal effects and because of the risk of serious toxicity and death from overdose.

Milieu Management

The milieu management of the borderline patient has two aspects: the patient and the unit staff. Any Unit which intends to regularly admit and treat borderline patients must attend to the treatment issues for the patient and provide ample and capable supervision and support for the staff.

The Patient

The essence of the milieu management of the hospitalized borderline patient is the capacity to ensure physical safety without compromising empathy.

The physical *safety* of the patient and of other patients and staff on the ward must always be the *first priority* of the milieu. Clear, consistent, and firm limits that contain the patient's regression and aggression must be established. All milieu decisions are then organized on the basis of these limits, which are derived from a fundamental *concern* for the patient's safety and well-being. It is this concern that allows for continuous *empathy,* which is integral to allying with the borderline patient and without which the healing process cannot occur. Empathy is not permissiveness. Empathy is the capacity of a person or group to experience and resonate with the affective state of another. It is an identification with another person without a loss of boundaries. It is the gift and the cultivated skill of an accomplished psychotherapist.[68, 69]

Abroms,[70] has prioritized the setting of limits. The milieu priorities he recommends apply particularly to borderline patients, though they have applicability to all patient types. They are as follows:
1. Destructive behavior
2. Disorganized behavior
3. Deviant behavior—rule breaking behavior or acting out
4. Withdrawn behavior
5. Dependent behavior

The following *procedural guidelines* allow for effective limit setting and make the process understandable to patients[71]:
1. Set few limits
2. Clearly define limits
3. The limits explained to the patient should not differ from the limits written in the order book
4. Limits should be realistic
5. Enforce limits promptly—failure to enforce limits promptly condones the pathological behavior and promotes further acting out
6. Give sound reasons for limits

The borderline patient will probably test the limits that the staff establish. It is important to recognize that this early *limit testing* represents the patient's effort to discover *whether the staff care enough to contain him* and *whether the staff has the capacity to do so.* Typically, limit testing occurs at a time when the patient is experiencing stress. It is also essential for the therapist and staff to be aware of the nature of the patient's distress and developmental vulnerabilities in order to maintain an empathic stance while firmly setting needed limits.

It is generally a mistake to wait for large infractions of the ward rules before responding. An *early response* to rule infractions allows for working with the patient while an alliance may still be present. Early intervention may also preclude further escalation of the pathological behavior. If a patient breaks a ward rule, immediate limit setting can be done by the available staff on the unit. Members of the staff, particularly those assigned to the patient, may then make time to meet to *review the incident.* The patient's history, the acuteness or chronicity of the behavior, the presence or absence of psychosis, the psychodynamics of the act, the gravity of the act, and the degree of therapeutic alliance must all be reviewed. On the basis of this review, an individually oriented treatment plan can be made.

The treatment plan that is developed must aim to contain the patient's pathology in a nonpunitive manner while maximally facilitating the patient's return to the tasks and goals of hospitalization. Often, ward restriction and observation may be adequate to accomplish these ends. At times, the judicious use of medication may enable the patient to control unbearable affects and impulses and, thereby, permit the patient to remain in treatment. On occasion, the need to provide safety for the patient and for those about him may demand that restraint or seclusion be ordered. Frequently, patients will later report that the firm containment of their aggression was, despite their verbal protestations, welcome.

Some patients will require transfer to a locked unit with its capacity to better manage destructive behavior. Time must be taken to help the patient understand why transfer has been decided upon and to inform the patient that once his violent impulses are under control he can be reevaluated for return to the open unit. Similarly, for some patients, a breach of ward rules will mark the end of their capacity to maintain a working treatment alliance. They would then be discharged, if considered safe to leave the hospital. The discharge process can be used therapeutically to help the patient understand what has happened and why.

Following the staff meeting that carefully examined the incident, a member of the staff can *meet with the patient to review the incident.* This meeting should enable the patient to understand the feelings that led to the behavior and to help the patient begin to organize alternate ways of managing his feeling state. The treatment plan that grew out of the staff meeting is also discussed with the patient at this time.

At times it will be important to *inform* a member of the *patient's family* of the incident. At other times it may be advisable to call the family in for a meeting, particularly if the family has played an instrumental role in the genesis of the rule-breaking behavior.

Some units have a readmission policy in which discharged patients are not allowed readmission for a specific period of time (e.g., 1 or 2 months). Alternatively, an evaluation of the circumstances surrounding discharge and the postdischarge course, rather than an established policy, may allow for greater fairness and better patient care. This evaluation would explore whether the work of the previous admission was completed and, if not, why not and who might bear responsibility (e.g., patient, family, staff). Why the posthospital regression occurred would also be considered in order to answer whether the unit can be helpful. Finally, questions surrounding whether the patient could be better managed by outpatient or partial hospital care would also be addressed. Through the mechanism of an evaluation for readmission the door can be left open for the patient (and outpatient therapist) thereby allowing for clinically appropriate readmission whenever this becomes necessary.[72, 73]

Managing Suicidality‡

The unlocked, voluntary psychiatric unit repeatedly confronts the problem of how to manage emergent suicidal ideas and impulses in hospitalized borderline patients. The gravity of this problem and its recurrent and time-consuming nature require special milieu attention.

The milieu management of suicidality begins with the critical *separation of idea from action.* From the beginning of hospitalization the patient is helped to understand that the unit staff accept and welcome the patient's talking about those feelings and ideas that disturb him and threaten his well-being. Simultaneously, the staff inform the patient that suicidal behavior cannot be tolerated. If the patient can come to staff to express and begin to understand his suicidal ideation, then the patient can be safely treated in an unlocked unit. If, however, the patient cannot behaviorally contain his self-destructive impulses (e.g., if the patient continues to burn himself with a cigarette) then the first priority of the milieu, namely, patient safety, cannot be met. The patient then requires transfer to a locked unit, where behavioral containment can be provided.

A further distinction that merits attention is that between *idea and threat.* A suicidal idea (or impulse) can be responded to by staff through a variety of psychotherapeutic, milieu, and pharmacological interventions, if the patient knows this idea will not be acted upon. If, however, the patient cannot state unequivocally that he can control his impulses, then staff experience this patient as a suicidal threat. As long as staff must attend to the threat of suicidal behavior they are subject to manipulation by the patient. Furthermore, their energies are marshalled around security measures which render the staff unable to attend to helping the patient understand and tolerate his grief and his pain. For these reasons, patients who become suicidal threats also require

transfer to a locked unit. Once suicidal activity or threat has abated, the patient can be evaluated for return to the unlocked unit.

With this foundation established, and idea distinguished from action and threat, the milieu can be highly effective in attenuating a patient's distress and consequent suicidal ideation. Psychoactive medications may play an important role, as discussed earlier in this chapter. Refuge within the shelter and support of a ward community, away from the stresses that had overwhelmed the patient, can also be palliative.

Further milieu management considerations are dependent on a thorough understanding of the patient's motives and his environmental reinforcers for suicidality.[74, 75] The wish to murder the self or another (carried out through the self), escape from pain, and reunion fantasies with a lost love object are common motives for suicide (see Chapter 1). Suicidality that empowers the patient, that enables him to transform his experience of himself from helpless victim to powerful controller, is a common environmental reinforcer.

Finally, many patients with chronic suicidal ideation will hold on to these ideas, as we see psychotic patients hold onto their delusions. Unit staff will need to see that this attachment satisfies a basic comforting need and represents a psychologically adaptive act on the patient's part.

The Staff

The staff of an Inpatient Unit has the complex and demanding therapeutic task of providing the patient with continuing concern and emotional availability while at the same time withstanding his angry and devaluing onslaughts and labile and primitive affects. In addition, limits must be set and promptly, firmly, and consistently maintained.

As the staff devotes itself to this endeavor, the patient is engaged in a set of verbal tactics and defensive operations that invite staff to retaliate or withdraw.[26, 61, 62, 76, 77] The patient goes about the unit making invidious comparisons between staff members as he repeatedly shifts attachments and alliances: today's favored staff member is apt to become the target of tomorrow's hos-

---

‡We are indebted to Drs. G. Jacobson and J. T. Maltsberger for the ideas expressed in this section.

tility. Legitimate authority is repeatedly assaulted by statements that suggest that if the staff really cared about the patient they would not be so rigid about rules. Fair staff expectations of cooperation become special favors in which the patient considers himself to be doing something for the staff for which he should be especially rewarded.

Through the defensive process of splitting, some staff members are idealized while others are seen as cruel and malevolent. Because of the borderline patient's sensitivity to minor frustration, those staff who are briefly idealized will soon become the focus of angry projections. The borderline's use of projective identification has him disown an aspect of himself and attribute it to a staff member, identify with it, and respond accordingly. Because these patients are particularly adept at sensing unconscious processes in those about them, their projections will frequently resonate with unconscious feelings in the staff. If, for example, the projected impulse is rage, as it often is, the completed process of projective identification has the patient responding with defensive fear, anger, or devaluation to staff rage which the patient evoked. If, for example, it is helplessness that is disowned, staff are apt to experience their own helplessness, in response to which the patient may respond with further anxiety and passivity.

The patient's defensive operations create the conditions for conflict among staff. Projected and split off good and bad affects and images can produce a subtle, elusive, and generally unconscious process among staff members. Because different staff may be viewed differently by the patient and come to feel differently about the patient, the potential for intrastaff strife is considerable. The same potential exists between the patient's therapist and the ward staff.

Furthermore, staff members are subject to personal and internal responses to the rage and helplessness that borderlines evoke. Highly capable therapists have reported the guilt, the intense personal doubt, the fears of criticism, and the masochistic submission that they and others have experienced in therapeutic work with borderline patients.[5, 78, 79]

A unit's staff needs encouragement by its supervisory group to understand and recognize the internal experiences and the group processes that borderline defenses generate in clinicians. In supervision, an agreement to examine staff feelings must be established and then consistently woven into the supervision. In staff meetings and case conferences, care must be taken not to ignore the day-to-day emotional life of the unit.[80, 81]

The capacity for staff to collaborate in this manner with each other and with supervisory personnel is based on *trust*. When trust is high and collaboration active, the staff has cohesion and zest. When trust breaks down, collaboration vanishes and demoralization pervades the unit. A demoralized staff finds work with patients enervating, and absenteeism and patient incidents tend to occur. The restoration of morale[82, 83] on a unit starts with trust. Staff must believe that they can safely talk about their emotional responses to patients as the first step in mastering them. Staff must also believe that the supervisory group values this process. In short, the unit's *supervisory group* is asked to work with staff in a manner that will serve as a *model* for the staff's approach to their patients. Active, empathic leadership becomes the basis for staff morale.

T. F. Main's [84] words support the clinician's and the patient's integrity in the difficult treatment process:

Sincerity by all about what can and what cannot be given *with good will* [italics ours] offers a basis for management that, however, leaves untouched the basic psychological problems, which need careful understanding, but it is the only way in which these patients can be provided with a reliable modicum of the *kind of love* [italics ours] they need, and without which their lives are worthless. More cannot be given or forced from others without disaster for all. . . .
It is important for such patients that those who are involved in their treatment and management be *sincere* with each other, in disagreement as well as agreement. . . .
Believing that sincerity in management is a *sine qua non* for the treatment of the patients I have described, I offer . . . one piece of advice. If at any time you are impelled to instruct others to be less hostile and more loving than they can truly be—*don't*!

Individual Psychotherapy

The psychiatric hospitalization of a borderline patient either occurs at a particular point in psychotherapy or offers the opportunity for therapy to begin. The hospital care of borderlines, which aims to contain and protect the patient from overwhelming affects and impulses and to understand why they are occurring at this time, must be distinguished from their psychotherapy. The hospital unit needs to see itself as providing evaluative and supportive backup to a patient and therapist who are engaged in a long-term, ongoing process. The hospital clinician will want to spend his meetings with the borderline patient gathering a history and providing an evaluation. A well-developed history should outline what is going on in the life of the patient and describe the people involved in the crisis or impasse. The understanding of the current difficulties is deepened by a thorough picture of the patient's family and by a formulation of what occurred early in his life that would render him vulnerable to his current difficulties. Finally, an assessment of previous and ongoing psychotherapy, if present, must be completed (see Psychotherapy Consultation).

Psychotherapy for the borderline naturally begins with such an evaluation. How psychotherapy should then proceed has been the subject of considerable debate, which has not resulted in a uniform or definitive psychotherapeutic treatment for the borderline patient. Treatment is, of course, based on a conviction about what heals. In this section, we will touch upon some of the major viewpoints about what heals and then discuss aspects of technique.

Winnicott[25] maintains that these patients are helped when they discover that their rage, no matter how intense or murderous, will not destroy the therapist. Adler,[26, 33, 61, 80] drawing upon Winnicott and other object relations theorists, emphasizes the healing power of a relationship with a caring and reasonable therapist who can tolerate the patient's rage and help him bear his grief and aloneness. Zetzel[85] has argued that it is stability, consistency, and realistic limitations with a therapist who does not present himself as inexhaustible or omnipotent that heals. Friedman[86] calls for an insight-oriented treatment based on a positive and realistic relationship with the therapist. He believes that regressions do not foster healing, and he stresses the use of limits and treatment interruptions whenever the ego is not able to observe and seek insight. Finally, Kernberg[59] states authoritatively:

What really strengthens the patient's ego is not the gratification of needs in the "here and now" that were denied in the "there and then" but a coming to terms with past frustrations and limitations in the context of an understanding of the pathological reactions, impulses, and defenses that were activated under those past traumatic circumstances and contributed importantly to the development and fixation of ego weakness.

Technically, in order for psychotherapeutic work to begin, the patient must experience the therapist as someone who is genuinely concerned and caring. The borderline patient's extremely limited capacity for a working alliance requires that this empathic presence be maintained and sustained at the limits of the therapist's capabilities and capacities.[87]

Within the empathic holding of the relationship with the therapist, the patient is gradually and gently expected to begin to explore his internal emotional life. Central to this exploration is the expectation that, with the therapist's help, the patient will contain his affects and impulses and begin to verbalize (rather than act upon) them. The therapist will need to assist the patient in learning to recognize when he is experiencing powerful internal feeling states and to differentiate the specific feelings involved. The patient can then start to lend words to these feelings. This commences a therapeutic process in which the patient understands his feelings as natural reactions to present and past experiences. Semrad[81] has outlined this process as "acknowledging, bearing, and putting into perspective."

From the opening moments of therapy, the therapist must remain keenly aware of the borderline patient's central belief that he will be abandoned by the therapist.

This belief is coupled with attendant feelings of panicky, desperate aloneness and rage and impulses for merger, destruction, and withdrawal. *Supervision* and professional *peer support* help the therapist to consistently maintain the essential therapeutic posture of accurate empathy and nonpunitive expectations that enables the patient to move beyond his fears and impulses. Supervision and peer support also help to minimize the therapist's countertransference reactions.

If the patient is to be *referred for psychotherapy* from the hospital, it is very important that the therapist and patient meet at least once, preferably more, prior to the patient's discharge. In all likelihood, the hospitalization occurred when the borderline patient felt bereft or alone. Discharge of this patient (who also lacks an inner sense of a comforting image of a supportive figure) to an unknown therapist stirs rageful fears of abandonment and creates a blank screen for primitive projections.

Recompensation from an acute borderline regression involves the reorganization, or coalescence, of the split ego in the presence of a constant and reliable object and setting.[21-25, 32, 58, 88-90] Crisis intervention, distance from an emotionally overwhelming relationship, containment of destructive impulses, limits, judicious use of medication, and the presence of supportive, durable professionals are all important elements in the recompensation.

To be supportive is not to be misunderstood as a call for the provision of unlimited support. Nor does it suggest license for all behavior or excessive sympathy. To be reliable, concerned, and empathic is different from being permissive and masochistically available. Gratification of past deprivations or replenishment of what has been exhausted in the self may be what these patients ask for but which, realistically, cannot be provided. Instead of the hospital attempting to provide a narcissistic nirvana, it can offer a reliable kind of care, with both limitations and gratifications, but truer to life in the real world.

With confidence in the likelihood of recompensation, the first order of business

for the clinician must be that of doing no harm. Indeed, however, this is exceedingly difficult, for these patients invite, through the process of projective identification, our most malicious or aversive responses. Inpatient staff providing psychotherapy to borderline patients appear vulnerable to a variety of treatment errors, errors which are often the product of countertransference difficulties. The technical errors discussed below will be recognized as technical errors that are products of countertransference difficulties.

Empathy

The suffering, isolation, and chaos so familiar to the borderline's experience, especially at the time of hospitalization, evoke in the therapist the special quality of emotional resonance called empathy.[91] Too much empathy expressed by the therapist induces an interpersonal intimacy that, though beneficial for some patients, is unbearable to the borderline patient. Clearly, this does not mean a heartless stance. Rather, we want to underline the danger of being vocally empathic with patients who are already fighting for affective modulation and interpersonal distance. Empathy can stimulate rapid, frighteningly intimate, and inevitably disappointing responses to so kindly and immediate an object as is the genuine and empathetic therapist. In other words, the therapist may feel genuinely and deeply moved by his patient, but must beware of saying so.

Transference

The borderline patient's proclivity toward intense and rapidly shifting transferences, often of psychotic proportions, and frequently beyond alliance and interpretation, makes cultivating the transference akin to wearing red in the bullring. For the therapist to be silent or to concentrate on the patient-therapist relationship during the acute phase of the patient's disorder fosters regression in the transference and its generally difficult-to-manage complications.

This position of eschewing a central focus on the therapist-patient dyad, and the transferences therein, is contrary to

Kernberg's position of the centrality of interpretation of the transference in the treatment technique he calls expressive psychotherapy (expressive therapy is differentiated from supportive therapy and traditional psychoanalysis).[92] Kernberg stresses that the transference, which is predominantly negative, should be systematically fostered and elaborated, beginning in the here-and-now, with genetic reconstruction occurring in the late phase of treatment. He states that interpretation is vital to integrating the split off parts of the internal world. This is, however, outpatient work, or extended inpatient work, which is different from short-term hospital treatment of regressed borderline patients which involves weeks, not months or years. In a short time frame, and on units with diverse clinical responsibilities, transference elaboration and interpretation is not the principal therapeutic mode. Instead, crisis intervention and psychological reconstitution within the container of a group and in the presence of reliable objects are the centerpieces of therapeutic healing.

Confrontation

Confrontation is an especially seductive therapeutic tack, for these patients quickly encourage us to surmise that no less a club than confrontation will soften their avoidant and irresponsible tendencies.[91-95] Short of confrontation of life-threatening impulses that are about to be acted upon, and which do not bow to everyday exploration, the technique of confrontation may do harm in a variety of ways. Especially provocative (and evocative of brewing transference feelings) is confrontation of the patient's rage.

Borderline patients are also well-known for their entitlement. Their expectation of special status and their, even if unsaid, readily observable stance of "Why haven't you done something for me lately?" are familiar. Confrontation of this ostensibly narcissistic position neglects an understanding that borderline patients cannot occupy a middle ground. To confront away overvaluation of the self is to leave the patient with its opposite, namely, devaluation of the self. Confrontation of entitlement may abruptly bring borderline patients into affective sight of their profound worthlessness and self-loathing. Stripping these patients of the thin, though entitled, robe of self-esteem in which they cloak themselves is to expose them to the potentially deadly bite of their most malevolent introjects. Even character work with higher order narcissistic personalities calls for a period of admiring and being admired, before allowing life's ironies, frustrations, and inevitable disappointments to foster character change.

Interpretation and Management

Interpretation is the psychotherapeutic technique of rendering the patient's unconscious conscious. Interpretation is accomplished by explaining to the patient the feelings, wishes, impulses, and conflict that exist out of awareness. The use of interpretations, especially the tendency of the therapist to be openly, that is vocally, intuitive, even if correct in his formulations, is yet another source of adverse consequence in working with borderline patients.

Case Example. A staff member informed a patient how his recent drug taking and fugue states were related to difficulties in the outpatient therapy. In fact, the staff member went on to say that these symptoms were an effort to run away from intense, even cannibalistic, longings for the therapist. On the unit, the patient became more passive and inactive; he reported he felt he could do very little without "checking it out with his therapist."

An interpretation offered in this manner is essentially therapeutic intolerance. The patient generally feels intruded upon, for the interpretation pre-empts the patient's willingness to reassess his position vis-à-vis himself and other people. When tempted to offer such bits of deft psychology, the therapist may be trying to soothe himself. Desperate behaviors and primitive feelings (like hate and destruction) on the part of our patients are a major test of skill and patience. At these times, one is vulnerable to a need to do something, to replace badness with goodness, hatred with brotherly love. It is indeed difficult to stand by and witness the savage and painful nature of some patients' lives. The power of the professional is challenged, for the force of their productions can be quite humbling. One can also feel tempted to compensate for the patient's early privations and try to give or replenish, in the form of words and understanding, what the patient did not receive in his early life. At such moments, interpretations are like sedatives, they quiet people down; they do not help to heal the wounds. They help the professional to feel potent at a time when he would otherwise feel the limits of his role.[95]

At times, management of a patient's activities, or lack of them, may serve the same purpose.

Case Example. A woman in her thirties was given a great deal of fine advice about how to plan vocationally and how to go about managing her home and finances. The more the staff said, the less she did. Before long, many staff were angry with her for not following through on all that they had said.

Therapeutic maneuvers, be they interpretation of unconscious processes, as with the first patient, or management of everyday life, as with the second, may neglect the patient in two ways. First, in soothing his distress with the patient's ailments and his relative impotence, the therapist fails to provide the patient with an opportunity to speak, without demand for change, about that which is most hateful and grievous in him. No one else is likely to provide this form of inquiry, which is so essential to healing the split ego. Second, when the therapist behaves with omniscience and omnipotence he invites magical fantasies on the part of his patients. Autonomy and initiative on the patient's part, through the struggle of trial, effort, and eventual mastery, are too easily curtailed by the "too-good, too able" therapist.

Pain

One infrequently challenged therapeutic assumption is that patients seek to be disentangled from their pain. Working by this assumption would have us encourage, cajole, and otherwise influence borderline patients to rid their lives of the pain begotten by their bodies, their environment, or their families and friends. Pain may be, however, a very particular experience for borderline patients whose early life and object experiences were not of the pleasurable sort that allows normal development to consolidate around trust and love.[96-98]

For borderline patients, early life was inconsistent and painful. For some, pain becomes a symbolic affect that represents the nature of (and perpetuation of) the relationship with mother. For these patients the attachment to pain is equivalent to their continued attachment to the primary object, namely, mother. Attachment to and identification with pain, pain as mother, is a far cry better than a barren inner world, devoid of human representation. For these patients, pain as the bad mother is better than no mother at all.

The inpatient therapist will find these patients exceedingly difficult, for their painful behaviors will not readily bend in the course of a short-term hospitalization. In the long run, the outpatient therapist faced with a patient who demonstrates this attachment to pain must early on settle into an interpretive, rather than a management, mode. Short of life-threatening behavior, painful behaviors and attachments cannot be managed away by containment or strict limits. The outpatient therapist must relentlessly pursue the meaning of the patient's agonized endeavors, without expecting to rid the patient of them. Over time the patient may gain some perspective and even obtain some measure of self-interest. Pleasure in relationships and work may, however, forever elude such a patient.

Psychotherapy Consultation

Many borderline patients are admitted to the Inpatient Unit upon referral from their outpatient therapist. In these cases, the unit can serve the patient and therapist by providing a psychotherapy consultation as part of the clinical services offered. Bernstein[99] has written on this process, from which we draw many of the comments that follow.

Hospitalization of a borderline patient in ongoing outpatient therapy does *not* signal a failure of treatment. An effective psychotherapy may mobilize feelings and drives that render the patient at risk to himself or require that he have the emotionally sustaining environment of a hospital to contain and limit a precipitous regression. Difficulties in therapy may also occur. They may reside in the patient's limitations or in the therapist's countertransference or technical difficulties.

Effective consultation to the referring therapist is a delicate procedure, for the therapist is threatened with feeling exposed. The difficulties he is having or, worse, a failure on his part may become apparent. The therapist should be encouraged to continue his meetings during hospitalization in order to counter the patient's fear of abandonment and to allow for the consultation to explore the ongoing treatment process.

Consultation to the referring therapist is best done after the unit's treatment team has had an opportunity to fully evaluate and then review the individual patient, the family, and the environmental situation, the nature of the current crisis, and the ongoing psychotherapy. The availability of a senior consultant at a case conference will allow the staff to present its formulation and recommendations for critical review before presenting this material to the referring therapist.

Frequently, the dilution of transference and the containing power of the hospitalization will be adequate to resolve the crisis that prompted admission and allow outpatient care to resume. In these instances the unit has been supportive to the referring therapist and can encourage his ongoing treatment of a difficult patient. At other times, consultation may enable the therapist to deepen or redirect the therapy in a manner more beneficial to the patient. If countertransference issues are the impediment, these can be supportively explored with the therapist in order to permit him access to feelings that may have been out of his awareness. In some cases termination or transfer is indicated and can be managed while the patient has the benefit of the holding environment of the inpatient unit. Clearly, when consultation is offered, it is provided in a sensitive manner that recognizes the difficulties experienced in working with borderline patients.

Evaluation and Treatment of the Family

The family evaluation of the borderline patient should include, whenever possible, the patient's parents, significant members of his family, and people with whom he is currently living. As discussed earlier, the families of borderline patients show marked psychopathology in their individual members or in the family's functioning as a group. The evaluator will want to assess the family and its members, as well as try to understand the role that the patient plays in the unconscious life of his parents and in the current psychic equilibrium of the family.

In addition to examining the family members, the clinician must carefully examine the patient's immediate living environment. Frequently, these patients have been living with friends, intimates, or in some informal or professionally managed living situation, e.g., a commune or halfway house. The patient's interpersonal environment must be assessed for the presence of toxic relationships or the absence of adequate structure and support.

The family evaluation is an opportunity to establish an alliance with individual members of the family and with the family as a whole. The working alliance with the borderline patient is tenuous at best.[87] This alliance may be strengthened by an effective working alliance with the family. Furthermore, when the family is negatively disposed to the hospital and its treatment staff, the working alliance with the individual borderline patient is seriously jeopardized.

Clinical opinion varies on how and when to provide family therapy for the families of borderline patients.[29, 34–36, 60] Though there seems to be uniformity about involving families in treatment, particularly when the patient is an adolescent or is living with the family, disagreement centers on when to begin therapy and whether the family should be seen separately from or together with the individual patient.

As Gunderson et al.[40] have suggested, an answer to these differences may emerge from the family assessment. Families of borderlines seem to segregate out into two types. In the first type (described by Gunderson), there is a tight parental bond with exclusion and even neglect of the child. Family treatment is contraindicated from the outset with this family structure. Instead, the patient and parents are seen separately. This appears to limit unconscious parental anxiety about the child's intruding upon their dyadic relationship. Excessive angry projections are also diminished by separating the child and family treatments.

In the second family type (described by Zinner, Shapiro, and Masterson), the family and borderline child are deeply enmeshed. In this type, the child and parents are overinvolved with each other and show mutual and marked dependent trends. In this family, separation is a fundamental fear. The appropriate treatment for these enmeshed families is to meet with the parents and child together. Structuring therapy in this manner minimizes fears of premature separation and allows the family, as a group, to begin to disengage and begin a process of progressive autonomy.

Though the design for treatment may differ, both family treatments aim to help all the family members begin to work through the separation-individuation issues that were inadequately mastered. In addition, the therapist works to minimize the family's use of projective identification and splitting as well as to help them begin to understand that autonomy is different from hateful abandonment. Finally, the therapist can serve as a model for a "good enough mother" for either parent to begin to emulate.[22]

Contact with Other Professional Agencies

Frequently, the borderline patient has established contact with several human service agencies. Diffuse, split, and disorganized caregiving, perhaps not unlike the care he received in his family, adds to the patient's difficulties. When multiple agencies have been involved in the care of a borderline patient, it is advisable for the clinician to arrange a meeting of the different caregivers. Wishnie[62] has suggested that the purposes of this meeting include clarifying roles, disengaging unnecessary helpers, and promoting patient autonomy.

MEDICOLEGAL CONSIDERATIONS

The hospital treatment of borderline patients does not occur without regular consideration of the staff's professional responsibilities and their risks of liability. The borderline patient's use of projection and the disavowance of personal responsibility that accompanies this defense, as well as the impulsive and self-destructive behaviors that typify this syndrome, are the principal factors in creating medicolegal problems for these patients.

Borderline patients are especially difficult to approach medicolegally because their dynamic interactions with hospital staff, and with the legal system, are not as clearly recognized as pathological, as would be the case with schizophrenic and depressed patients.[100, 101] Patients feelings of entitlement can result in the conviction that the hospital is offering less than optimal care, or even negligence. Splitting may result in certain staff becoming devalued and depicted as agents of professional malfeasance. Finally, transferences of psychotic proportions can cast physician and nurses, in particular, as the source of maintenance of all the patient's difficulties.

Borderline dynamics of entitlement, splitting, and psychotic transference in themselves would not necessarily present medicolegal difficulties were it not for the essential treatment intervention of limit setting and the impulsive self-destructive behavior that these patients engage in when in their most desperate and regressed states. The importance of limits has been addressed clinically. From a medicolegal perspective, however, limits may be seen as punitive, arbitrary, or as a deprivation of right to treatment. Furthermore, when patients respond to limits with suicidal threats or behavior, the hospital and its staff may appear to be responsible for inducing problems, rather than seeking to remedy them. Discharge from a hospital, as a form of limit setting, is most problematic medicolegally when the patient continues to be at risk for suicide.

In all medicolegal dilemmas, as Gutheil has emphasized,[102, 103] the solution lies in a well-considered *treatment plan that is clinically, not legally, based.* Careful docu-

mentation of the patient's pathology and the thinking by which decisions for limits (including curtailment of privileges, transfer, or discharge) were developed is critical: in the mind of the court, if it is not documented it did not occur. Finally, *consultation* (evidence that the professional staff were concerned enough to review the case with peers or supervisor) should be sought and documented for complicated or worrisome patients.

COURSE AND PROGNOSIS

Poor prognosis for borderline patients appears related to the following clinical and historical parameters.[5]

1. Poor motivation for treatment
2. Severe limitations in the capacity to tolerate anxiety and to control impulses
3. A history of poor object relationships
4. Antisocial trends
5. An inability to experience concern, sadness, or guilt

Prognosis is also dependent on the capabilities of the psychotherapist. Psychotherapeutic work with the borderline patient requires highly refined empathic and technical skills. A highly skilled psychotherapist may be able to work effectively with a poor prognostic borderline; yet, a better prognostic borderline patient may not do well in the hands of an unskilled and unempathic therapist.

REFERENCES

1. American Psychiatric Association. *Diagnostic and Statistical Manual of Mental Disorders,* ed. 3, Washington, D.C., American Psychiatric Association, 1980.
2. Jacobson G: Personality disorders, in Lazare A (ed): *Outpatient Psychiatry, Diagnosis and Treatment,* Baltimore, Williams & Wilkins, 1979.
3. Kernberg OF: Borderline personality organization. J Am Psychoanal Assoc, *15:* 641–682, 1967.
4. Schmideberg M: The borderline patient, in Arieti S (ed): *American Handbook of Psychiatry,* vol. 1, pp. 398–416, New York, Basic Books, 1959.
5. Kernberg OF: *Borderline Conditions and Pathological Narcissism,* esp. pp. 111–152, New York, Jason Aronson, 1975.
6. Gunderson JG, Kolb JE: Discriminating features of borderline patients. Am J Psychiatry, *135:* 792–796, 1978.
7. Andrulonis PA, Glueck BC, et al.: Borderline personality subcategories. J Nerv Ment Dis, *170:* 670–679, 1982.
8. Andrulonis PA, Donnelly J, et al.: Preliminary data on ethosuximide and the episodic dyscontrol syndrome. Am J Psychiatry, *137:* 1455–1456, 1981.
9. Andrulonis PA, Glueck BC, et al.: Organic brain dysfunctions and the borderline syndrome. Psychiatr Clin North Am, *4:* 47–66, 1981.
10. Akiskal HS, Rosenthal TL, et al.: Characterological depressions: Clinical and sleep EEG findings separating "sub-affective dysthymias" from "character spectrum disorders." Arch Gen Psychiatry *37:* 777–783, 1980.
11. Stone MH: Contemporary shift of the borderline concept from a subschizophrenic disorder to a subaffective disorder. Psychiatr Clin North Am: 577–594, 1979.
12. McGlashan TH: The Borderline Syndrome: II. Is it a variant of schizophrenia or affective disorder? Arch Gen Psychiatry, *40:* 1319–1323, 1983.
13. Perry CJ: Depression in borderline personality disorder. Am J Psychiatry, *142:* 15–21, 1985.
14. McNamara E, Reynolds CF, et al.: EEG sleep evaluation of depression in borderline patients. Am J Psychiatry, *141:* 182–186, 1984.
15. Gunderson JG, Elliot GR: The interface between borderline personality disorder and affective disorder. Am J Psychiatry, *142:* 277–288, 1985.
16. Soloff PH, Millward JW: Psychiatric disorders in the families of borderline patients. Arch Gen Psychiatry, *40:* 37–44, 1983.
17. Klein DF, Davis JM, et al.: *Diagnosis and Drug Treatment of Psychiatric Disorders,* ed. 2, pp. 243–250, 440–441, Baltimore, Williams & Wilkins, 1980.
18. Rifkin A, et al.: Lithium carbonate in emotionally unstable character. Arch Gen Psychiatry, *27:* 519–523, 1972.
19. Meissner WW: *The Borderline Spectrum,* esp. pp. 301–331. New York, Jason Aronson, 1984.
20. Rochlin G: Personal communication.
21. Mahler MS: *On Human Symbiosis and the Vicissitudes of Individuation,* New York, International Universities Press, 1968.
22. Winnicott DW: The theory of the parent-infant relationship. Int J Psychoanal, *41,* 585–595, 1960.
23. Mahler MS, et al.: *The Psychological Birth of the Human Infant,* New York, Basic Books, 1975.
24. Winnicott DW: Ego distortion in terms of the true and false self, in *The Maturational Process and the Facilitating Environment,* New York, International Universities Press, 1965.
25. Winnicott DW: The use of an object. Int J Psychoanal, *41:* 585–594, 1969.
26. Adler G: Helplessness in the helpers. Br J Med Psychol, *45:* 315–326, 1972.
27. Modell AH: "The holding environment" and the therapeutic action of psychoanalysis. J Am Psychoanal Assoc, *24:* 285–307, 1976.

28. Mahler MS, et al.: The mother's reaction to her toddler's drive for individuation, in Anthony EJ, Benedek T (eds): *Parenthood,* Boston, Little Brown & Co., 1970.

29. Masterson JF: *Treatment of the Borderline Adolescent: A Developmental Approach,* New York, John Wiley & Sons, 1972.

30. Masterson JF: *Psychotherapy of the Borderline Adult: A Developmental Approach,* New York, Brunner/Mazel, 1976.

31. Masterson JF: The borderline adult: Therapeutic alliance and transference. Am J Psychiatry, *135:* 437–441, 1978.

32. Kernberg OF: *Object Relations Theory and Clinical Psychoanalysis,* New York, Jason Aronson, 1976.

33. Adler G, Buie DH: Aloneness and borderline psychopathology: The possible relevance of child development issues. Int J Psychoanal, *60:* 83–96, 1979.

34. Shapiro ER, Shapiro RL, et al.: The borderline ego and the working alliance: Indications for family and individual treatment in adolescence. Int J Psychoanal, *58:* 77–87, 1977.

35. Zinner J, Shapiro ER: Splitting in families of borderline adolescents. In Mack JE (ed): *Borderline States in Psychiatry,* New York, Grune & Stratton, 1975.

36. Shapiro ER, et al.: The influence of family experience on borderline personality development. Int Rev Psychoanal, *2:* 399–411, 1975.

37. Bion WR: *Experiences in Groups,* London, Tavistock Publications, 1961.

38. Rioch MJ: The work of Wilfred Bion on group, in Colman AD, Bexton WH (eds): *Group Relations Reader,* Sausalito, Calif., Grex Publishers, 1975.

39. Masterson JF, Rinsley DB: Borderline syndrome: The role of the mother in the genesis and psychic structure of the borderline personality. Int J Psychoanal, *56:* 163–177, 1975.

40. Gunderson JG, et al.: The families of borderlines: A comparative study. Arch Gen Psychiatry, *37:* 27–33, 1980.

41. Walsh F: Family study: 1976: 14 new borderline cases, in Grinker RR, Werble B (eds): *The Borderline Patient,* pp. 158–177, New York, Jason Aronson, 1977.

42. Feldman RB, Guttman HA: Families of borderline patients: Literal-minded parents, borderline parents, and parental protectiveness. Am J Psychiatry, *141:* 1392–1396, 1984.

43. Nemiah JC, Sifneos FE: Affect and fantasy in patients with psychomatic disorders, Hall DW (ed): in *Modern Trends in Psychosomatic Medicine,* London, Butterworths, 1970.

44. Lesser IM: A review of the alexithymia concept. Psychosom Med, *43:* 531–543, 1981.

45. Gunderson JG, Singer MT: Defining borderline patients: An overview. Am J Psychiatry, *132:* 1–10, 1975.

46. Perry JC, Klerman GL: The borderline patient: A comparative analysis of four sets of diagnostic criteria. Arch Gen Psychiatry, *35:* 141–150, 1978.

47. Perry JC, Klerman GL: Clinical features of the borderline personality disorder. Am J Psychiatry, *137:* 165–173, 1980.

48. Gunderson JG, Siever LJ, et al.: The search for a schizotype: Crossing the border again. Arch Gen Psychiatry, *40:* 15–22, 1983.

49. McGlashan TH: The borderline syndrome: Testing three diagnostic systems. Arch Gen Psychiatry, *40:* 1311–1318, 1983.

50. Zilboorg G: The problem of ambulatory schizophrenias. Am J Psychiatry, *113:* 519–525, 1956.

51. Shapiro D: *Neurotic Styles,* New York, Basic Books, 1965.

52. Spitzer RL, Endicott J, et al.: Crossing the border into borderline personality and borderline schizophrenia. Arch Gen Psychiatry, *36:* 17–24, 1979.

53. Adler G: The borderline-narcissistic personality disorder continuum. Am J Psychiatry, *138:* 46–50, 1981.

54. Kohut H, Wolf HS: The disorders of the self and their treatment: An outline. Int J Psychoanal, *59:* 413–425, 1978.

55. Kohut H: *The Restoration of the Self,* New York, International Universities Press, 1977.

56. Vaillant GE: *The Natural History of Alcoholism,* Cambridge, Mass., Harvard University Press, 1983.

57. Bean M: Clinical implications of models for recovery from alcoholism, in Shaffer H (ed): *The Addictive Behaviors,* New York, Haworth Press, 1984.

58. Kernberg O: A psychoanalytic classification of character pathology. J Am Psychoanal Assoc, *18:* 800–822, 1970.

59. Kernberg O: Technical considerations in the treatment of borderline personality organization. J Am Psychoanal Assoc, *24:* 795–829, 1976.

60. Friedman HJ: Some problems of inpatient management with borderline patients. Am J Psychiatry, *126:* 299–304, 1969.

61. Adler G: Hospital treatment of borderline patients. Am J Psychiatry, *130:* 32–36, 1973.

62. Wishnie HA: Inpatient therapy with borderline patients, in Mack, JE (ed): *Borderline States in Psychiatry,* pp. 41–62. New York, Grune & Stratton, 1975.

63. Sadavoy J, et al.: Negative responses of the borderline to inpatient treatment. Am J Psychothe, *33:* 404lc4–417, 1979.

64. Hackett TP: Alcoholism: Acute and chronic states. In Hackett TP, Cassem NH (eds): *MGH Handbook of General Hospital Psychiatry,* pp. 15–28, C.V. Mosby, St. Louis, 1978.

65. Renner JA: Drug addiction, in Hackett TP, Cassem NH (eds): *MGH Handbook of General Hospital Psychiatry,* pp. 29–40, C.V. Mosby, St. Louis, 1978.

66. Brinkley JR, et al.: Low-dose neuroleptic regimens in the treatment of borderline patients. Arch Gen Psychiatry, *36:* 319–326, 1979.

67. Spitzer RL, Williams JBW: Hysteroid dysphoria: An unsuccessful attempt to demonstrate its syndromal validity. Am J Psych *139:* 1286–91, 1982.

68. Rogers CR: The necessary and sufficient con-

ditions of therapeutic personality change. J Consult Psychol, *21:* 95–103, 1957.

69. Truax CB, Carkhuff RR: *Toward Effective Counselling and Psychotherapy: Training and Practice,* Chicago, Aldine Publishing Co., 1962.

70. Abroms GM: Setting limits. Arch Gen Psychiatry, *19:* 113–119, 1968.

71. MacDonald DM: Acting out. Arch Gen Psychiatry, *13:* 439–443, 1965.

72. Henisz JE: *Psychotherapeutic Management on the Short Term Unit,* pp. 122–130, Springfield, Ill., Charles C Thomas, 1981.

73. Pirdis MJ, Soverow GJ, et al.: Day hospital treatment of borderline patients: A clinical perspective. Am J Psychiatry, *135:* 594–596, 1978.

74. Buie DH, Maltsberger JT: *The Practical Formulation of Suicide Risk.* Cambridge, Mass., Firefly Press, 1983.

75. Havens LL: Anatomy of a suicide. N Engl J Med, *272:* 401–1c4406, 1964.

76. Pollack IW, Battle WC: Studies of the special patient: The sentence. Arch Gen Psychiatry, *9:* 56–62, 1963.

77. Groves JE: Taking care of the hateful patient. N Engl J Med, *298:* 883–887, 1978.

78. Maltsberger JT, Buie DH: Countertransference hate in the treatment of suicidal patients. Arch Gen Psychiatry, *30:* 625–633, 1974.

79. Winnicott DW: Hate in the countertransference. Int J Psychoanal, *30:* 69–74, 1949.

80. Adler G: Hospital management of borderline patients and its relation to psychotherapy, in Harticollis P (ed): *Borderline Personality Disorders: The Concept, The Syndrome, The Patient,* New York, International Universities Press, 1977.

81. Semrad EV: *Teaching Psychotherapy of Psychotic Patients,* New York, Grune & Stratton, 1969.

82. Sederer LI: Morale therapy and the problem of morale. Am J Psychiatry, *134:* 267–272, 1977.

83. Weisman A: Morale and the human condition. Unpublished manuscript. Presented at Hunter College, New York, March 28, 1977.

84. Main TF: The ailment. Br J Med Psychol, *30:* 144–145,1957.

85. Zetzel ER: A developmental approach to the borderline patient. Am J Psychiatry, *127:* 867–871, 1971.

86. Friedman HJ: Psychotherapy of borderline patients: The influence of theory on technique. Am J Psychiatry, *132:* 1048–1052, 1975.

87. Adler G: The myth of the alliance with borderline patients. Am J Psychiatry, *136:* 642–645, 1979.

88. Gedo JE, Goldberg A: *Models of the Mind,* Chicago, University of Chicago Press, 1973, esp. pp. 153–168.

89. Buie D, Adler G: The definitive treatment of the borderline patient, Int J Psychoanal Psychother *9:* 51–87, 1982.

90. Ogden TH: On projective identification. Int J Psychoanal *60:* 357–373, 1979.

91. Havens L: Explorations in the uses of language in psychotherapy: Counterprojective statements. Contemp Psychoanal, *16:* 53–67, 1980.

92. Kernberg OF: *Severe Personality Disorders: Psychotherapeutic Strategies,* New Haven, Yale University Press, 1984.

93. Buie DH, Adler G: The uses of controntation with borderline patients. Int J Psychoanal Psychother *1*(3): 90–108, 1972.

94. Adler G, Buie DH: The misuses of controntation with borderline patients. Int J Psychoanal Psychother *1*(3): 110–120, 1972.

95. Adler G: Helplessness in the helpers. Br J Med Psychol, *45:* 315–326, 1972.

96. Valenstein AF: On attachment to painful feelings and the negative therapeutic reaction. Psychoanal Study Child *28:* 365–392, 1973.

97. Guntrip H: *Schizoid Phenomena, Object Relations and The Self,* New York, International Universities Press, 1969, esp. 310–365.

98. Herzog JM: *A Neonatal Intensive Care Syndrome: A Pain Complex Involving Neuroplasticity and Psychic Trauma,* New York, Basic Books, 1981, pp. 291–300.

99. Bernstein SB: Psychotherapy consultation in an inpatient setting. Hosp Community Psychiatry, *31:* 829–834, 1980.

100. Gutheil TG: Medicolegal pitfalls in the treatment of borderline patients. Am J Psychiatry, *142:* 9–14, 1985.

101. Gutheil TG, Appelbaum PS: *Clinical Handbook of Psychiatry and the Law,* New York, McGraw Hill, 1982.

102. Gutheil TG, Magraw R: Ambivalence, alliance and advocacy: Misunderstood dualities in psychiatry and law. Bull Am Acad Psychiatry Law, *12:* 51–58, 1984.

103. Gutheil TG: *Malpractice liability in suicide: Legal aspects of psychiatric practice. 1*(2): 1–4, 1984.

anorexia nervosa

Gordon Harper, M.D.

DEFINITION

Anorexia nervosa is a disorder of unknown etiology marked by self-imposed dieting, weight loss of at least 25% of body weight, disturbed perception of body or appetite, and amenorrhea (in females), with no known medical illness to account for the weight loss.

Associated features include[1]: other eating disorders [bulimia (see Diagnosis and Differential Diagnosis)], vomiting, obsessive food preparation for others, hoarding food, eating rituals (including crumbling); denial of illness and rejection of treatment; delayed psychosexual development; and compulsive behavior including handwashing.

The disorder was defined and the name "anorexia nervosa" coined by Gull in the 1870's. The large numbers seen today make it appear to be an illness of modern times (see Epidemiology). On the other hand, sporadic cases of what would today probably be called anorexia nervosa appear in earlier records, like the report written by Morton[2] in 1689.

DIAGNOSIS AND DIFFERENTIAL DIAGNOSIS

Diagnosis

The Diagnostic and Statistical Manual of Mental Disorders (Third Edition) (DSM-III)[1] provides the following diagnostic criteria for Anorexia Nervosa*:

---

*The omission of anorexia from the DSM-III criteria reflects the recognition that "anorexia nervosa" is a misnomer. Many patients demonstrate an increased, but vigorously resisted appetite.

A. Intense fear of becoming obese, which does not diminish as weight loss progresses.

B. Disturbance of body image, e.g., claiming to "feel fat" even when emaciated.

C. Weight loss of at least 25% of original body weight, or, if under 18 years of age, weight loss from original body weight plus projected weight gain expected from growth charts may be combined to make 25%.

D. Refusal to maintain body weight over a minimal weight for age and height.

E. No known physical illness that would account for the weight loss.

Feighner et al.[3] offer the following diagnostic criteria for research purposes (A through E are required):

A. Age of onset prior to 25.

B. Anorexia with accompanying weight loss of at least 25% of original body weight.

C. Distorted, implacable attitude towards eating, food, or weight.

D. No known medical illness to account for anorexia and weight loss.

E. No other known psychiatric disorder.

F. At least two of the following:
amenorrhea
lanugo
bradycardia ($P < 60$)
periods of overactivity
episodes of bulimia
vomiting.

At Children's Hospital in Boston, Rollins and Piazza[4] found that the following psychopathology more precisely described their patients:

A. A weight phobia and/or distorted body image at any time
B. A pervasive sense of inadequacy.

One of the following physical criteria:

A. Self-induced starvation of 20% or more of body weight
B. Weight loss to 20% or more below expected weight for height or age.

Rollins' and Piazza's work has particular clinical relevance because patients who have lost less than 25% body weight but who otherwise show the characteristic features of the disorder are effectively treated if managed as if they had anorexia nervosa, even if they do not meet DSM-III or research criteria.

The patient's apparent *intent* to lose weight, or to maintain emaciation, and refusal to gain weight or maintain a normal weight are important clinical signs. Yet these matters defy simple definition. Volition and self-determination are very complicated matters in these patients. Some patients vigorously deny any intent to lose weight and appear to be dissembling (lying). What appears to be dissembling may be described more accurately as confusion as to the nature of wishes and intent and possibly about personal boundaries as well. In some of these patients, outspoken willfullness may represent an attempt to experience as volitional those behaviors which are beyond conscious control (pseudovolitionalization).

The relationship of vomiting disorders to anorexia nervosa is unclear. Vomiting, almost always covert, and sometimes to the point of dehydration or hypokalemia, develops in as many as 50% of patients with anorexia nervosa, especially in those with more chronic course. There is also a large group of patients with *bulimia,* a chronic vomiting disorder usually associated with bingeing, in which weight is maintained in the normal range, with or without evidence of metabolic compromise. Opinion differs as to whether bulimia and anorexia nervosa are more usefully considered as aspects of the same disorder or as separate disorders.[5-7] Presence of vomiting, especially vomiting as part of a daily routine, worsens prognosis in anorexia nervosa. On the other hand, vomiting and other aberrant eating behaviors occur in large numbers of women of normal weight who are not patients and who are functioning well socially, in the general population.[8]

Schwabe et al.[9] have argued that the etiological and clinical heterogeneity of patients with anorexia nervosa is so great as to justify a concept of *anorexia nervosa spectrum disorders,* implying a variety of subgroups and mechanisms. This would be analogous to the schizophrenia spectrum disorders (see Chapter 3).

For three decades, the late psychiatrist Hilde Bruch[10-12] was a leading figure in the study and treatment of anorexia nervosa. She described impaired *ego development* in anorectic patients. Perceptual and cognitive function, the experience of the self as authentic, and a personal sense of effectiveness are all affected. Her work, hypothesizing the origin of this disorder in defects in mirroring relationships in early life, clearly has connections to that, earlier, of Winnicott[13] and later, of Kohut.[14] Bruch introduced the terms *primary anorexia nervosa* and *atypical anorexia nervosa.* The latter refers to patients in whom the refusal to eat and weight loss are not due to the particular psychological finding that Bruch has described as a relentless pursuit of thinness. This nosology has been difficult to validate and has been discarded in favor of considering primary anorexia nervosa as that disorder *not* associated with any other psychiatric disorder (e.g., schizophrenia or depression). Secondary anorexia nervosa is diagnosed in patients with a primary psychiatric disorder who also evidence anorexia nervosa.

A careful diagnostic examination must be performed because diagnosis may be missed due to denial of the problem by parents and patient, even when emaciation is severe; by the extraordinary lengths to which patients will go to conceal the degree of weight they have lost (e.g., wearing bulky or loosefitting clothes, concealing weights on their bodies, or gorging on water just before weighing); and by the degree to which parents also conceal their preoccupations with body and appetite.

DIFFERENTIAL DIAGNOSIS

Medical Disorders

1. Brain tumor, especially tumors of the hypothalamus or third ventricle
2. Inflammatory bowel disease
3. Hyperthyroidism
4. Panhypopituitarism (Simmond's disease)

None of those patients with these medical disorders show the intense fear of becoming obese seen in anorexia nervosa. They accurately perceive the degree of malnutrition they suffer. If they vomit, they usually do so openly. Finally, they usually willingly seek treatment.

Psychiatric Disorders

1. Schizophrenia. Patients with schizophrenia show generalized impairment of thinking rather than the specific delusion related to body image and eating seen in anorexia nervosa.
2. Depression. Patients with depression are not determined to lose weight, even if they do lose weight because of lack of appetite or because of a specific depressive delusion.
3. Somatization disorder. Patients with somatization disorder may lose weight but may have other physical symptoms which patients with anorexia nervosa do not.
4. Bulimia. Patients with bulimia do not lose weight.

EPIDEMIOLOGY

The epidemiological study of anorexia nervosa has been difficult. Patient and family concealment and denial keep many patients from medical attention. Furthermore, because most studies are hospital-based, even though many patients are never hospitalized, incidence and prevalence figures probably are not representative of the total population.

Anorexia nervosa begins most frequently between the ages of 13 and 20. Latency and adulthood cases are, however, not uncommon. Patients are predominantly females, with males comprising only 4–10% in large series. Incidence estimates range from 0.24 to 1.6 new cases per hundred thousand population per year.[15, 16] Prevalence may be much higher (up to 1%) in selected populations.[17] Upper socioeconomic classes are most affected. The disorder is rare in nonwhites and nearly unknown in blacks. Anorexia nervosa has been considered a disorder of affluence. It is rare in populations where food is scarce.

The relationship of anorexia nervosa to the affective disorders has been the subject of considerable study. Such a relationship has been suggested by the presence of many depressive and manic-like symptoms in anorexia nervosa patients (up to 50% of anorexia nervosa patients meet criteria for major depressive disorder), by the occurrence of depressive episodes in such patients, and because of reports of positive response to antidepressant agents in anorexia nervosa.[18] In addition, there are similarities between the endocrine abnormalities seen in anorexia nervosa and affective disorders, particularly in the relative underactivity of the hypothalamic-pituitary-thyroid and gonadal axes, and the apparent relative increase in activity of the hypothalamic-pituitary-adrenal cortical axes.[19] This relationship has been investigated most fruitfully to date by family history studies of the prevalence of affective disorder in relatives of anorexia nervosa patients and of controls.[20, 21] Winokur et al.[20] found primary affective disorder to occur in 22% of the relatives of anorexia nervosa patients with affective disorder and twice as often as in relatives of controls (10%). Twinship studies have been inconclusive.

Despite difficulties in estimating true incidence from the number of diagnosed cases, a practice obviously influenced by referral patterns and changing "fashions" in illnesses, it seems clear that incidence is increasing.[22] This secular change is one of the fascinating and unexplained aspects of the disorder, particularly since most of the etiological theories proposed as bases for treatment postulate causal factors whose frequency we would have no reason to believe would increase as dramatically as has the frequency of anorexia nervosa.[23] Secular changes in culture and society (for example, the "slimness culture" or the changing status of women) are implicated.[24] Perhaps there are as-yet-unknown toxic or infectious environmental factors. The concept of an anorexia nervosa-spectrum disorder has bearing here as the final common pathway that expresses changes in multiple systems occurring to different degrees in different individuals.

THEORIES OF ETIOLOGY

Biological Hypotheses

Historical

Although anorexia nervosa since its definition in the 1870's has been regarded as a psychological disorder, interest in finding organic etiologies for a disease with such striking physical findings has never been absent. In fact, from the first description of pituitary cachexia in 1914 to its differentiation from anorexia nervosa in the 1930's, anorexia nervosa was regarded as an endocrine deficiency disease. This view is no longer held.

Contemporary

There are three areas of interest in the biological basis for anorexia nervosa: (1) predisposing physical factors; (2) psychophysiological effects, especially those affecting the hypothalamus and anterior pituitary; and (3) the physiological effects of starvation and their reversibility with refeeding.

1. Possible Predisposing Factors. Older parental age, genetic predisposition, occult hypothalamic dysfunction, and neurotransmitter dysfunction have all been proposed, though none have been substantiated.[22] One-third of patients are mildly overweight premorbidly. Most patients with anorexia nervosa have been perfectionistic overachievers.[25] The predominance of females is unexplained.

2. Psychophysiological Effects In attempts to separate the effects of starvation from possible primary psychological effects, amenorrhea has been of particular interest. It is well-established that amenorrhea may be of psychogenic origin.[26] In as many as one-third of cases of anorexia nervosa, menses stop prior to the onset of weight loss. The significance of such an event is that the amenorrhea is clearly not an effect of emaciation. This finding and the lack of evidence of a primary hypothalamic lesion, amid much evidence of hypothalamic dysfunction, stir hypotheses about possible direct cortical effects on the hypothalamus. These hypotheses must be regarded as occupying the level of speculation.[9]

3. Physiological Effects of Weight Loss. Mental alertness and normal or excessive physical activity are preserved in anorexia nervosa, despite weight loss. Though these patients selectively avoid calories, they preserve their intake of protein and vitamins.[27] Normal levels of protein, amino acids, and vitamins probably account for the mental brightness seen in anorexia nervosa, except terminally, which contrasts markedly with the mental torpor seen in victims of protein-calorie malnutrition. Anemia, when present, is generally less striking than the degree of emaciation would suggest. Susceptibility to infection is not increased, again in contrast to other forms of malnutrition. When present, potassium deficiency reflects emetic losses and renal compensation, rather than nutritional deficiency.

Other physiological functions are not preserved but return to normal when weight is regained. These include a lowered metabolic rate that is reflected by a lowered pulse and temperature, depressed thyroid function (especially marked by a low T_3), decreased production of somatomedin C, decreased bone marrow activity with leukopenia and a relative lymphocytosis, hypercholesterolemia and hypercarotenemia, and electrocardiographic changes (flattened T wave, ST segment depression, lengthened QT interval).[22]

The one physiological change that does not consistently return to normal with weight recovery is gonadotropin function and menses. Psychogenic factors may be involved, as noted earlier, but this has not been established. It is clear that the cause of gonadotropin insufficiency is not localized at the level of the anterior pituitary (the adequacy of which can be demonstrated with synthetic releasing factors). The hypothalamus or higher centers are therefore implicated.[28]

Psychodynamic (Developmental) Hypotheses

The first psychodynamic theories on anorexia nervosa were offered by Waller et al.[29] about 40 years ago. They postulated the disorder to be a defense against unconscious oral impregnation fantasies. Current theorists agree that this model is too simple, though they disagree about which model should replace it. Some emphasize an individually oriented psychopathological model, some a social learning model, some a family systems model, and all attempt, to some degree, to form an integrated model.

Bruch[10] emphasizes defects in ego development that are based on empathic failures in the mother-child relationship in the first 2 years of life. In her view, the child, lacking validation and mirroring of her own inner feelings and drives, fails to integrate these as her own and grows up living according to others' expectations. Bruch describes a child who has premorbidly papered over her inner deficiencies by adopting an overcompliant stance to the world. In doing so she fails to develop a sense of herself as a separate and autonomous person. Bruch postulates that this occult psychopathology existed before the onset of the anorexia. The clinical emergence of the syndrome reflects the breakdown of this adaptation under maturational pressures. As evidence, Bruch cites inaccurate body and appetite perceptions in patients with anorexia nervosa and their "paralyzing sense of ineffectiveness" which she feels to be at the core of this disorder.[11, 12]

Crisp,[27] without postulating the extent of early pathology cited by Bruch, offers a similar view of the adolescent with anorexia nervosa. His term "weight phobia" captures a sense of fleeing into this disorder in order to gain control of a rapidly approaching adolescent world. Deeply insecure with her emerging sexuality, which is represented in several ways by adolescent fullness, the adolescent develops a "weight phobia" and, in time, the clinical syndrome of anorexia nervosa.

Sours[30] differentiated two main subtypes in the group of patients with anorexia nervosa. One consists of early adolescents with relatively healthy previous development who, as in Crisp's model, flee phase-specific drive conflicts (fear of sexuality) by developing anorexia nervosa. This group, in keeping with relatively better early psychological development, carries a better prognosis. The other group develops anorexia nervosa in late adolescence or young adulthood. Its members are more typically like those described by Bruch, with pervasive ego defects. Male patients most often resemble this group.

Sours' emphasis on differentiating personality types *within* the anorexia nervosa population is important. Despite lip service paid to the idea of individual psychological assessment, the tradition of psychosomatic *specificity*,[31] that is, the assumption that there is a characteristic core conflict, if not a typical personality, associated with each psychosomatic disorder, is very strong in the anorexia nervosa literature. Surely there are striking similarities seen in the behavior of patients with this disorder, but there are several unanswered questions. Is this pattern a *universal,* or a *modal* pattern in patients with anorexia nervosa? To what extent is this pattern diagnostic of the premorbid personality, and to what extent is it "merely" a part of the psychobiology of the disorder itself? And, if the pattern described so often (including here) as if it were the *only* psychological and family profile in anorexia nervosa is in fact only the most frequent mode, what are the other modes? And what are the associated features and predisposing factors linked to each?

Family and Social Learning Hypotheses

Minuchin and his group[32] have proposed anorexia nervosa to be the paradigmatic psychosomatic disorder in which a *family dysfunction* is expressed by the symptomatic child. They find affected families to be *enmeshed* (family members are overinvolved in each other's lives) and *rigid* (their limited communications are stereotyped, inflexible, and maladaptive), and to *detour* conflict (especially between the parents) into struggles about the child's illness. Minuchin's system perspective locates the cause of the disorder in the family rather than in the patient. From this theoretical viewpoint, when clinicians diagnose and treat individual patients, they "scientifically" validate the family's pathological view that the problem is in the identified patient. Such practice threatens to provide an iatrogenic factor in the family's maintenance of the disorder.

Selvini Palazzoli's work[24] provides a sociocultural and historical dimension to the family assessment. Although based on clinical work with patients and families in northern Italy, her work integrates clinical and theoretical work by English language authors. Further, her work has been found useful by North American clinicians. She sees anorexia nervosa occurring in the daughters of traditional families (with patriarchal, collectivist, and self-sacrificial mores) who are caught in a transition to industrial society. In this society, opportunities beckon women. Those women whose personal and family resources cannot meet this call are vulnerable to anorexia nervosa. From another point of view, the anorexic patient may be seen as acting as the secret family rebel, challenging the inherited but obsolete mores.

THE BIOPSYCHOSOCIAL EVALUATION

The Biological Evaluation

The patient with anorexia nervosa is usually referred for inpatient care because of her compromised physical condition. The first tasks are to assess her degree of physical compromise and to rule out any possible organic factors.

The assessment of the degree of physical compromise has important psychotherapeutic as well as medical implications because of the critical role which autonomy and oral control struggles have come to play in the life of the patient. Most patients with anorexia nervosa expect those who care for them to try to control what they eat and weigh; their emaciation obviously invites the physician to fulfill medically this role long familiar at home. Long-term treatment outcome depends on the doctor's making an alliance with the patient's own wish to recover and grow and to make her own choices; the weight loss which "requires" coercive intervention therefore sets the stage for a relationship which can easily become regressive and antitherapeutic. Some experienced clinicians, in fact, while acknowledging to the outpatient that she has a potentially fatal disorder, deliberately disavow, at the outset of treatment, any aim, wish, or capacity to control the patient's weight, leaving this to the patient, while offering help in exploring the psychological circumstances which would bring a person to such a point.[33] Not all clinicians share this perspective by any means. Because this aspect of the relationship is so predictably loaded from the beginning, however, the physician needs knowledge of this regressive aspect of the healing relationship, very clear information about the patient's actual physical status, and a clear sense of how he will manage the patient and the patient's body.

History

It is essential that separate histories be taken from the patient and the family. We can expect that the patient will distort and conceal and that the family's reaction to the patient's illness is itself an important subject to assess. Distortions by the patient should not be taken as a moral failing, but as a key clinical sign, influenced by the patient's distorted perception of her body size, her eating and vomiting habits, and her very limited and guarded ability to entrust these aspects of her experience to a new doctor.

The history should quickly locate where the patient is in *the course of her illness*. Is this a first major weight loss with prior good health or is it a chronic eating disorder?

Similarly, the patient's *growth and maturation* must be assessed. Puberty and physical growth are both important. The importance of the growth history cannot be overemphasized. In plotting the patient's weight and height over her entire life on a standard growth curve, one obtains (1) a basis for comparison of the patient's present weight to her premorbid weight which, extrapolated, can be taken as "normal" for her, and (2) an indication whether linear growth (which stops whenever significant weight loss exists for more than a few months) ceased *before* significant weight loss. If linear growth stopped before significant weight loss, a primary organic disorder (pituitary or other brain tumor, or chronic inflammatory disease) is quite likely.

A history of *affective* disorder in first and second degree relatives and of depressive symptoms in the patient must be sought.

The *history of the present illness* should include the date and circumstances of the onset of weight loss; the patient's ideation since that time about body size, desired weight, and means used to lose weight (dieting, purging); the subsequent course of her weight; the occurrence or cessation of menses; and a complete inventory of prior treatments and interventions attempted by the family and by the patient.

A *dietary history* is particularly important. Unusual food preferences, such as vegetarian or macrobiotic diets or diets composed of only one or two foods, are common and should be explored. The clinician needs to be concerned with both the dietary extremes to which the patient's psychopathology has driven her and with the possibility of malnutrition. An *eating history* is important and should examine the *context* of eating, e.g., some patients eat only in isolation while others have complicated eating and purging rituals.

The clinician should always inquire about vomiting, laxative abuse, and exercising, even though it may be very difficult for the patient to be an accurate observer, let alone a reporter, of these parts of her life.

The *review of systems* should look specifically for sequelae of malnutrition and/or vomiting: fatigue, lightheadedness, dental erosion (from vomited gastric acid); poor wound healing or frequent infections; abdominal pain or constipation; change in quality of skin; and numbness, paresthesias, or other signs of peripheral neuropathy.

Physical Examination

Height and weight quantify the emaciation and, as noted, should be plotted on standard growth charts. Weighing the patient requires particular attention: weighing should be done at the same time each day (e.g., after the first morning voiding) and in standard dress (preferably in hospital gown), and careful attention should be paid to the likelihood that the patient will conceal objects on her body to increase her weight. Vital signs include pulse, blood pressure, respiration and, especially, temperature. Quality of skin, including yellowish color and presence of lanugo (soft, downy body hair), muscle wasting, presence of edema, and integrity of dentition and mucus membranes should all be noted. Any signs of congestive heart failure should be noted. Thyroid and abdomen should be carefully palpated. Degree of sexual maturation should be assessed. In the extremities, adequacy of circulation should be assessed by warmth and color. The neurological examination should include special attention to any signs of peripheral neuropathy and to cranial nerves and visual fields.

Laboratory Studies

Regular Studies. Complete blood cell count (CBC), urinalysis, serologic test for syphilis, BUN, electrolytes, blood sugar, thyroxine (T_4), triiodothyronine (T_3), total protein and albumin, B_{12}, and folate. Potassium deficiency is the best measure of the severity of occult vomiting and is screened and followed via serum electrolytes; electrocardiography may be used to confirm the physiological significance of low serum potassium, which may change faster than intracellular levels. An H_2 breath test will put to rest concerns about lactose intolerance.

Special Studies. If abdominal signs or symptoms are present, a gastroenterology consultation and possible contrast studies may be indicated. For any patient with an atypical growth history or with CNS signs, skull films, EEG, computerized tomography, and neurological consultation are indicated.

The Psychodynamic Evaluation

The psychological assessment of the patient must proceed from the beginning of hospital treatment, despite the temptation to focus on dilemmas about administration (privileges, need for bed rest), relations with family (especially regarding family ambivalence about participation in therapy), and somatic therapy (weight, content and route of refeeding, weight goal).

The Place of Anorexic Ideation in the Patient's Mental Life

The clinician will immediately be confronted by the degree to which the patient's mental life is dominated by concerns with eating, food, actual or desired body weight, and the details of her treatment program. The degree of preoccupation reflects the extent to which the patient has, from a psychological point of view, "resorted" to eating obsessions in an effort to control her panic about her life situation. As a general rule, the patient's capacity for alliance and her prognosis vary inversely with the degree of this preoccupation.

Anorexic ideation may be occult. Not only may the patient deny concern with weight or appetite and state that she wishes to gain weight, but also she may appear highly sophisticated about insight-oriented therapy and appear remarkably ready to "talk the therapist's language." This verbal behavior may gratify the therapist, but it must be evaluated in light of the patient's history of overcompliance and her current *somatic* behavior (Is she gaining weight?). The patient is as likely to be compliant with the therapist as elsewhere. Progress in psychotherapy must be discounted in the presence of persistent emaciation. It represents an example of what Kohut[14] called "vertical splitting," in which borderline patients experience different aspects of their lives in isolation from each other.

The Developmental Assessment

The developmental assessment begins with the history of the circumstances of the patient's conception and the mother's experience of the pregnancy and the child's birth and infancy. The patient's temperament as an infant and the degree of mutuality and enjoyment, especially in feeding, as recalled by both mother and daughter are important information. Conventional development milestones (age of first sitting, walking, talking, etc.) are likely to be remarkable only for the precocity of these high-achieving girls. On

the other hand, the acquisition of assertiveness and of the capacity to have an opinion of her own, even forcefully, may have been a problem. Attention must be paid to the possibility that compliance, pseudoautonomy, and the development of a *false self*[13] (a sense of self based not on an integration of one's own inner feelings but on responses to external demands) occurred instead. A good history in this area will help distinguish those patients who are fleeing from higher level phase-specific sexual and developmental conflicts in adolescence from those with the more deep-seated ego and self-pathology described by Bruch.

The clinician must also examine the *current* situation of the patient, with specific attention to the developmental impasse in which she is ensnared. The goal of this examination is not, however, a diagnosis in the classificatory or taxonomic sense, nor is it just a formulation of developmental arrest or fixation. The goal is to provide the patient with an empathic statement in everyday language of why her developmental progress has been brought to a halt (for example, "You seem to have managed your questions about being a woman by deciding for the time being that you would slow down your body and your life.")

The Capacity for Autonomous Alliance versus the Need for External Controls

As noted earlier the therapist is sailing through difficult waters in his effort to form an alliance with a patient who skillfully complies while she fails to grow as an individual. It is for this reason, in particular, that an assessment be made of the patient's capacity to ally in a manner that is autonomous and free of her need for external controls. The test occurs, of course, in regard to her somatic behavior, that is, her weight gain. Verbal and social behavior alone are inadequate to judge a patient's progress. Some degree of external control, specifically, clinical decision-making for the patient with regard to eating and weight rehabilitation, is almost always necessary with a hospitalized patient. The eventual goal is, of course, that the patient function autonomously, though some ego functions (such as perception of caloric needs and choice of amount and type of foods to be eaten) may have to be taken over for her temporarily. As Dr. Nancy Rollins used to say, with kindness but firmness, "I'm interested in your making your own choices, too, but right now you've got some screwy ideas about eating, so we've got to decide this for you for a while."[34]

Assessment of the Patient's Strengths

An assessment of strengths in the patient is critical because of her deep feelings of worthlessness and emptiness. Talent and mastery may be in athletics or in the arts. It is particularly important for patients who experience their prior academic excellence as something "done for mother" to develop strengths which they can identify more deeply as a part of themselves, even (sometimes especially) if discordant with family ideals.

The Family Evaluation

The hospital treatment of the anorexia nervosa patient requires family participation, even in ostensibly "emancipated" young adults. Even those using an individual model of anorexia nervosa, that is, who postulate no ongoing family dysfunction, recognize that the patient whose anorexia nervosa is severe enough to warrant hospitalization will need family assistance in her recovery. In married patients, the spouse occupies a role similar to that of the parents. In the paragraphs that follow, "spouse" can, therefore, be added to or interchanged with "parents" for such patients.

Systems Approach

The systems point of view looks at the family as a whole. The clinician must assess the degree to which enmeshment and rigidity are present as well as the family's capacity for adaptability. The possibility that the patient, via her illness, is serving a function of quieting conflict in the family system must be given special attention.[32]

Maternal and Paternal Relationships

The patient's relationship with her parents deserves special emphasis. The degree of warmth between patient and mother (often too cold) and the degree of distance between patient and father (often too close) require assessment, as does the extent of rapport or latent schism in the marriage. The possibility that the patient serves, partly by her own characteristics and partly by qualities attributed to her in habitual family transactions, to stabilize some aspect not just of the family, but of one or both parents, must be considered. By such *projective identification*[35] an emotionally unacceptable but highly invested aspect of the parent is psychologically located and cultivated in the child. In the following example, projective identification was seen to operate in one parent and displacement in both.

A 14-year-old girl with anorexia nervosa had, somewhat atypically, been the most outspoken, headstrong, and volatile of three daughters. While constitutional endowment certainly played a role in the development of this personality in this girl, such a role in the family functioned in a way which stabilized aspects of both parents. For example, the mother chastised the girl for losing her temper over a trivial domestic privilege, while the mother lost an opportunity to empathize with the girl's deeper unhappiness. On inquiry, the mother felt she had missed her daughter's unhappiness because a habitual stereotype of the girl in the family ("She's just being her stubborn self") discouraged exploration of what the girl was actually angry about. As the mother expanded on "stubborn" she mentioned "nonpliable," and "can't get her to do what I want," which led her to recognize the displacement of her anger from her husband, whom she experienced similarly. She also related her lack of empathy for the self-assertive daughter to her own upbringing, which emphasized that a woman never enjoys privileges comparable to those of men, but should honor men's dominance. Keeping the daughter in the position of the defiant, headstrong woman permitted the mother both to keep in emotional touch with this repudiated part of herself and to condemn it. The girl played a parallel role for the father. He felt unduly angry at her because, he said, she was working nonstop, having no pleasure, and damaging her health as a result. His wife pointed out the distortion—the girl was in fact enjoying herself more than before. The husband, it seemed, was displacing resentment from his wife, who had recently exacerbated past injuries by strenuous work, thereby inconveniencing the rest of the family. He had never experienced, much less expressed, resentment toward his wife for her conscientious self-neglect. The girl became a "safer" repository for this affect.

Empathy and Parenting

Given the modal patient's difficulty knowing her own experience and taking care of herself, attention must be focused on the kind of empathy and parenting she received from her parents. This, in turn, would lead to an exploration of the nature and quality of the parenting that the parents themselves received.

The parents of a 15-year-old girl with a history of severe weight loss and hypokalemia repeatedly concealed from the doctor, at follow-up weighings, their daughter's vigorous drinking of water before visits in order "to pass the doctor's test." "She's had so much trouble, we wanted to give her a break," they said later in reviewing this phase of their daughter's illness, which was fatal soon thereafter.

Women's Role in the Family

The feminist movement, by focusing on the economic and political bases of interpersonal relationships and on the way women are raised, has provided a new perspective from which to view psychiatric disorders commonly found in women.[36] These considerations can be applied as well in the assessment of families with anorexia nervosa.[37] What are the power relationships, the sex role stereotypes, and the valued sex roles? What are the overt and covert tensions between the sexes? Identifying sexuality, sex roles, and gender-related psychopathology can be useful to therapy. The case of the 14-year-old illustrates, in addition to the mechanisms of projective identification and displacement, the *theme* of occult male-female tension as a factor in maintaining the patient's illness in the family. From a technical point of view, it may be useful to help the patient who tends to be unconsciously self-blaming and devaluing of women to externalize by identifying with the feminist movement in formulating her

developmental impasse as due at least in part to socially determined male-female sex role differences.

HOSPITAL TREATMENT

Hospital treatment occurs in three sequential but overlapping phases—nutritional, family, and individual rehabilitation. How much of this work may be undertaken during any given admission usually depends on factors external to the patient, namely, limits by most insurers on length of hospital stay covered and limits by many hospitals on the number of patients with eating disorders who may be admitted. Many critically ill patients, especially those with chronic disorders, lack insurance altogether; others have insurance but cannot obtain admission. The following sections describe treatment of the patient with coverage for acute-to-intermediate length hospital treatment.

Nutritional Rehabilitation

Refeeding

A variety of paradigms can be used. They all tend generally to exclude the family from the patients refeeding; to employ a form a operant conditioning in which privileges are contingent on weight gain; to assume that nutritional recovery usually must precede meaningful psychological changes (though it does not guarantee it); and to provide the patient with concrete structuring of normal eating habits by companioned eating, preselected meals of perscribed size, or artificial caloric supplements (e.g., Sustacal, Ensure). Some patients who are intolerant of food may accept artificial supplements, though staff must recognize this as a way station toward overcoming of a food phobia.

Regardless of the paradigm or protocol chosen, the outcome appears most dependent on the experience and cohesion of the nursing staff and on their degree of comfort with the particular protocol. Unresolved staff differences are quickly exposed by the patients and result in staff splitting. This occurs particularly when one group of staff is seen as too indulgent and another group as unempathic and cruelly depriving.

For these reasons, a routine approach to nutritional rehabilitation is crucial. If a ward does not have a clear, cohesive approach, case by case, kilo by kilo, obsessive negotiations of every detail of the program will occur. Treatment will be stalled. The patient will not be helped to undo her own obsessions with food, weight, and her body so that she may begin to come to terms with her life situation.

A sample protocol is provided in the appendix. The protocol must specify the level of vital signs at which bed rest will be required (e.g., P < 60, BP < 70, T < 97). Except in rare cases (for example, the patient who is a highly trained athlete and is normally bradycardic), these parameters should be the same for all patients.

When an experienced, cohesive staff is working with an etablished protocol, voluntary patient compliance with refeeding (by food or supplement) is the rule. Recourse to nasogastric intubation is a sign of undisclosed staff anxiety, discord, or exhaustion, or it may suggest that the primary diagnosis is not anorexia nervosa but another medical or psychiatric disorder, e.g., Crohn's disease or schizophrenia.

Dietary counseling, both for parents and patients, is important to address the misinformation and food phobias present.

Other Nutritional Therapy

Vitamins are indicated. It is important to remember, particularly for the severely emaciated patient with the mental status changes of starvation, that *calories and amino acids* are the psychoactive drugs that are immediately needed. For some patients with weight loss greater than 35-40% of ideal body weight, *central hyperalimentation* has been used, in coordination with individual and family therapy.[38] Indications for such an approach include life-threatening weight loss and failure of alternate (i.e., oral and enteric) routes of refeeding. The obvious advantage of hyperalimentation is that of bypassing a gastrointestinal tract which may be functioning in a physiologically abnormal manner as well as being highly conflicted psychologically for the patient. In doing so, the patient is quickly brought out of the negativism, apathy, and clouded sensorium associated with advanced degrees of starvation which obviously interfere with psychosocial therapy. Risks include all of the risks normally associated with central venous lines (sepsis, venous thrombosis, and fluid overload) as well as the dangers particular to patients with anorexia nervosa (including manipulation of the line with resulting air embolus or sepsis, both of which can be fatal). Experience with regard to patients' tolerance of and use of this modality has been mixed: several patients with a history of poor toleration of enteric refeeding have tolerated this approach well; line interruption and air embolus have occurred in a minority.[38, 39] Those experienced with hyperalimentation emphasize that it cannot be used as a panacea, nor as the sole treatment in anorexia nervosa, but rather as part of a combined medical and psychiatric program.

Bulimia and Laxative Abuse

Bulimia and laxative abuse are seen more and more frequently, both in patients with concurrent anorexia nervosa ("bulimarexia") and in women of normal weight, maintained despite gorging only by vomiting and purging. Their presence in anorexia nervosa makes prognosis worse. Bulimia has been considered both a habit disorder (like cigarette smoking) and a compulsive disorder. Little consensus exists about treatment,[22] though social modalities (self-help groups, social reinforcements, even intense environmental control, e.g., having college students spend the entire evening in a food-bare study-cum-infirmary) appear of more promise than exploratory therapy. The range of approaches used with cigarette smoking (including hypnosis) may usefully be applied here. Laxative abuse, particularly in the underweight patient, may be life-threatening and taxes the skill of the physician and ward team just as does self-destructive, control-inviting behavior by borderline patients (see Chapter 4).

When to "Panic"

Urgent intervention is indicated when a patient (in or out of hospital) falls below a critical weight, previously set in collaboration with a medical colleague; in the presence of severe potassium deficiency (serum [K] < 3.0 mEq/L); when the patient is in an "eating disorder panic," with uncontrolled bingeing, purging, or fasting; and when the physician lacks reliable information about the patient's condition. Intervention may consist of hospitalization, increased supervision or restriction of the hospitalized patient, or a less autonomous approach to feeding. It may also include limit-setting on parents.[40]

Family Rehabilitation

Hospitalization per se generally accomplishes the first goal of interrupting the negative cycle of pleading and guilt-exchanging interaction between the patient and her family. The second goal of hospitalization is to enlist the family, often against considerable resistance, in treatment. Families will often deny or conceal family pathology, even of severe degree. Engaging previously noncooperative family members in treatment is, with nutritional rehabilitation, perhaps the most important accomplishment of hospitalization.

The goals of family treatment during hospitalization incude the shifting of the family focus from the patient as the problem toward previously unacknowledged problems elsewhere in the family or to the family system as a whole. Clinical administrative limit-setting on life-threatening failures of parenting may be necessary before the patient can respond to treatment.[40] Because communication in anorectic families is often disturbed with diffuse, detoured patterns and lack of conflict resolution, initial work at improving communication is also essential. Furthermore, dysfunctional alliances in which one parent is paired with the patient against the other parent are common. Treatment must aim to reunite the parents and allow the child to separate. Finally, family treatment should identify and begin to ventilate and work through any salient, unresolved family events, such as deaths, moves, or transitions.

Relabeling the patient's behavior from "sick" to "stubborn" may be a short-term goal, but must be approached with caution, since the shedding of the sick role without other concurrent change in the family will expose the patient to the family's resentment, generated over the years, of her domination-through-weakness.

As discussed in Women's Role in the Family, the feminist perspective may be useful in catalyzing (and normalizing) change in many of these families.

The family is ready to have the patient back home when family and individual treatment are underway, and some shift towards a more facilitating home environment has occurred, particularly when demonstrated by the patient's maintaining her weight on weekend passes home.

After discharge, the goals of family treatment are the continued working through of the dysfunctional patterns impeding the patient's recovery. As indicated below, for some patients, overall treatment will be coextensive with family therapy; for others, family therapy will be only a necessary prelude to longer-term individual psychotherapy.

Individual Rehabilitation

Some patients with relatively circumscribed adolescent disorders with generally healthy preadolescent development may do well with short-term family work. However, for those patients with severe long-term developmental pathology, individual psychotherapy is essential and represents the long-term phase of treatment. Hospital and family treatment constitute only a beginning for these patients, with the hospital goals dependent on individual pathology, ability to use therapy, and length of stay available.

Milieu Therapy

On the ward, all patients have much to gain from activities, structured therapy groups, and free time with fellow patients and ward staff. Patients may later recall peer friendships made on the ward as the most helpful part of the hospitalization.[41] Most patients are hungry for relationships that are different from those they have experienced at home. They generally benefit from seeing fellow patients and staff model a wider variety of emotionality and self-assertion than they have known in their family.

A particularly important benefit of intermediate-length hospitalzations (60–150 days) for patients with anorexia nervosa is the opportunity to have a corrective emotional experience through mirroring and empathy (functions postulated by so many authors to have been deficient both in their early childhood and ongoing family relationships).[12, 30, 32] In contrast to their previous experience, these patients find hospital nurses and fellow patients generally quite eager to empathize and to pay close attention to their feelings and ideas. Over a period of weeks to months in the hospital, experiences of this kind tend to support the growth of the rudimentary authentic and autonomous sense of self.

Activities, especially in the arts and in music, and community planning groups are useful places for patients to experiment. In these groups they can discover strengths different from the narrow range of academic achievement in which they have traditionally excelled.

This mention of the benefits of milieu therapy for patients with anorexia nervosa should not suggest that this therapy is consistently easy or smooth-running. On the contrary, a psychiatric ward, because it is a powerful therapeutic agent in anorexia nervosa, is thereby vulnerable to expectable complications. One complication is that of *excessive preoccupation with the details of refeeding*. This can be recognized by the predominance (in rounds and team meetings) of discussions of calories and weight to the neglect of the consideration of the psychological aspects of individual and family therapy. Protocol is changed and changed again; soul-searching and mutual devaluation occur among staff; and the patient does not gain weight. The ward staff has unwittingly recreated a pathological aspect of the child's relationship with the mother in which the child reproaches the parent for not being a good caretaker or nurturer. The reproach may be expressed verbally or silently (failing to gain weight). The patient's message is: "Your milk stinks and my wasted body is the evidence." If not recognized as transference, this unspoken reproach may in-

duce the staff to feel guilty, respond with one effort after another, just as the parents did at home, to provide the "right" food (or care, or medication, or therapy), and thereby be set up for frustration with and rage at the patient. Along the way, covert competition among staff to be the "good mother" may occur and may cause further regression in the patient.

A second complication is that of *exhaustion*. Staff feel great emotional demands when relating to a patient who is frequently fragmented, who is often elusive, and always needy, and who is often in a life-threatening condition yet frustrates and may openly mock her doctors and nurses as they try to help her. The resulting countertransference rage, if recognized and sympathetically shared, can provide (among other things) a good basis for empathy with patient's parents. Unrecognized, it contributes to the arrest of therapeutic progress.

Finally, the *iatrogenic risks of psychiatric hospitalization* itself must be considered. Some resist altogether psychiatric hospitalization of patients with anorexia nervosa,[32, 33] citing the danger either of validating the family's (pathological) view of the child as the sole problem, or of confirming a vulnerable teenager seeking an idea of who she is in the role and identity of "the anorectic." Both are real dangers, particularly given the poor development of herself as a whole person from which the *modal* patient with anorexia nervosa suffers painfully. On a ward with several patients with anorexia nervosa, it is striking how avidly the old patients define the newcomer as "one of us," and with what relief the newcomer reports she has found "people who are like me: at last I'm not alone."

On balance, it seems psychiatric hospitalization can be useful for patients with anorexia nervosa if the above dangers are borne in mind; if the attitudes conveyed in the habit of referring to the patient as "an anorectic," and the usage itself, are avoided; and if one remembers that for many patients who have extremely limited ideas of themselves as people, and who seem to have received from family only identities they cannot use, totalistic identification with people who feel safe (and safely "like me") may be crucial to recovery, as long as it is seen as a stage in treatment (as in development), and not as the final goal of personal growth.

Pharmacotherapy

The role of pharmacotherapy is controversial. Drugs are generally used as adjuncts to other treatment; few would treat a patient with medication alone. Some of the most experienced clinicians in anorexia nervosa, Bruch[12] and Crisp,[42] regard the use of drugs in anorexia nervosa as ineffective and even dangerous, because of their adverse effect on the required psychological rehabilitation of the patient. Despite this, a disorder with such obviously physiological components has consistently drawn clinicians to attempt to discover a "magic bullet" to undo its symptoms. Short-lived flurries of interest have attended the use of chlorpromazine,[43] cyproheptadine,[44] amitriptyline,[18] and lithium.[45] In all these studies, the focus was on the short-term intervention, with the outcome parameters primarily those of weight and eating. The effect on the underlying psychopathology and longer-lived effects have yet to be investigated. The one drug studied in a good design with significant numbers is the antihistamine cyproheptadine. In that study, Goldberg et al.[46] found no significant effect on weight and eating, except in a subgroup of patients characterized by a history of birth trauma, great emaciation, and previous treatment failures. Amitriptyline is now the study of double blind trials.[47, 48] Naloxone has also stirred current interest, based on the hypothesis that endorphins may be involved in anorexia nervosa.[49]

Despite the appeal of pharmacotherapy in this disorder, the present use of drugs in anorexia nervosa remains experimental. While the current expansion of knowledge of neurotransmitters and brain chemistry makes it possible that a single pharmacological approach to a central mechanism of anorexia nervosa may be found, it appears more likely that clinical pharmacologic investigations will be more useful in distinguishing physiological subgroups than in playing a definitive role in therapy.

Individual Psychotherapy

Individual therapy seeks to give the patient an experience of nonpossessive empathy in which accurate identification of her inner states, including confusion and feelings of emptiness, can occur.[12] The therapist tries to understand the nature of the patient's experience and to help her to articulate and share her inner life. This focus is deliberately emphasized to contrast with the unstated expectation of patient and family that psychotherapy should be primarily insight-oriented meaning, to them, aimed at "finding the secret" of the patient's self-starvation. The danger is that insight or expressive therapy might become another intellectualized game in which the patient again feels isolated, coerced, and compliant.

A 16-year-old hospitalized patient had hardly anything to say about her own feelings, while preoccupied with feeding other patients and struggling with staff over what she took to be their expectations of what she was to do. She was puzzled and annoyed at having twice weekly "talking" therapy appointments since she felt she herself had nothing to say. She was surprised to find that having nothing to say was a feeling her therapist could understand, and shared that she in fact felt this way a good deal of the time. In concurrent work in individual therapy, ward groups, and unscheduled conversations with ward nursing staff, and with support from family as the family changed in family therapy, she gradually came to feel that perplexity, sadness, loneliness, anger and hunger could all be identified, articulated, and even shared.

It is important to help the patient understand her experience because she frequently does not experience affect in a clearly defined form. The therapist must be careful not to be fooled by her outward maturity and verbal expression of feelings. In a later phase of psychotherapy, more defined ego states such as depression may be experienced. The following case shows the gain in ego development that depression may represent (cf., M. Klein[50]).

A 17-year-old college-bound high school senior and the youngest of four children presented for hospitalization with 25% weight loss and social withdrawal. Her fear of normal body size and her covert efforts to avoid weight gain gradually became apparent. The family background was notable for paternal defection at an early age and for subsequent singlehanded raising of the family by the mother, who appeared chronically depressed, distant, and self-absorbed.

The patient's mental status was notable for pervasive feelings of lack of direction, blandness, and poorly articulated neediness. There was no depression; in fact, she showed little clearly felt affect. Specific people seemed to mean little to her. Developmentally, the patient appeared to have major and early defects in self-development, characterized by interpersonal avoidance, poorly differentiated object relations, and poorly developed self-concept and capacity for self-regulation.

After several months in hospital with combined behavioral, individual, and family treatment, the patient returned home and continued in psychotherapy with a senior therapist. She graduated from high school and went on to college. Upon the anniversary of her first hospitalization and during holiday vacations both from college and therapy, a brief hospitalization was necessary to contain the patient's panic and self-harming ideation. Her weight and eating were normal. Psychotherapeutic exploration revealed specific intense pain over losses of people, actual or feared, with concomitant depression. "A year ago, I never felt depressed, then I just had the anorexia," was the patient's comment. "Now it really hurts."

The Central Dilemma: Coercion versus Reconstruction

As the above discussion makes clear, the psychiatrist treating the patient with anorexia nervosa operates between the horns of a dilemma shaped by the nature of the disease itself. On the one hand, life-reserving, or health-restoring, action, including some coercive action, is necessitated by the patient's physical emaciation and her inability to act autonomously on her own behalf. And the patient, to get well, must comply. At the same time, the most compelling formulation of developmental pathology places excessive compliance to others' demands close to the heart of the patient's disorder and, without too great a leap, sees the anorexic stance as one last, ill-chosen but desperate attempt to be in control of something, namely, the body and its drives. This hy-

pothesis helps explain the inner satisfaction the patient has, even while denying it, with her emaciation.

For the clinician, the dilemma takes the form of a thousand choices between and among health-restoring interventions of varying degrees of coerciveness versus an approach which lets the patient get well and grow "at my pace." To the extent that this formulation is an accurate description of developmental psychopathology and not simply a psychological reflection of disordered brain chemistry to be set aright by refeeding and drugs, the most telling critique of behavioral, pharmacologic, and other short-term, coercively-oriented, hospital-based treatments is that alone they do nothing for, and in fact may exacerbate, the patient's difficulties in finding herself.[51] Indeed it is likely that the striking decrease in mortality in recent series (see Course and Prognosis of Anorexia Nervosa) has occurred because most contemporary treatment programs treat the patient as a person whose eating disorder is located in an understandable existential and developmental impasse, and not just as a nutritional or endocrinological case in need of physical rehabilitation.

A pharmacological study highlighted inadvertently the patient's capacity to resist and undo even the most plausible-appearing changes "from outside." In a trial[52] of the gastrokinetic drug metoclopramide, the delay in gastric emptying characteristic of anorexia nervosa responded dramatically to the drug, with decreased emptying time and, one would think, decreased subjective bloating, of which patients frequently complain. Most patients transiently gained some weight. Despite this, most of the patients rejected continued drug therapy, and a fair number were lost to follow-up.

There are considerable differences between existing treatment programs on this dimension of coercion versus reconstruction. Resolution of the dilemma will wait on long-term, comparative follow-up studies that look at total, long-term biopsychosocial functioning, not just weight recovery and maintenance and eating behavior.[53]

COURSE AND PROGNOSIS OF ANOREXIA NERVOSA

The course of anorexia nervosa is extremely variable. Some patients may have a single, short-lived episode of anorexia nervosa in early- or mid-teenage years. Other patients may go on to develop a severe, chronic disorder with restricted eating (with or without vomiting), continued emaciation, recurrent crises with hospitalization, poor social adjustment and, not infrequently, death. Associated with poor prognosis are late onset, longer duration of illness, obsessive personality style, vomiting, laxative abuse, poor premorbid psychosocial adjustment, a family resistant to treatment, and late arrival to treatment.[22]

In a large series, the mortality from anorexia nervosa ranged from 1 to 21% with an average of 8%.[51] More recent series report much lower mortality,[41] suggesting either sampling differences, a secular trend toward a less severe form of the disease, or the results of the more comprehensive view of rehabilitation referred to earlier (see Nutritional Rehabilitation). One series found about half of patients eventually cured of their eating and weight disorder; another series found less than a third attain normal eating behavior.[53]

Vocational adjustment seems to be the best area for these patients, with two-thirds showing good outcome. Some, remarkably, even worked as their health declined and death ensued. While more than half of the patients marry or live in stable relationships, the quality of the relationships is poor (little mutual satisfaction).[53] Menses may return, though irregularly, in 70%,[54] and there are reports of several patients becoming pregnant and bearing children after weight gain, although still underweight (around 41 kilos).

The Physician and the Patient with Anorexia Nervosa

Few disorders offer the challenges or elicit the range of emotional reaction from physicians that anorexia nervosa does. At one extreme are the cynicism and anger often evident when clinicians talk about patients' "tricks" to conceal weight loss, and the disparagement implicit in the habit of referring to patients as "anorectics" or "anorexics," an attitude which expresses both the frustration felt by the clinician caught in a control struggle with the patient and also the realistic fear that a patient may die of a "functional" disorder. Among those with more equanimity about such patients, one hears several themes. One is that of coming to terms with being scared, with the possibility that the patient may die, and with the limitations of medical omnipotence implicit in being a therapist, not an administrator to the patient.[33] Others experience a psychotherapeutic challenge in trying to find and make alliance with the part of the patient which wants to be well and to recover.[12, 34, 55] Others experience a high degree of empathy for the existential dilemma of the person who resorts to self-starvation as a solution to understandable life dilemmas, as Crisp put it, crying out, "Let me be."[42] For all, the challenge of a disorder with great potential morbidity and some mortality, in individuals with considerable talents and potential "if only . . .," and in which physical, psychological, and family function are so inextricably interwoven, will continue to exert a strong pull on clinicians.

REFERENCES

1. American Psychiatric Association: *Diagnostic and Statistical Manual of Mental Disorders*, ed. 3, Washington, D.C., American Psychiatric Association, 1980.
2. Morton R: *Phthisiologia—or a Treatise on Consumption*, London, Smith & Walford, 1694, quoted in Woodruff RA Jr., Goodwin DW, Guze SB, *Psychiatric Diagnosis*, p. 166, New York, Oxford University Press, 1975.
3. Feighner JP, Robins E, Guze SB, Munoz R: Diagnostic criteria for use in psychiatric research. *Arch Gen Psychiatry*, 26: 57–73, 1972.
4. Rollins N, Piazza E: Diagnosis of anorexia nervosa. *J Am Acad Child Psychiatry*, 17: 126–137, 1978.
5. Casper RC, Eckert ED, Halmi KA, et al.: Bulimia: Its incidence and clinical importance in patients with anorexia nervosa. *Arch Gen Psychiatry*, 37: 1030–1035, 1980.
6. Fairburn CG: Self-induced vomiting. *J Psychosom Res*, 24: 193–197, 1980.
7. Russell G: Bulimia nervosa: An ominous variant of anorexia nervosa. *Psychol Med*, 9: 429–428, 1979.
8. Thompson MG: Life adjustment of women with anorexia nervosa and anorexic-like behavior. *Int J Eating Disorders*, 1: 47–60, 1982.

9. Schwabe AD, Lippe BM, Chang RJ, et al.: Anorexia nervosa: UCLA Conference. Ann Intern Med, *94:* 371–381, 1981.

10. Bruch H: *Eating Disorders: Obesity, Anorexia Nervosa, and the Person Within,* New York, Basic Books, 1973.

11. Bruch H: Perceptual and conceptual disturbances in anorexia nervosa. Psychosom Med, *24:* 187–194, 1962.

12. Bruch H: Anorexia nervosa, in Arieti S (ed): *American Handbook of Psychiatry,,* vol. 4, New York, Basic Books, 1975.

13. Winnicott DW: Ego distortions in terms of true and false self, in *The Maturational Process and the Facilitating Environment,* New York, International Universities Press, 1965.

14. Kohut H: *The Analysis of the Self,* New York, International Universities Press, 1975.

15. Theander S: Anorexia nervosa. Acta Psychiatr Scand Suppl, *214:* 29, 1970.

16. Kendell RE, Hall DJ, Harley A, Babigian HM: The epidemiology of anorexia nervosa. Psychol Med, *3:* 200–203, 1973.

17. Crisp AH, Palmer RL, Kalucy RS: How common is anorexia nervosa? A prevalence study. Br J Psychiatry, *128:* 549–554, 1976.

18. Needleman H, Waber D: Use of amitriptyline in anorexia nervosa, in Vigersky R (ed): *Anorexia Nervosa,* New York, Raven Press, 1977.

19. Halmi KA: Anorexia nervosa: Recent investigations. Annu Rev Med, *29:* 137–148, 1978.

20. Winokur A, March V, Mendels J: Primary affective disorder in relatives of patients with anorexia nervosa. Am J Psychiatry, *137:* 695–698, 1980.

21. Cantwell RD, Sturzenberger S, Burroughs J, et al.: Anorexia nervosa: An affective disorder? Arch Gen Psychiatry, *34:* 1087–1093, 1977.

22. Herzog DB, Copeland PM: Eating disorders (medical progress). N Engl J Med, *313:* 295–303, 1985.

23. Harper G: Anorexia nervosa: What kind of a disorder? The Consensus Model, myths, and clinical implications. Pediatr Ann, *13:* 812–828, 1984.

24. Selvini Palazzoli M: *Self-Starvation: From Individual to Family Therapy in the Treatment of Anorexia Nervosa,* New York, Jason Aronson, 1978.

25. Strober M: Personality and symptomatological features in young, nonchronic anorexia nervosa patients. J Psychosom Res, *24:* 353–359, 1980.

26. Lachelin GC, Yen SS: Hypothalamic chronic anovulation. Am J Obstet Gynecol, *130:* 825–831, 1978.

27. Crisp AH: Anorexia nervosa: "Feeding disorder," "nervous malnutrition," or "weight phobia?" World Rev Nutr Dietectics, *12:* 452–504, 1970.

28. Mecklenburg RS, Loriaux DL, Thompson AE, et al.: Hypothalamic dysfunction in patients with anorexia nervosa. Medicine (Baltimore), *53:* 147–159, 1974.

29. Waller JV, Kaufman R, Deutsch F: Anorexia nervosa: A psychosomatic entity. Psychosom Med, *2:* 3–16, 1940.

30. Sours JA: *Starving to Death in a Sea of Objects: The Anorexia Nervosa Syndrome,* New York, Jason Aronson, 1980.

31. Alexander F, French TM, Pollock G (eds): *Psychosomatic Specificity: Experimental Study and Results,* vol. 1, Chicago, University of Chicago Press, 1968.

32. Minuchin S, Rosman BL, Baker L: *Psychosomatic Families: Anorexia Nervosa in Context,* Cambridge, Harvard University Press, 1978.

33. Reinhart JB: Personal communication, 1983.

34. Rollins N: Personal communication, 1978.

35. Grotstein JS: *Splitting and Projective Identification,* New York, Jason Aronson, 1981.

36. Weissman M, Paykel ES: *The Depressed Woman: A Study of Social Relationships,* Chicago, University of Chicago Press, 1974.

37. Harper G: Anorexia nervosa and the women's movement. Unpublished paper.

38. Maloney MJ, Farrell MK: Treatment of severe weight loss in anorexia nervosa with hyperalimentation and psychotherapy. Am J Psychiatry, *137:* 310–314, 1980.

39. Maloney MJ: Personal communication.

40. Harper G: Varieties of parenting failure in anorexia nervosa: Protection and parentectomy, revisited. J Am Acad Child Psychiatry, *22:* 134–139, 1983.

41. Rollins N, Piazza E: Anorexia nervosa: A quantitative approach to follow-up. J Am Acad Child Psychiatry, *20:* 167–183, 1981.

42. Crisp AH: *Anorexia Nervosa: Let Me Be,* London, Academic Press, 1980.

43. Dally PN, Sargent WA: A new treatment of anorexia nervosa. Br Med J, *1:* 1770–1773, 1960.

44. Zubiate TM: Tratamiento de la anorexia nervosa con una asociacion cyproheptadina-vitaminas. Rev Med Caja Nac Seguro Soc, *19:* 147–153, 1970.

45. Barcai A: Lithium in adult anorexia nervosa. Acta Psychiatr Scand, *55:* 97–101, 1977.

46. Goldberg SC, Halmi KA, Eckert ED, et al.: Cyproheptadine in anorexia nervosa. Br J Psychiatry, *134:* 67–70, 1979.

47. Halmi KA: Personal communication, 1983.

48. Biederman J: Personal communication, 1983.

49. Moore R, Mills IH, Forster A: Naloxone in the treatment of anorexia nervosa: Effect on weight gain and lipolysis. J R Soc Med, *74:* 129–131, 1981.

50. Klein M: *Writings of Melanie Klein,* vol 3, pp. 1–24, London, Hogarth Press, 1975.

51. Bruch H: Perils of behavior modification in treatment of anorexia nervosa. JAMA, *230:* 1419–1422, 1974.

52. Saleh GW, Lebwohl P: Metoclopramide-induced gastric emptying in patients with anorexia nervosa. Am J Gastroenterol, *74:* 127–132, 1980.

53. Schwartz DM, Thompson MG: Do anorexics get well? Current research and future needs. Am J Psychiatry, *138:* 319–323, 1981.

54. Crisp AH, Hsu LKG, Harding B, Hartshorn J: Clinical features of anorexia nervosa. J Psychosom Res, *24:* 179–191, 1980.

55. Lucas AR: Personal communication, 1983.

56. Liebman R: Personal communication, 1983.

appendix

guidelines for clinical management of anorexia nervosa

It has been found in the treatment of patients with *anorexia nervosa* (AN) that it is very important that much of the protocol for nutritional rehabilitation be relatively standard for all patients on the ward, and *not* require frequent and subjective individualized decision-making. It is equally important that everyone caring for the patient feel comfortable with and supportive of the regimen chosen—the solidarity and the firm but kindly atmosphere around the patient are more important than the particular approach taken.

This protocol treats the nutritional disorder in AN, which is usually the first phase of treatment. It is not aimed at the associated eating disorder, family disorder, or personality disorder.

Measurements

1. The patient is weighed every morning by staff, in night clothes, after voiding.
2. Vital signs (VS—T, BP, P, R) are taken each morning by a nurse or child care worker.
3. *Low VS* means T < 97; P < 60; or SBP < 70. *Normal VS* means all three greater than these figures.

Bed Rest and Lounge Rest

4. If any VS are low, charge nurse notifies house officer, and patient is put on *Bed Rest*. The patient on Bed Rest stays in bed, in night clothes, has meals in bed and has no bathroom privileges.
5. On Bed Rest, VS are taken every 4 hours.
6. When VS are normal for 4 hours (i.e., on two determinations), patient is on Lounge Rest. The patient on Lounge Rest stays in lounge, in eyesight observation, in street clothes, but attends individual and group meetings, has meals in cafeteria, and bathroom privileges.
7. When VS are normal for another 4 hours, patient has full privileges except
8. After any period of Bed Rest or Lounge Rest, patient has no outside or vigorous activity for 48 hours.

Caloric Supplementation

9. Weight gain is at least 0.1 kg/day and at least 0.5 kg/week.
10. Sustacal (or, for patients with lactose intolerance, Ensure) is used for calorid supplementation. Each Sustacal supplement is 1 can = 360 cc = 360 kcal. For Ensure, 1 can = 250 cc = 250 kcal. A supplement level (= number of supplements) for each patient is determined at team meeting; usual starting number is 4 per day.
11. Supplements are given at 4 prescribed times per day.
12. The assigned number of supplements will be given on any day requiring bed rest for low vital signs, and on any day that weight is not at least 0.1 kg above previous highest inhospital weight, beginning with the first a.m. weight on the ward.
13. Supplements are given per nasogastric tube if not taken voluntarily in 15 minutes.
14. Patient is observed without bathroom privileges for 60 minutes following each administration of supplements.
15. If the net gain for the week is less than 0.5 kg, the number of supplements administered on each indicated day is raised by one.

16. Whether and how to administer supplements when patients are on LOA home will be decided at team meeting.

Weight Goal

17. The weight goal for each patient is decided at team meeting.

Activity Regulation and Eating Supervision

18. Patients attend meals together with other patients. Nutritional consultation a routine part of the program.
19. Except as in 8 above, surveillance and regulation of patient physical activity is not a part of the program.

Working Together

20. It is incumbent on all those working with anorexia nervosa patients to maintain a high level of self-observation, because our feelings about their care and about the others working with them are so critical to their ability to organize coherently their own inner experiences. Any questions or misgivings about the protocol should be promptly brought to rounds or team meetings.

chapter 6

delirium

Eugene V. Beresin, M.D.

DEFINITION

Organic Mental Disorders: An Overview

Organic mental disorders constitute an important part of psychiatric medicine because of their association with significant morbidity and mortality. Moreover, in recent years their incidence has steadily increased. The growing frequency of organic mental disorders has been attributed to a variety of influences, including the expanding number of aged in the population, the prolonged survival of brain-damaged patients, the cerebral consequence of modern medical and surgical therapeutics, and the abuse of alcohol and drugs.[1] Despite this trend, no other area of psychiatry has been more neglected.[2] The field suffers from insufficient empirical research, little knowledge of epidemiology and pathogenesis and, above all, terminologic confusion. In response to this unfortunate state, efforts have been made to establish more precise definitions and diagnostic criteria of organic mental disorders with the hope that this will stimulate new research and improve diagnosis and treatment.[3, 4]

Classification

According to the *Diagnostic and Statistical Manual of Mental Disorders*, ed. 3 (DSM-III), organic mental disorders are a heterogeneous class of disorders caused by transient and/or permanent cerebral dysfunction.[5] Each syndrome represents a cluster of psychological and behavioral abnormalities that tend to occur together.[1] The underlying cerebral disorder may be diffuse, focal, or both. It may be *primary* (i.e., originating in the brain) or *secondary*

to systemic illness.[1] Although each syndrome has specific diagnostic criteria, individual clinical presentations vary widely due to pathology-related variables such as localization, mode of onset and progression, duration, and the nature of the pathophysiologic process.[5] In addition, the clinical picture for any patient is influenced by intrapersonal, interpersonal, sociocultural, and environmental factors.[6] Intrapersonal variables include biological attributes such as age, sex, and constitution and psychological attributes such as personality traits, psychodynamic features, education, and intelligence. Interpersonal and sociocultural characteristics encompass the quality and nature of social supports, cultural attitudes, beliefs, and values. Features of the environment such as sensory overload or deprivation, social isolation, and unfamiliarity of the surroundings may also influence the clinical presentation.[7]

The DSM-III classification of organic mental disorders consists of seven sets of psychological and behavioral signs and symptoms designated "organic brain syndromes." The seven syndromes are organized into three groups[1]: (1) those with *global cognitive* impairment (Delirium, Dementia); (2) those with *selective cognitive* impairment (Amnestic syndrome, Organic hallucinosis); and (3) those with *primarily noncognitive* impairment manifested by personality disturbances or resembling so-called functional disorders (Organic personality syndrome, Organic affective syndrome, organic delusional syndrome). It is noteworthy that these are *descriptive*, not etiologic, syndromes. The diagnosis of an organic brain syndrome must, therefore, initiate a thorough search for one or more definable organic causes.

Biopsychosocial Model

In the biopsychosocial model, all illnesses are viewed as the product of biological, psychological, and social codeterminants. This perspective, positing the multicausality of disease,[8, 9] advocates an integrative and holistic approach to clinical medicine and requires the study of people as biological organisms in a social and environmental context. The multiaxial diagnostic system of DSM-III represents the pragmatic clinical application of this concept. All patients, including those with delirium must, therefore, have a multiaxial formulation and treatment plan.

Delirium and Dementia

Delirium and dementia differ from other organic brain syndromes by their common feature of global cognitive impairment. Both disorders display deficits in the acquisition, storage, and retrieval of information necessary for purposeful behavior, problem solving, and decision making.[4] Though the syndromes overlap, it is important to distinguish them clinically, if possible.

Delirium signifies *acute, widespread cerebral dysfunction and is the clinical correlate of acute brain failure.*[10] Prompt therapeutic intervention is essential for preventing serious medical complications of the underlying disorder (such as permanent brain damage) and for controlling behavior which is potentially life-threatening.[11]

History of Delirium

Ancient Views

Clinical descriptions of delirium can be found in medical literature since the Greeks and Romans.[10-13] Hippocrates was the first to delineate a mental disorder, which he called "phrenitis"[1] and which was usually associated with a febrile illness and featured restlessness, excitement, and "wandering of the wits."[10] The ancient writers distinguished phrenitis from its opposite, "lethargus,"[10] also associated with organic illness but was characterized by reduced awareness and somnolence. The term delirium was coined by Celsus in the 1st century A.D.[1] He equated delirium with phrenitis, but in later works of other authors it applied both to phrenitis and lethargus.

Modern Views

Lipowski, in his scholarly review of the history of delirium,[10] points out that until the 19th century delirium referred to insanity in general and to an acute, temporary derangement of intellect and behavior. The latter, and our modern conception of delirium, was formulated as early as the 17th century by Thomas Willis, who recognized that delirium is not a disease but a symptom complex produced by infections, intoxications, visceral disorders, and malnutrition.[14] In the early 20th century, Bonhoeffer rejected the prevalent Kraepelinian view that each noxious agent affecting the brain causes a specific psychiatric syndrome[3] and, consistent with Willis, postulated that entirely different physical illnesses can lead to identical psychiatric syndromes.[15]

Wolff and Curran,[16] in their descriptive study of delirium, observed that the variability in clinical presentation arises from distinctive personal traits, past history, intelligence, and age. Freud later commented that the form and content of the delirious experience is partly related to the individual's experience and unconscious conflicts.[13]

Between 1940 and 1946 Engel and Romano[17] systematically investigated delirium, correlating clinical, metabolic, psychological, and encephalographic data. These authors concluded that delirium is a syndrome of cerebral insufficiency associated with cognitive impairments and a characteristic general slowing of the electroencephalogram. (The only exception to this rule is seen in delirium tremens displaying EEG fast activity.[18]) Engel and Romano argue that the common denominator in all deliria is a cerebral metabolic derangement which may result in a spectrum of behaviors ranging from hyperactivity to stupor and coma.

Adams and Victor,[19] in contrast with

Engel and Romano, regard delirium as a special type of acute confusional state characterized by vigilance, disorders of perception, overactive psychomotor and autonomic functions, and a variable EEG pattern which may be normal. They see delirium tremens as the paradigm of this syndrome.

Lipowski stands out as the most important recent contributor to our understanding of delirium. In his comprehensive monograph,[10] Lipowski upholds a unitary conception of delirium as a distinct psychopathological state representing the final common pathway for dysfunctions of cortical and subcortical structures subserving arousal, alertness, attention, information processing, and the sleep-wakefulness cycle.[10] He suggests that an imbalance of cerebral noradrenergic and cholinergic neurotransmitters, particularly in the medial reticular activating and medial thalamic projection systems, underlies reduced alertness and concomitant EEG changes.[10, 20] Clinically, Lipowski views delirium as a psychosomatic condition with biological, psychological, and environmental determinants.

Definition of Delirium

The medical and psychiatric literature is filled with many terms used synonomously with delirium. Among these are acute confusional state; acute brain syndrome; metabolic encephalopathy; toxic psychosis; and infective-exhaustive syndrome. Such clinical entities are defined variably by disturbances in cognition, alterations of consciousness, or mental confusion. For the purpose of this discussion the following terms must be defined.

Cognition. Cognition refers to the processes of perceiving, thinking, and remembering.

Consciousness. Consciousness may be defined as awareness of self and environment.[21] Two aspects of consciousness are to be distinguished, the content of consciousness and arousal. The former depends upon the integrity of the cerebral hemispheres, while the latter is controlled by brain stem structures, specifically, the ascending reticular activating system.[21] "Clouding of consciousness" denotes a glo-

bal impairment of cognitive processes which varies in degree.

Confusion. Confusion refers to an incapacity to think with one's customary speed, clarity, and coherence.[3, 19] It has been accepted as the hallmark of organic brain syndromes,[3] despite the term's ambiguity in the literature. Plum and Posner[21] consider a confusional state to be an advanced form of clouding of consciousness. Because of long-standing imprecision, it may be best to delete the term from psychiatric nosology.[3] Delirium is herein defined as a *transient organic brain syndrome characterized by acute onset, global impairment of cognitive functions, and widespread derangement of cerebral metabolism.*[1, 10]

The DSM-III[5] diagnostic criteria for delirium are:

1. Clouding of consciousness with decreased ability to shift, focus, and sustain attention
2. At least two of the following:
   a. Perceptual disturbance: misinterpretations, illusions, or hallucinations
   b. Incoherent speech
   c. Disturbance of sleep-wakefulness cycle
   d. Increased or decreased psychomotor activity
3. Disorientation and memory impairment
4. Clinical features that develop acutely (hours to days) and fluctuate over the course of a day
5. Demonstration from the history, physical examination, or laboratory tests of an organic etiology

CLINICAL FEATURES

Variability

There is considerable variability in the clinical presentation of delirium. All patients will show evidence of widespread cognitive impairment and a defective ability to integrate stimuli with past experience and learning and thus to act rationally.[10]

Individual variability is the rule, with deficits due to cognitive fluctuations which are often most severe at night. Lucid intervals, in which the patient is more alert, attentive, and in touch with the environment, may last from minutes to hours.

Another source of variability is attributed to individual differences in personality, ego strength, and emotional response to the illness.[17] Thus, one patient may appear withdrawn, perplexed, and mute; another may exhibit agitation, hostility, and frantic attempts to flee hallucinations; and still another becomes overtly despondent and contemplates suicide.

Prodromal Phase

The onset of delirium is usually rapid. At first, the patient may report mild and transient symptoms such as headaches, vague feelings of uneasiness, malaise, anxiety, or depression. He may lose interest in activities and become easily fatigued, irritable, and restless.[11, 14, 22] Sustained concentration diminishes; thinking loses clarity; and focused attention becomes difficult. Hypersensitivity to light and sounds may occur. Misinterpretation of sensory stimuli may herald the onset of illusions and hallucinations. Drowsiness, daytime somnolence, insomnia, and vivid dreams or nightmares are not uncommon.[3, 10, 14] Awareness is dulled as the patient drifts between sleep and wakefulness. Upon awakening he may be disoriented and unable to judge the passage of time. As cognitive impairment worsens, the patient has trouble distinguishing dreams from valid perceptions.

Delirium may first appear at night. Often the patient wakes up from a vivid dream grossly disoriented, fearful, agitated, and hallucinating. Typically, the night nurse is alerted to appraise the situation. In general, disturbances in the sleep-wakefulness cycle with nocturnal episodes of cognitive disorganization are the most sensitive index of incipient delirium and warrant serial mental status examinations, close supervision, and a search for organic causes.

Sometimes a patient will acknowledge he is having difficulties thinking or remembering. Other times this will become evident to the physician, who observes clear changes in mentation or notices expressions of puzzlement and confusion, hesitancy in speech, or errors of fact that the patient does not realize.[17] When a patient is aware of his cognitive impairment he may react with feelings of anxiety, embarrassment, anger, guilt, or depression. Ego mechanisms (such as denial, projection, conversion, or withdrawal[14]) may be wielded to defend against the insult. Many patients will feign normalcy and evade questions aimed at assessing cognition. Some may blatantly refuse testing, confabulate, or respond with abusive language and angry outbursts.[10] The variety of reactions are as protean as the diversity of personality structures among affected patients.

Delirium may be limited to the prodromal phase or may progress to a more florid picture. The following sections describe common elements seen in later stages of delirium.

Attention and Wakefulness

The delirious patient is unable to maintain, focus, and shift attention voluntarily in response to internal and external stimuli. Many authors contend that this deficit is the primary abnormality giving rise to all other cognitive impairments.[23-26] When a patient cannot maintain or focus attention, he will be distractible and unable to concentrate. Thinking, therefore, loses its clarity and direction.[25] Conversation may become fragmented. The patient may stop in midsentence and interpose a completely different idea. Failures in the selectivity of attention allow environmental stimuli, such as sounds or lights, to interfere with other tasks. Moreover, inability to consistently attend to surroundings may account for disorientation to time and place.[25] When attention shifts rapidly and unintentionally the registration of new information is impaired, leading to recent memory defects. Internal stimuli, such as somatic sensations or memories, may intrude into consciousness and disrupt goal-directed thinking. Hence, associations may appear loose. Involuntary fluctuations in attention, along with deficits in screening incoming stimuli, promote sensory misinterpretations. A patient may mistake a sound in the corridor for a human conversation.[25]

Disturbances in the sleep-wakefulness cycle are the rule in delirium. There is often a reversal in the cycle with daytime drowsiness and insomnia at night.[26] Patients commonly refer to this delirious experience as "dreamlike," feeling they hover in a state between full wakefulness and sleep.[1, 16]

Lipowski proposes that delirium is primarily a disorder of wakefulness.[10] In his view, all properties of wakefulness, viz., alertness, arousal, activation, vigilance, and attention are to some degree disturbed in delirium. Hence, he postulates that delirium represents disorganization of the cerebral systems subserving these functions: the reticular activating system (wakefulness and arousal), the basal ganglia (perceptual expectancy and motor readiness), the limbic system (voluntary attention), and the frontal lobes (onset and duration of arousal).[10]

Thinking

Thought disorders are prominent in delirium. The flow, form, and content of thinking are all commonly affected. The delirious patient may present with slowed or accelerated thinking.

A formal thought disorder is an abnormality in the organization, logic, and coherence of thinking. In delirium, thinking is often fragmented, undirected, incoherent, and illogical.[27]

The content of thought may be impoverished, stereotyped, and banal[3] or, conversely, rich in imagery and fantasies filled with personal meaning.[26] Abstract thinking is often absent.[18] Delusions are common. They differ from the delusions of functional disorders (e.g., schizophrenia) in that they are poorly systematized, transient, vague, easily forgotten, inconsistently reported, and influenced by features of the environment.[3, 16] Paranoid delusions are especially common.[28]

Speech and language functions are almost always abnormal in delirium. Speech is variable in rate and volume but is often slurred.[23] There may be verbigeration or echolalia. Chedru and Geschwind[23] noted mild word-finding difficulties, verbal paraphasias, slowed word fluency, and poorly organized spontaneous speech. Moreover, they discovered that writing is defective in almost all delirious patients, with poorly drawn and spatially aligned letters, reluctance to write, syntactical mistakes, and spelling errors.[29] The authors remark that dysgraphia is the most sensitive indicator of delirium.

Memory

Memory disturbances are found in every delirious patient. With clouding of consciousness there is defective registration, retention, and recall. Registration of information is hindered by diminished arousal and attention. Impairments in retention lead to difficulties with new learning. This, in Lishman's view,[3] is a good indicator of delirium in mild stages. It is generally agreed that recent memory is more severely affected than remote memory.[10] Both retrograde and anterograde amnesia occur in delirium.[10]

Confabulation may also be present in delirium.[16, 28] According to Lipowski,[10] confabulations are typically simple, shifting, and merging with delusions. Most commonly, confabulations refer to familiar activities and discussions with friends.[16]

Perception

Perceptual abnormalities may be dramatic in delirium. Although they are quite common and often signal an organic process, they are not essential for the diagnosis. Perceptual disturbances are either distortions, illusions, or hallucinations. Perceptual *distortions* refer to changes in the quality, form, or intensity of a real experience. Visual distortions include alterations in the size of objects (micropsia and macropsia), distortions of shape and position, and apparent movement of stationary objects.[3, 16] The patient may also lose the perceptual discrimination of boundaries between inner experience and the environment and between self and others.[3]

Illusions are misinterpretations of stimuli arising from external objects. Abnormalities may occur in visual, auditory, tactile, and kinesthetic modalities. Visual illusions are by far the most common. Environmental objects are the usual basis for misinterpretations; such disturbances are fostered by low light situations. Examples of illusions are: mistaking a sound in the hall for a gunshot, seeing folds in sheets as a snake, and identifying spots on the floor as crawling insects. Misidentification of people is common in delirium. In most cases the patient will "recognize" familiar people among the hospital staff.[16] It has been observed that illusions are frequently projections of personally meaningful fantasies onto the surroundings.[16]

Hallucinations are perceptions without an external sensory origin. They, too, may involve any sensory modality, but visual ones are most common. Patients over age 60 tend to hallucinate much less than younger patients.[30]

Visual hallucinations may be simple, consisting of geometric forms, flashes of light, and bright colors. More complex ones include inanimate objects, animals, insects, human figures, or ghost-like forms.[16] Auditory hallucinations are the next most common after visual hallucinations.[16] They present as simple noises, music, perceived voices, and conversations. Tactile hallucinations are less common[10] and may involve sensations of crawling insects, pain, or burning.[16] Olfactory and gustatory hallucinations are rare in delirium. Usually they are reported as unpleasant smells such as burning rubber, decaying food, or feces.[16]

Most delirious patients perceive their hallucinations as real and respond with fear.[16, 28, 31] Some patients will attempt to interact with their hallucinations by talking to them, screaming, reaching out, or trying to escape. States of panic, especially coupled with hopelessness or despair, may significantly increase a patient's risk of unintentional physical harm or even suicide.

Delirious hallucinations differ from those found in schizophrenia in that delirious hallucinations usually occur at night. Visual hallucinations are most common; one or two modalities may occur simultaneously, but rarely three or more, and there is less likely to be an element of self-reference.[31, 32]

Orientation

Orientation refers to correct knowledge of time, person, and place. In mild delirium, orientation may remain intact, but as delirium progresses orientation becomes defective.[16, 22, 28, 33-35] The patient loses orientation for time before failing to recognize the place or correctly identify people around him. Rarely does the patient mistake his own identity.

Psychomotor Behavior

The behavioral manifestations of delirium are extraordinarily diverse. Lipowski[7, 10] distinguishes three clinical variants: hypoactive, hyperactive, and mixed forms. The preponderance of descriptions of hyperactive delirium in the literature may be due to the fact that this variety uniformly comes to medical attention. However, Morse and Litin[22] found approximately equal numbers of agitated and retarded cases. Lipowski[10] states that the mixed form is most common.

Emotion

Expressions of emotion are highly variable in delirium. In early stages and hypoactive states, mild depression, irritability, and apathy are often observed. Affect may be shallow, constricted, or flat. The most common emotional reactions are fear and depression.[16, 28] A majority of patients will also experience anxiety and anger, with euphoria or elation rarely present. Lability of affect may be striking. Patients enraged or terrified may react with fight or flight, at times resulting in serious accidents. More depressed patients have been known to attempt suicide.

Affective changes in delirium are multidetermined. They are influenced by personality, current interpersonal relationships, beliefs about the disease process, and recent life events, among other psychosocial variables. An obsessive patient, for example, who prizes control and intellectual mastery may panic with growing awareness of cognitive dissolution. Schizoid patients may become more withdrawn, while patients with paranoid traits defend against illusions with increased suspicion, mistrust, and anxiety.

EPIDEMIOLOGY

Little is known about the incidence and prevalence of delirium. It is estimated that 10–15% of hospitalized medical and surgical patients manifest delirium at some time during their admission.[10, 36, 37] Lipowski[10] believes that this figure is deceptively low since data has usually been obtained from patients requiring psychiatric consultation for grossly disturbed behavior. Hypoactive delirium is probably not reflected in the sample populations.

The reported incidence is considerably higher after open-heart surgery, among severely burned patients, and in intensive care units. In the general hospital and psychiatric inpatient settings the most common causes are related to *alcohol* (withdrawal and cerebral damage after chronic abuse predisposing to increased susceptibility to delirium) and *drugs* (toxic reactions to medications, drug abuse, and withdrawal).[27, 36, 38, 39] Although delirium is seen in all age groups, it is most frequent in children and the elderly.[11] Delirium is probably the most common and serious mental disorder in geriatric patients[20] (see Course and Prognosis). Among patients over 60 years of age, the prevalence is about 40%.[27, 30]

The current medical literature is entirely silent on the incidence of delirium in psychiatric inpatient units. However, one can expect an upward trend on the basis of progressive aging of the population with increasing geriatric admissions (many of these patients have chronic metabolic, cardiovascular, respiratory, and cerebral disease); rises in drug and alcohol abuse; and more widespread use of psychoactive medications with potential adverse cerebral side effects.

ETIOLOGY AND PATHOGENESIS

Pathogenesis

Delirium can be caused by a host of systemic and cerebral diseases. The most commonly associated illnesses are outlined in Table 6.1.

A *necessary* condition for the syndrome is a widespread disturbance of cerebral metabolism. This may result from varying disease-related pathophysiological processes which[10]:

1. Interfere with the supply, uptake, or utilization of substrates for oxidative metabolism (e.g., oxygen, glucose)
2. Disrupt or destroy functional anatomic pathways in the CNS.
3. Alter the milieu of the brain (e.g., changes in pH, concentration of electrolytes)
4. Have direct toxic effects on the brain (e.g., poisons, drugs, endotoxins)
5. Directly or indirectly modify normal neurosynaptic transmission

The systems underlying attention and wakefulness appear to be most adversely affected, i.e., the brainstem reticular activating system-hippocampal-frontal circuits.[10, 24] Though deranged cerebral metabolism is a necessary condition for the syndrome, it is not always *sufficient*. For example, all patients with a blood glucose of 50 will not be delirious. What makes one person delirious and another not is a function of the interaction of biological, psychological, and environmental vectors.

Biological Variables

Biological characteristics of the noxious stimulus and the host may increase the likelihood of delirium.[7, 10, 20, 39, 40] Such features of the *organic disorder* include:

1. Absolute strength of the noxious agent(s)
2. Acuity of onset (rapid change in the chemical milieu)
3. Degree of invasiveness
4. Presence of more than one pathogenic factor

Traits of the *host* that predispose to delirium are:

1. Age (children, patients aged over 60 years)
2. Pre-existent cerebral damage and disease (especially vascular and degenerative)
3. Addiction to alcohol and/or drugs
4. Nonspecific individual susceptibility
5. Presence of chronic illness
6. Use of multiple medications
7. Impaired metabolism, reduced excretion and protein binding of drugs (the norm in geriatric patients)
8. Impaired vision and/or hearing

Table 6.1.
Etiology of Delirium[3, 10, 13, 45]

INTOXICATIONS

a. *Medications*—Anticholinergics, tricyclic antidepressants, lithium, sedative-hypnotics, antihypertensive agents, antiarrhythmic drugs, digitalis, anticonvulsants, antiparkinsonian agents, steroids and anti-inflammatory drugs, analgesics (opiates and nonnarcotic), disulfiram, antibiotics, antineoplastic drugs, cimetidine
b. *Drugs of abuse*—phencyclidine and hallucinogenic agents
c. *Alcohol*
d. *Poisons*—heavy metals, organic solvents, methyl alcohol ethylene glycol, insecticides, carbon monoxide

WITHDRAWAL SYNDROMES

a. *Alcohol*
b. *Sedatives and hypnotics*

METABOLIC

a. *Hypoxia*
b. *Hypoglycemia*
c. *Acid-base imbalance*—acidosis, alkalosis
d. *Electrolyte imbalance*—elevated or decreased sodium, potassium, calcium, magnesium
e. *Water imbalance*—inappropriate antidiuretic hormone, water intoxication, dehydration

f. *Failure of vital organs*—liver, kidney, lung, pancreas
g. *Inborn errors of metabolism*—porphyria, Wilson's disease, carcinoid syndrome
h. *Remote effects of carcinoma*
i. *Vitamin deficiency*—thiamine (Wernicke's encephalopathy), nicotinic acid, folate, cyanocobalamin

ENDOCRINE

a. *Thyroid*—thyrotoxicosis, myxedema
b. *Parathyroid*—hypo- and hyperparathyroidism
c. *Adrenal*—Addison's disease, Cushing's syndrome
d. *Pancreas*—hyperinsulinism, diabetes
e. *Pituitary hypofunction*

CARDIOVASCULAR

a. *Congestive heart failure*
b. *Cardiac arrhythmia*
c. *Myocardial infarction*

NEUROLOGICAL

a. *Head trauma*
b. *Space-occupying lesions*—tumor, subdural hematoma, abscess, aneurysm
c. *Cerebrovascular disease*—thrombosis, embolism, arteritis, hemorrhage, hypertensive encephalopathy
d. *Degenerative disorders*—Alzheimer's disease, multiple sclerosis

e. *Epilepsy*
f. *Migraine*

INFECTION

a. *Intracranial*—encephalitis and meningitis (viral, bacterial, fungal, protazoal)
b. *Systemic*—pneumonia, septicemia, subacute bacterial endocarditis, influenza, typhoid, typhus, infectious mononucleosis, infectious hepatitis, acute rheumatic fever, malaria, mumps, diphtheria, etc.

HEMATOLOGICAL

a. *Pernicious anemia*
b. *Bleeding diatheses*
c. *Polycythemia*

HYPERSENSITIVITY

a. *Serum sickness*
b. *Food allergy*

PHYSICAL INJURY

a. *Heat*—hyperthermia, hypothermia
b. *Electricity*
c. *Burns*

Psychological Variables

Although psychological factors may determine the manifestations of and predisposition to delirium, they are not sufficient to cause the syndrome. The effects of personality styles on delusions, perceptual disturbances, and emotional responses to illness have been mentioned. Psychological influences that may facilitate cognitive disorganization include:

1. Stress—psychological stress may be related to the psychosocial setting in which illness develops,[14] the symbolic meaning of the disease,[6] and the emotional reaction to cognitive changes. Consequent autonomic arousal may exacerbate delirium.[10]
2. Ego weakness[17, 41]
3. Lack of social supports
4. Poor relationship between the patient and health care team[14]
5. Low intelligence[16]

Environmental Variables

Characteristics of the surroundings have long been recognized to impact on cognitive functioning. Negative variables are:

1. Sensory overload or deprivation ("sundowning" is the well-known

syndrome of cognitive dysfunction in the evening or low light situations)[42, 43]

2. Immobilization[14]
3. Social isolation[7]
4. Unfamiliarity with the environment[14, 41]
5. Sleep deprivation[44]

Etiology

A thorough discussion of all potential organic causes of delirium listed in Table 6.1 is tantamount to reviewing a textbook of internal medicine. The following outline attempts to highlight the more important etiologies encountered on psychiatric inpatient units.

Intoxications

Anticholinergic Drugs. Anticholinergic medications are ubiquitous in medical and psychiatric practice. They cause delirium more than any other prescribed drug.[10] This class includes antihistamines, antispasmodics, antiparkinsonian agents (benztropine, trihexyphenidyl, procyclidine), cyclopegics and mydriatics (atropine, scopolamine, cyclopentolate), low potency antipsychotics (thioridazine, chlorpromazine), and tricyclic antidepressants (amitriptyline, doxepin). Signs of peripheral toxicity include: dry mouth, blurred vision, constipation, urinary retention, dilated pupils, flushed skin, tachycardia, and hyperpyrexia.[46-51]

The diagnosis of anticholinergic delirium can be confirmed and the delirium treated by using *physostigmine*, an anticholinesterase agent.[46, 52] The drug is given in a 1–2 mg test dose (slow I.V. push). Pulse, mental status, and bowel motility should change within a few minutes. Additional doses may be used in intervals of 30 minutes to 2 hours.[46] Complications of physostigmine include: precipitation of asthmatic episodes, heart block, respiratory arrest, or seizures. Toxicity due to physostigmine, first exhibited by nausea, vomiting, or diarrhea, may be reversed by using atropine (0.5 mg) for each milligram of physostigmine administered.[53] Physostigmine is relatively contraindicated in patients with respiratory distress, current

history of asthma, or cardiac conduction defects.[46]

Lithium. Lithium toxicity usually occurs at high serum levels, but may appear at normal or even low levels.[53-57] Symptoms include confusion, neuromuscular irritability, generalized seizures, stupor, and coma. Treatment consists of reducing the dose or eliminating the drug, correcting electrolyte imbalance, and occasionally using saline infusions or dialysis.[56]

Recently a number of cases of delirium have been reported in patients receiving lithium and concurrent electroconvulsive therapy (ECT). In these instances, lithium levels were well below toxic values.[59, 60]

Cardiac Drugs. *Digitalis* toxicity is a common medical problem. CNS intoxication occurs in one of five patients treated with digitalis.[61, 62] Delirium may appear in the absence of other clinical toxic features or electrolyte disturbances.[63] The elderly are particularly at risk.[64]

Antiarrhythmic drugs, including quinidine, procainamide, and lidocaine, occasionally produce delirium.[10] *Propranolol* may also cause delirium in high or low doses.[65-67]

Neurological Drugs. Diphenylhydantoin, the most commonly used anticonvulsant, has been reported to cause cognitive disturbances acutely and chronically at toxic doses or with therapeutic blood levels.[68]

Antiparkinsonian agents besides anticholinergic compounds can cause delirium (e.g., levodopa, carbidopa, and amantadine).[69-71]

Anti-inflammatory Drugs. Steroid psychoses may appear manic, depressive, schizophreniform, or delirious, singly or in combination.[72, 73] *Indomethacin* and *salicylates* can also cause delirium.[10]

Analgesic Drugs. Morphine rarely produces delirium. However, *meperidine* causes disorientation, bizarre feelings, hallucinations, or psychosis in 0.5% of patients receiving it orally and 0.4% of patients given parenteral administration.[74] *Pentazocine* precipitates delirium in about 2% of patients.[75] Clouding of consciousness is a common side effect of *propoxyphene*.[76]

Disulfiram. Employed for the treatment of alcoholism, disulfiram induces psychotic symptoms in 2–20% of patients.[77] The clinical symptoms may present as delirium, anxiety states, affective disorders, paranoia, or catatonia.[78, 79]

Sedative-Hypnotic Drugs. Delirium is only rarely caused by sedative and hypnotic intoxication. The elderly seem more sensitive to this adverse reaction than do younger patients. Delirium, however, is seen in withdrawal syndromes (see below).

Other Medical Drugs. *Antibiotics* (penicillin, sulfonamides, streptomycin, gentomycin, cephalexin), *antituberculous agents* (isoniazid), and *antimalarial drugs* (quinacrine, chloroquine) occasionally engender delirium.[10]

Recently a number of reports have indicated that *cimetidine,* in normal or high dosage, can cause delirium.[80, 81]

Drugs of Abuse. *Phencyclidine* deserves special mention because of its upsurge during the last 15 years. This drug characteristically causes a distortion of body image, depersonalization, disorganization of thought, disorientation, hallucinations, hostility, and agitation.[82, 83] Treatment should involve a quiet setting and use of diazepam or haloperidol.[83]

Withdrawal Syndromes

Alcohol. Mild abstinence symptoms present as irritability, positional nystagmus, sleep disturbances, and hallucinations.[84–86] They may abate or progress to more severe reactions such as major motor seizures ("rum fits") or delirium tremens. True delirium tremens consists of extreme autonomic hyperactivity, hallucinations, global cognitive impairment and, usually, agitation.[85]

Sedative and Hypnotic. Withdrawal syndromes following cessation of habitual sedative and hypnotic use are virtually identical with alcohol abstinence syndromes. Mild symptoms of anorexia, weakness, insomnia, and irritability may be followed by autonomic arousal, hyperreflexia, full-blown delirium, and seizures. These reactions have been described following withdrawal from barbiturates,[87] chlordiazepoxide,[88] diazepam,[89–91] lorazepam,[92] ethchlorvynol,[93, 94] meprobamate,[95] methaqualone,[96] and glutethimide.[97] The customary treatment entails substituting and gradually reducing a cross-tolerant sedative medication, usually pentobarbital or phenobarbital.[98]

Cardiovascular Disorders

Myocardial infarctions, congestive heart failure, and cardiac arrhythmias cause delirium by acute, subacute, or chronic cerebral hypoxia. It is very important to realize that among geriatric psychiatric patients as many as 40% with acute confusional episodes may have "silent" myocardial infarctions, without complaints of pain.[39] Clark found that a very common presentation of paroxysmal tachycardias in the elderly is mental confusion and abnormal behavior.[99] Another source of delirium, particularly in the aged, is postural hypotension. This may appear symptomatically as lightheadedness, as dizziness, or as confusional episodes.[100] Many psychotropic drugs produce postural hypotension, such as phenothiazines, monoamine oxidase inhibitors (MAOI), and tricyclic antidepressants. Dangers increase with coexistent dehydration or use of diuretics.

Neurological Disorders

Cerebrovascular Disease. Strokes and transient ischemic attacks can cause delirium as the presenting feature without primary sensory or motor impairment.[23, 101, 102] Intracranial hemorrhage and hypertensive encephalopathy also induce delirium. These are sudden, catastrophic events, usually accompanied by severe headache and often unconsciousness.

Head Trauma. In chronic subdural hematoma, classical signs of increased intracranial pressure (i.e., headache, vomiting, focal neurological deficits, meningeal irritation) are often absent in the aged.[103, 104] Many geriatric patients will only show confusion, disorientation, and personality changes.[104]

Epilepsy. Seizure disorders induce periods of delirium in the following conditions.[105]

1. Petit mal status epilepticus
2. Psychomotor (complex partial) status epilepticus

3. Postictal states
4. Interictal states

All but interictal confusional states demonstrate EEG abnormalities. Interictal delirium is associated with temporal lobe epilepsy. Recently, Ellis and Lee[106] described a condition of acute prolonged confusion in later life due to generalized seizure activity that was responsive to parenteral diazepam.

Delirium *following ECT* has been reported in 10% of patients.[107] This may be a postictal state or prolongation of seizure activity. Concurrent lithium therapy appears to predispose to post-ECT delirium in some cases.[108]

Metabolic Disorders

Next to intoxications and withdrawal syndromes, metabolic disorders are by far the most important cause of delirium.[10] It is beyond the scope of this chapter to discuss each of the entities listed in Table 6.1. However, some issues relevant to inpatient psychiatry should be mentioned.

Hypoglycemia. Islet cell tumors are rare. A more common cause of hypoglycemia is related to improper use of insulin in diabetes or inadequate food intake following insulin administration.

Vital Organ Failure. Many patients with hepatic, renal, pancreatic, cardiac, or pulmonary failure will have histories of chronic disease that alert the physician to likely sources of metabolic dysfunction.

Fluid and Electrolyte Imbalance. Delirium in psychiatric patients should always raise suspicion of hyponatremia. Dilutional hyponatremia results from failure of the kidneys to excrete a water load, i.e., produce dilute urine. It may be caused by compulsive water drinking (psychogenic polydipsia) and/or inappropriate secretion of antidiuretic hormone (ADH). Some psychotic patients are compulsive water drinkers.[109, 110] Psychoactive drugs such as amitriptyline, thioridazine, haloperidol, thiothixene, fluphenazine, and carbamazepine may induce dilutional hyponatremia.[111, 112] Unexplained worsening of psychosis in a schizophrenic patient, for example, should suggest cognitive examination and a search for organic causes before increasing neuroleptic medications.

Vitamin Deficiency. Wernicke's encephalopathy is a syndrome caused by thiamine deficiency most often found in association with chronic alcoholism. It consists of nystagmus, ataxia, ophthalmoplegia (abducens and conjugate gaze palsies), and delirium.[113]

Vitamin B deficiencies are not infrequent among the elderly.[114, 115] They are potential causes of both delirium and dementia. Geriatric psychiatric patients with poor nutritional intake and chronic disease should have serum B_{12} and folate levels checked. It is always a good idea to prescribe supplemental multivitamins.

Abnormal Temperature Regulation. Some medications, such as phenothiazines, butyrophenones, and anticholinergic agents, compromise the hypothalamic mechanisms of heat preservation and heat loss. Both hyperthermia and hypothermia are associated with delirium. These conditions may be fatal.[116]

Infection

Almost any infection can cause delirium.[117, 121] Although fever has classically been linked with confusional states, delirium may arise in an afebrile infected patient. A list of infections often complicated by delirium appears in Table 6.1.

DIAGNOSIS AND DIFFERENTIAL DIAGNOSIS

Diagnosis

The diagnosis of delirium is establshed when the DSM-III criteria are met. Clinical data may be obtained from the history, direct observation, relatives and friends, and the medical record. It is always wise to have a high index of suspicion in patients at risk, e.g., the young, the elderly, substance abusers, patients using multiple medications, and patients with major medical or surgical illnesses.

Direct observation is the mainstay of clinical assessment. Though ancillary laboratory and psychological tests have value, delirium is primarily diagnosed at the bedside. In most hospital settings the nurses have the greatest contact with the patient. Hence, reviewing nursing notes, particularly those indicating fluctuations of the sensorium and nocturnal exacerbation of symptoms, may lead the way toward a diagnosis. It cannot be overemphasized that *delirium is an emergency.* Diagnosis must be rapid and thorough.

The diagnostic process has two components[10]: (1) Recognizing the syndrome and differentiating it from other psychiatric disorders; and (2) determining the organic etiology. Thus, *two* differential diagnostic exercises are required.

Sources of error on a psychiatric inpatient unit are:

1. Looking exclusively for psychological reasons to explain "psychological" phenomena[39]
2. Considering a syndrome functional because of an apparent precipitating event[122]
3. Overuse of Occam's Razor—one existent psychiatric disorder does not preclude the presence of another, either functional or organic.
4. Abandoning the search for an organic diagnosis when physical and neurological examinations are normal.

Differential Diagnosis

Etiological Differential Diagnosis

Once the diagnosis of delirium is made clinically, an extensive search for organic causes must begin (see Table 6.1).

Psychiatric Differential Diagnosis

Other Organic Brain Syndromes. Organic hallucinosis, personality disorder, and delusional syndrome differ from delirium by their lack of global cognitive impairment. Distinguishing delirium from *dementia* may be difficult since they both feature widespread intellectual disorganization. Moreover, delirium is often superimposed on dementia. Finally, some disorders initially causing delirium progress to chronic cerebral disease.

Dementia is an organic brain syndrome usually characterized by an insidious onset and a chronic deteriorating course.[123] It is also manifested by memory deficits, impaired abstract thinking, poor judgment and impulse control, labile affect, and personality change.[5] Social and occupational functioning is compromised. Delirium differs from this picture by its acute onset, brief duration, and fluctuations in cognition (see Table 6.2).

The demented patient is more likely to exhibit a poverty of thought as opposed to the rich fantasies and vivid perceptual disturbances of the delirious patient.[3] Many demented patients, particularly those with longstanding disease, exhibit cortical release phenomena such as grasp, glabellar, palmomental, sucking, and Babinski reflexes.[124] Whereas the EEG is always abnormal in delirium, it is often normal or borderline in dementia. A CAT

Table 6.2.
Delirium versus Dementia[10, 125]

Features	Delirium	Dementia
Onset	Acute	Usually insidious
Duration	Brief	Chronic, unless reversible
Consciousness	Fluctuation	Static
Orientation	Abnormal; mistake familiar for unfamiliar	May be normal in mild cases
Memory	Recent defective (registration, retention, and recall)	Recent and later remote defective
Attention	Always impaired	May be intact
Perception	Frequently disturbed; contents vivid	Misperceptions may be absent; contents less florid
Thinking	Disorganized; contents rich	Impaired; contents empty and stereotyped
Judgment	Poor	Poor; frequent inappropriate social behavior
Insight	May be present in lucid intervals	Absent
Sleep	Always disturbed	Usually normal
EEG	Invariably abnormal (slow; fast in withdrawal)	Normal or mild slowing

scan may reveal cortical atrophy in some demented patients.[123]

Schizophrenia. Occasionally schizophrenic patients demonstrate attentional deficits, memory impairments, sleep disturbances, and confusion.[126, 127] However, that is the atypical case, and the two syndromes can be differentiated on a number of grounds. Hallucinations in schizophrenia are generally auditory, as opposed to typically visual perceptual abnormalities in delirium. The schizophrenic patient's delusions are often paranoid, self-referential, bizarre, longstanding, and highly systematized, whereas delusions in delirium are fleeting, poorly systematized, and usually related to environmental stimuli.[3, 128] In contrast to the acute nature of delirium, schizophrenia is a chronic disorder with insidious onset. Few delirious patients present with thought broadcasting, delusions of control, or flat affect. Finally, delirium is manifested by global cognitive impairment with severe attentional disturbances. The schizophrenic usually has a clear sensorium.

Catatonia may occur in schizophrenia, in other functional disorders, and in a variety of organic mental disorders, including delirium.[129] This syndrome obviously raises diagnostic problems. Recent investigators have found that a *sodium amytal interview* is useful in distinguishing functional from organic causes of catatonia and confusion.[130, 131] Patients suffering from functional states generally show mental clearing under the influence of amytal, while delirious patients exhibit increased cognitive impairment. The interviewing technique involves administering amobarbital (75 mg/ml) at a rate of 1 ml/minute for the first 2 minutes. Each additional 1 ml is delivered over 1 minute, followed by a 1-minute interruption to evaluate the effects. The patient should be kept awake and talking during the procedure.[130]

An EEG can also be helpful in the differential diagnosis of functional and organic catatonia.

Atypical or Brief Reactive Psychoses. These psychotic states are acute episodes of emotional turmoil involving delusions, incoherent thinking, hallucinations, and disorganized behavior.[5, 132, 133] Clouding of consciousness may also be present.

Affective Disorders. Both manic and depressive disorders may present with cognitive disturbances that raise differential diagnostic problems. Mania, in its severe stages, has been known to manifest confusion, attentional deficits, and disorientation.[134, 135] In fact, some authors recognize "acute delirious mania" as a specific clinical entity possessing features of both mania and delirium.[136] Mania, however, can be distinguished from hyperactive delirium by a history of affective disorder in the patient and/or family; signs of euphoria, grandiosity, religiosity, etc.; characteristic stages during the course of illness[134]; and response to antimanic medications. Retarded depression, with slowed thinking, impaired concentration, and memory deficits, can simulate hypoactive delirium or dementia ("pseudodementia").[137, 138]

Depression differs from delirium by a history of affective disorder; predominance of depressive feelings, self-reproach, blame, etc.; absence of fluctuating gross impairments of cognition; and response to antidepressants. Cognitive deficits in affective disorders usually clear under the influence of amytal. The EEG should be normal.

Amnestic States. *Fugue states, psychogenic amnesia,* and *hysterical psychosis* are usually characterized by sudden onset, inability to recall important personal information and past history, and occasionally assumption of a new identity. Memory loss is spotty. Delirium differs in its global rather than selective cognitive impairment and its disorientation to time and place rather than person. The *Ganser syndrome*[139] is a rare, dramatic phenomenon consisting of paralogia, approximate answers, and clouding of consciousness. It is often highlighted by ludicrous responses (e.g., "How many legs does a three-legged stool have?" Answer: "Four").[37] Again, memory deficits are not generalized and personal identity may be lost.

Factitious disorders, e.g., malingering, Munchausen syndrome, may also present with apparent confusion, disorientation, and memory impairments. Careful investigation will generally reveal voluntary control of symptoms and the importance of secondary gain.

In cases of malingering, fugue states, and syndromes with a substantial component of hysteria, the amytal interview may *not* produce clinical improvement.[130] However, the EEG should be normal.

Neurotic Disorders. Patients with neurotic anxiety and depression may complain of irritability, insomnia, difficulty concentrating, and poor memory.[128] The history will often disclose an intrapsychic basis for such problems. However, organic brain syndromes commonly begin with hypochondriacal, phobic, and obsessive symptomatology.[3] Obsessive-compulsive behavior may be a defensive response to early cognitive disorganization. A useful clinical axiom is: Any new neurotic (or psychotic) behavior beginning after age 40 implicates organicity and necessitates a medical evaluation.[3, 122]

BIOPSYCHOSOCIAL EVALUATION

Biological Evaluation

The biological assessment of delirium is a challenging task, requiring a fluid integration of medical and psychiatric skills. The goal of this evaluation is to acquire a data base necessary for developing an etiological differential diagnosis. Assessment must be comprehensive, yet swift. The delirious patient is in need of urgent treatment and cannot wait for the outcome of a leisurely clinical investigation.

History

History-taking has five essential components, listed below (social history is considered under sociocultural evaluation). Since delirious patients are often unable to provide clear factual data, ancillary sources must be utilized. The examiner should consult family members or friends, review the medical record, speak with outpatient physicians, and read notes in the chart.

1. *Present illness.* Nature of symptoms, their onset, course and duration; current medications; use of alcohol or drugs; active medical problems; recent injuries
2. *Past medical history.* Serious illnesses; history of surgery; past injuries; previous medications; allergic reactions; history of delirium; dietary history
3. *Past psychiatric history.* History of psychosis, depression, anxiety states; hospitalizations
4. *Family history.* Hereditary diseases; medical, surgical and psychiatric disorders
5. *Review of systems.* General health; neurological symptoms; cardiorespiratory symptoms; gastrointestinal function; fever; sleep; appetite

Mental Status Examination

The diagnosis of delirium is made primarily on the basis of the mental status examination. Although some formal testing is required, delirium can generally be recognized during the course of taking the routine history. The examiner, by carefully observing the patient and listening to his verbal responses, should notice distractibility, attentional deficits, irritability, hypersensitivity to lights and sounds, incoherent thinking, fluctuations in consciousness, etc. Abnormal movements, mood, and affect can also be appreciated. During the interview, the clinician must ask about delusions, hallucinations, and suicidal, homicidal, and paranoid ideation.

If the patient reacts negatively to or refuses testing, the physician can assess cognitive functioning by asking for data such as home address, telephone number, dates of births in the family, etc. Difficulties attending to such questions or inconsistent answers are indicative of disturbances in consciousness. In addition to examining the patient in a nonthreatening manner, it is always important to reassure the patient that questioning is a routine procedure.

The cornerstone of the evaluation of delirium is the cognitive examination. Traditionally, this has included assessment of alertness, attention, memory (recent and remote), orientation, judgment, abstractions, fund of knowledge, and insight. While there are many standard clinical tests of the sensorium that are designed to appraise these functions, it is best to use an instrument that is reliable, valid for differentiating functional from organic conditions, and quantifiable. The *Mini-Mental State Examination* designed by Folstein and colleagues[140] is an excellent example of a simple test that meets these criteria and takes only 5–10 minutes to administer. This test should be given routinely and *repeated at regular intervals* during the hospitalization. By recording the results in the form of a flowsheet, the physician can keep an accurate account of the patient's progress. An adaptation of the mini-mental state appears in Table 6.3.

Physical Examination

The physical examination must be meticulous. Routine vital signs include temperature, pulse, respirations, and *orthostatic* blood pressure measurements. Keep in mind that a normal temperature does not rule out infection, particularly in the elderly. In one study of acute brain syndromes, 29% of patients with systemic infections were afebrile.[28] The physician must be alert for autonomic hyperactivity and must pay careful attention to organ systems implicated by the history.

The neurological examination deserves special emphasis. The physician should check for signs of elevated intracranial pressure, meningeal irritation, cranial nerve palsies, visual field defects, and unilateral motor and sensory disturbances. All focal signs and any abnormal reflexes (e.g., grasp, snout, glabellar, palmomental, and Babinski) must be noted.

Table 6.3.
Mini-Mental State Examination[a]

Patient _____
Examiner _____
Date _____

MAXIMUM SCORE	SCORE	
		ORIENTATION:
5	( )	What is the (year) (season) (date) (day) (month)?
5	( )	Where are we (state) (county) (town) (hospital) (floor)?
		REGISTRATION:
3	( )	Name 3 objects: 1 second to say each. Then ask the patient all 3 after you have said them. Give 1 point for each correct answer. Then repeat them until he learns all 3. Count trials and record.
		TRIALS _____
		ATTENTION AND CALCULATION:
5	( )	Serial 7's: 1 point for each correct. Stop after 5 answers. Alternately spell "world" backwards.
		RECALL:
3	( )	Ask for 3 objects repeated above. Give 1 point for each correct.
		LANGUAGE:
2	( )	Name a pencil and watch (2 points)
1	( )	Repeat the following: "no ifs, ands or buts" (1 point)
3	( )	Follow a 3-stage command: "Take a paper in your right hand, fold it in half, and put it on the floor." (3 points)
1	( )	Read and obey the following: "Close your eyes." (1 point)
1	( )	Write a sentence. (Must contain subject and verb and be sensible). (1 point)
		VISUAL-MOTOR INTEGRITY
1	( )	Copy design (2 intersecting pentagons. All 10 angles must be present and 2 must intersect). (1 point)
30		TOTAL SCORE _____
		Assess level of consciousness along a continuum

Alert   Drowsy   Stupor   Coma

[a]Adapted from Folstein MF, Folstein SE, McHigh PR: Mini-mental state: A practical method for grading the cognitive state of patients for the clinician. J Psychiatr Res, *12:* 189–198, © 1975, Pergamon Press.

Cerebellar function must also be evaluated. Finally, abnormal movements, including tremor, twitching, and asterixis should be documented.

Laboratory Studies

There are a vast number of laboratory tests and procedures that may be ordered to evaluate the delirious patient. The choice of studies for a given patient always depends on sound clinical judgment. As a rough guide, investigations may be divided into routine and special studies (see Table 6.4).

The EEG is a valuable tool in the diagnosis of delirium.[141-143] Slowing is the most common abnormality indicative of delirium. Low voltage fast activity may be present in withdrawal syndromes. Since EEG changes parallel the clinical state, serial recordings are often a quantitative way of monitoring progress or decline.

Psychodynamic Evaluation

It is a serious error to focus exclusively on the biological aspects of delirium and to discard a psychodynamic formulation. Hackett and Weisman[144, 145] point out that appraisal of the intrapsychic dimension is crucial in establishing an effective doctor-patient relationship and in planning necessary therapeutic interventions. The formulation is a systematic expression of predominant defense mechanisms, emotional patterns, object relationships and core unconscious drives, fears, wishes, and conflicts.[144] Above all, the formulation should be operational. Once the patient is understood dynamically, the physician will know how to form a working alliance, how to strengthen the most adaptive defenses, how to communicate unambiguously, and how to provide comfort and support in a tangible way. Part of every psychodynamic assessment is a determination of suicide and homicide potential.

Sociocultural Evaluation

Since reality orientation is an important part of managing the delirious patient, it is essential to know about meaningful relationships, customary daily routines, habits, familiar household objects, hobbies, and occupational activities. In addition, the impact of the hospital environment should be appreciated: Is sensory input excessive or deficient? Is the patient immobile or isolated? Is communication clear and simple? What are the patient's

Table 6.4.
Laboratory Studies to Investigate Delirium

ROUTINE PROCEDURES

1. Complete blood count
2. Blood chemistries—electrolytes (Na, Ca, Cl, CO_2), calcium, phosphate, glucose, BUN, liver enzymes
3. Serologic test for syphilis
4. Urinalysis
5. Erythrocyte sedimentation rate
6. Chest x-ray
7. Electrocardiogram
8. Electroencephalogram

SPECIAL PROCEDURES

1. Blood chemistries: creatinine, magnesium, B_{12}, folate, thyroxine, ammonia, serum proteins, osmolality, arterial blood gasses
2. Blood levels of medications
3. Blood and urine toxic screens (drugs and poisons)
4. Blood cultures
5. LE preparation and antinuclear antibody (ANA) levels
6. CSF examination—cells, protein, glucose, culture, serology, pressures
7. Urine—osmolality, porphobilinogen
8. Skull films
9. CAT scan
10. Brain scan
11. Sodium amobarbital interview (functional versus organic differential)

cultural attitudes toward doctors, treatment, and the hospital?

HOSPITAL TREATMENT

General Medical Management

Once the diagnosis of delirium is made, treatment begins. Management has two major components which occur simultaneously: (1) identification and treatment of the organic cause; (2) general management of symptoms, which involves psychotherapeutic, environmental, and pharmacologic interventions. Thus, support, reassurance, and sedation may be necessary to calm a patient while metabolic disturbances are being corrected. While the causal treatment will vary with each particular disease, certain universal principles of medical management include the following[11, 146–148]:

1. If the etiological diagnosis is unknown, rule out or treat life-threatening conditions first (e.g., decreased cerebral oxygenation due to any cause, meningitis, toxic states, hypertensive encephalopathy, hypoglycemia, severe electrolyte imbalance, intracranial hemorrhage).[122]
2. Discontinue all medication if medically permissible.
3. Closely monitor vital signs (at least every 2 hours).
4. Maintain adequate fluid and electrolyte balance. An intake-and-output chart should be kept.
5. Ensure proper nutrition and vitamin supply. B vitamin supplements are always in order for a delirious patient.
6. Protect the patient from physical harm. Although physical restraints are liable to exacerbate fear and agitation, they may be required in extreme cases. Low beds, guard rails, and constant supervision are first-line measures.
7. Periodic physical and mental status examinations must be charted to document progress or decline.
8. Anticipate the need for cardiopulmonary resuscitation and immediate transfer to an intensive care unit. Basic life support systems must be present on the unit.
9. Never hesitate to obtain medical or surgical consultation.

Milieu Management

The key to effective symptomatic management of delirium is a carefully planned ward program. Milieu management must be tailored to the patient's clinical state, personality, education, intelligence, and sociocultural background. A comprehensive approach should address the following areas[35, 41, 42, 124, 149–156]

Environment

1. Sensory input should not be excessive, sparse, inadequate, or ambiguous. The room should be quiet and well-lit and have a night light. A radio or television may be useful.
2. The patient should be presented with one stimulus or task at a time.
3. Medication schedules should not interrupt sleep.
4. Atmosphere should be calm and orderly. Tests and procedures should be spaced throughout the day.

Orientation

1. Each room should have a calendar, clock, and chart of the day's schedule.
2. Attempt to keep the patient in the same surroundings.
3. Verbal cues regarding the time, date, and place should be used consistently.
4. Evaluate the need for eyeglasses, hearing aids, or foreign language interpreters.

Familiarity

1. Obtain familiar possessions from home to help orient the patient.
2. Family members should be asked to stay with the patient. They provide the most important basis for orientation, reassurance, and support. Also, their active participation in ward management will facilitate adequate after-care planning at home.

3. Find familiar areas of interest to discuss with the patient, e.g., occupation, family status, hobbies.
4. The same staff members should routinely care for the patient.

Communication

1. Instructions and explanations should be simple, clear, repetitive, and slow-paced.
2. Face-to-face contact is important.
3. Convey warmth and an attitude of kind firmness.
4. Determine how the patient likes to be addressed and use this name consistently.
5. Begin each contact with orienting and identifying information.
6. Acknowledge the patient's emotional status and encourage verbal and nonverbal expression.

Activities

1. Movement should be unrestrained if the patient is not in danger of self-harm.
2. Self-care and participation in ward activities (e.g., occupational therapy, community meetings) should be encouraged as tolerated to strengthen self-esteem and sense of competence.

Psychotherapy

Hackett and Weisman advocate a supportive, noninterpretive psychotherapeutic approach in treating the delirious patient.[144, 145, 157] As opposed to traditional dynamic therapies, this method is not aimed at insight or resolving underlying conflicts. The clinician is not a neutral observer, but rather is an active participant. It should be stressed that noninterpretive intervention depends on a dynamic understanding of the patient.

The goal of psychotherapy is to facilitate ego stabilization, mastery, adequate coping mechanisms, and reality testing, which are promoted by the doctor-patient relationship. The clinician should be experienced as a real person who provides instructions, explanations, guidance, comfort, and reassurance. It is important for the clinician to find areas of common interest and "speak the patient's language."[144, 145] Reviewing past accomplishments and periods when reality testing was at an optimum enable the patient to reorient himself. When the clinician is seen as an ally and not as a stranger, he can effectively clarify misperceptions, convey optimism, and prevent unnecessary oscillations in affect. In effect, he becomes an ancillary ego for the patient.

Sessions should be frequent and brief. The patient must know that the clinician is interested in him as a person and is available. Once an alliance has developed, even a late night phone call may be all that is necessary to calm an agitated patient. It is essential to continue therapy after delirium has cleared. The patient must have the opportunity to understand and assimilate the experience of this highly stressful life event.[158]

An alternative approach is the confrontation problem-solving technique.[159] This therapy involves presenting the patient with a statement followed by a question. The statement confronts the patient with a symptom or maladaptive behavior that he exhibits. The statement is followed by a question: "What do you think or feel about what I told you?" This technique is claimed to foster goal-directed thinking, increase self-awareness, and enhance reality testing and adaptive behavior.

In either therapeutic approach, a vital role of the clinician is to explain the nature of the delirious episode to the patient and family. The patient should be told he is not "going crazy," but rather that he is suffering from a reversible condition with a specific medical cause. Working closely with the family ensures adequate social supports and helps pave the way for family involvement after discharge.

Psychopharmacological Management

Symptomatic treatment of delirium may include the use of medications when a patient is agitated, restless, sleepless, belligerent, or excessively fearful. In order to avoid any hazardous consequences, no pharmacological agent should be given until the cause of delirium is determined. An anticholinergic delirium treated with chlorpromazine may become worse, or a patient with hepatic failure given a sedative-hypnotic may lapse into coma. The choice of tranquilizing agent, its dosage, and its route of administration must depend on the patient's medical disorder, age, weight, and level of arousal.[10] Care must be exercised not to compromise cardiac or respiratory functions. The goal of pharmacological management is to keep the patient relaxed and comfortable without further clouding consciousness. Drugs are most useful in helping the patient get a good night's sleep. The physician may employ the following classes of medications.

Benzodiazepines

Diazepam and chlordiazepoxide are most beneficial in treating withdrawal syndromes. Though they may be given as antianxiety agents in delirium, they can cause paradoxical excitement in the elderly,[42] and they are not effective in quelling hallucinations or delusions. Moreover, they are poorly absorbed when given I.M. Oral administration may be impossible if a patient is agitated and uncooperative. Diazepam (5–10 mg orally t.i.d.) or chlordiazepoxide (10–25 mg t.i.d.) with double doses at bedtime are recommended to provide mild sedation during the day and correct nighttime insomnia.[144] For insomnia alone, flurazepam 15–30 mg h.s. is often effective. If a sedative-hypnotic agent is indicated, the newer short-acting benzodiazepines, such as temazepam (15–30 mg at bedtime) are preferable for most delirious patients.[20]

Phenothiazines

These medications have been used to manage excitement and psychosis. Low potency phenothiazines such as chlorpromazine have both antipsychotic and sedative properties. There are many disadvantages when prescribing phenothiazines in delirium: the low potency sedative agents are highly anticholinergic; there is risk of tachycardia, cardiac arrhythmias, and orthostatic hypotension; and, they are poorly tolerated by the elderly and patients with cardiac, pulmonary, and hepatic disease.

Butyrophenones

The drug of choice in treating delirium pharmacologically is *haloperidol*.[146, 147, 160–162] Its advantages include relatively minimal sedation, antipsychotic activity, low toxicity, mild anticholinergic effects, safety in patients with cardiac and pulmonary disease, and P.O. or I.M. administration. The most common side effects are anticholinergic and extrapyramidal.

For a severely agitated adult without hepatic disease under 60 years old, the physician may use a "rapid tranquilization" method.[10, 160, 161] The patient is given 5–10 mg I.M. every hour until mild sedation is achieved. The drug may then be given in oral doses one-half to two times the total I.M. doses on a divided daily schedule.[10] The total daily oral dose rarely exceeds 40 mg. For some patients h.s. doses alone are sufficient. Geriatric patients should receive lower initial doses, e.g., 2–5 mg I.M. In cases of milder excitement, oral haloperidol is preferable. The patient should receive 5–15 mg in the morning and at bedtime.[10] Again, smaller doses should be used for the elderly. Extrapyramidal side effects can be controlled with benztropine 1–2 mg P.O., b.i.d. As the delirium improves, medication should be gradually tapered.

Electroconvulsive Therapy (ECT)

ECT has been shown to be an effective, safe, therapeutic modality for intractable cases of delirium.[10, 163, 164] It should be used only when the organic etiology is defined (and not a contraindication for ECT), when hyperactivity is life-threatening, and when all other conventional interventions have failed.

COURSE AND PROGNOSIS

The definition of delirium stipulates that it is an acute disorder. It may last for a few days to a few months. Usually the duration of delirium is 1 week.[10] Its course will depend upon the treatment of the underlying medical illness. In chronic diseases, intermittent delirium may be a characteristic feature. Correction of the organic cause, too, determines the prognosis. For most patients, delirium terminates in full recovery. The scope of possible outcomes includes[10, 15]:

1. Full recovery
2. Progression to stupor, coma, and death
3. Progression to dementia or another irreversible organic brain syndrome

Little information is available regarding mortality rates in delirium. Henker found that approximately 7% of 409 cases of acute brain syndrome died.[38] The mortality rate in another study was 12%.[28] In a third study, 262 patients referred for psychiatric consultation in a general hospital setting with a diagnosis of "organic brain syndrome" were compared with controls matched for age, sex, and medical diagnosis. The mortality rate of the former group was 11%, nearly twice that of the control group.[165] It was not noted, however, whether the psychiatric diagnosis was delirium or dementia. In all of these studies, patients were referred for consultation from medical and surgical services because of a severe behavioral disturbance. Thus, sample populations were somewhat selective. It is estimated that between 15% and 30% of geriatric patients with delirium will progress to stupor, coma, and death.[164] One study demonstrated that 25% of delirious elderly patients died within a month of admission to the psychiatric ward of a general hospital.[27] It can be inferred that delirium in a medical patient, particularly an elderly patient, can have grave prognostic implications. The prognosis in psychiatric patients among all age groups is not known.

REFERENCES

1. Lipowski ZJ: Organic mental disorders: Introduction and review of syndromes, in Kaplan HI, Freedman AM, Sadock BJ (eds): *Comprehensive Textbook of Psychiatry/III*, Baltimore, Williams & Wilkins, 1980.
2. Lipowski ZJ: Organic brain syndromes: A reformulation. Compr Psychiatry, *19:* 309–322, 1978.
3. Lishman WA: *Organic Psychiatry: The Psychological Consequences of Cerebral Disorder*, Oxford, Blackwell Scientific Publications, 1978.
4. Lipowski ZJ: A new look at organic brain syndromes, Am J Psychiatry, *137:* 674–677, 1980.
5. American Psychiatric Association: *Diagnostic and Statistic Manual of Mental Disorders*, ed. 3, Washington, D.C., American Psychiatric Association, 1980.
6. Lipowski ZJ: Psychiatry of somatic diseases: Epidemiology, pathogenesis, classification. Compr Psychiatry, *16:* 105–124, 1975.
7. Lipowski ZJ: Organic brain syndromes: Overview and classification, in, Benson DF, Blumer DB (eds): *Psychiatric Aspects of Neurologic Disease,* New York, Grune & Stratton, 1975.
8. Engel GL: The clinical application of the biopsychosocial model. Am J Psychiatry, *137:* 535–544, 1980.
9. Lipowski ZJ: Psychosomatic medicine in the seventies: An overview. Am J Psychiatry, *134:* 233–244, 1977.
10. Lipowski ZJ: *Delirium: Acute Brain Failure in Man,* Springfield, Ill., Charles C Thomas, 1980.
11. Henry WD, Mann AM: Diagnosis and treatment of delirium. Can Med Assoc J, *93:* 1156–1166, 1965.
12. Hankoff LD: Ancient description of organic brain syndrome: The "kordiakos" of the Talmud. Am J Psychiatry, *129:* 147–150, 1972.
13. Heller SS, Kornfeld DS: Delirium and related problems, in Reiser MF (ed): *American Handbook of Psychiatry,* vol. 4, New York, Basic Books, 1975.
14. Lipowski ZJ: Delirium, clouding of consciousness and confusion. J Nerv Ment Dis, *145:* 227–255, 1967.
15. Bleuler M: Acute mental concomitants of physical diseases, in Benson DF, Blumer DB (eds): *Psychiatric Aspects of Neurologic Disease,* New York, Grune & Stratton, 1975.
16. Wolff HG, Curran D: Nature of delirium and allied states. The dysergastic reaction. AMA Arch Neurol Psychiatry, *33:* 1175–1215, 1935.
17. Engel GL, Romano J: Delirium: A syndrome of cerebral insufficiency. J Chronic Dis, *9:* 260–277, 1959.
18. Romano J, Engel GL: Delirium. I. Encephalographic data. AMA Arch Neurol Psychiatry, *51:* 356–377, 1944.
19. Adams RD, Victor M: Delirium and other acute confusional states, in Isselbacher KJ, Adams RD, Braunwald E, Petersdorf RG, Wilson JD (eds): *Harrison's Principles of Internal Medicine,* ed. 8, New York, McGraw-Hill, 1980.
20. Lipowski ZJ: Transient cognitive disorders (delirium, acute confusional states) in the elderly. Am J Psychiatry, *140:* 1426–1436, 1983.
21. Plum F, Posner JB: *Diagnosis of Stupor and Coma,* Philadelphia, F. A. Davis, 1972.
22. Morse RM, Litin EM: The anatomy of a delirium. Am J Psychiatry, *128:* 111–115, 1971.
23. Mesulam M-M, Waxman SG, Geschwind N, Sabin TD: Acute confusional state with right middle cerebral artery infarctions. J Neurol Neurosurg Psychiatry, *39:* 84–89, 1976.
24. Chedru F, Geschwind N: Disorders of higher cortical functions in acute confusional states. Cortex, *8:* 395–411, 1972.
25. Seltzer B, Frazier SH: Organic mental disorders, in Nicholi AM (ed): *The Harvard Guide to Modern Psychiatry,* Cambridge, Mass., Harvard University Press, 1978.

26. Lipowski ZJ: Delirium updated. Compr Psychiatry, 21: 190–196, 1980.
27. Simon A, Cahan RB: The acute brain syndrome in geriatric patients. Psychiatr Res Rep, 16: 8–21, 1963.
28. Farber IF: Acute brain syndrome. Dis Nerv Syst, 20: 296–299, 1959.
29. Chedru F, Geschwind N: Writing disturbances in acute confusional states. Neuropsychologia, 10: 343–353, 1972.
30. Robinson, WG: The toxic delirious reactions of old age, in Kaplan OJ (ed): Mental Disorders in Later Life, Stanford, Calif., Stanford University Press, 1956.
31. Frieske DA, Wilson WP: Formal qualities of hallucinations: A comparative study of the visual hallucinations in patients with schizophrenic, organic and affective psychoses, in Hoch PH, Zubin J (eds): Psychopathology of Schizophrenia, New York, Grune & Stratton, 1966.
32. Goodwin DW, Alderson P, Rosenthal R: Clinical significance of hallucinations in psychiatric disorders. Arch Gen Psychiatry, 24: 76–80, 1971.
33. Levin M: Varieties of disorientation. J Ment Sci 102: 619–623, 1954.
34. Levin M: Spatial disorientation in delirium. Am J Psychiatry, 113: 174–175, 1956.
35. Folstein MF, McHugh PR: Phenomenological approach to the treatment of "organic" psychiatric syndromes, in Wolman BJ (ed): The Therapist's Handbook, New York, Van Nostrand Co., 1976.
36. DeVaul RA: Acute organic brain syndromes: Clinical considerations. Tex Med, 72: 51–54, 1976.
37. Engel GL: Delirium, in Freedman AM, Kaplan HI (eds): Comprehensive Textbook of Psychiatry, Baltimore, Williams & Wilkins, 1967.
38. Henker FO: Acute brain syndromes. J Clin Psychiatry, 40: 117–120, 1979.
39. Varsamis J: Clinical management of delirium. Psychiatr Clin North Am, 1: 71–80, 1978.
39a. Romano J, Engel GL. Physiologic and psychological considerations of delirium. Med Clin North Am, 28: 629–638, 1944.
40. Liston EH: Diagnosis and management of delirium in the elderly patient. Psychiatr Ann, 14: 109–118, 1984.
41. Nadelson T: Sending the patient home. Psychother Psychosom, 30: 68–75, 1978.
42. Davidhizar R, Ganden E, Wehlage D: Recognizing and caring for the delirious patient. J Psychiatr Nurs, 16: 38–41, 1978.
43. Steinhart MJ: Treatment of delirium—A reappraisal. Int J Psychiatry Med, 9: 191–197, 1979.
44. Morris GO, Singer MT: Sleep deprivation: The context of consciousness. J Nerv Ment Dis, 143: 291–304, 1966.
45. Aita JA: Everyman's psychosis—The delirium. Nebr Med J, 53: 424–427, 1968.
46. Granacher RP, Baldessarini RJ: Physostigmine. Arch Gen Psychiatry, 32: 375–380, 1975.
47. Safer DJ, Allen RP: The central effects of scopolamine in man. Biol Psychiatry, 3: 347–355, 1971.
48. Greenblatt DJ, Shader RI: Anticholinergics. N Engl J Med, 288: 1215–1219, 1973.
49. Dysken MW, Merry W, Davis JM: Anticholinergic psychosis. Psychiatr Ann, 8: 452–456, 1978.
50. Spiker DG, Weiss AN, Chang SS, et al.: Tricyclic antidepressant overdose: Clinical presentation and plasma levels. Clin Pharmacol Ther, 18: 539–546, 1975.
51. Davies RK, Tucker GJ, Harrow M, Detre TP: Confusional episodes and antidepressant medications. Am J Psychiatry, 128: 95–99, 1971.
52. Heiser JF, Wilbert DE: Reversal of delirium induced by tricyclic antidepressant drugs with physostigmine. Am J Psychiatry, 131: 1275–1277, 1974.
53. Jenike MA: Anticholinergic delirium: Diagnosis and treatment. Topics Geriatr 1: 6–7, 1982.
54. Baldessarini RJ, Lipinski JF: Lithium salts: 1970–1975. Ann Intern Med, 83: 527⅓533, 1975.
55. Johnson GF: Lithium neurotoxicity. Aust NZ J Psychiatry, 10: 33–38, 1976.
56. Reisberg B, Gershon S: Side effects associated with lithium therapy. Arch Gen Psychiatry, 36: 879–887, 1979.
57. West AP, Meltzer HY: Paradoxical lithium neurotoxicity: A report of five cases and a hypothesis about risk for neurotoxicity. Am J Psychiatry, 136: 963–966, 1979.
58. Appelbaum PS, Shader RI, Funkenstein HH, Hanson MA: Difficulties in the clinical diagnosis of lithium toxicity. Am J Psychiatry, 136: 1212–1213, 1979.
59. Hoenig J, Chaulk R: Delirium associated with lithium and electroconvulsive therapy. Can Med Assoc J, 116: 837–838, 1977.
60. Mandel MR, Madsen J, Miller AL, Baldessarini RJ: Intoxication associated with lithium and ECT. Am J Psychiatry, 137: 1107–1109, 1980.
61. Reus VI: Behavioral side effects of medical drugs. Primary Care, 6: 283–294, 1979.
62. Shear MK, Sacks M: Digitalis delirium: Psychiatric considerations. Int J Psychiatr Med, 8: 371–381, 1978.
63. Shear MK, Sacks MH: Digitalis delirium: Report of two cases. Am J Psychiatry, 135: 109–110, 1978.
64. Portnoi VA: Digitalis delirium in elderly patients. J Clin Pharmacol, 19: 747–750, 1979.
65. Voltolina EJ, Thompson SI, Tisue J: Acute organic brain syndrome with propranolol. Clin Toxicol, 4: 357–359, 1971.
66. Kuhr BM: Prolonged delirium with propranolol. J Clin Psychiatry, 40: 198–199, 1979.
67. Kurland ML: Organic brain syndrome with propranolol. N Engl J Med, 300: 366, 1979.
68. Trimble MR, Reynolds EH: Anticonvulsant drugs and mental symptoms: A review. Psychol Med, 6: 169–178, 1976.
69. Sweet RD, McDowell FH, Fiegenson JS, et al.:

Mental symptoms in Parkinson's disease during chronic treatment with levodopa. Neurology, *26:* 305–310, 1976.

70. Lin J T-Y, Ziegler DK: Psychiatric symptoms with initiation of carbidopa-levodopa treatment. Neurology, *26:* 699–700, 1976.

71. Hausner RS: Amantadine-associated recurrence of psychosis. Am J Psychiatry, *137:* 240–242, 1980.

72. Hall RCW, Popkin MK, Stickney SK, Gardner ER: Presentation of the steroid psychoses. J Nerv Ment Dis, *167:* 229–236, 1979.

73. The Boston Collaborative Drug Surveillance Program: Acute adverse reactions to prednisone in relation to dosage. Clin Pharmacol Ther, *13:* 694–698, 1972.

74. Miller RR, Jick H: Clinical effects of meperidine in hospitalized medical patients. J Clin Pharmacol, *18:* 180–189, 1978.

75. Miller RR: Clinical effects of pentazocine in hospitalized medical patients. J Clin Pharmacol, *15:* 198–205, 1975.

76. Bernstein JG: Medical-psychiatric drug interactions, in Hackett TP, Cassem NH (eds): *Massachusetts General Hospital Handbook of General Hospital Psychiatry,* St. Louis, C. V. Mosby, 1978.

77. Knee ST, Razani J: Acute organic brain syndrome: A complication of disulfiram therapy: Am J Psychiatry, *131:* 1281–1282, 1974.

78. Weddington WW, Marks RC, Verghese JP: Disulfiram encephalopathy as a cause of the catatonia syndrome. Am J Psychiatry, *137:* 1217–1219, 1980.

79. Hotson JR, Langston JW: Disulfiram-induced encephalopathy. Arch Neurol, *33:* 141–142, 1976.

80. McMillen MA, Ambis D, Siegel JH: Cimetidine and mental confusion. N Engl J Med, *298:* 283–285, 1978.

81. Barnhart CC, Bowden CL: Toxic psychosis with cimetidine. Am J Psychiatry, *136:* 725–726, 1979.

82. Allen RM, Young SJ: Phencyclidine-induced psychosis. Am J Psychiatry, *135:* 1081–1083, 1978.

83. Showalter CV, Thornton WE: Clinical pharmacology of phencyclidine toxicity. Am J Psychiatry, *134:* 1234–1238, 1977.

84. Sellers EM, Kalant H: Alcohol intoxication and withdrawal. N Engl J Med, *294:* 757–762, 1976.

85. Thompson WL: Management of alcohol withdrawal syndromes. Arch Intern Med, *138:* 278–283, 1978.

86. Gross MM, Lewis E, Hastey J: Acute alcohol withdrawal syndrome, in Kissin H, Begleiter H (eds): *The Biology of Alcoholism,* vol. 3, New York, Plenum Press, 1973.

87. Wilker A: Diagnosis and treatment of drug dependence of the barbiturate type. Am J Psychiatry, *125:* 758–765, 1968.

88. Essig CF: Addiction to non-barbiturate sedative and tranquilizing drugs. Clin Pharmacol Ther, *5:* 334–343, 1964.

89. Maletzky BM, Klotter J: Addiction to diazepam. Int J Addict, *11:* 95–115, 1976.

90. DeBard ML: Diazepam withdrawal syndrome: A case with psychosis, seizure and coma. Am J Psychiatry, *136:* 104–105, 1979.

91. Winokur A, Rickles K, Greenblatt DJ, et al.: Withdrawal reaction from long-term, low-dosage administration of diazepam. Arch Gen Psychiatry, *37:* 101–105, 1980.

92. Stewart RB, Salem RB, Springer PK: A case report of lorazepam withdrawal. Am J Psychiatry, *137:* 113–114, 1980.

93. Flemenbaum A, Gunby B: Ethchlorvynol (Placidyl) abuse and withdrawal. Dis Nerv Syst, *32:* 188–192, 1971.

94. Heston LL, Hastings D: Psychosis with withdrawal from ethchlorvynol. Am J Psychiatry, *137:* 249–250, 1980.

95. Haizlip TM, Ewing JA: Meprobamate habituation. N Engl J Med, *258:* 1181–1186, 1958.

96. Ewart RBL, Priest RG: Methaqualone addiction and delirium tremens. Br Med J, *3:* 92–93, 1967.

97. Essig CF: Newer sedative drugs that can cause states of intoxication and dependence of the barbiturate type. JAMA, *196:* 126–129, 1966.

98. Shader RI, Caine ED, Meyer RE: Treatment of dependence on barbiturates and sedative-hypnotics, in Shader RI (ed): *Manual of Psychiatric Therapeutics,* Boston, Little, Brown & Co., 1975.

99. Clark ANG: Ectopic tachyarrhythmias in the elderly. Gerontol Clin, *12:* 203–212, 1970.

100. Fine W: Postural hypotension. Practitioner, *220:* 698–701, 1978.

101. Mesulam M-M: Acute behavioral derangements without hemiplegia in cerebrovascular accidents. Primary Care, *6:* 813–826, 1979.

102. Medina JL, Rubino FA, Ross E: Agitated delirium caused by infarctions of the hippocampal formation and fusiform and lingual gyri. Neurology, *24:* 1181–1183, 1974.

103. Fogalholm R, Heiskanen O, Waltimo O: Chronic subdural hematoma in adults. J Neurosurg, *42:* 43–46, 1975.

104. Potter JF, Fruin AH: Chronic subdural hematoma—The "great imitator." Geriatrics, *32:* 61–66, 1977.

105. Helmchen H: Reversible psychic disorders in epileptic patients, in Birkenmayer W (ed): *Epileptic Seizures-Behavior-Pain,* Bern, Huber, 1976.

106. Ellis JM, Lee SI: Acute prolonged confusion in later life as an ictal state. Epilepsia, *19:* 119–128, 1977.

107. Abrams R: Technique in ECT. Convulsive Ther Bull, *2:* 37–38, 1977.

108. Weiner RD, Whanger AD, Erwin CW, Wilson WP: Prolonged confusional state and EEG seizure activity following concurrent ECT and lithium use. Am J Psychiatry, *137:* 1452–1453, 1980.

109. Rosenbaum JF, Rothman JS, Murray GB: Psychosis and water intoxication. J Clin Psychiatry, *40:* 287–291, 1979.

110. Jose CJ, Perez-Cruet J: Incidence and morbidity of self-induced water intoxication in state mental hospital patients. Am J Psychiatry, *136:* 221–222, 1979.

111. Moses AM, Miller M: Drug-induced dilutional hyponatremia. N Engl J Med, *291:* 1234–1239, 1974.
112. Weitzel WD, Shraberg D, Work J: Inappropriate ADH: The role of drug re-challenge. Psychosomatics, *21:* 771–779, 1980.
113. Victor M, Adams RD, Collins GH: *The Wernicke-Korsakoff Syndrome,* Philadelphia, F. A. Davis Co., 1971.
114. Mitra ML: Confusional states in relation to vitamin deficiencies in the elderly. J Am Geriatr Soc, *19:* 536–545, 1971.
115. Strachan RW, Henderson JG: Psychiatric syndromes due to avitaminosis B12 with normal blood and marrow. Q J Med, *34:* 303–317, 1965.
116. Newsletter: Hyperthermia encore. Biol Ther Psychiatry, *1:* 39–40, 1978.
117. Dunn T, Arie T: Mental disturbance in the ill old person. Br Med J, *2:* 413–416, 1972.
118. Polly SM, Sanders WE: Surgical infections in the elderly: Prevention, diagnosis and treatment. Geriatrics, *32:* 88–97, 1977.
119. Editorial: Organic psychosis. Br Med J, *2:* 214–215, 1974.
120. Wilson LG: Viral encephalopathy mimicking functional psychosis. Am J Psychiatry, *133:* 165–170, 1976.
121. Stewart RM, Baldessarini RJ: Viral encephalopathy and psychosis. Am J Psychiatry, *133:* 717, 1976.
122. Anderson WH: The emergency department, in Hackett TP, Cassem NH (eds): *Massachusetts General Hospital Handbook of General Hospital Psychiatry,* St. Louis, C. V. Mosby Co., 1978.
123. Wells CE: Diagnosis of dementia. Psychosomatics, *20:* 517–522, 1979.
124. Murray GB: Confusion, delirium and dementia, in Hackett TP, Cassem NH (eds): *Massachusetts General Hospital Handbook of General Hospital Psychiatry,* St. Louis, C. V. Mosby Co., 1978.
125. Keller MB, Manschreck TC: Disorders of higher intellectual functioning, in Lazare A (ed): *Outpatient Psychiatry: Diagnosis and Treatment,* Baltimore, Williams & Wilkins, 1979.
126. Freedman BJ: The subjective experience of perceptual and cognitive disturbances in schizophrenia. Arch Gen Psychiatry, *30:* 333–340, 1974.
127. Vaillant GE: Prospective prediction of schizophrenic remission. Arch Gen Psychiatry, *11:* 509–518, 1964.
128. Peterson GC: Organic brain syndrome: Differential diagnosis and investigative procedures in adults. Psychiatr Clin North Am, *1:* 21–36, 1978.
129. Gelenberg AJ: The catatonic syndrome. Lancet, *1:* 1339–1341, 1976.
130. Ward NG, Rowlett DB, Burke P: Sodium amylobarbitone in the differential diagnosis of confusion. Am J Psychiatry, *135:* 75–78, 1978.
131. Santos AB, Manning DE, Waldrop WM: Delirium or psychosis? Diagnostic use of the sodium amobarbital interview. Psychosomatics, *21:* 863–864, 1980.
132. Manschreck TC, Petri M: The atypical psychoses. Cult Med Psychiatry, *2:* 233–268, 1978.
133. McCabe MS, Stromgren E: Reactive psychoses. Arch Gen Psychiatry, *32:* 447–454, 1975.
134. Carlson GA, Goodwin FK: The stages of mania. Arch Gen Psychiatry, *28:* 221–228, 1973.
135. Taylor MA, Abrams R: The phenomenology of mania. Arch Gen Psychiatry, *29:* 520–522, 1973.
136. Bond TC: Recognition of acute delirious mania. Arch Gen Psychiatry, *37:* 553–554, 1980.
137. Wells CE: Pseudodementia. Am J Psychiatry, *136:* 895–900, 1979.
138. Cavenar JO, Maltbie AA, Austin L: Depression simulating organic brain disease. Am J Psychiatry, *136:* 521–523, 1979.
139. Whitlock FA: The Ganser syndrome. Br J Psychiatry, *113:* 19–29, 1967.
140. Folstein MF, Folstein SE, McHugh PR: Minimental state. A practical method for grading the cognitive state of patients for the clinician. J Psychiatr Res, *12:* 189–198, 1975.
141. Pro JD, Wells CE: The use of the electroencephalogram in the diagnosis of delirium. Dis Nerv Syst, *38:* 804–808, 1977.
142. Obrecht R, Okomina FOA, Scott DF: Value of EEG in acute confusional states. J Neurol Neurosurg Psychiatry, *42:* 75–77, 1979.
143. Fenton G: The straightforward EEG in psychiatric practice. Proc R Soc Med, *67:* 911–919, 1974.
144. Hackett TP, Weisman AD: Psychiatric management of operative syndromes. I. The therapeutic consultation and the effect of noninterpretive intervention. Psychosom Med, *22:* 267–282, 1960.
145. Hackett TP, Weisman AD: Psychiatric management of operative syndromes. II. Psychodynamic factors in formulation and management. Psychosom Med, *22:* 356–372, 1960.
146. Lipowski ZJ: Delirium, in Conn HF (ed): *Current Therapy,* 27th ed., Philadelphia, W. B. Saunders, 1975.
147. Kiely WF: Psychiatric syndromes in critically ill patients. JAMA, *235:* 2759–2761, 1976.
148. Fauman MA: Treatment of the agitated patient with an organic brain disorder. JAMA, *240:* 380–382, 1978.
149. Gerdes L: The confused or delirious patient. Am J Nurs, *68:* 1228–1233, 1968.
150. Morris M, Rhodes M: Guidelines for the care of confused patients. Am J Nurs, *72:* 1630–1633, 1972.
151. Trockman G: Caring for the confused or delirious patient. Am J Nurs, *78:* 1495–1499, 1978.
152. Drummond L, Kirchhoff L, Scarbrough DR: A practical guide to reality orientation: A treatment approach for confusion and disorientation. Gerontologist, *18:* 568–573, 1978.
153. Bayne JRD: Management of confusion in elderly persons. Can Med Assoc J, *118:* 139–141, 1978.
154. Stedeford A: Understanding confusional states. Br J Hosp Med, *20:* 694–698, 1978.
155. Nadelson T: The psychiatrist in the surgical

intensive care unit. Arch Surg, *111:* 113–117, 1976.

156. Rynearson EK: The acute brain syndrome: A family affair. Psychiatr Ann, *7:* 77–83, 1977.
157. Weisman AD, Hackett TP: Psychosis after eye surgery. N Engl J Med, *258:* 1284–1289, 1958.
158. Mackenzie TB, Popkin MK: Stress response syndrome occurring after delirium. Am J Psychiatry, *137:* 1433–1435, 1980.
159. Godbole A, Falk M: Confrontation-problem solving therapy in the treatment of confusional and delirious states. Gerontologist, *12:* 151–154, 1972.
160. Moore DP: Rapid treatment of delirium in critically ill patients. Am J Psychiatry, *134:* 1431–1432, 1977.
161. Oldham AJ, Bott M: The management of ex-citement in a general hospital psychiatric ward by high dosage haloperidol. Acta Psychiatr Scand, *47:* 369–376, 1971.
162. Ayd FJ: Haloperidol: Twenty years' clinical experience. J Clin Psychiatry, *39:* 807–814, 1978.
163. Heshe E, Roeder E: Electroconvulsive therapy in Denmark. Br J Psychiatry, *128:* 241–245, 1976.
164. Roberts AH: The value of ECT in delirium. Br J Psychiatry, *109:* 653–655, 1963.
165. Guze SB, Daengsurisri S: Organic brain syndromes. Arch Gen Psychiatry, *17:* 365–366, 1967.
166. Liston EH: Delirium in the aged. Psychiatr Clin North Am *5:* 49–66, 1982.

chapter 7

dementia

Andrew E. Slaby, M.D., Ph.D., M.P.H.

DEFINITION

Dementia, like depression or mania, is a clinical syndrome, rather than a diagnostic entity. It has multiple etiologies. Dementia is defined as a chronic deterioration of intellectual ability secondary to malfunctioning of cerebral cortical or subcortical cells. The cardinal features of dementia are disturbances of memory (dysmnesia), disorientation, impairment of judgment, alteration in personality, and deterioration of other intellectual functioning.[1-18] The degree of reversibility depends on the extent, the location, and the character of CNS damage. Dementia may be classified as primary and secondary and as treatable and untreatable.[11]

The primary dementias are illnesses in which cognitive deterioration is a predictable part of the course of the disease state. Examples of primary dementias are Huntington's chorea, Alzheimer's disease, and Pick's disease. Secondary dementias are those illnesses in which cognitive deterioration is not a predictable predominant feature of an illness. Examples of secondary dementia are multiple sclerosis and meningiomas. The term "treatable" is used to refer to those dementias in which a therapeutic intervention, if propitiously timed, may reverse the course of cognitive deterioration or at least arrest further change. Examples of treatable dementias include normal pressure hydrocephalus, pernicious anemia, and hypothyroidism. Diseases in which the dementia associated with them may not be arrested or reversed are called untreatable. These include Alzheimer's disease, Pick's disease, Marchi-afava-Bignami disease, and multi-infarct dementia.

Case Example. Primary Dementia. Mrs. D., a 67-year-old widow, was referred for consultation because of increased seclusiveness, lack of personal hygiene, failure to eat regular meals, and increased concern that her family was plotting to take her property from her. A consulting psychiatrist was called by the family, and after some discussion it was felt that, given the patient's reluctance to leave her house, he should see her in her own home at teatime. On evaluation, she appeared to be a woman of faded elegance who spoke well but was disheveled and wore decidedly inappropriate clothing for her education and social background. She wore a torn dressing gown over a food-stained nightgown, nylons with runs, tattered bedroom slippers, and some old family jewelry. Mrs. D. had an excellent memory for the early years of her marriage and for the location of many shops, churches, and schools in the neighborhood where she had resided for her entire life. She did not, however, know the date, month, or year of the evaluation and did not recognize her own daughter (whom she referred to as her "godchild"). When family members left the room, she was more comfortable and expressed considerable concern over the fate of her property.

The consulting psychiatrist felt that admission to an inpatient psychiatric unit was indicated for full evaluation of the patient's deteriorating mental status, with a goal of identifying potentially treatable causes. This was discussed with family members, who concurred with the decision, but when plans were presented to her, the patient refused to follow the suggestion. The psychiatrist then spoke with her internist of several years' duration and with her family members and learned that Mrs. D. had maintained a close personal relationship with an old college friend, who saw her on a daily basis. This friend was contacted and asked to facilitate implementation of the treatment plan, since the patient was not certifiable by existing criteria, and the family preferred not to go through the courts if at all possible. The friend was able to get the patient to the hospital and, once she was there, Mrs. D. was persuaded to sign in.

In the hospital, Mrs. D. was more fearful but less paranoid. She was markedly disoriented to time, place, and person. Both recent and past memory were impaired, and her judgment was poor. Mrs. D. was unable to subtract serial sevens and provided concrete interpretations to all proverbs presented. Current knowledge of recent events was virtually nonexistent in the patient, although she was able to give considerable information about government changes and government policy in the 1930's and 1940's. She exhibited poor judgment and had difficulty with all calculations except those involving multiplication tables (e.g., "9 × 8 = 72") which are more a test of past remote memory than of an ability to calculate. Mrs. D. was concerned that people were trying to take things away from her but did not admit to any hallucinations, illusions, or other delusions. Physical examination was within normal limits except for mild elevation of blood pressure and frontal lobe signs (viz., palmomental reflex, snout reflex, and grasp reflex) on neurologic examination.

Skull films, serum electrolytes, triiodothyronine (T3), thyroxine (T4) and thyroid-stimulating hormone (TSH), complete blood cell count (CBC), serology, electrolytes, EKG, serum B12 level, serum protein, BUN, creatinine, serum glucose, liver studies, cerebrospinal fluid studies, and urine studies were all within normal limits. Electroencephalography showed diffuse generalized slowing bilaterally over the skull. A computerized axial tomography (CAT) scan provided evidence of symmetrical cerebral atrophy bilaterally. Neuropsychologic testing revealed marked evidence of organic impairment, which was most apparent in the Wechsler-Bellevue Adult Intelligence Scale (WAIS) and the Bender Visual-Motor Gestalt Test. Responses to the Rorschach Test included perseveration, confusion, prolonged reaction times, stereotypic responses, and a paucity of associations. Treatment focuses on the unit were (1) evaluation of patient's maximum level of functioning

and (2) work toward appropriate placement in a community health care facility. No treatable cause was identified. The patient was given low doses of an activating antipsychotic agent (i.e., perphenazine, 2 mg P.O. t.i.d.), with amelioration of the paranoid ideation and assuagement of the patient's agitation. Because of the patient's limitations, the social worker on the unit and the patient's primary nurse met with the family to plan appropriate placement and to help the family understand the patient's compromised functioning and need for a structural, nonstressful environment. A guardian of person was chosen with the aid of the patient's attorney, and appropriate placement was made in a nursing home staffed by members of a religious order whom the patient had known as a child and felt especially comfortable with.

PSEUDODEMENTIA

Pseudodementia is a term that refers to those disorders for which there are no identifiable neuropathologic changes apparent at necropsy.[11, 17, 18] These include hysteria, Ganser's syndrome ("pseudostupidity"), mania, depression, and schizophrenia. All these disorders may be mistaken for dementia, particularly if a patient is of advanced age. It is possible that some of what is now felt to be pseudodementia may someday prove to be organic in origin. Bleuler[19] astutely suggested early in this century, when he spoke of the "group of schizophrenias," that the thought disorders in all likelihood are not a monolithic entity. The form of schizophrenia sometimes referred to as "dementia praecox" may indeed be shown to have an organic basis. Depression can coexist with dementia, causing a greater apparent cognitive deficit than actually present. Studies indicate that a substantial number (viz., 8%–15%) of individuals initially diagnosed as demented are suffering from depressive illness.[20] Abrupt onset and previous depressive episodes, combined with a normal EEG, suggest coexistence of affective illness. Sodium amytal interviews may bring about verbalization of material of markedly depressive content without significantly increasing the manifestations of cognitive impairment and may serve to corroborate the diagnosis of functional illness.[21]

DIAGNOSIS AND DIFFERENTIAL DIAGNOSIS

Primary Dementia

In the dementias referred to as "primary," cognitive impairment is often a presenting symptom. The etiology of most of these diseases is uncertain, although in some, such as Huntington's chorea, there is a well-documented genetic trend. The symptoms seen are a result of cellular damage, the patient's attempt to adapt to these changes, other concurrent psychophysiologic processes, the patient's premorbid defenses, and the character of the patient's sociocultural matrix.

Diagnosis

In most patients with primary dementia the following symptoms are seen:

1. There is an insidious onset of cognitive changes of months' to years' duration that persists with variation when the environment is manipulated or when the patient is stressed.
2. Consciousness is not impaired except in extreme instances.
3. Disturbance of memory (dysmensia) is the principle feature. At first, the defect may be written off as "absentmindedness," and careful testing may be needed to document it. Recent memory goes before remote memory. Registration of new information, retention, and recall eventually become so impaired that acquisition of new skills becomes impossible. The individual increasingly relies on earlier learned sets of behavior.[1]
4. The patient is disoriented, first to time, then to place, and finally to person. At first a patient may skillfully hide the deficit by avoiding allusion to it, but as the dementia progresses, close friends and family go unrecognized, and the patients fail to know their own names.[13]
5. Judgment is impaired, and the patient loses a critical perspective on his own behavior, which is particularly upsetting to family and friends. Conduct may be totally incongruous with that seen premorbidly. Attention is no longer paid to the appropriateness of behavior. A patient may be careless with both money and dress. Judgment is a complex process entailing comprehension of data presented, weighing of alternatives, and formulation of appropriate plans of action. Individuals in positions in which decision-making has far-reaching implications are more likely to show impairment earlier than individuals with less demanding lives.
6. Personality change is often seen with dementia but alone cannot be construed as having an organic basis without the attendant changes in cognition. Affect may be altered, and a patient's premorbid defenses more pronounced. Someone who employs projection frequently (e.g., "Look what you made me do!") may become more paranoid. Tolerance to environmental changes is reduced, and the catastrophic reaction[20, 22] is observed. The latter is an unconscious defense against awareness of compromised intellectual capacities. The patient, when confronted with a task he cannot perform, responds with anxiety or rage despite initial affability.
7. A patient may be unable to abstract. Response to the test of similarities or interpretation of proverbs on mental status examination is concrete.
8. There is difficulty with calculations, such that the patient cannot subtract serial 7's or 3's. An examiner must be aware that asking simple addition or multiplication is often a test more of remote rote memory than ability to calculate.
9. Fund of knowledge is compromised. The patient does not usually know who the current presi-

dent is, nor does he know of recent newsworthy events. Again, caution must be exerted against testing in an area of a patient's own expertise, as one may be testing remote memory.

10. Attention may be impaired but not clouded. If a patient is delirious, one sees a fluctuating level of consciousness or clouded sensorium.[23] A demented person may just be so agitated that he is unable to register material at all. If so, the finding tends to be constant and not change over time.[24, 25]

Differential Diagnosis of Primary Dementia

Simple Dementia. This term is used for patients with a chronic organic mental syndrome without focal neurologic signs, primary psychotic symptoms, or evidence of one of the other dementias. On autopsy there is little evidence to support the diagnosis of another recognizable form of dementia such as Alzheimer's disease, Pick's disease, or Creutzfeldt-Jakob's disease. Onset of cognitive deterioration is insidious over the years with no other evidence of neurologic dysfunction.

Alzheimer's Disease.[11, 26–32] Clinical presentation of patients with Alzheimer's disease varies dependent upon the location and density of the pathologic lesions. Subtle changes in personality and insidious deterioration of memory occur early in the illness. The patient may present as depressed or flippant or superficial in conversation. Eventually, patients become disoriented and confused, with increasing lack of concern for appearance, work, and social propriety. Comprehension is diminished, and the patient may have difficulty finding words, calculating, and writing. Slurred speech, dysphagia, weakness, difficulty in sleeping, and seizures may also occur. Patients may wander from home. In the terminal stages, hallucinations, delusions, apraxia, extrapyramidal signs, and incontinence are common. Reductions in cortical choline acetyltransferase activity are reported[33] in biopsy and autopsy samples of brain in specific association with the classical neuropathological changes of Alzheimer's disease. This is not found consistently in multi-infarct dementia, as there appears to be no reduction in the number of muscarinic cholinergic receptors in Alzheimer's disease, suggesting that those intrinsic cortical cells which are postsynaptic to the dysfunctional or degenerating cholinergic afferents remain in tact. This raises the therapeutic possibility that the presynaptic deficit in cholinergic neurotransmission may be rectified with drugs that potentiate residual synaptic function (such as choline or acetylcholinesterase inhibitors) or that directly activate muscarinic receptors.[33]

Pick's Disease.[11, 32, 35] Some authors feel that clinically it is impossible to distinguish patients with Pick's disease from those with Alzheimer's disease. Those who contend that a separation is possible emphasize the fact that Pick's patients exhibit more apathy or insouciance, ostensibly because of the predominant involvement of the frontal lobes, while patients with Alzheimer's exhibit more irritability, agitation, and diffuse symptoms, given the more widespread cerebral atrophy and dissemination of lesions. In any event, the onset of Pick's disease is similar to that of Alzheimer's. Changes may be so subtle that they go unnoticed, with slight memory loss, loss of spontaneity, and difficulty in concentrating. At times, patients may appear euphoric. Aphasia is common, and memory for words may be less. Patients attempt to compensate by use of paraphrases. There is a marked diminution of initiative. Neurologic changes include visual and tactile agnosia, agraphia, spasticity, rigidity, and alexia. In the final state, cachexia, contractures, incontinence, bed sores and, sometimes, seizures are seen. Confabulation, delusions, and hallucinations are rare.

Creutzfeldt-Jakob's Disease.[11, 36–49] Cognitive deterioration coupled with pyramidal and extrapyramidal symptoms are the prominent features of this disease. The course is much more rapid than that of Alzheimer's or Pick's disease, with patients frequently dead in less than 12 months. The onset tends to be the middle years, earlier than for Alzheimer's or Pick's, and the clinical picture is more diffuse. The disease begins with patients presenting with vague complaints of odd or painful sensations, fatigue, difficulty concentrating, and memory loss, accompanied by nystagmus, ataxia, vertigo, dysarthria, and motor incoordination. There is a decreasing alertness and ability to attend to and to function in daily activities. After several weeks, signs of more severe mental impairment are coupled with other evidence of cortical, pyramidal, and extrapyramidal involvement. Muscle weakness, spastic ataxia, hyperactivity of deep tendon reflexes, extensor plantar responses, tremors, chorioathetotic movements, dysarthria, rigidity, and Parkinson-like symptoms are seen. Muscle wasting resembles that of amyotrophic lateral sclerosis. The patient is bedridden with urinary and fecal incontinence in the final stages.

Huntington's Chorea.[50-52] Marked mental deterioration may precede the onset of the movement disorder by years in patients with Huntington's chorea. An autosomal dominant affecting both sexes equally, this disease is characterized by personality changes, dementia, and chorioathetotic movements. Facial grimacing and involuntary twitches seen earlier, which tend to disappear when the patient is aware he is being observed, give way to explosive speech, athetosis, bizarre grimacing, and jerky choreiform movements first appearing in the upper extremities and neck. Gait is eventually impaired and takes on a grotesque dancing character due to the unpatterned movement of the lower extremities. Abnormal movements usually disappear with sleep and are enhanced when a patient is stressed. Swallowing is impaired as the disease progresses. In the final stages, the patient is bedridden.

Marchiafava-Bignami Disease (Primary Degeneration of the Corpus Callosum).[53, 54] This rare complication of alcoholism presents with dementia and signs of generalized or focal neurologic involvement. Personality changes, dysarthria, seizures, tremors, paraparesis, aphasia, and transitory hemiparesis are common. Terminally, there is wasting.

Schilder's Disease.[55] While children characteristically show dementia with cortical blindness with this rare disease,

adults may only show dementia or behavioral changes. This finding causes some to be misdiagnosed as having the "dementia praecox" form of schizophrenia.

Normal Pressure Hydrocephalus.[56-64] Dementia, ataxia, and fecal and/or urinary incontinence make up the triad of symptoms characterizing this disease. Sometimes there is a history of cerebral trauma or infection. The course is usually rapid over months, necessitating early diagnosis and treatment (with an atrioventricular shunt) if the cognitive deterioration is to be reversed.

Bechet's Disease.[11]

Kuf's Disease.[11]

Myoclonus Epilepsy and Subacute Dementia.[11]

Parkinsonism-Dementia Complex of Guam.[65-67]

Primary Parenchymatous Cerebellar Atrophy with Dementia.[11]

Progressive Supranuclear Palsy.[11]

Wilson's Disease.[68, 69]

Secondary Dementia

The secondary dementias, as mentioned earlier, are a group of diseases of known etiology in which dementia may, but not always, occur. Because a number of these are imminently treatable, it is incumbent upon the clinician to investigate the possibility of their occurrence and initiate appropriate therapy where possible.

Differential Diagnosis of Secondary Dementia[70-110]

Alcohol Encephalopathy.

Angioma.

Anoxia.

Arteriosclerosis.[77]

Barbiturate Abuse.

Bromide Intoxication.

Carbon Monoxide Intoxication.[104]

Cardiorespiratory Failure.

Cerebral Abscess.

Cerebral Concussion with Glial Scars.[70]

Cerebral Tuberculosis.

Cerebrovascular Syphilis.[80, 82, 98, 110]

Chronic Subdural Hematoma.[70, 108, 109]

Collagen Disease.[90]

Dementia Pugilistica.[70, 95, 99]

Electrolyte Imbalance.[81, 94]

Endocrinopathies.[86, 91, 105]

Epidemic Encephalitis.
General Paresis.[79, 80, 82, 98]
Hepatic Failure.
Hypoglycemia.
Intracranial Aneurysms.[86, 107]
Meningiomas.[74, 84]
Meningovascular Syphilis.[87]
Metastatic Tumors.
Multiple Myeloma.
Multiple Sclerosis.
Other Cerebral Infections.[78, 89]
Other Cerebral Trauma.[86, 93]
Postconcussion Syndrome.
Primary Cerebral
    Tumor.[72, 73, 92, 100, 101,102, 103]
Pseudodementia.
Renal Failure.[94]
Sarcoidosis.[96, 97]
Subacute Bacterial Endocarditis.
Vitamin Deficiencies.[71, 81, 88]

Case Example. Pseudodementia. A 76-year-old man with a history of alcohol abuse and mild liver dysfunction was transferred to the psychiatric unit for evaluation of the extent of his dementia and consideration of referral to a nursing home. The patient was reported to be fine until 5 days previous, when he fell and was admitted to the orthopedic service of a hospital. Shortly after admission he was noted to be confused, and it was assumed he had a stroke. History revealed he was somewhat forgetful but lived alone, making his own meals and doing his own shopping. A physical examination was relatively normal for his age, save for some liver enlargement and a fracture of his left ankle. On mental status, however, he was confused, disoriented to time, place, and person, and had impaired recent memory. He could not abstract and had a poor fund of knowledge. He denied hallucinations, delusions, illusions, and ideas of reference. He was on no medication save diazepam (Valium, 5 mg t.i.d.), which was prescribed to help manage him. The receiving clinician called the unit from which the patient was transferred as to his condition on arrival. The primary nurse who had been assigned to him stated that he was mildly disoriented on admission but became more markedly confused one day after. By checking the patient's medication record, it was discovered that the diazepam was ordered on the day of admission. It was discontinued, and 2 days later the patient became oriented to place and person but not to time. He had moderately good recent memory and excellent past memory. He was no longer confused and was able to give the last five Presidents' names and to perform simple calculations. A more extensive evaluation of the patient failed to render any major medical or psychiatric problems, except for mild dementia and elevated liver enzymes. He was discharged home with a diagnosis of mild organic mental syndrome and impaired liver function, both attributed to excessive alcohol use.

EPIDEMIOLOGY[111–131]

There are few epidemiologic studies of dementia per se. Dementia is not a disease in itself but rather a symptom of many diseases, some of which are incompletely understood, such as Pick's and Alzheimer's diseases, and others, like Huntington's chorea, which are fairly well defined clinically. The principle difficulty in detailing the natural history of forms of dementia is that they are confused clinically early, and accurate diagnosis is possible in many cases only by cerebral biopsy prior to death or at autopsy. Not all cases come to autopsy and/or are identified later in their course, making a definition of their early onset and natural history difficult, if not impossible, at the time.

Incidence and Prevalence

The actual incidence and prevalence of dementia in the general population is difficult to estimate epidemiologically. Many cases go unreported because impairment is minimal or because a primary diagnosis of another disorder is tendered. Furthermore, there still exists considerable confusion clinically as to the exact nature of a cause of an organic mental syndrome. Alzheimer's disease, once thought to be "presenile dementia" (i.e., dementia occurring before the senium, viz., the period of life after age 65) is now known to be a disease itself, characterized by specific neuropathologic changes that may occur at any age. Seventy-five percent of geriatric patients admitted to a public psychiatric institute for the first time are said to have a chronic organic mental syndrome,[112] or 10–20% of the elderly in general. Of these, dementia of the Alzheimer's type accounts for at least 50% of the cases seen[111, 132] with each decade in life and is, in fact, more frequent in the senium than in the presenium. It is fortunately quite rare but nevertheless more common than Pick's disease, from which it is clinically difficult to distinguish. The ratio between the two is about 5:2 (Alzheimer's disease/Pick's disease) at post-mortem. Huntington's chorea and Creutzfeldt-Jakob's disease are even more rare. In the former instance, save for sporadically occurring aberrant cases, only those with a family history of it would be expected to develop it, as the gene for Huntington's chorea is an autosomal dominant. Creutzfeldt-Jakob's disease is quite rare. The incidence of normal pressure hydrocephalus is probably underestimated. It may develop following occult cerebral infections as well as trauma. It should be considered in every evaluation of patients with dementia as cognitive, and other changes may be entirely reversible if the disease is diagnosed and patients are given a ventriculoatrial shunt.

Age

Alzheimer's and Pick's diseases are rare before age 40. The evidence of both increases with each decade of life. The mean age of onset of Creutzfeldt-Jakob disease is in the middle adult years, remarkably earlier than Pick's or Alzheimer's. Huntington's chorea has its onset in the mid-30's, thereby making genetic counseling difficult, as many individuals have children prior to its onset. The age of onset of normal pressure hydrocephalus correlates with that of cerebral trauma in the young adult years, although cases also result from cerebrovascular accidents later in life and from infections at any time.

Sex

Alzheimer's disease, Creutzfeldt-Jakob's disease, and Huntington's chorea are said to affect men and women equally. Pick's disease is different, in that women are affected more frequently than men. Normal pressure hydrocephalus is said to occur more frequently with men because of their more frequent exposure to cerebral trauma at work and in athletic endeavors.

Race

Alzheimer's disease, Pick's disease, Creutzfeldt-Jakob's disease, normal pressure hydrocephalus, and Huntington's chorea are seen in all ethnic and racial groups.

Socioeconomic Status

Although the dementias are seen in all social classes, the lack of proper nourishment and attendant medical problems seen in the lower social economic class contribute to both exaggerating symptoms when they exist and to increasing the likelihood of the illnesses in an almost arithmetic way. An individual who is mildly impaired cognitively because of Alzheimer-related changes in his or her brain may show more rapid deterioration if vitamin deficiencies due to lack of proper nourishment occur, or if he has infections and other illnesses, such as unattended hearing or visual loss, superimposed. Alcoholism is seen in all social classes and may alone cause a chronic organic mental syndrome, as well as be a contributing factor in others.[133, 134]

THEORIES OF ETIOLOGY

Biologic Factors

There are no specific laboratory tests to confirm the diagnosis of dementia. Studies of indoleamine and catecholamine metabolism have suggested that the concentrations of homovanillic acid (the o-methylated acid metabolite of dopamine) and 5-hydroxyindoleacetic acid (the principle metabolite of serotonin) are diminished in patients with senile and presenile dementias.[11, 135–139] Scores on a number of psychological rating scales, in fact, have been found to negatively correlate with the concentration of these two metabolites. The greater the deterioration, the lower the concentrations. Decreased homovanillic acid has also been found at necropsy in the brains of some demented patients.

Blood flow studies are not practical as diagnostic tools but, overall, cerebral blood flow has been found to be reduced, together with gray matter weight, in patients with dementia, regardless of cause. The reduction is proportional to the level of intellectual deterioration and is usually accompanied by decreased total mean cerebral oxygen uptake.[140, 141]

There are a number of identifiable neuropathologic changes specific to the various dementias that are useful in diagnosing a patient when a cerebral biopsy is taken or in confirming a diagnosis at autopsy. These include the following.

Alzheimer's Disease

This disease is characterized by the presence of numerous miliary cortical lesions. These silver-staining lesions are called Alzheimer plaques. Alois Alzheimer, who first described the disease in 1907, thought it was an example of early onset senility. Today we know this is not true. While the diseases (i.e., senile dementia and Alzheimer's disease) resemble each other clinically, Alzheimer's differs from the former by having a higher concentration of plaques and neurofibrillary tangles, especially in areas such as the hippocampus, which is associated with recent memory.[11, 27, 31] The brain shows diffuse cortical atrophy, and there is dilation of the entire ventricular system. Reduction in brain weight is greater than in senile dementia. Both neuronal loss and glial proliferation are present. Although the argentophilic plaques and neurofibrillary tangles are found predominantly in the cerebral cortex, they also occur to a lesser degree elsewhere in the brain. On electronmicroscopic examination, the neurofibrillary tangles are found to be composed of large numbers of tightly packed, normal neurofilaments coursing through the cytoplasm, displacing other cytoplasmic organelles. The plaques themselves contain a central core composed of amyloid fibrils and are found in the gray matter of the cerebral cortex.

Pick's Disease

Atrophy in Pick's disease tends to be well-circumscribed and limited to the frontal and temporal regions of the brain. Enlarged, balloon-shaped cell bodies with round globular argentophilic intraneuronal inclusions are found together with gliosis and neuronal degeneration. Neuronal loss is particularly great in the outer layers of the cortex. The etiology of these changes is unknown.

Creutzfeldt-Jakob's Disease

Creutzfeldt-Jakob's disease is characterized by moderate symmetrical cerebral atrophy, diffuse neuronal loss, glial proliferation, and a spongy appearance to the cerebral cortex referred to as status spongiosus. Comparable changes are found in the thalamus, cerebellum, basal ganglia, bulbar motor neurons, and anterior horn cells. Electronmicroscopic studies indicate that the status spongiosus is due to dilation of cell bodies of both neurons and astrocytes and their processes without expansion of the extracellular space. The exact etiology of the illness remains, but it appears a slow virus is the pathogen. Creutzfeldt-Jakob's disease can be transmitted to laboratory animals, and virus-like particles resembling certain myxoviruses have been demonstrated by electronmicroscopy.[11, 96]

Marchiafava-Bignami Disease

Bilateral symmetrical demyelination of the corpus callosum, anterior and posterior commissures, and other areas of white matter with sparing of the gray matter characterize the disease first described by Marchiafava and Bignami in 1903.[54] The etiology is unknown. Ingestion of a crude red Italian wine may play a role.

Huntington's Chorea

Huntington's chorea is characterized pathologically by widespread changes in the cerebral cortex and basal ganglia.[142] The caudate, putamen, and frontal and precentral cortex are especially involved. The brain appears atrophic, and the ventricles are dilated. Replacement gliosis and neuronal loss are found histologically. The disease may be due to a genetically determined deficiency of gamma aminobutyric acid (GABA) in the basal ganglia. In addition to GABA, homocarnosine and glutaric acid-decarboxylase are reduced, and glycerophosphoethanolamine is increased in the substantia nigra, putamen, globus pallidus, and caudate nucleus.[51, 52]

Summary

Alzheimer's disease accounts for nearly 50% of chronic organic mental syndromes seen in older people. The other clinical syndromes presenting with dementia, except for those associated with atherosclerotic cerebrovascular disease and alcohol use, are seen considerably less frequently. Diagnosis can usually be made at postmortem if not premorbidly by characteristic neuropathologic changes. The etiology of most dementias remains obscure. A slow virus has been posited as the putative etiologic agent in Creutzfeldt-Jakob's disease and a genetically determined deficiency of GABA in the basal ganglia in Huntington's chorea.

Genetic Factors

With the exception of Huntington's chorea and the Parkinsonism-dementia complex of Guam,[66] most of the dementias occurring in the presenium and senium do not have a major genetic component in their etiology.[11] Huntington's disease is inherited as a Mendelian dominant. Sporadic cases without a family history have been reported but are rare. The original patients described by Huntington[142] in his practice in East Hampton, Long Island, were found to descend from three men who immigrated from Suffolk, England, in about 1630. Most cases of Pick's and Alzheimer's diseases are believed to occur sporadically.[11] A variant of Pick's may be inherited as an autosomal dominant, and in some families there appears to be some genetic inclination for the occurrence of Alzheimer's disease. Alzheimer changes in the brain have been reported in some patients with mongolism[26, 143, 144] who survive to adulthood. It is uncertain whether these cases are instances in which the two diseases occur together or whether Alzheimer-like changes in the brain are a predictable part of mongolism in adults.

Summary

The most frequently occurring dementias, with the exception of Huntington's chorea, are not felt to have a major genetic component in their etiology. Huntington's disease is transmitted as an autosomal dominant such that nearly 50% of men and women in affected families are expected to manifest some form of the disease during their life.

Psychological Factors

No instances of true dementia are caused by purely psychological factors.[116] Psychosocial variables do influence the intensity[120, 121, 145, 146] and frequency of symptoms in affected individuals. Depression, schizohrenia, Ganser's syndrome, and malingering may present as pseudodementia. Individuals respond unconsciously to an internal biological threat to the integrity of their person much as they do to an external psychological or social threat.[17] Defenses become more rigid and pronounced. In extreme instances, such as with the catastrophic reaction,[22] management becomes difficult without the use of family counseling, consultation to attending staff, and/or psychotropic medication.[11, 145] A previously fairly orderly and neat individual may become severely obsessive-compulsive as he deteriorates. Individuals who projected a good deal in their premorbid state (e.g., attributed to others the cause of difficulties they were primarily responsible for bringing onto themselves) become paranoid. Structure, routine, and reduction of environmental tension allow a patient to function at maximal capacity.

Familial/Environmental Factors

Nongenetic familial environmental factors enhance or diminish manifest symptoms.[11, 17, 22, 120, 121, 126, 147, 148] Families often feel threatened psychologically, financially (due to the loss of a wage earner as well as due to cost of care of a chronic debilitating illness) and, sometimes, physically, if the patient has violent outbursts. Suicide is greater in families with Huntington's chorea, both in individuals affected with the illness, as well as in nonaffected relatives. Support of families and education as to the nature of patients' illness and as to how environmental changes and tension affect symptoms adversely are an integral part of any inpatient treatment program. Ventilation of feelings of anger, frustration, loss, and depression by nonaffected members reduce tension and facilitate the creation of a structured environment with sufficient routine and minimal tension to allow the patient to operate at the highest level he can.

BIOPSYCHOSOCIAL EVALUATION

Biologic Evaluation[11, 17]

The first step in the evaluation of a patient with dementia is an attempt to identify treatable causes of the chronic organic mental syndrome.[149]

History

The acquisition of a reliable and accurate case history from patients with dementia presents a challenge to the clinician. In addition to the obvious fact that someone with impairment of memory cannot be relied upon to give a detailed history, obtaining a history from close relatives is also often difficult.[11, 17] Cognitive deterioration, with the exception of more rapidly progressing lesions such as subdural hematomas and fast-growing tumors, is usually insidious. Denial of impairment by patients is reinforced by a family's need to deny that a cherished relative is deteriorating, often at a relatively young age. Rapid change in environment eliciting a catastrophic reaction or superimposition of trauma, aspiration, infection, or other physical insult may draw attention to the impairment. Etiologic status may be attributed to events that merely expose the handicap of a patient.[11] Relatives may find it easier to accept an intercurrent traumatic insult that does not imply continued deterioration as the cause of a patient's difficulty, rather than to accept the fact that they must face the inexorable deterioration of someone they love.

It is helpful to obtain an impression of a patient's premorbid personality from friends, relatives, and employers in order to understand the psychodynamic basis of a patient's response pattern to the loss (e.g., a suspicious person becoming increasingly paranoid) and also to obtain clues as to etiology (e.g., history of remissions and exacerbations in patients with multiple sclerosis).

Information which may be helpful to the examiner includes a history of dementia in the family as well as a personal history of seizures, cerebrovascular disease, infections (e.g., tuberculosis and syphilis), subacute bacterial endocarditis, pulmonary disease, nutritional deficiency, foreign travel, tumor elsewhere in the body (especially in the lungs or breasts[73]), craniotomy, pernicious anemia, alcoholism,[133, 134] drug addiction,[150] and transient ischemic attacks.[11, 17] Patient's relatives should be queried as to a family or personal history of schizophrenia and affective illness which may have presented as pseudodementia. Documentation of changes that occurred in an individual's behavior provide indicia of the rate of deterioration and clues to etiology. Dates of onset of symptoms such as convulsions and memory lapses allow evaluation for duration of illness.[11] In order to obtain this type of information, it is often necessary to question people such as employers who are not as close as the patient's immediate family members, who themselves may have a vested interest in denying the illness.[11, 17] In addition to the history of the present illness and personal and family histories, a review of systems should be undertaken. This serves both to reveal the primary nature of the disease as well as coexisting conditions which may exaggerate the patient's impairment. Information regarding any changes in the patient's vision or hearing should be obtained from the patient or his relatives. Sleep disturbance, depressed mood, anorexia, constipation, psychomotor retardation, and impotence suggest an affective component.

Is there a history of sinusitis or mastoiditis (a possible source of infection that may give rise to a brain abscess) or of recurrent infections, especially respiratory (a not unusual site for origin of a septic embolus to the brain). Symptoms such as weight loss, hemoptysis, cough, or night sweats may indicate tuberculosis or carcinoma of the lungs, which may have metastasized before the primary is diagnosed. Urinary symptoms may indicate the presence of a renal tumor such as a hypernephroma, which can metastasize widely to the CNS. Pedal edema and dyspnea suggest cardiovascular disease, which influences the status of the cerebral circulation.

Clues as to the possible role of drugs, metals, and toxins such as carbon monoxide, heavy metals, or even alcohol may be obtained in an occupational history.[149] Medications a patient is currently taking or has been using in the past (e.g., bromides) are also important to document. Older people are vulnerable to effects of toxic and metabolic disorders. A mild organic mental syndrome may be exaggerated by relatively minor fluctuations in metabolic status.[149]

Mental Status Examination

The mental status examination of a demented person entails both general observation of mien and style of interacting with the examiner as well as specific diagnostic techniques to bring out focal deficits.

Memory is assessed indirectly by observation of the coherence and consistency of patients' statements. Attention should be paid to recall of both recent and remote events. Organic deterioration of cerebral functioning is first reflected in the inability to recall recent material, with remote memory remaining intact.[1, 70] Retention can be evaluated by giving the patient three objects to remember and asking him a few minutes later to recall them.

Attention and immediate recall are evaluated by asking a patient to repeat forward and backward a string of digits stated at the rate of 1 per second.

Orientation is evaluated by directly asking the patient the date, where he is, and who he and the examiner are. If correct answers are proffered for all three, the individual is said to be oriented to time, place, and person. Deterioration affects the three in order of the foregoing sequence, with disorientation to person generally being the last affected.

Fund of knowledge is educationally dependent. Information, least dependent on formal education, should, therefore, be used. Most people, regardless of level of formal education, will be able to name five large cities or give the significance of major holidays. Insight is evaluated by a patient's awareness of why he is being examined and by the appropriateness of his behavior.

Judgment is assessed by standard questions as to what the patient would do if he found a stamped, addressed envelope or detected smoke in a movie theater. Similarities and proverbs are used to evaluate the ability to abstract.

Evidence of mood changes and other symptoms indicative of nonorganic psychopathology should be sought. Severe retarded depression presents with apathy, paucity of thought, psychomotor retardation, and impairment of concentration and memory suggestive of dementia.

Specific deficits may enable localization and thereby facilitate diagnosis.[2] Lesions of the major hemispheres may produce impairment of language or conceptualization, while minor hemispheric lesions tend to produce symptoms limited to the contralateral field such as neglect of the left side.[11] Gerstmann's syndrome (acalculia, agraphia, finger agnosia, and right-left confusion) is said to indicate a lesion of the angular and supramarginal gyri of the dominant hemisphere. Neglect of the left side, as seen in lesions of the right parietal lobe, may be documented by asking a patient to draw the face of a clock. The left side of the clock face (numbers 6 through 12) may be distorted or absent in the presence of a right parietal lesion.[11]

Subtlety of changes in the early stages of some dementias cannot be overstated. Detection of impairment in individuals who have developed a great repertoire of skills which have since become nearly automatic in behavior is more difficult than recognizing impairment in relatively simple people with a limited number of acquired skills or verbal facilities. As people grow older, speed of thinking may slow down, but performance is maintained because years of experience have minimized the need for innovation in thinking.

Physical Examination

Frequent physical examination is needed to provide clues to etiology, to document change, and to provide evidence of rapidity of course of illness.[4, 8] Subtler signs of cerebral deterioration should be sought, in addition to the usual examination of cranial nerves, reflexes, gait and station, and sensory and motor function.[149] As demented patients deteriorate, they begin to display reflexes often referred to as "developmental" or "primitive."[11, 17] These reflexes are usually found early in life but disappear as the nervous system matures. With age or presence of disease, these reflexes may recur. They include the grasp reflex, the palmomental reflex, gegenhalten (hypertonia), the snout reflex, the sucking reflex, and the corneomandibular reflex. These reflexes are thought to represent release phenomena, as they appear to be present only in the presence of higher cortical dysfunction. Stereognosis, graphesthesia, texture discrimination, weight discrimination, two-point discrimination, sensory extinction, and aphasia indicate changes in specific higher central functions.[24] Focal deficits suggest an intracranial mass. Normal pressure hydrocephalus should be considered with spasticity or ataxia of the lower limbs. A toxic or metabolic disorder is indicated by coexistence of peripheral neuropathy and dementia. Resting tremor, choreoathetosis, and rigidity are seen with extrapyramidal disorders. Myoclonus, postural tremor, and asterixis suggest a toxic-metabolic disorder.

Laboratory Studies

Routine Studies. CBC and differential; urinalysis; erythrocyte sedimentation rate; serum test for syphilis; blood glucose; serum electrolytes; liver function studies; creatinine; calcium and phosphorus; BUN; T_3; T_4 and TSH; and bilirubin.

Special Studies. Screen of urine for potential toxins (e.g., bromides, lead) serum vitamin B_{12} level; lumbar puncture; protein electrophoresis; serum cholesterol; serum levels of copper and ceruloplasmin; urine porphobilinogen; urinary copper; urine 17-hydroxysteroids; and serum folate.

Radiologic Studies

Routine Studies. Chest film.
Special Studies. Skull series; CT.[151–153]

Special Studies

EEG (with wake and sleep tracings)[154–156] EKG; audiometry; visual field examination; cerebral angiography[141]; and cerebral biopsy.

Psychological Evaluation[11]

The presence of and change in intellectual impairment can be documented by standard tests of cognitive capacity such as the Bender-Gestalt Test, the Wechsler-Bellevue Intelligence Test, the Porteus Maze Test, and the Vigotsky Test. Projective examinations such as the Rorschach and Thematic Apperception Test provide information as to the extent to which psychological factors contribute to the picture of mental impairment. Patients with organic brain disease taking the Rorschach Test show confusion, perseveration, stereotypic responses, a low number of responses due to paucity of associations, an increased number of pure form responses, and the presence of color-naming responses. On the Goodenough Draw-a-Man Test, in which an individual's ability to draw a picture of someone of the same and of the opposite sex is compared to that of other people, a patient with a defect such as blindness in one eye omits a drawing of that eye. As with other tests, patients with brain damage exhibit perseveration, tremulousness, and loss of control while attempting to perform.

Social Evaluation

While familial dynamics do not serve as primary etiologic factors in the development of dementias, interviews with family members are important in ascertaining:

1. An understanding of the degree of and rate of deterioration of a patient
2. The role family members may play in enhancing or diminishing intensity of symptoms
3. An understanding of whether there is a family history of affective illness or schizophrenia which may alone or in addition to organic disease cause dementiform symptoms.

HOSPITAL TREATMENT

Specific Treatment

In addition to general approaches that may be used in the management of all patients with a dementiform illness, there are a number of specific measures that are applicable in specific cases.[11] For example, vitamin B complex, withdrawal of alcohol, and appropriate diet are used in the management of dementia, presenting as part of alcoholic encephalopathy. Amantidine[36, 45] and vidarabine[157] have been suggested in the management of Creutzfeldt-Jakob's disease because of their slow virus etiology. Ventriculoatrial shunting is used for normal pressure hydrocephalus,[57] and penicillin is used for dementia secondary to syphilis.[82, 98, 158] Thyroid replacement therapy[105] is used for myxedema and vitamin B_{12} for pernicious anemia.[71, 87, 88]

Individual Psychotherapy

Any attempt at verbal intervention with patients later in the course of the dementia is thwarted because of the patient's deteriorated cognitive functioning. Supportive psychotherapy with less emphasis on exploration of intrapsychic conflict and more on reinforcement of adaptive defenses early in the course of the illness, however, may be and often is useful. Patients and families benefit from emotional support provided at a time when options seem limited and from the direction provided by a skillful therapist in helping them to prioritize their needs and to separate the realities of the illness from the fantasies. A patient's awareness of inevitable doom in diseases such as Huntington's chorea may lead to a severe depression early that will act synergistically with dementia and further compromise the little capacity the patients may have to function at work or at home. Thoughts of suicide are not infrequent in patients who become aware of the meaning of the early mental and neurological changes. Because psychiatric symptoms may precede crippling neurologic dysfunction, active supportive psychotherapy and use of appropriate psychotropic drugs may facilitate functioning for months or years.

Family Therapy

Active counseling and supportive psychotherapy are important in enabling families to adjust to patients' illnesses. Senile dementias may be anticipated in the elderly, but the occurrence of dementia in early and middle years is usually unexpected, except in instances such as Huntington's chorea in which there are family histories of the illness. It is extremely difficult to see someone you have loved deteriorate before your eyes. While much of the behavior seen may be considerably different from that of the premorbid personality, enough of the old personality usually remains the same or is exaggerated, so as to cause family and friends to be at the same time drawn toward the person and yet unable to accept some of his uncharacteristic behavior. Spouse and children may, with time, be overcome with a sense of abandonment. This is especially true when the dementia occurs in the presenium. A wife may be distraught with the thought or reality of being left with a family to raise and no source of income. Spouses may be concerned over the fate of young children if a young parent is affected. The financial drain on the family of having a patient with a chronic illness is a further source of anxiety.

It is necessary, if an illness is only partially treatable, as in a resectable tumor or syphilis, to help patients and their families to adjust to residual impairment. Where deterioration is inevitable, it is helpful to work with family members to deal realistically with patients' behaviors (e.g., urinary or fecal incontinence) and to offer assistance in future planning. Ultimately, it is usually necessary to help families to plan for terminal care at home or elsewhere.

Food Intake

Demented patients are negligent of food intake, particularly if they have lived alone. Vitamin deficiencies may develop and contribute to mental impairment primarily caused by another disease process. Frequent weighing may be necessary to determine food intake. Hydration is sometimes a problem. Skin turgor and other clinical signs of hydration should be monitored. Supplementing vitamins (e.g., thiamine, vitamin B complex) may be helpful. When dysphagia is present, a semisoft or soft diet may be needed. Tube feedings with a liquid diet may be necessary if swallowing is markedly impaired.

Physical Therapy

Vigorous physiotherapy combined with muscle relaxants enhances patients' comfort and maximizes functioning. Spasticity to the extent of spontaneous clonus may be a prominent sign and may be mitigated by range of motion exercises or muscle relaxants. Efforts should be made to minimize sensory stimuli, such as distention of the bladder or abrasions to the skin, which may precipitate spasms. Supplementary devices, such as footdrop braces, are helpful for patients with weakness of the hands, jaws, neck, feet, etc. Patients having difficulty talking while retaining a certain modicum of cognitive functioning may be enabled to continue to function by communicating with the use of a writing pad. Dysarthria can be particularly frightening to a patient who remains alert, for it creates a frustrating isolation for those about him which need not exist if other forms of communication, such as touching and writing, are developed.

Environmental Engineering

Demented patients do poorly when sensory input is decreased or environments are changed. It is important, therefore, that the individual have glasses of the correct prescription and hearing aids if required. Quiet dark nights are especially frightening to patients. A small night lamp helps in keeping a patient oriented and in reducing anxiety. If placement in an institutional setting becomes necessary, the introduction of familiar objects from home, such as a family photograph, a favorite bed lamp, a religious statue, and other cherished items from a patient's own bedroom or house, facilitates functioning in a new environment. Finally, frequent visits by well-recognized and often seen relatives and friends minimizes the fear of abandonment which is enhanced by paranoia in some patients as they deteriorate. Reality therapy aimed at reorienting a demented person and returning him to current reality has been employed with equivocal success.[158, 159] Comparable questions have been raised concerning the efficacy of other behavior modification techniques.[158] Gains, when made, appear to be modest, unrelated to the degree of dementia, specific, not maintained after termination of treatment, and dependent on active patient involvement. When misemployed, reality-oriented therapy and other behavioral techniques can cause more problems than they can solve.[159]

Management of Intercurrent Infections

Debilitated patients are particularly prone to infection. Demented patients must be observed carefully. Early signs of changes may be harbingers of fatal infection. Intermittent physical examinations as dictated by a patient's condition, and appropriate laboratory studies are needed. Careful attention to nutritional needs,

changing of a patient's catheters, pulmonary toilet, and development of decubiti reduce the incidence of infection.

Genetic Counseling

In families riddled by hereditary forms of dementia, individuals who are contemplating having children might find genetic counseling helpful regarding the likelihood that they or their offspring will develop the illness. This is difficult with family members who are about to marry and who are still below the age when the disease is likely to manifest itself. For instance, the mean age of onset of Huntington's chorea is estimated to be 35 years, 10–15 years beyond the usual age most individuals marry for the first time (i.e., at 20–25 years), and the risk of getting the disease caused by an autosomal dominant is approximately 50%.

Human genetic counseling is in a nascent phase. There are many ethical and religious issues raised that increase knowledge of how genetic illnesses are transmitted. These are not easy or even always answerable. Indeed, as our knowledge becomes greater, these issues may become more difficult.

Bed Care

The usual precautions must be taken to avoid bedsores, hypostatic pneumonia, macerations secondary to soiling, and other problems secondary to limited ambulation once a patient becomes bedridden. The nursing staff directly involved in daily care shoulders this responsibility in most nursing homes and hospitals. Little may be done to arrest or reverse the course of many dementias but much can be done in a patient's last days to make him comfortable and to maintain a certain modicum of human dignity.[160]

Where arrest or some reversal of a course of a dementiform process is possible (e.g., by atrioventricular shunting in cases of normal pressure hydrocephalus), it is necessary to help patients maximize remaining functioning capacity. Education of patients and relatives may be required to direct individuals to employment, that they may be able to cope with, given the compromised level of functioning. Continued efforts should be made to enhance level of cognitive functioning. Increase in self-esteem along with what may appear to be only miniscule progress to those around a patient is an important part of therapy.

Custodial Care

Institutionalization is often necessary in the final stages of a dementia because of the constant attention a patient needs. Friends and family members need help in how to logistically effect this (e.g., Where should one send a patient? How is such care paid for?) and with their own feelings of guilt, helplessness, and despair when such a turn becomes necessary.

Psychopharmacotherapy[145–169]

No specific medications have been identified which are helpful in reversing or controlling the course of dementia in general. Psychotropic agents, however, provide symptomatic relief. Small doses of activating phenothiazines and drugs such as haloperidol (e.g., 1 mg b.i.d. or t.i.d.), thiothixene (e.g., 1–2 mg b.i.d. or t.i.d.), molindone (e.g., 5 mg b.i.d. or t.i.d.), perphenazine (e.g., 2 mg b.i.d. or t.i.d.) and loxapine (i.e., 5 mg b.i.d.) may bring about remarkable improvement in a patient's mental status.[3, 11, 161, 163, 164, 169] Neuroleptics are effective in managing emotional lability, uncooperativeness, anxiety, and excitement. Patients with the most severe symptoms appear to benefit the most.[161, 164, 167] Liquid medication or a decanoate form may be needed to enhance compliance.[169] Antidepressants such as amitriptyline, imipramine, desipramine, trazodone, and doxepin in appropriate doses (e.g., 10–25 mg b.i.d.) may be used with patients presenting with signs of depression (e.g., difficulty in falling asleep, early morning awakening, sleep interruption, anorexia, weight loss, and psychomotor retardation).[162, 165] Special care must be exercised in using psychotropic medications in demented patients, especially when older or wasted, as they are more vulnerable to side effects such as urinary retention, hypotension, confusion, and extrapyramidal symptoms. A sudden change in mental status may occur in such a population due to a number of effects,

including sedation (the so-called "paradoxical effect"), hypotension leading to decreased cerebral flood flow, atropine psychosis, changes in cardiac rhythm with inconstant cerebral blood flow and anxiety, and urinary retention or constipation leading to increased anxiety and confusion. Treatment of mood and personality change is especially important in patients in whom mental changes may precede neurological deterioration by several years, such as in patients with Pick's disease or Huntington's chorea. The impact of effects of the physiology of aging on pharmacokinetics and the likelihood of severe side effects dictate that lower dosages should be employed.[162] If increase in medication is required, it should be done gradually, using serum levels coupled with clinical response as a guide.

Psychostimulants, such as methylphenidate (10 mg twice per day), have been suggested for use in demented patients who are depressed, in situations in which medical condition, intolerance to anticholinergic side effects, or patient or family preferences militate against the use of tricyclic antidepressants or electroconvulsive shock. Adverse side effects such as palpitations, hypertension, cardiac arrhythmias, nervousness, headaches, insomnia, precipitation of paranoid ideation or overt psychosis, rapid tolerance to euphoriant effects, and abuse of the agents is not seen when low doses of psychostimulants are used. Response is usually reported within 3 days.[170, 171]

Barbiturates and other CNS depressants used as sleeping medication or for sedation should be avoided in patients with symptoms of a chronic mental syndrome because they increase confusion and agitation.

Lithium, where required to stabilize fluctuations in mood or to augment treatment response to antidepressant medication, may be used. Neither the presence of dementia nor of aging appears to alter the decline of plasma lithium following cessation of lithium treatment. There is an increased tendency toward lithium-induced toxicity in patients with organic mental syndromes.[168] Lithium treatment of Alzheimer patients may lead to a marked accentuation of extrapyramidal symptoms in patients with pre-existing basal ganglia disease.[166]

Special care must be provided for clear, simple instruction on how medication should be taken.[150] It may be necessary, especially later in the course of the illness, to have a patient's relatives or friends either guide the taking of or actually administer medication. Failure to do so may result in drug autonomism, a state whereby a patient in a semitoxic state repeats dosages and becomes more confused and sedated. In the extreme, such behavior can lead to death by nonintentional overdose.

Antispasmodic and Antiparkinsonism Drugs

Extrapyramidal symptoms and uncomfortable spasms seen with many of the diseases associated with dementia, for which there are no specific therapies, may be helped by the usual pharmacologic agents recommended for symptomatic relief of these conditions.[172]

Anticonvulsant Medication

Seizures are seen in a number of the diseases associated with dementia (e.g., cerebral neoplasia, Alzheimer's disease). The use of appropriate doses of anticonvulsant medication will minimize occurrence.

Nursing Care

It is the nursing staff which in most instances coordinates treatment of demented patients on an inpatient psychiatric unit and anticipates their needs. The nurses are in a position to first notice a change in the status and are, therefore, able to minimize effects of progressive impairment. When patients have difficulty swallowing, the nursing staff is responsible for suctioning the patients or, if patients are able, teaching them to remove excess salivary secretions that are in most people unconsciously disposed of. Where tracheotomies are indicated, day care again falls in most instances into the nursing staff's hands. This activity is often frustrating and seemingly unrewarding with patients who are no longer able to express any overt appreciation for that which makes patients in the final stages of

their illnesses as comfortable as one may expect under such conditions.

Nonspecific Modes of Treatment

Various agents have been suggested for alleviating symptoms in patients with various dementias not affected by more specific modes. These include ribonucleic acid, magnesium, pemoline, L-Dopa, steroids, bishydroxycoumarin, lecithin,[173-178] choline, chloride,[179-181] vasodilators,[182] lysine vasopressin,[183] and tryptophan.[184] Use of lecithin[173-178] and choline[179-181] has been prompted by the lower choline acetyltransferase and higher monoamine oxidase levels found in severe dementia of the Alzheimer variety.[186] Most treatment techniques aimed at rectifying this problem have led to equivocal or negative results.[173] Choline lecithin seems to have limited value. Postsynaptic treatments such as physostigmine hold more hope of longer-acting oral preparations being developed.[186] ACTH, vasopressin,[183] and piractam may have value, but their role needs to be defined.[186] One pilot study has suggested that an increase in tryptophan absorption is a necessary condition for improvement in cognitive states when it occurs.

Betahistine, papaverine, hexobendine, and possibly cyclandelate and vincamine appear to be effective cerebral vasodilators when given in single parenteral doses, but their efficacy with regular oral administration has not been documented.[182] The risk of intracerebral steal makes cerebral vasodilator therapy contraindicated in all patients with *acute* stroke.[182] In patients with Alzheimer's dementia, ergoloid mesylates and nafronyl have been consistently found to improve cognitive performance.[182] Neither of these drugs increases cerebrovascular blood flow. In addition to their peripheral vasodilator activity, both appear to have metabolic effects.

Appropriate double-blind controlled studies with a sufficient number of subjects are needed before any conclusive statements may be ventured in regard to the efficacy of these treatments.[185, 186]

COURSE AND PROGNOSIS

The course and prognosis of the dementias are determined by their etiology.[187] If the dementia is one of the nontreatable forms, such as Alzheimer's disease, Pick's disease, or Huntington's chorea, the course is unremitting deterioration until death. In the final stages, the patient is entirely disoriented to person, place, and time and is bedridden and incontinent of feces and urine. Death is usually due to intercurrent infection. If the disease is potentially treatable, as in instances of pernicious anemia, normal pressure hydrocephalus, or syphilis, the level of functioning remaining depends upon the point in the trajectory of a patient's illness when the disease was arrested.

Acknowledgements. Mr. Ari Solomon helped in identifying literature relevant to this chapter.

REFERENCES

1. Brain WR: Disorders of memory, in Brain WR, Wilkinson M (eds): *Recent Advances in Neurology and Neuropsychiatry,* ed. 8, Boston, Little, Brown & Co., 1969.
2. DeJong RN: *The Neurological Examinations,* ed. 3, New York, Harper & Row, 1967.
3. Detre TP, Jarecki HG: *Modern Psychiatric Treatment,* Philadelphia, Lippincott, 1971.
4. Gilroy J, Meyer JS: *Medical Neurology,* ed. 2, New York, MacMillan, 1975.
5. Gooddy W: Introduction to the problems of dementia. Proc Aust Assoc Neurol, *6:* 9–11, 1969.
6. Karp H: Dementias in adults, in Baker AB, Baker LH (eds): *Clinical Neurology,* New York, Harper & Row, 1973.
7. McMenemey, WH: The dementias and progressive diseases of the basal ganglia, in Blockwood W, McMenemey WH, Norman RM, Russell DS (eds): *Greenfield's Neuropathology,* ed. 2, London, Arnold, 1963.
8. Merritt HH: *A Textbook of Neurology,* ed. 4, Philadelphia, Lea & Febiger, 1970.
9. Raskin NH: Dementia. Calif Med, *111:* 227–228, 1969.
10. Salmon JH: Senile and presenile dementia. Geriatrics, *24:* 67–72, 1969.
11. Slaby AE, Wyatt RJ: *Dementia in the Presenium,* Springfield, Ill., Charles C Thomas, 1974.
12. Vijayan N, Duanang JR, Dreyfus PM: Dementia: Current concepts. Calif Med, *111:* 208–216, 1969.
13. Wells CE: *Dementia,* Philadelphia, F. A. Davis, 1971.
14. Terry RD: Dementia: A brief and selective review. Arch Neurol, *33:* 1–44, 1976.
15. Wang HS: Dementia in old age, in Wells CE (ed): *Dementia,* ed. 2, *Contemporary Neurology Series,* pp. 15–26, Philadelphia. F. A. Davis, 1977.
16. Wells CE: Dementia: Definition and description, in Wells CE (ed): *Dementia,* ed. 2, *Contemporary Neurology Series,* pp. 1–14, Philadelphia, F. A. Davis, 1977.
17. Slaby AE, Tancredi LR, Lieb J: *General Clinical Psychiatry,* New York, Harper & Row, 1981.
18. Wells CE: Pseudodementia. Am J Psychiatry, *136:* 895–900, 1979.
19. Bleuler E: *Dementia Praecox or the Group of Schizophrenias,* Zimkin J (trans), New York, International Universities Press, 1950.
20. McAllister T, Price T: Severe depressive pseudodementia with and without dementia. Am J Psychiatry, *139:* 626–629, 1982.
21. Snow S, Wells C: Case studies in neuropsychiatry: Diagnosis and treatment of coexistent dementia and depression. J Clin Psychiatry, *42:* 439–441, 1981.
22. Goldstein K: *After-Effects of Brain Injuries in War,* New York, Grune & Stratton, 1942.
23. Lipowski ZJ: Delirium, clouding of consciousness and confusion. J Nerv Ment Dis, *145:* 227, 1967.
24. Locke S: *Neurology,* Boston, Little, Brown & Co., 1966.
25. Lipowski ZJ: A new look at organic brain syndromes. Am J Psychiatry, *137:* 674–678, 1980.
26. Solitare GB, Lamarache JB: Alzheimer's disease and senile dementia as seen in mongoloids: Neuropathological observations. Am J Ment Defic, *70:* 840–848, 1966.
27. Sourander P, Sjogren H: The concept of Alzheimer's Disease and its clinical implications, in Wolsterholm GWW, O'Connor M (eds): *Alzheimer's Disease and Related Conditions,* London, Churchill, 1970.
28. Alzheimer A: Ueber eine eigenartige erkrankung der hirnrinde. Zentralbl Nervenheilk Psychiatry, *30:* 177–179, 1907.
29. Field EJ: Amyloidosis, Alzheimer's disease and aging. Lancet, *2:* 781, 1970.
30. Hughes W: Alzheimer's disease. Gerontol Clin, *12:* 129–148, 1970.
31. Sin M, Susman J: Alzheimer's disease: Its natural history and differential diagnosis. J Nerv Ment Dis, *135:* 489–499, 1962.
32. Sjogren H: Alzheimer's disease—Pick's disease. A clinical analysis of 72 cases. Acta Psychiatr Neurol Scand (Suppl), *74:* 189–192, 1951.
33. Deakin J: Alzheimer's disease: Recent advances and future prospects. Br Med J, *287:* 1323–1324, 1983.
34. Wisniewski HM, Coblentz JM, Terry RD: Pick's disease. A clinical and ultrastructural study. Arch Neurol, *26:* 97–108, 1972.
35. Ernst B, Dalby MA, Dalby A: Aphasic disturbances in presenile dementia. Acta Neurol Scand (Suppl 46), *43:* 99–100, 1970.
36. Bratan J: Jakob-Creutzfeldt disease: Treatment by amantadine. Br Med J, *4:* 212–213, 1971.
37. Burger LJ, Rowan HJ, Goldensohn ES: Creutzfeldt-Jakob disease. An electroencephalographic study. Arch Neurol, *26:* 428–433, 1972.
38. Friede RL, DeJong RN: Neuronal enzymatic

failure in Creutzfeldt-Jakob disease: A familial study. Arch Neurol, *10:* 181–195, 1964.

39. Gajdusek DC: Slow virus diseases of the central nervous system. Am J Clin Pathol, *56:* 320–332, 1971.

40. Gajdusek DC, Gibbs CJ: Transmission of two subacute spongiform encephalopathies of man (kuru and Creutzfeldt-Jakob disease) to New World monkeys. Nature, *230:* 588–591, 1971.

41. Gibbs CJ, Gajdusek DC: Infection as the etiology of spongiform encephalopathy (Creutzfeldt-Jakob disease). Science, *165:* 1023–1025, 1969.

42. Gibbs CJ, Gajdusek DC, Asher DM, et al.: Creutzfeldt-Jakob disease (spongiform encephalopathy). Transmission to the chimpanzee. Science, *161:* 388–389, 1968.

43. Kirschbaum WR: *Jakob-Creutzfeldt Disease (Spastic Pseudosclerosis: A Jakob-Heidenhain Syndrome: Subacute Spongiform Encephalopathy),* New York, American Elsevier, 1968.

44. Lampert PW, Gajdusek DC, Gibbs CJ: Experimental spongiform encephalopathy (Creutzfeldt-Jakob disease) in chimpanzees. J Neuropathol Exp Neurol, *30:* 20–32, 1971.

45. Sanders WL, Dunn TL: Creutzfeldt-Jakob disease treated with amantadine. J Neurol Neurosurg Psychiatry, *36:* 581–584, 1973.

46. Vernon MI, Horta-Barbosa L, Fucillo DA, et al.: Virus-like particles and nucleoprotein-type filaments in brain tissue from two patients with Creutzfeldt-Jakob disease. Lancet, *1:* 964–966, 1970.

47. Jakob A: Uber eigenartige erkrankungen des zentranervensystems mit berkenswerten anatomischen befunde (Spastische pseudosklerose-encephalomyelopathic mit disseminierten degenerationsherden). Deut Z. Nervenheilk, *70:* 132–146, 1921.

48. Jervis G: Sheep, minks, savages, and presenile dementia: The story of the slow viruses. Psychiatr Q (Suppl), *42:* 371–375, 1968.

49. Siedler H, Malamud N: Creutzfeldt-Jakob's disease. Clinicopathological report of 15 cases and review of the literature (with special reference to a related disorder designated as subacute spongiform encephalopathy). J Neuropathol Clin Neurol, *23:* 381–402, 1963.

50. Klawans HL, Jr: A pharmacologic analysis of Huntington's chorea. Eur Neurol, *4:* 148–163, 1970.

51. Perry TL, Hansen S, Kloster M: Huntington's chorea. Deficiency of gamma-aminobutyric acid in the brain. N Engl J Med, *288:* 337–342, 1973.

52. Bird ED, Mackay AVP, Royner CN, Iversen LL: Reduced glutamic-acid-decarboxylase activity of post-mortem brain in Huntington's chorea. Lancet, *1:* 1090–1092, 1973.

53. Ironside R, Bosanquet FD, McMenemy WH: Central demyelination of the corpus callosum (Marchiafava-Bignami disease) with report of a recent case in Great Britain. Brain, *84:* 212–230, 1961.

54. Marchiafava E, Bignami A: Sopra un'alterazione del corpo calloso osservata in soggetti alcoolisti. Riv Patol Nerv Ment, *8:* 544–549, 1903.

55. Poser CM, van Bogaert L: Natural history and evolution of the concept of Schilder's diffuse sclerosis. Acta Psychiatr Neurol Scand, *31:* 285–293, 1956.

56. Adams RD: Further observations on normal pressure hydrocephalus. Proc R Soc Med, *59:* 1135–1140, 1966.

57. Adams RD, Fisher CM, Hakin S, et al.: Symptomatic occult hydrocephalus with "normal" cerebrospinal fluid pressure: A treatable syndrome. N Engl J Med, *273:* 117–126, 1965.

58. McCullough DC, Harbert JC, DiChiro G, et al.: Prognostic criteria for cerebrospinal fluid shunting from isotope cisternography in communicating hydrocephalus. Neurology, *20:* 584–598, 1970.

59. McHugh PR: Hydrocephalic dementia. Bull NY Acad Med, *42:* 907–917, 1966.

60. Jarpe S: Presenile dementia and hydrocephalus: Therapeutic experiences. Acta Neurol Scand (Suppl), *46:* 89, 1970.

61. Jensen F, Malmros R, Hansen HH: Isotope encephalography in low-pressure hydrocephalus. Acta Neurol Scand (Suppl), *46* 93, 1970.

62. Bannister R, Gilford E, Kocen R: Isotope encephalography in the diagnosis of dementia due to communicating hydrocephalus. Lancet, *2:* 1014–1017, 1967.

63. Geschwind N: The mechanism of normal pressure hydrocephalus. J Neurol Sci, *7:* 481–493, 1968.

64. Tator CH, Fleming JFR, Sheppard RH, et al.: A radioisotopic test for communicating hydrocephalus. J Neurosurg, *28:* 327–340, 1968.

65. Schnur JA, Chse TN, Brady JA: Parkinsonism-dementia of Guam: Treatment with L-dopa. Neurology, *21:* 1236–1242, 1971.

66. Hirano A, Kurland LT, Krooth RS, et al.: Parkinsonism-dementia complex: An endemic disease on the island of Guam. I. Clinical features. Brain, *84:* 642–661, 1961.

67. Lessell S, Hirano A, Torres J, et al.: Parkinsonism-dementia complex. Arch Neurol, *7:* 377–385, 1962.

68. Bearn AG: A genetical analysis of thirty families with Wilson's disease (hepatoilenticular degeneration). Ann Hum Genet, *24:* 33–43, 1960.

69. Walshe JM: Wilson's disease: The presenting symptoms. Arch Dis Child, *37:* 253–256, 1962.

70. Brooks DN: Memory and head injury. J Nerv Ment Dis, *155:* 350–355, 1972.

71. Burvill PW, Jackson JM, Smith WG: Psychiatric symptoms due to vitamin B12 deficiency without anemia. Med J Aust, *2:* 388–390, 1969.

72. Cancer and the nervous system. Br Med J, *3:* 193–194, 1969.

73. Cushing H: *Intracranial Tumors, Notes Upon a Series of Two Thousand Verified Cases with Surgical Mortality Percentages Pertaining Thereto.* Springfield, Ill., Charles C Thomas, 1932.

74. Cushing H, Esenhardt L: *Meningiomas: Their Classification, Regional Behavior, Life History, and Surgical End Results,* New York, Hafner, 1962.

75. Daniels AC, Chokroverty S, Barron KD: Thalamic degeneration, dementia, and seizures. Arch Neurol, *21:*15–24, 1969.

76. Davies DL: Psychiatric changes associated with Friedreich's ataxia. J Neurol Neurosurg Psychiatry, *12:* 246–249, 1949.

77. Dayan AD: Presenile dementia: Some pathological problems and possibilities. Proc R Soc Med, *64:* 829–831, 1971.

78. Edwards, VE, Sutherland JM, Tyrer JH: Cryptococcosis of the central nervous system. Epidemiological clinical and therapeutic features. J Neurol Neurosurg Psychiatry, *33:* 415–425, 1970.

79. Binder BL, Dickman WA: Psychiatric manifestations of neurosyphilis in middle-aged patients. Am J Psychiatry, *137:* 741–742, 1980.

80. Hooschmand J, Escobar MR, Kopf SW: Neurosyphilis. JAMA, *219:* 726–728, 1971.

81. Jose CJ, Cruet-Perez J: Incidence and morbidity of self-induced water intoxication in state mental hospital patients. Am J Psychiatry, *136:* 221–222, 1979.

82. Sparling PF: Diagnosis and treatment of syphilis. N Engl J Med, *284:* 642–655, 1971.

83. Wells CE: Chronic brain disease: An overview. Am J Psychiatry, *135:* 1–12, 1978.

84. Fisher A: On meningioma presenting with dementia. Proc Aust Assoc Neurol, *6:* 29–38, 1969.

85. Fodor IE: Impairment of memory function after acute head injury. J Neurol Neurosurg Psychiatry, *35:* 818–824, 1972.

86. Ford CV, Bray GA, Swerdloff RS: A psychiatric study of patients referred with a diagnosis of hypoglycemia. Am J Psychiatry, *133:* 290–294, 1976.

87. Shuylman R: Vitamin B_{12} deficiency and psychiatric illness. Br J Psychiatry, *113:* 252–256, 1967.

88. Shulman R: A survey of vitamin B_{12} deficiency in an elderly psychiatric population. Br J Psychiatry, *113:* 241–251, 1967.

89. Johnson KR, Rosenthal MS, Lerner, PI: Herpes simplex encephalitis: The course in five virologically proven cases. Arch Neurol, *27:* 103–108, 1972.

90. O'Connor JF, Musher DM: Central nervous system involvements in systemic lupus erythematosus. Arch Neurol, *14:* 157–164, 1966.

91. Olivarius B. de F, Roeder E: Reversible psychosis and dementia in myxedema. Acta Psychiatr Scand, *46:* 1–13, 1970.

92. Paillas JE, Legre J, Alliez B, et al: Diagnosis and treatment of tumors of the basal ganglions. Anatomicoclinical data from 50 cases. Neurochirurgie, *16:* 89–115, 1970.

93. Parker N: Post-traumatic dementia. Proc Aust Assoc Neurol, *6:* 39–44, 1969.

94. Mahurkar SD, Dhar SK, Slata R, et al.: Dialysis dementia. Lancet, *1:* 1414–1424, 1973.

95. Martland HS: Punch drunk. JAMA, *91:* 1103–1107, 1928.

96. Matthews WB: Sarcoidosis of the nervous system. J Neurol Neurosurg Psychiatry, *28:* 23–29, 1965.

97. Mayock RL, Bertrand P, Morrison CE: Manifestations of sarcoidosis. Analysis of 145 patients with a review of nine series selected from the literature. Am J Med, *35:* 67–89, 1963.

98. Idose O, Guthe T, Willcox RR: Penicillin in the treatment of syphilis. Bull WHO (Suppl), *47:* 1972.

99. Johnson J: Organic psychosyndromes due to boxing. Br J Psychiatry, *115:* 45–53, 1969.

100. Anderson PG: The clinical picture in middle-aged psychiatric patients with intracranial tumors. Acta Neurol Scand (Suppl 43), *46:* 79–80, 1970.

101. Anthony JJ: Malignant lymphoma associated with hydantoin drugs. Arch Neurol, *22:* 450–454, 1970.

102. Avery TL: Seven cases of frontal tumor with psychiatric presentation. Br J Psychiatry, *119:* 19–23, 1971.

103. Frazier CH: Tumor involving the frontal lobe alone. A symptomatic survey of one hundred and five verified cases. Arch Neurol Psychiatry, *35:* 527–571, 1936.

104. Ginsburg R, Romano J: Carbon monoxide encephalopathy: Need for appropriate treatment. Am J Psychiatry, *133:* 317–320, 1976.

105. Sanders V: Neurologic manifestations of myxedema. N Engl J Med, *266:* 547–552, 1962.

106. Haberland C: Alzheimer's disease in Down's syndrome. Clinical neuropathological observations. Acta Neurol Belg, *69:* 360–380, 1969.

107. Hafken L, Leichter S, Reich T: Organic brain dysfunction as a possible consequence of postgastrectomy hypoglycemia. Am J Psychiatry, *132:* 1321–1329, 1975.

108. Lavy S, Herishianu Y: Chronic subdural hematoma in the aged. J Am Geriatr Soc, *17:* 380–383, 1969.

109. Lennox WG: Brain injury, drugs, and environment as causes of mental decay in epilepsy. Am J Psychiatry, *99:* 174–180, 1942.

110. Beerman H, Nicholas L, Schamberg II, et al.: Syphilis: Review of the recent literature 1960–1961. Arch Intern Med, *109:* 324–344, 1962.

111. Fisch M, Goldfarb A, Shahinian S, et al.: Chronic brain syndrome in the community aged. Arch Gen Psychiatry, *18:* 739–745, 1968.

112. Wang HS, Obrist WD, Busse EW: Neurophysiological correlates of the intellectual function of community elderly. Presented at the 122nd Annual Meeting of the American Psychiatric Association, Miami Beach, Fla., May 5–9, 1969.

113. Myers JM, Sheldon D, Robinson SS: A study of 138 elderly first admissions. Am J Psychiatry, *120:* 244–247, 1963.

114. Amster LE, Krauss HH: The relationship between life crises and mental deterioration in old age. Int J Aging Hum Dev, *5:* 51–55, 1974.

115. Bergmann K: Chronic brain failure—Epidemiologic aspects. Age Aging (Suppl), *6:* 4–8, 1977.

116. Blumenthal MD: Psychosocial factors in reversible and irreversible brain failure. J Clin Exp Gerontol, *1:* 39–55, 1979.

117. Bollerup TR: Prevalence of mental illness among 70-year-olds domiciled in nine Copenhagen suburbs. Acta Psychiatr Scand, *51:* 327–329, 1975.

118. Jarkvik LF, Ruth V, Matsuyama SS: Organic brain syndrome and aging: A six-year follow-up of surviving twins. Arch Gen Psychiatry, *37:* 280–286, 1980.

119. Kay DWK, Beamish P, Roth M: Old age mental disorders in Newcastle upon Tyne. Part I: A study of prevalence. Br J Psychiatry, *110:* 146–158, 1964.

120. Aldrich C: Personality factors and mortality in the relocation of the aged. Gerontologist, *4:* 92, 1964.

121. Blenkner M: Environmental change in the aging individual. Gerontologist, *7:* 101, 1967.

122. Facts About Older Americans—1977, DHEW Pub No (OHD) 78-20006, 1978.

123. Susser M: *Community Psychiatry: Epidemiologic and Social Themes,* New York, Random House, 1968.

124. Gruenberg E: A Mental Health Survey of Older Persons, in Hoch PH, Zubin J (eds): Comparative Epidemiology of the Mental Disorders, New York, Grune & Stratton, 1961.

125. Gruenberg EM, Turns DM: Epidemiology, in Friedman AM, Kaplan HI, Sadock BJ (eds): *Comprehensive Textbook of Psychiatry II,* ed. 2, vol. 1, Baltimore, Williams & Wilkins, 1975.

126. Lieberman M: Relationships of mortality rates to entrance to a home for the aged. Geriatrics, *16:* 515, 1961.

127. Teetor RB, et al.: Psychiatric disturbances of aged patients in skilled nursing homes. Am J Psychiatry, *133:* 1430, 1976.

128. Kay DWK, Beamish P, Roth M: Old age mental disorders in Newcastle-upon-Tyne. Part I: A study of prevalence. Br J Psychiatry, *110:* 146, 1964.

129. Kay DWK, Beamish P, Roth M: The old age mental disorders in Newcastle-upon-Tyne. Part II: A study of possible social and medical courses. Br J Psychiatry, *110:* 668, 1964.

130. Larsson T, Sjogren T, Jacobson G: Senile dementia. A clinical, sociomedical and genetic study. Acta Psychiatr Scand (Suppl 39), *167:* 1–259, 1963.

131. Sim M, Turner E, Smith WR: Cerebral biopsy in the investigation of presenile dementia. Br J Psychiatry, *112:* 119–125, 1966.

132. Tomlinson BE, Blessed G, Roth M: Observation on the brains of demented old people. J Neurol Sci, *11:* 205–242, 1970.

133. Wilkinson P: Alcoholism in the aged. J Geriatr: 59, 1971.

134. Zimberg S: Elderly alcoholics. Gerontology, *14:* 221, 1974.

135. Gottfries CG, Gottfries I, Roos BE: Disturbance of monoamine metabolism in the brains from patients with dementia senilis and Mb. Alzheimer. Excerpta Med Int Congr, *180:* 310–312, 1969.

136. Gottfries CG, Gottfries I, Roos BE: Homovanillic acid and 5-hydroxy-indoleacetic acid in the cerebrospinal fluid of patients with senile dementia, presenile dementia, and Parkinsonism. Acta Psychiatr Scand, *46:* 99–105, 1970.

137. Gottfries CG, Gottfries I, Roos BE: Homovanillic acid and 5-hydroxy-indoleacetic acid in the cerebrospinal fluid of patients with senile dementia, presenile dementia, and Parkinsonism. J Neurochem, *16:* 1341–1345, 1969.

138. Gottfries CG, Gottfries I, Roos BE: The investigation of homovanillic acid in the human brain and its correlation to senile dementia. Br J Psychiatry, *115:* 563–574, 1969.

139. Belendiuk K, Belendiuk GW, Freedman DX: Blood monoamine metabolism in Huntington's disease. Arch Gen Psychiatry, *37:* 325–332, 1980.

140. Yesavage JA, Tinlenberg JR, Hollister LE, et al.: Vasodilators in senile dementias: A review of the literature. Arch Gen Psychiatry, *36:* 220–223, 1979.

141. Bower HM, Andrews JT, Pope RA: Dementia and cerebral blood flow. Med J Aust, *1:* 207–211, 1970.

142. Huntington G: On chorea. Med Surg Rep, *26:* 317–321, 1972.

143. Haberland C: Alzheimer's disease in Down's syndrome. Clinical neuropathological observations. Acta Neurol Belg, *69:* 360–380, 1969.

144. Neumann MA: Langdon Down syndrome and Alzheimer's disease. Neuropathol Exp Neurol, *16:* 149–150, 1967.

145. Hollister LE: *Clinical Use of Psychotropic Drugs,* Springfield, Ill., Charles C Thomas, 1973.

146. Blummer D: Organic personality disorder, in Lion J (ed): *Severe Personality Disorders*, Baltimore, Williams & Wilkins, 1974.

147. Reifter B, Esidorfer C: A clinic for the impaired elderly and their families. Am J Psychiatry, *137:* 1399–1403, 1980.

148. Bower HM: The differential diagnosis of dementia. Med J Aust, *2:* 623–626, 1971.

149. Cummings J: Treatable Dementias, in *The Dementias,* New York, Raven Press, 1983.

150. Pascarelli EF, Fischer W: Drug dependence in the elderly. Int J Aging Hum Dev, *5:* 347, 1974.

151. Tsai L, Tsuang MT: Computerized tomography and skull x-rays: Relative efficacy in detecting intracranial disease. Am J Psychiatry, *135:* 1556–1557, 1978.

152. Ambrose J: Computerized x-ray scanning of the brain. J Neurosurg *40:* 679–695, 1974.

153. Engeset A: Radiological considerations of the aetiological and anatomical background of the presenile dementias. Acta Neurol Scand (Suppl 43), *46:* 32–41, 1970.

154. Stensman R, Ingvar DH: EEG and cerebral circulation in presenile dementia. Electroencephalogr Clin Neurophysiol, *30:* 255–274, 1971.

155. Gorden EB: Serial EEG studies in presenile dementia. Br J Psychiatry, *114:* 779–780, 1968.
156. Gordon EG, Sim M: The EEG in presenile dementia. J Neurol Neurosurg Psychiatry, *30:* 285–291, 1967.
157. Furlow T, Whitley R, Wilmes F: Repeated suppression of CJD disease with vidabarine. Lancet: 564–565, 1982.
158. Sparling PF: Diagnosis and treatment of syphilis. N Engl J Med, *284:* 642–653, 1971.
159. Leng N: Behavioral treatment of the elderly. Age Aging, *11:* 235–243, 1982.
160. Buckholdt D, Gubrium J: Therapeutic pretense in reality orientation. Int J Aging Human Development, *16:* 167–87, 1983.
161. Hermann H: Ethical dilemmas intrinsic to the care of the elderly demented patient. J Am Geriatr Soc, *32:* 655–656, 1982.
162. Barnes R, Veith R, Okinoto J, Raskind M, Gumbrecht G: Efficacy of antipsychotic medications in behaviorally disturbed dementia patients. Am J Psychiatry, *139:* 1170–4, 1982.
163. Gerner R: Antidepressant selection in the elderly. Psychosomatics, *25:* 528–34, 1984.
164. Gilleard CJ, Morgan K, Wade BE: Patterns of neuroleptic use among the institutionalized elderly. Acta Psychiatr Scand, *68:* 419–425, 1983.
165. Gotestam K, Ljunghall S, Olsson B: A double blind comparison of the effects of haloperidol and ciz(Z)-clopenthixol in senile dementia. Acta Psychiatr Scand (Suppl), *294:* 46–53, 1981.
166. Haryadi T: Mental health issues in the elderly. Primary Care, *9:* 143–159, 1982.
167. Kelwala S, Pomara N, Stanley M, Sitaram N, Gershon S: Lithium-induced accentuation of EPS in individuals with Alzheimer's disease. J Clin Psychiatry, 45: 342–344, 1984.
168. Noel G, Jeanmart M, Reinhardt B: Treatment of the organic brain syndrome in the elderly. Neuropsychobiology, *10:* 90–93, 1983.
169. Pomora N, Block R, Domino E, Gershon S: Decay in plasma lithium and normalization in red blood cell choline following cessation of lithium treatment in two elderly individuals with Alzheimer-type dementia. Biol Psychiatry, *19:* 919–923, 1984.
170. Viukari M, Salo H, Lamminsivu U, Gordin A: Tolerance and serum level of haloperidol during parenteral and oral haloperidol treatment in geriatric patients. Acta Psychiatr Scand, *65:* 301–308, 1982.
171. Kaplitz SE: Withdrawn apathetic geriatric patients' responses to methylphenidate. J Am Geriatr Soc, *23:* 271–276, 1975.
172. Katon W, Raskind M: Treatment of depression in the medically ill elderly with methylphenidate. Am J Psychiatry, *137:* 963–965, 1980.
173. Swash M, Roberts AH, Zakko H, Heathfield KWG: Treatment of involuntary movement disorders with tetrabenazine. J Neurol Neurosurg Psychiatry, 35: 186–191, 1972.
174. Brinkman S, Smith R, Myer J, Vroulis G, Shaw T, Gordon J, Allen R: Lecithin and memory training in suspected Alzheimer's disease. J Gerontol, *37:* 4–9, 1982.
175. Canter N, Hollet M, Growdon J: Lecithin does not affect EEG spectral analysis or P300 in Alzheimer disease. Neurology, *32:* 1260–1266, 1982.
176. Dysken M, Fovell P, Harris C, Davis J, Noronha A: Letter to the editor. Neurology, *32:* 1203–1204, 1982.
177. Etieme P, Dastoor D, Gouthier S, Ludwick R, Collier B: Alzheimer's disease; lack of effect of lecithin treatment for three months. Neurology, *31:* 1552–1554, 1981.
178. Fishman M: Clinical pharmacology of senile dementia. Prog Neuropsychopharmacol, *5:* 447–454, 1981.
179. Levy R: Lecithin in Alzheimer's disease. Lancet: 671–672, 1982.
180. Pomara N, Stanley M: Cholinergic precursors in Alzheimer's disease. Lancet: p. 1049. 1984.
181. Roberts E: Potential therapies in aging and senile dementias. Ann NY Acad of Sci, *366:* 165–176, 1982.
182. Thal LJ, Rosen W, Sharpless NS, Crystal H: Choline chloride fails to improve cognition in Alzheimer's disease. Neurobiol Aging, *2:* 205–208, 1981.
183. Koch W, Cook P, James I: Drug therapy—Cerebral vasodilators (second of two parts). N Engl J Med, *305:* 1560–1564, 1981.
184. Durso R, Fedio P, Brouwers P, Cox C, Martin AJ, Ruggieri SA, Tamminga CA, Chase TN: Lysine vasopression in Alzheimer's disease. Neurology, *32:* 674–677, 1981.
185. Lehmann J, Perrson S, Walinder J, Wallin L: Tryptophan malabsorption in dementia. Improvement in certain cases after Try therapy as indicated by mental behavior and blood analysis (a pilot study). Acta Psychiatr Scand, *64:* 123–131, 1981.
186. Fisman M: Clinical pharmacology of senile dementia. Prog Neuro-Psychopharmacol, *5:* 447–457, 1981.
187. Goodnick P, Gershon S: Chemotherapy of cognitive disorders in geriatric subjects. J Clin Psychiatry, *45:* 196–209, 1984.
188. Katona C, Lowe D, Jack R: Prediction of outcome in psychogeriatric patients. Acta Psychiatr Scand, *67:* 297–306, 1983.

chapter 8

alcoholism

John A. Renner, Jr., M.D.

Alcoholism frequently complicates the treatment of patients admitted for inpatient psychiatric care. This chapter focuses on the evaluation and treatment of this common problem.

In some cases, alcoholism may be one of the primary reasons for recommending inpatient treatment. Indications for admission include symptoms of a major psychiatric illness in patients whose drinking is so out of control that it prevents effective outpatient psychiatric treatment. Since alcohol is primarily a depressant drug, alcohol abuse often exacerbates a preexisting depressive illness and may lead to suicide attempts, marital breakdown, and marked social deterioration, necessitating inpatient treatment. Alcoholics may also develop dementia or acute psychotic symptoms secondary to their drinking, e.g., alcohol hallucinosis, and thus may require hospitalization. Patients may also be admitted if they have been repeated failures in outpatient treatment.

In other cases, the patient's alcohol problem may not be directly related to his psychiatric admission, yet it will be a factor complicating inpatient treatment. This is particularly true for patients with schizophrenia or bipolar affective disease. Hospitalization may present a good opportunity to deal more effectively with both the drinking and the psychiatric illness.

Inpatient psychiatric treatment is not necessary for alcholics requiring routine detoxification with no complicating psychiatric problems. Such patients should be referred to specialized alcoholism treatment units. Correspondingly, admission to an inpatient unit is contraindicated when no physiological addiction is present

or when the patient is primarily a binge drinker. These patients can usually be managed in an outpatient treatment program.

DEFINITION

Alcoholism is a group of syndromes with multiple etiologies that may involve strong genetic, psychological, or sociological components. The clinical presentations are variable, and the course is unpredictable. Some patients will present intoxicated, with clear evidence of marked physical and social deterioration. Binge drinkers may show no physical signs of alcoholism, yet their drinking may have produced severe marital, economic, legal, or medical problems. Professionals may be particularly successful in masking their problem, despite an advanced stage of alcoholism.

Despite this variability, chronic alcoholism tends to have a life of its own and often develops along a remarkably consistent course. Most chronic patients drink on a daily basis and present with a constellation of easily recognizable physical symptoms, psychiatric complaints, and maladaptive behaviors. It is important to realize that these physical and psychiatric complaints are the consequence of chronic alcoholism. Rarely are they the cause of the patient's drinking.[1]

Clinicians have found it difficult to agree on diagnosis and have advanced a number of systems for defining and explaining alcoholism, each with a varying degree of functional application.

Chafetz[2] used the concept of "problem drinking" essentially to avoid the controversy over whether alcoholism was a moral aberration, a physical disease, or a psychological illness. This proved to be a very functional approach because of its usefulness in work with patients. The stigma of the label "alcoholism" was avoided with the problem drinking concept, thus reducing semantic, yet often real, barriers to some patients' entry into treatment.

Chafetz described alcoholism as a chronic behavior disorder manifested by repeated drinking in excess of social use. This is accompanied by an undue preoccupation with alcohol and a loss of control when drinking that interferes with physical, mental, social, or economic functioning.

More recently, Edwards and Gross[3] offered a provisional description of the "alcohol dependence syndrome." Based on solid clinical observations, they gave practical guidance to clinicians and avoided the controversy surrounding the etiology and pathological processes involved in problem drinking. Edwards noted that not all elements are present in every patient and that they vary in intensity. The elements of the alcohol dependence syndrome include:

1. Narrowing of the drinking repertoire. The social drinker's choice of beverage and pattern of consumption vary widely depending on internal cues and social circumstances. As alcoholism develops, drinking becomes more stereotyped, often involving one preferred beverage. Eventually this is consumed on a daily time-table primarily designed to avoid symptoms of alcohol withdrawal. The alcoholic's mood or social situation may have little impact on this drinking pattern.
2. Salience of drink-seeking behavior. Drinking gradually becomes the most important priority in a person's life. It overshadows interest in and obligations to family, friends, job, and even health.
3. Increased tolerance to alcohol. The alcohol-dependent person can tolerate and function relatively normally with a blood-alcohol level that would render a nontolerant person drowsy or comatose. Cross tolerance extends to minor tranquilizers, barbiturates, and other nervous system depressants.
4. Repeated withdrawal symptoms. Eventually the person experiences daily, severe withdrawal symptoms upon awakening. These continue until he ingests a "morning eye opener." Mild symptoms, including tremor, nausea, sweating, and mood disorder, occur frequently whenever there is a drop in the blood alcohol level.
5. Relief or avoidance of withdrawal by further drinking. The alcohol-dependent person has learned that almost continuous drinking is necessary to maintain steady blood alcohol levels and thus avoid even mild symptoms of withdrawal. The longer a person is able or willing to go between drinks and to tolerate withdrawal symptoms, the less advanced is the dependence.
6. Subjective awareness of compulsion to drink. The person may wish *not to drink*. He may recognize that he is struggling with an irrational compulsion. Yet, despite numerous conscious efforts to avoid drinking, he will nonetheless proceed to drink.
7. Reinstatement after abstinence. In moderately dependent persons, it may take one or more months for the syndrome to redevelop after a period of abstinence has ended. The more severely dependent person usually finds that the syndrome, complete with minor withdrawal symptoms, can be fully reinstated after a few days of drinking.

Primary vs. Secondary Alcoholism

For purposes of treatment planning, it is useful to distinguish between primary and secondary alcoholism. Following the disease classification model suggested by Woodruff and Guze at Washington University in St. Louis, a distinction is made based on which symptoms developed earliest in the patient's history.[4]

Primary Alcoholism

In primary alcoholism, the drinking problem begins before the development of any other specific psychiatric condition. Such patients may present with concurrent psychopathology, but a careful history will document that there were no serious psychiatric symptoms prior to the start of abusive drinking. The only exception to this rule is men with a history of childhood hyperactivity and/or conduct disorder. Family studies suggest that a genetic predisposition to both alcoholism and antisocial behavior is inherited independently in males in some families.[5]

For practical purposes, primary alcoholism is often equivalent with familial alcoholism. A strong family history suggests a major genetic component in the etiology of this form of alcoholism. These patients are usually men; they show signs of abusive drinking at an earlier age than nonfamilial alcoholics, and they have a rapid, more severe course of illness.[6] It can be expected that most of their psychiatric complaints will resolve once these patients have achieved stable sobriety.

Secondary Alcoholism

In these cases, a detailed longitudinal history will establish that the patient's alcoholism developed after the start of some other specific psychiatric illness. It is often clear that the patient is self-medicating with alcohol. In some cases, unfortunately, it is extremely difficult to obtain an adequate history, or to perform diagnostic interviews at the time of admission. It may not be possible to clarify the relationship between drinking and psychiatric symptoms until the patient has sustained an extended period of sobriety. When dealing with a case of secondary alcoholism, treatment must focus on *both* the alcoholism and the primary psychiatric problem.

DIAGNOSIS

Jellinek

Jellinek's[7] categorization of alcoholic syndromes represents an initial effort to separate groups of alcoholics according to the severity of the illness.

"*Alpha*" alcoholics are characterized by occasional excessive use when under stress, without loss of control.

"*Beta*" alcoholics demonstrate a drinking pattern with physical complications (such as cirrhosis) but display no physiological or psychological dependence.

"*Gamma*" alcoholics are physically dependent and manifest tolerance and loss of control.

"*Delta*" alcoholics are daily drinkers who are both physically and psychologically dependent.

National Council on Alcoholism

A focus on the signs and symptoms of alcoholism rather than its etiology is proposed by the National Council on Alcoholism.[8] A Major and Minor Criteria System evaluates the development of alcoholism on two Tracks.

Track I measures Physiological and Clinical Indicators; Track II measures Behavioral, Psychological, and Attitudinal Indicators. There are major and minor criteria in each track. Valid diagnosis requires evidence from both tracks to adequately describe the syndrome.[8] Examples of these criteria follow.

Major Criteria

Track I: Physiological
1. Withdrawal syndrome
2. Tolerance
3. Blackout periods
Clinical
1. Alcoholic hepatitis
2. Laennec's cirrhosis
3. Wernicke-Korsakoff syndrome

Track II: Behavioral, Psychological, and Attitudinal
1. Drinking despite medical contraindications
2. Drinking despite social contraindications
3. Subjective complaint of loss of control
Minor Criteria

Track I: Physiological and Clinical
1. Odor of alcohol on the breath
2. Alcohol facies
3. Abnormal liver function tests
4. Blood-alcohol level over 300 mg/100 ml at any time

Track II: Behavioral
1. Gulping drinks
2. Morning drinking
3. Missing work
4. Frequent automobile accidents

Psychological and Attitudinal
1. Frequent talk about drinking
2. Drinking to relieve stress
3. Spouse complains about drinking
4. Family disruption

The Diagnostic and Statistical Manual of Mental Disorders of the American Psychiatric Association, edition 3, (DSM-III)

DSM-III divides alcohol-related conditions into two general groups. The first is an alcohol section under "Substance Induced Organic Mental Disorders" and the second is grouped under "Substance Use Disorders."[9]

Substance Induced Organic Mental Disorders include:

Alcohol Intoxication (300.00)
Alcohol Idiosyncratic Intoxication or Pathological Intoxication (291.40)
Alcohol Withdrawal (291.80)
Alcohol Hallucinosis (291.00)
Alcohol Amnestic Syndrome or Korsakoff's Syndrome (291.10)
Dementia Associated with Alcoholism (291.2X)

Substance Use Disorders include:
Alcohol Abuse (305.0X)*
A. A pattern of pathological alcohol use: daily use, inability to stop drinking, binges, blackouts, etc.
B. An impairment in social or occupational functioning due to alcohol use.
C. Duration of disturbance of at least 1 month.

Alcohol Dependence (or alcoholism) (303.9X)*
A. A pattern of pathological alcohol use or an impairment in social or occupational functioning due to alcohol use (Criteria A or B above)
B. Either tolerance or withdrawal.

---

*Code fifth digit as: *1* = continuous; *2* = episodic; *3* = in remission; and *0* = unspecified.

The Substance Induced Organic Mental Disorders contain those conditions that are primarily due to the chemical effects of alcohol. The Substance Use Disorders reflect the psychological rather than the organic aspects of alcoholism. The primary distinction made between alcohol "abuse" and "dependence" is that the latter requires either tolerance or withdrawal.

DIFFERENTIAL DIAGNOSIS

Major problems in the differential diagnosis of alcoholism usually fall into two areas. The first problem is the confusion between symptoms of alcohol abuse and symptoms caused by the abuse of other drugs. The second problem is the distinction between symptoms secondary to alcoholism and symptoms related to other psychiatric diseases.

More than 40% of today's alcoholics also abuse other drugs, obtained both illicitly and by prescription. This percentage is even higher in individuals under 30. Clinicians therefore need to be alert to the signs of the abuse of other drugs. A careful workup should include questions about other drugs, and the physical examination should include a check for track marks caused by opiate injections and nasal ulcerations secondary to cocaine abuse. If the picture is unclear, as it often is, urine samples should be analyzed for the presence of other drugs. Withdrawal seizures occurring more than 48 hours after the last drink suggest addiction to barbiturates or benzodiazepines. Any intoxicated individual with signs of nystagmus, ataxia, or slurred speech, with no alcohol on his breath, is likely to be abusing other sedative-hypnotic drugs. Because of the similarity between the signs of intoxication and withdrawal for both alcohol and other sedative-hypnotic drugs, diagnosis can only be confirmed by a careful history and urine analysis for drugs.

The confusion between symptoms of alcoholism and other psychiatric diseases is a more difficult problem. Most alcoholics complain of depression and anxiety. Until proven otherwise, such complaints should be assumed to be secondary to alcohol abuse. In most cases, these symptoms clear a few days after completion of detoxification. However, complaints of depressed affect and mood disturbances secondary to alcoholism can continue up to 2 months after detoxification, and insomnia can last 4–6 months. In cases of severe alcoholism, anxiety and tremors have been reported up to 6–9 months after detoxification. To diagnose a primary affective disease, the clinician should look carefully for symptoms of depression (or mania) that may have preceded the drinking behavior. The diagnosis is also suggested by a positive family history, vegetative signs of depression, and symptoms of psychosis and/or suicidal preoccupation that persist after both acute intoxication and detoxification.

Similar diagnostic problems exist regarding schizophrenia and alcohol-related syndromes. Again, a careful history to identify symptoms that preceded the episode of alcohol abuse is quite important, as is a thorough family history. Borderline individuals can appear psychotic and paranoid when intoxicated, though these symptoms usually disappear promptly when the patient is sober. The hallucinations of delirium tremens are characteristically visual and tactile, though they can also be auditory. One's seeing small animals or bugs in the room or crawling on the person is typical. Paranoid delusions are also common. All of these symptoms are associated with the very obvious physical signs of alcohol withdrawal, usually clearing promptly with appropriate detoxification treatment, and are relatively uncharacteristic of schizophrenia and other psychoses. If symptoms of psychosis persist after the completion of detoxification, it is likely that they are *not related to the patient's alcoholism*. The patient may, however, be suffering from alcohol hallucinosis. Although this condition may be difficult to differentiate from schizophrenia, the treatment in either case is similar.

In alcohol hallucinosis, the patient characteristically has auditory hallucinations of a paranoid, often homosexual nature. He sometimes can identify the voice he hears as belonging to a specific person. Such specificity rarely occurs in schizophrenia, where the patient is more likely to be unable to identify the specific voice or may report hearing thoughts rather than voices. If the patient's symptoms persist for more than 30 days, or if they recur, with no recurrence of drinking, the diagnosis of alcohol hallucinosis is unlikely.

Confusion also exists between the minor and major symptoms of alcohol withdrawal (delirium tremens, DT's). This syndrome develops after a drop in blood alcohol in someone with a 3-to-5 year history of heavy drinking. It is characterized by nightmares, mental confusion, tremor, hyperactivity, elevated vital signs, and hallucinations (usually visual). These symptoms can be divided into early and later appearing symptoms (Table 8.1).

The delirium sometimes associated with alcohol withdrawal can also be confused with alcohol hallucinosis. The latter condition occurs infrequently and always with a clear sensorium (no disorientation) and no tremor. The hallucinations are usually auditory and persecutory in nature, as contrasted with the visual hallucinations typical in alcohol withdrawal delirium. Both conditions can occur after either cessation or reduction of drinking. Alcohol hallucinosis, however, occurs more frequently when drinking is reduced but not eliminated.

Table 8.2 details the differences in these conditions.

Confusion sometimes exists regarding the various types of cognitive impairments associated with alcoholism. In the alcohol amnestic syndrome (Korsakoff's syndrome), there is impairment of short- and long-term memory occurring in a normal state of consciousness and associated with neurological disturbances such as peripheral neuropathy, myopathy,

Table 8.1.
Stages of Alcohol Withdrawal

Minor (Early) Withdrawal Symptoms
(Start 8–9 hr after last drink)—tremors, sweating, flushed face, insomnia, hallucinations (25%), grand mal seizures (rum fits), mild or no disorientation
Major (Later) Withdrawal Symptoms
(Start 48–96 hr after last drink)—tremors, elevated psychomotor activity, vivid hallucinations, profound disorientation, elevated autonomic activity, fever, no seizures

Table 8.2.
Delirium Tremens vs. Alcohol Hallucinosis

	Sensorium	Tremor	Hallucinations	Pupils	Vital Signs	Onset	Duration (Days)
DT's	Confused	Yes	Visual	Dilated, slow to react	↑	Gradual	3–10
Alcohol hallucinosis	Clear	±	Auditory	Normal	↑	Rapid	5–30

or cerebellar ataxia. Immediate memory (digit span) is *not impaired* by this condition.

In dementia associated with alcoholism, there is memory impairment, significant loss of intellectual abilities, and impairment of abstract thinking, judgment, or other disturbances of higher cortical functions. (see Wet Brain).

Delirium can be distinguished from dementia by a clouding of the state of consciousness (normal in dementia), and symptoms of intellectual impairment which fluctuate over time (relatively stable in dementia). The differential diagnosis of dementia also includes Alzheimer's disease, chronic schizophrenia, and the normal aging process. Individuals with a severe depression may complain of problems with concentration, memory, and other intellectual abilities. This phenomenon is termed "pseudodementia"; it usually clears when such depressed patients are sufficiently motivated to perform routine intellectual functions.

EPIDEMIOLOGY

Incidence

There are no accurate figures available on the incidence of alcoholism (the number of new cases in a given population over the course of 1 year). This is explained in part because of the gradual onset of alcohol dependence and the extreme reluctance of many clinicians to record this diagnosis because of their concern that such a "label" will prejudice the patient's future medical care.

Prevalence

Depending on the definition used, there are 6–9 million (4.5% of the population) Americans at any given time suffering from alcoholism. One out of every 10

Americans who drinks is likely to experience symptoms of alcoholism. Alarmingly, it has recently been reported that 3 out of 10 high school students are moderate to heavy drinkers and that drinking among young high school girls is increasing.[10]

Per capita consumption of beer, wine, and spirits also continues to rise. Per capita consumption reached 2.7 gallons per year in 1978, up from 2.5 gallons in 1970 and 2.0 gallons in 1960. Interestingly, while consumption increased, the rate of increase over the years has slowed, suggesting that consumption patterns may eventually stabilize.[11]

Age, Sex, and Race

Changes in age, sex, and racial usage of alcohol reflect the current shift in drinking patterns in the United States. The percentage of Americans who drink increased from 58% in 1939 to 71% in 1978, with significant increases in drinking among women and teenagers.[12] Adult drinking habits in the United States reveal that, in the heavier drinking category, males (14%) outnumber females (4%). Furthermore, 25% of males reported abstaining from beverage alcohol, as opposed to 40% of females. While some ethnic groups have traditionally had a high (Irish) or low (Italian) prevalence of alcoholism, the more these groups have become integrated into American society, the more their drinking patterns have changed and become more consistent with the general population.[13] Blacks continue to have a higher prevalence than whites, but this may be primarily due to socioeconomic rather than genetic factors.[14]

SOCIOECONOMIC STATUS

Alcoholism shows no respect for social class. It is widely distributed among all groups. Traditionally, the upper classes have been better able to hide the evidence of their problem drinking. This concealment has been aided by physicians who are reluctant to record the diagnosis because they fear the effect of such a stigma on middle class or upper class patients. Obviously, this makes for difficulty obtaining accurate epidemiological data. It is clear, however, that the stereotyped skid row alcoholic represents less than 3% of the alcoholic population and is a minor, though highly visible, part of the problem. For many alcoholics, chronic drinking has severe economic consequences and leads to a downward drift on the socioeconomic scale. Others, however, continue to work and function, despite their drinking—often protected from the consequences of their drinking by their higher socioeconomic status. The more alcoholism is studied, the more apparent it is that the widely held view of alcoholism as a problem of the lower classes is not substantiated by fact.

Families

Alcoholism is clearly a familial disease. Persons reporting a liquor-related problem in their family rose from 12% in 1962 to 33% in 1983.[12, 15] A family history of alcoholism suggests a high potential for the disease, especially in the sons and brothers of alcoholics (see Genetic Theories). Winokur's[16] studies of alcoholic families demonstrated that 46% of the brothers of male alcoholics were alcoholic, as were 50% of the brothers of female alcoholics. Females tend to manifest the disease at a later age than males.

Health Problems

Alcoholism is the third ranking cause of death in the United States, following cancer and heart disease. Ten percent of all deaths in the United States are alcohol-related, including up to 80% of all suicides.[11] One in ten adults who drink is likely to become a heavy drinker or an alcoholic.

The Hospital Discharge Survey (U.S. Department of Health, Education and Welfare) estimated an almost 10% increase in the number of alcoholism-related discharges between 1975 and 1977. The number of alcohol discharges from Veterans Administration Hospitals doubled between 1970 and 1977.[11]

A recent longitudinal study reported mortality rates in a group of alcoholics to be 2½ times greater than expected. For all ages, mortality due to cirrhosis is nearly twice as high for blacks as for whites. For urban black males (age 25–34), the rates for mortality due to cirrhosis are 10 times higher than for white males of the same age.[11]

Brain atrophy is reported in 50–100% of alcoholics. New evidence suggests that heavy social drinking may also result in brain atrophy.[17] Numerous studies have also shown that chronic ingestion of alcohol may cause sexual impotence, loss of libido, breast enlargement, loss of facial hair, and testicular atrophy.[11]

About half of the 55,000 highway deaths per year can be attributed to alcohol.

ETIOLOGY

The confusion over an exact definition of alcoholism reflects the lack of agreement over the etiology of this condition. Many theories have been proposed. The major ones are outlined below.

Genetic Theories

It has been recognized that alcoholism tends to recur in certain families. Numerous studies in various countries have shown higher rates of alcoholism among relatives of alcoholics than among the general population.[18] However, it was previously assumed that these findings were due to environmental factors rather than heredity, though the role of genetic influences was never adequately explored.

Recent studies have been very helpful in clarifying the etiology of some forms of alcoholism and have demonstrated the relative importance of both environmental and genetic factors. Alcoholism in males, particularly in its most severe form, is most likely a genetically transmitted disease. In women and in men with milder forms of alcoholism, the etiology is less clear and may involve a combination of genetic and environmental factors.

One way to study the varying effects of heredity and environment has been to compare the drinking patterns of identical and nonidentical twins raised in the same family. Kaij[19] studied 174 pairs of twins in Sweden, where one member of each pair had been listed on the Swedish National Register of Alcohol Abusers. The importance of heredity was demonstrated by the finding that when one twin was a serious alcohol abuser, the other twin was also an alcohol abuser in 54% of the identical twins but only in 28% of the nonidentical twins.

A more effective study to separate the influences of genetics and environment was carried out by Goodwin et al.[20] using the Danish Adoption and Psychiatric Register. Sons of alcoholics separated in early life from alcoholic parents were almost four times more likely to become alcoholics than were adoptees without alcoholic biological parents. The increasing severity of the biological father's alcoholism increased the likelihood that the son would be alcoholic.

Similar studies did not document a clear genetic transmission pattern in adopted daughters of alcoholics.[21]

Winokur et al.[22] have hypothesized that there is a genetic link between alcoholism, unipolar depression, and antisocial personality. He studied 259 alcoholics and 507 of their relatives and concluded that female relatives of alcoholics have an increased incidence of unipolar depression and that male relatives have an increased incidence of both alcoholism and antisocial personality, *but not depression.*

Other studies, however, have not documented a clear genetic link between alcoholism and other psychiatric diseases. Goodwin's[23] Danish Adoption Studies found that the increased risk for alcoholism did not involve an increased risk for depression, antisocial personality, or other psychopathology.

Cloninger and Guze[24] found a link between sociopathy and alcoholism in their study of American prison inmates, though no linkage between criminality and alcoholism exists in the general population. In a study in the United States of adopted-away children of criminals, Crowe[25] found an increased risk of criminal activity among the adoptees but no increased risk

for alcoholism or other psychiatric disorders. After reviewing the literature in this area, Cloninger and associates[26] concluded that there were genetic contributions to the susceptibility to alcoholism, antisocial personality, and depressive illness, and that these conditions sometimes appear in the same family and in the same individual. However, these conditions were considered etiologically and clinically separate and not as alternative manifestations of the same underlying etiological mechanism.

In a further effort to clarify the impact of environment and heredity in the development of alcoholism, Cloninger et al.[27] studied 862 Swedish men adopted by nonrelatives at an early age. They were able to identify two different types of alcoholism that have distinct genetic and environmental causes.

The more frequent "milieu-limited" type is usually mild in symptomatology and is associated with histories of mild alcohol abuse in one or both biological parents. More severe alcoholism in the adopted son is related to a postnatal environment characterized by low economic status of the adoptive father and a history of extensive institutional care of the adoptee prior to the final placement. In contrast, the other type of alcoholism ("male-limited type") is associated with moderate to severe symptoms of alcoholism, severe alcoholism and criminality in the biological father, but not in the biological mother, and is unrelated to any problems in the postnatal environment.

While much work remains to be done to clarify the etiology of alcoholism, it is now apparent that genetic factors are a major determinant, particularly in the most severe cases of alcoholism. Family studies have shown that the incidence of alcoholism for first degree and second degree relatives of alcoholics is the same, thereby ruling out a single recessive or dominant gene pattern of Mendelian inheritance.[28] It is therefore probable that several gene locations are involved in the inheritance of alcoholism. In less severe cases, it is also probable that environmental factors play a significant role. Whatever the mechanism of inheritance, it appears specific for alcoholism (at least in males) and unrelated to any personality disorder or other psychiatric illness.

Psychodynamic Theories

Early analysts emphasized the libidinal (instinctual) gratification and the "regressive" aspects of alcohol use.[29, 30] Knight noted the connection between alcoholism and a passive-dependent personality structure and described a particular family environment that he believed predisposed individuals to these disorders.

Knight outlined these factors: (1) an overindulgent mother; (2) a cold, severe, inconsistently supportive father; (3) an oral-dependent son who demands oral affection while feeling rejected once it is received, and who drinks to overcompensate for feelings of inferiority, passivity, and effeminacy and to overcome inhibitions on the expressions of rageful and sexual feelings.[31]

In the last three decades, there has been a shift in emphasis in analytic theory away from the view that alcohol abuse is "regressive" behavior. Contemporary analysts now focus more on the "progressive" aspects of the "abuse" of alcohol and other drugs. Glover[32] noted that drugs (alcohol) could be used adaptively to cope with and defend against powerful drives of rage and aggression.

Kernberg[33] has connected borderline pathology to alcoholism, but it is not clear whether he believes that alcoholism is caused by borderline symptomatology or whether there are similar processes that affect both conditions. He theorizes that individuals with these conditions suffer from an "ego defect" with a lack of impulse control and anxiety intolerance. He suggests that they manifest primitive ego defenses, including splitting of introjects, rigid walling off of good and bad introjects, and denial in the service of preventing the individual from experiencing anxiety associated with aggressive drives.

More recently Khantzian[34] has related alcohol abuse problems to disturbances in ego functions involving self-care (avoidance of harmful activities and situations) and the ability to identify, verbalize, and regulate affects.

After comparing the drinking patterns of Italians and Italian-Americans, Jessor[13] concluded that Americans, unlike Italians, use alcohol to cope with frustration and alienation. Tyndel,[35] in a sample of 1,017 alcoholics admitted to a medical ward, found that all of the individuals in this sample had major pyschiatric disorders. In this group, 58% (591) suffered anxiety and other neurosis; 36% (365) displayed personality disorders; and 6% (61) were diagnosed as psychotic or suffering from affective disorders.

Further breakdown of the sample showed that many of these alcoholic patients had symptoms of depression, organic memory deficiencies, and a history of DT's or hallucinations. This study further documented the connection, in North American drinking habits, between psychological distress and excessive drinking.

Sociocultural Theories

Peer pressure has been identified as a factor in the etiology of alcoholism, primarily in adolescents. Although decidedly a dangerous activity to prove adulthood, adolescent drinking continues to increase in popularity as a means of attaining acceptance.

There is also ample evidence of cultural acceptance and prohibition of deviant drinking behavior. The Irish have an alcoholism rate that is two to three times that of other groups. Sociological theories conclude that this is derived from the cultural suppression of aggression and sexuality coupled with the enforced dependence of most males, both of which produce a high degree of inner tension in the individual. The general acceptance of drinking and drunkenness in the pubs and a profound tolerance of "poor boy" syndromes further reinforces alcoholic behavior.

Jews, by comparison, who ritualize the early use of alcohol, have an extreme prohibition against drunkenness and a low rate of alcoholism, attesting to the potent impact of a consistent social attitude on group behavior. In addition, Jewish culture permits alternate (other than alcohol) means of tension release and satisfaction.

Most theories on the sociocultural etiology of alcoholism support the following conclusions: social drinking is a sociological variable that correlates with sex, age, religion, class, and urbanization; heavy drinking correlates with psychological variables and is linked to psychological stress.[36]

Learning Theories

Behavioral theory holds that drinking and drunkenness are learned behaviors that are repeated because they are rewarded. Alcohol use can be strongly reinforcing because it reduces anxiety.[37] Conger[38] hypothesized that alcoholism can reduce sexual and aggressive drives and is therefore reinforcing.

Learning theory regards drinking as leading to immediate positive reinforcement in the form of euphoria and tension reduction. These immediate reinforcements are more powerful than the delayed, negative reinforcement of a hangover. Furthermore, alcohol intake lowers inhibitions, thereby permitting the expression and consequent reduction of sexual and aggressive drives.

BIOPSYCHOSOCIAL EVALUATION

Interviewing the Patient

There are few areas in modern psychiatry in which the hypotheses testing approach to diagnosis is more useful. Lazare noted that during the clinical assessment process, clinicians utilize a number of common, but often unarticulated, perspectives. He suggested that more effective assessment can be accomplished by directing specific attention to the four most common perspectives, namely, the biological, sociological, psychodynamic, and behavioral models. Viewing the patient from each of these perspectives permits the clinician to develop a number of clinical hypotheses regarding the nature of the patient's difficulty. By further questioning and data collection, the clinician can test the various hypotheses and thus reach a more accurate and comprehensive understanding of the patient's problems.[39]

In psychiatry, the primary tool used in this clinical assessment process is the patient interview. Since the patient is often unaware of, or denies, the role of alcohol is his problem, direct questioning about drinking may be highly unproductive. Once the clinician has picked up clues suggesting a drinking problem, he can respond by formulating a variety of hypotheses that relate the drinking to the patient's symptoms.

The clinician soon learns, however, that the questioning necessary to elicit information and to develop various clinical hypotheses can sometimes be carried out only by avoiding a direct confrontation of the drinking problem. Many patients, particularly those feeling guilty about their alcohol problems, will distort and lie about the amount of alcohol consumed and its effect on their lives.

One useful approach to data gathering that does not generate hostility or defensiveness is the CAGE system developed by Drs. Ewing and Rouse at the University of North Carolina. CAGE is a mneumonic for four questions which Ewing and Rouse intersperse in the medical and psychiatric history.

C—Have you ever thought you should CUT DOWN on your drinking?

A—have you ever felt ANNOYED by others' criticism of your drinking?

G—have you ever felt GUILTY about your drinking?

E—Have you ever had a morning EYE OPENER?

These questions will elicit positive responses in a very high percentage of alcoholics, without confronting the patient's denial. Two or more "yes" answers are correlated with serious alcoholism in more than 90% of the patients tested.[40]

Another helpful method for evaluation has been suggested by Hanna.[41] She recommended collecting a detailed drinking history for the full 7 days prior to admission. Inquiry should be made regarding the type of alcohol consumed, the exact quantity and form, the frequency, setting, reason for drinking, and any evidence for loss of control. Such detailed questioning also helps less aware patients realize the full magnitude of their drinking problem.

The clinician must remember that alcoholism is one of those areas of psychiatry wherein conflict between the patient and the clinician can become a major impediment to effective treatment. The difficulty begins over the definition of the problem. Negotiating a mutually acceptable definition of the problem is the most difficult task and may require an ongoing effort during most of the early stages of therapy. One may have to begin with a simple agreement to thoroughly evaluate the patient's medical and psychological status. Even reluctant patients may cooperate with this, as long as they are not prematurely forced to acknowledge an alcohol problem or make a committment to treatment.

Alcoholism can be understood using a variety of conceptual models. The biological, psychological, behavioral, and social models are not competing ideological explanations for the condition, but rather reflections of the complex factors interacting in the alcoholic patient. In developing hypotheses to evaluate the alcoholic, it is helpful to use all four of these conceptual models.

Biological-Medical Evaluation

Because of the medical complications of chronic alcohol abuse, the alcoholic usually requires a more thorough admission evaluation than many other psychiatric patients. The minimal workup should include: medical history, physical examination, chest x-ray, EKG, complete blood cell count (CBC) with differential, hemocrit, glucose, BUN, sodium, calcium, prothombin time, VDRL, amylase, magnesium, and liver function tests.

If there is a history of seizures, a neurological consultation is indicated. The most important and pressing need is usually for detoxification or treatment to prevent DT's. This will be described in a later section.

Adequate evaluation of the patient requires a knowledge of the metabolism of alcohol and its effect on the body. Alcohol is rapidly absorbed through the stomach mucosa with a measurable blood-alcohol level in 15–20 minutes. One ounce of alcohol can be metabolized per hour by metabolic breakdown in the liver and excretion by the lungs and kidneys.

Blood alcohol levels of 0.05% are associated with decreased inhibitions and impaired judgment. A level of 0.10% affects motor and speech functions; 0.20% is characterized by motor impairment; 0.30% usually produces stupor; and levels of 0.40–0.60% result in coma and/or respiratory paralysis. In most cases, five beers or three double shots in 1 hour produce a blood alcohol level of 0.10%; it would take 3 hours for the patient to revert to a level of 0.05%.

Alcohol has a paradoxical effect on the central nervous system (CNS). It both excites and depresses. The sedative effect occurs first and usually lasts for 3 hours. This is followed by a period of psychomotor hyperactivity that can last up to 12 hours after the initial drinking episode. During this period individuals may start to drink again in an effort to counteract the feelings of tension produced by the CNS hyperactivity. For chronic alcoholics, this means repeated cycles of sedation, followed by hyperactivity, followed by more drinking to restore the desired sense of sedation.

Metabolically, alcohol (C_2H_5OH) is first broken down to acetaldehyde, then to acetic acid, and eventually to $CO_2 + H_2O$. Disulfiram (Antabuse) inhibits the enzyme acetaldehyde dehydrogenase which acts to catalyze the metabolism of acetaldehyde to acetic acid.

When this metabolism is severely retarded by disulfiram, the patient becomes ill because of toxic blood levels of acetaldehyde.

Being alcoholic is no protection against the development of other psychiatric conditions such as depression, mania, or schizophrenia. Appropriate medications are indicated in these conditions. It may be impossible to evaluate and treat the problem of alcoholism without adequate control of any concurrent medical or psychiatric disorder.

Psychological Evaluation

In assessing the psychological aspects of the patient's condition, many problems are obvious. Are there specific psychodynamic and psychological issues that have permitted the drinking to continue and have fostered the intensification of the illness? How will the patient respond to treatment?

Because alcoholism is a chronic condition, plans must be started early to develop a long-term after-care program. How will the patient's particular personality type or style affect the type of treatment he may find acceptable and believe to be effective? Will he accept Alcoholics Anonymous (A.A.) or another group-oriented therapy? Does a particular treatment program need to be developed to compensate for the patient's special psychological problems? Does the patient's denial make referral to A.A. or other alcohol rehabilitation programs impossible? It is also important to consider what particular psychological stress or problem may have precipitated the patient's request for treatment at this time.

Behavioral Evaluation

In assessing alcoholism from a behavioral perspective, it is clear that there can be strong behavioral reinforcements for excessive drinking. Alcohol, particularly in lower doses, relieves tension and anxiety and may permit the expression of otherwise guilt-ridden or conflicted impulses. Such drinking behavior can be reinforcing. Because the patient usually focuses on the more immediate relief-giving aspects of the drinking rather than on its long-term negative consequences, the drinking tends to recur. Careful questioning about the circumstances when the patient drinks or, more importantly, when he loses control of his drinking, may pinpoint particular stresses or conflicts that the patient resolves by drinking. How does he act when drunk? Are certain conflicted impulses acted out during drinking spells? Does drinking or being sick and hung over bring out reinforcing responses from the patient's family, friends, or employer?

Social Evaluation

When assessing the patient, it is important to recognize that cultural norms regarding drinking patterns, type of alcohol consumed, the social situation, and the quantities consumed may differ from one social group to another. The alcoholic's drinking pattern must be assessed in comparison with the normal pattern of his own social group. In early stages, the social impact of drinking may be apparent only in terms of decreased economic functioning. In later stages of alcoholism, the social consequences of drinking become obvious. When alcohol becomes the focus for the individual's total social life, the drinking problem clearly is in an advanced stage. Are all of your patient's relationships determined by a common interest in drinking? Has the patient lost friends or changed social groups because of his drinking? In severe cases, alcohol becomes a substitute for all meaningful interpersonal relationships. Some patients will verbalize that they have turned to alcohol to replace painful and disappointing interpersonal relationships.

The patient's family must be involved in the admission and the evaluation process and must be actively engaged in the treatment process. Alcoholism may be an outgrowth of destructive patterns of family interaction. Alcoholism always has a negative impact on family life.

Family members should be interviewed as a group and individually. The evaluation should focus on individual and family drinking patterns. How does the patient's drinking effect the family? How does the family respond to the patient when he is drunk, sober, hung over, or about to drink? Are patterns of family interaction reinforcing the drinking behavior? What problems does the drinking cause? What family problems does the drinking resolve? What problems does it hide? It is not unusual to discover that the spouse or other family members are also alcoholic. Alcoholism may be a family secret that can only be confronted with the assistance of the treatment staff.

A similar inquiry must also be made in regard to the patient's circumstances at work and in his primary social and recreational activities. In alcoholism, there is no area of the patient's life that is not affected. For treatment to succeed, the patient may require assistance in every major area of his life.

HOSPITAL TREATMENT

Initial Treatment Goals

Uncomplicated alcohol detoxification rarely requires hospitalization on a psychiatric unit. However, it is not uncommon to discover that alcoholism is a major problem for patients admitted for treatment of other psychiatric conditions. Suicide attempts, severe marital conflict, and other emotional crisis may mask underlying problems with alcohol. The diagnosis of alcoholism is often missed, even by competent physicians, if the patient is married, employed, has insurance, or is a voluntary admission with some other illness.

Even when there is little question about the presence of a drinking problem, the patient may continue to deny it and may resist the idea of hospitalization. It may be necessary for the staff to take a flexible attitude on admission and not insist that the patient admit he is an alcoholic or agree that sobriety is necessary as a treatment goal. Excessive initial demands by staff may drive the patient away from badly needed treatment.

With patients who deny their alcoholism, it is often best that initial treatment goals focus on the patient's need to accept hospitalization to fully "evaluate a problem." After a treatment relationship is established and the basic evaluation is completed, it may be possible to confront the patient about the reality of his drinking problem. Confrontation can begin by emphasizing the consequences of the patient's drinking; namely, the medical, social, and economic costs associated with his destructive drinking pattern. It is often helpful to involve the family in this confrontation process.

It is wise not to argue over the quantity of alcohol consumed or the label of "alcoholism" but rather to focus on the need to do something about a "problem." Ultimately, the therapist's initial goal is to negotiate a treatment contract that the patient will accept. This may involve an agreement that the patient has a drinking problem while avoiding use of the word alcoholism. The patient may be willing to accept reduced drinking as an initial treatment goal, whereas he may refuse to accept total sobriety as a goal. As treatment progresses, the patient may be more willing to accept the reality of his alcoholism and to define more realistic treatment goals.

Medical Management

The Intoxicated Patient

Occasionally patients may be mildly intoxicated on admission. Ordinarily this situation requires no special treatment, other than to ensure that the patient does not injure himself, fall out of bed, etc. In cases of moderate agitation, 25 or 50 mg chlordiazepoxide P.O. can be given to assist the inebriate in sleeping it off.[42]

Treatment of the Alcohol Withdrawal Syndrome

More frequently, the alcoholic patient has stopped drinking immediately prior to admission and will show signs of early alcohol withdrawal (see Table 8.1). Prompt sedation is necessary to reduce the severity of the withdrawal syndrome and to avoid the life-threatening sequelae of delirium tremens. Benzodiazepines are the preferred class of drugs, because of both effectiveness and safety.[43] They produce minimal respiratory and cardiovascular depression. They also act without depressing REM sleep, which permits more rapid dream recovery following the prolonged dream suppression caused by alcohol.[44] The standard treatment is chlordiazepoxide (100 mg P.O.) on admission, with hourly repeats until adequate sedation is accomplished. It is rarely necessary to exceed 600 mg in the first 24 hours. Detoxification can be completed by gradually tapering the dose over 5–6 days. Individual doses should be withheld if the patient shows any signs of excessive sedation.

If there is any evidence of hepatic disease, oxazepam is the drug of choice because of its short duration of action and its lack of hepatic toxicity. Oxazepam is available only in oral form. Chlordiazepoxide and diazepam are available I.M., but absorption is unreliable, always making oral administration preferable. In case of vomiting, or other gastrointestinal upset, sedation may be initiated with a dose of diazepam (10 mg I.V.). This can usually be followed with oral medications as described above.

Ancillary Medication

Thiamine: 100–200 mg I.M. or I.V. on admission; the same dose should be repeated orally for the next 3 days.

Folic acid: 1–5 mg I.M. or P.O. daily while hospitalized.

Multivitamins: 1 capsule P.O. daily while hospitalized.

Magnesium sulfate (50% solution): 2–4 ml I.M. q. 8 hours for three doses). Regardless of serum concentrations, most alcoholics are magnesium depleted. Hypomagnesia may lower the seizure threshold and can contribute to the alcoholic's symptoms of lethargy and weakness.

Optional Medications

Vitamin K: 5–10 mg I.V. as a single dose, *if the prothrombin* time is greater than 3 seconds beyond control.

Diphenylhydantoin (100 mg P.O. t.i.d.) if the patient has any history of seizures.

Note: Diphenylhydantoin will not prevent alcohol withdrawal seizures, but it will provide control of seizures in patients with a pre-existing seizure disorder (see If Withdrawal Seizures Occur for treatment of withdrawal seizures).

Pharmacological Treatment of Concurrent Psychiatric Problems

Despite frequent complaints on admission of anxiety and depression, alcoholics who are not suffering from other psychiatric diseases do not require long-term psychopharmacological treatment. The use of minor tranquilizers (particularly benzodiazepines) is to be avoided after detoxification because of problems with habituation and poly-drug abuse. In a prospective study of alcohol use and mental health, Vaillant[45] has demonstrated that depression and an inability to cope are a consequence, not a cause, of the alcoholic's inability to control alcohol consumption.

Vaillant's study showed that among high social status problem drinkers, personality changes occurred (development of oral-dependent personality traits; pessimism, self-doubt, passivity, etc.) after the individual lost control of the drinking. Anecdotal information from Alcoholics Anonymous members tends to confirm this information, along with the observation that symptoms of depression and anxiety disappear and personality changes reverse after an individual maintains sobriety.

Regardless of these findings, it is clear that alcoholism confers no immunity to other psychiatric illness. Furthermore, there is a subset of individuals who may self-medicate with alcohol in an effort to control pre-existing psychological distress. Such cases of *secondary alcoholism* can be identified through a careful examination and history with an emphasis on symptoms that predated the patient's drinking.

There have been many reports of studies done to establish the efficacy of various psychopharmacological drugs in the treatment of *primary alcoholism.* Reviews of the literature[46–48] have shown disappointing results. Most of the studies have been uncontrolled and poorly designed and hence have not adequately documented the effectiveness of the agents tested. At the present time, there is insufficient evidence to recommend the pharmacological treatment of *primary alcoholism.*

However, in patients with secondary alcoholism who show clear-cut evidence of other psychiatric conditions, various recommendations for psychopharmacologic treatment can be made:

Schizophrenia

Routine treatment with neuroleptics is recommended. This often leads to marked improvement in drinking patterns.

Affective Disorders

Various studies of depression in alcoholics have shown an incidence ranging from 3% to 98%.[49] These studies are difficult to compare because of imprecise diagnosis and the wide variety of diagnostic tests utilized. The only clear evidence for the effectiveness of tricyclic antidepressants is in those patients with a psychotic depression (3%–8.6% of the sample of alcoholics, depending on which study is used).

Schuckit[50] has also reviewed the literature on the use of antidepressants in alcoholics and does not recommend routine use of tricyclics in *primary alcoholism.* He notes that alcohol in high doses will cause depressed affect in normals and alcoholics and that the depression will clear a few days after drinking ceases.

Nonpsychotic patients with unipolar depression have been noted to decrease, increase, or stabilize their drinking while depressed. Treatment with tricyclics may improve their depression, but it has no predictable effect on their drinking.

Bipolar patients tend to increase their drinking during manic phases and often reduce their drinking when treated with lithium. Lithium has also been reported to be effective in reducing the drinking of patients with *secondary alcoholism* who show symptoms of depression. Interestingly, the lithium was effective in reducing drinking without eliminating the subject's depression. Kline suggests that lithium may reduce the euphoric effects of alcohol and thus discourage drinking. This drug had no beneficial effect on alcoholics who were not depressed. The results in this patient group also suggest that their depression was not the direct cause of their drinking.[51-53]

Studies by Judd et al. and Fawcett et al. have suggested that treatment with lithium will increase abstinence in alcoholics, unrelated to any history of affective disease.[54, 55] However, these findings must be re-evaluated in larger controlled trials before one can recommend the use of lithium for treating *primary alcoholism*.

Anxiety States

Some patients continue to complain of anxiety after the completion of detoxification. In most cases this is a prolonged withdrawal effect from alcohol, and the symptoms will gradually disappear if the patient refrains from the use of alcohol and minor tranquilizers. If complaints of anxiety are extreme and continue beyond 2 weeks of sobriety, the patient should be evaluated carefully for the presence of a "primary" anxiety disorder. Hyperthyroidism and caffeine intoxication must also be ruled out. Agoraphobia and panic disorder are distinct clinical entities generally associated with recurrent but time-limited episodes of anxiety. These conditions respond well to antidepressants (tricyclics or monoamine oxidase inhibitors) or behavior therapy. Specific symptoms of anxiety and agoraphobia were impressively relieved in some alcoholics by treatment with imipramine in a study reported by Quitkin et al.[56]

In generalized anxiety disorder one looks for a history of chronic complaints, autonomic hyperactivity, motor tension, apprehensive expectation, vigilance, and scanning. There is often a family history of anxiety disorders. Treatment should be very conservative. *There is no evidence that minor tranquilizers are effective for the long-term management of chronic anxiety in the alcoholic or in other patients.* Because of the potential for abuse, these drugs should be used with extreme caution in this patient population.

Treatment alternatives include relaxation therapy, biofeedback, and/or psychotherapy. If the patient's complaints are extreme, one might consider the use of beta-blockers or low doses of a neuroleptic, such as thioridazine (25 mg P.O. t.i.d.). Overall et al. have reported the effectiveness of amitriptyline (25 mg P.O. t.i.d.) in treating symptoms of anxiety and depression in the recently detoxified alcoholic.[57]

Special Syndromes

On occasion some special syndromes related to alcohol abuse will occur and will require appropriate management.

Hangover

The usual symptoms which occur 8–12 hours after intoxication are a severe headache (made worse by sounds, bright lights, and movement), heartburn, nausea, and vomiting. Severe thirst, dry mouth, dizziness, sweating, and insomnia may also be present.

Moderate symptoms do not require treatment, though a mild analgesic may be given. Tranquilizers and sedatives should be avoided.

Pathological Intoxication

Following ingestion of a small quantity of alcohol (one to three drinks), which is not enough to produce intoxication, there occurs a marked behavioral change with confusion, unpredictable violent behavior, and disorganized thought processes and speech. The episode may last minutes or several hours and is followed by deep sleep and total or partial amnesia for the incident.

Patients with pathological intoxication usually have a history of some type of significant head injury. Incidents of pathological intoxication are often precipitated by severe stress.

Sedation is required in cases of extreme agitation. The patient must also be counseled on the serious risks of even moderate drinking.

Alcohol-Induced Coma

On rare occasions, patients have attempted suicide by the ingestion of large quantities of alcohol. Such situations represent a medical emergency. The patient should immediately be transferred to an intensive care unit.

The poison unit at Guy's Hospital in London has recently reported complete reversal of alcohol-induced coma. Twenty percent of cases treated with naloxone (up to 1.2 mg I.M. or I.V.) improved within 10 minutes.[58]

Withdrawal Seizures

Prophylactic Treatment. In patients with no history of seizures except during prior alcohol withdrawal, there is no evidence that prophylactic diphenylhydantoin will prevent withdrawal seizures. Routine detoxification treatment with benzodiazepines provides adequate anticonvulsant coverage and will greatly reduce the incidence of seizures.

Patients with Known Seizure Disorders. Individuals with a history of grand mal seizures unrelated to alcohol withdrawal are at increased risk during detoxification. If they have been on regular maintenance diphenylhydantoin, this should be continued at its normal dosage. If diphenylhydantoin was stopped 5 or more days prior to admission, then total body stores have been depleted and a loading dose of 1 g in 500 ml of 5% dextrose in water should be given by continuous infusion over 1–4 hours. Regular maintenance doses can be reinstituted the following day.[48]

If Withdrawal Seizures Occur. Seizures usually occur within 48 hours of cessation of drinking and are characteristically grand mal and nonfocal in nature. There are rarely more than two seizures, and they cease without specific treatment. No additional care is indicated other than to protect the patient from self-injury and to observe carefully during the postictal period.

If seizures are repeated, then treatment for status epilepticus should be instituted. Diazepam (5 mg I.V. per minute) can be given until the seizures cease, with a ceiling of 25 mg. An alternative is phenobarbital (120 mg I.M.). If there is any evidence of focal seizures, focal neurological signs, increased intracranial pressure, head injuries, or metabolic disturbance, the patient should have an immediate and complete neurological workup.

Abuse of Other Drugs

It is not uncommon to encounter alcoholics who also abuse other sedatives, marijuana, or stimulants, including cocaine. Although the patient may require specialized medical treatment for detoxification, the long-term clinical management should be no different from that outlined here for the alcoholic. Once an individual has become addicted to any drug, it is unlikely that he will ever be able to use other psychoactive drugs without abuse or dependency. The goal of treatment should therefore be abstinence from *all* psychoactive drugs. Participation in A.A. or similar group support programs, as outlined below, should be the major treatment modality.[59]

Wet Brain

Chronic alcoholics may be suffering from more extensive neurological impairment than is apparent on routine physical and mental status examination. In contrast to the traditional view that Korsakoff's syndrome has a sudden onset, Ryback[60] has proposed that alcoholics manifest distinctive neuropathological and cognitive changes that develop gradually, correlated with the severity and duration of alcohol use and avitaminosis.

Deficits in short-term memory and learning ability have been documented in a group of detoxified chronic alcoholics. These patients had *no complaints of memory loss* and did not differ from controls on standard clinical memory tests, yet showed significant impairment on more demanding experimental tests. Alcoholics complaining of memory problems showed even greater impairment on clinical and experimental tests when compared to controls and other alcoholics. This group bordered on the marked impairment seen in Korsakoff patients.[61]

These findings have important clinical implications. Even in early stages of alcoholism, it may take weeks of sobriety before a patient regains full higher level intellectual capacities. In chronic alcoholics it may take months, or even years, of sobriety and adequate diet before normal capacities are regained. Patients with any significant memory deficit are unlikely to attain any lasting benefit from formal psychotherapy until the memory deficit is improved. This must be kept in mind when developing treatment plans.

If there is any doubt regarding a patient's capacities, a thorough neurological evaluation, including psychoneurological testing, should be obtained (Table 8.3).

Table 8.3.
Recommended Psychoneurological Tests

1. Comprehensive Cognitive and Intellectual
   Functions
   Wechsler Adult Intelligence Scale-Revised
   (WAIS-R)
   Wechsler Memory Quotient
   Memory-for-Design Tests;
   Bender-Gestalt
   Benton Visual Retention Test
   Graham-Kendall
2. Personality Functions
   Minnesota Multiphasic Inventory (MMPI)
   Rorschach
   Thematic Apperception Test (TAT)
   (using 5 to 7 cards)
3. Cognitive, Educational, and Occupational Skills
   Holland's Self Directed Search Test
   Strong-Campbell Interest Inventory
   Jastak Wide Range Achievement Test (WRAT)
   Minnesota Importance Questionnaire
   General Aptitude Test Battery (GATB)

Borderline cases of impairment may be missed because such patients may appear to function normally in social settings and less demanding jobs and usually show no impairment of intelligence on routine I.Q. tests. Their problems may only be apparent in tasks requiring learning of new material, recent memory, and judgment. Testing should not be attempted until 1–2 weeks after the completion of detoxification.

Milieu Management

Treatment for the patient's alcoholism should be carried out concurrently with the treatment of other psychiatric problems. The management approaches suggested in this section are recommended as supplementary to the basic inpatient milieu program and do not supplant other needed psychiatric treatment.

There are two primary goals in the inpatient treatment of the alcoholic. The first is to safely detoxify the patient from alcohol. The second and more important is to break through the patient's denial about his illness and to effectively engage him in a long-term outpatient therapy program. The inpatient milieu can be especially helpful in achieving this second goal. Indeed, there is evidence that a peer-oriented approach is more successful and is certainly more cost effective than a staff intensive individual therapy model for the treatment of alcoholics.[62]

The milieu approach should be modified in certain ways to best manage some of the specific problems of the alcoholic. Ideally, a special group just for alcoholic patients can be established, just as some wards set up specialized groups for women's issues, or men's issues, etc. The group should meet three times weekly. Since Alcoholics Anonymous (A.A.) will be a primary referral for most patients following discharge, orientation and involvement in this program should begin as early as possible.

The primary problem encountered early in hospitalization usually is the patient's denial and reluctance to commit himself to ongoing treatment. Some patients will be particularly opposed to A.A. For this reason, it is recommended that the inpatient group be co-led by a staff member who is sympathetic to A.A. and a volunteer A.A. member, ideally a former patient. The group work should include education about alcohol and its effects on physical and psychological health, A.A. and other community treatment resources, and confrontation about the patient's specific drinking problem. It is important, however, that these groups *specifically not be A.A. meetings.*

In addition to these groups, the alcoholic patient should be required to attend two A.A. meetings per week. The hospital can invite an outside A.A. group to hold one open A.A. meeting per week at the hospital. Attendance should be mandatory for alcoholic inpatients and voluntary for other interested patients or visitors. As soon as a patient is stable, he should also be required to attend one A.A. meeting per week outside of the hospital, escorted by an A.A. volunteer.

Alcoholics Anonymous

It is important that the unit staff become familiar with the program and philosophy of A.A. The staff should learn about specific A.A. groups in their community and how to make appropriate referrals to these groups.

A.A. is basically a group process. Individuals are comfortable in A.A. only if they can successfully identify with other group members. A.A. does not officially acknowledge that particular groups have special economic or social orientations and often insist that the common identity of being an alcoholic is all that is necessary for an individual to fit into any A.A. group. Unfortunately, this is not always the case. Some individuals drop out of A.A. not because of their difficulty acknowledging a drinking problem nor because of conflict with the basic philosophy of A.A., but because they were never able to feel comfortable with the social aspects of the particular group they had joined.

A.A. is basically a middle-class program. Individuals of the lower, upper middle, and upper classes often have difficulty adjusting to A.A., unless they make contact with a group whose membership matches their social class. Information regarding the makeup of specific groups is available informally from A.A. members in the community.

To get the most out of A.A., an effort should be made to refer patients to A.A. groups that are comparable with their sex, race, social class, and employment background. In all metropolitan areas, there are a variety of A.A. groups. There often is an A.A. Central Service that will help with referrals. A.A. is the original self-help program in which the active drinker is helped to achieve sobriety through the support of sober alcoholics. A major part of their approach is the emphasis on remaining sober "one day at a time." The alcoholic is required to acknowledge his disease and his inability to control it. Total abstinence is the only acceptable treatment goal. Many would-be social drinkers find it difficult to accept this philosophy and often use this to justify their refusal to join A.A. The program is based on frequent, often daily, group meetings at which members spell out in great detail how alcohol negatively affected them and how they have learned to gain control over their illness. Strong group support is available for any member making a genuine effort to achieve sobriety.

It is important to recognize that patients participating in A.A. sometimes experience conflict with the guidance and direction given in their psychiatric treatment. Many A.A. members are leery about all forms of medication and may encourage a patient to stop taking medically prescribed drugs. A.A. itself takes no official position on these matters, but many A.A. members have difficulty differentiating mood-altering and other potentially abusive drugs from those medications necessary to control major psychoses or seizures, or from other necessary medication. Often, the physician will have to give very direct instruction and support the A.A. member to encourage him to continue taking such needed medication.[63]

To make A.A. work, the inpatient unit staff must establish an effective working relationship with A.A. volunteers from the community. A.A. members who have maintained at least 2 years sobriety should be sought. Over time, the unit should be able to develop a group of former patients, now active in A.A., who are willing to volunteer time on a regular basis.[64]

Family Therapy

Alcoholism almost invariably has devastating effects on the patient's spouse and children. Weekly or, more frequently, family meetings should be initiated as soon as the patient has completed detoxification.

The goals of these family meetings should be to:

1. Provide emotional support to all family members
2. Educate the family about alcoholism and treatment resources, particularly Alanon and Alateen;
3. Confront the patient about his denial and rationalizations about drinking.

Successful treatment often requires that other family members become active in Alanon. This should be encouraged even when the patient continues to drink or signs out of the hospital prematurely. Alanon is a group support program run by A.A. and designed for spouses or other persons closely involved with the alcoholic. Similar services and support are available in Alateen for the children of the alcoholic. Both of these programs are helpful in relieving the guilt and anger family members often feel regarding their relative's drinking problem. Group support and helpful guidance are given on how to respond to an active drinker in ways that encourage sobriety and do not foster, directly or indirectly, continued drinking. Both of these groups are open to family and friends, even when the alcoholic himself refuses to participate in A.A. or any other form of therapy.

If there is a strong family history of alcoholism, family members should be counseled about the possible hereditary nature of alcoholism and should be warned about possible alcohol problems in children and siblings of the patient.

In some cases, it may also be appropriate to include "significant others," even employers, in the family meetings. The more people in the patient's life who become aware of the problem and become involved

in helping the patient avoid denial or rationalization, the more likely the patient is to sustain sobriety.

Individual Psychotherapy

Individual psychotherapy need not be a major treatment focus for most patients with *primary alcoholism*. In fact, the period immediately following detoxification is inappropriate for intensive uncovering psychotherapy. The patient's intellectual capacities may be diminished at this time, and confrontation may best be done in milieu and family meetings. Psychotherapy is also of little benefit for individuals with memory deficits secondary to chronic alcoholism.

Psychotherapy works best with individuals in the early stages of alcoholism who have not yet lost control over their drinking and have not restructured their lives to make alcohol their primary focus. Individual psychotherapy is particularly recommended for patients with obvious psychological problems that *antedate their drinking*. Psychotherapy can also be recommended for patients who have been involved in A.A. but who have not found that approach adequate in achieving sobriety.

Psychotherapy can begin with the acknowledgment of the diagnosis of alcoholism, the existence of an "alcohol problem," or at least the willingness to explore the possibility of an alcohol-related problem. In any case, the therapist needs to understand that the initial task of therapy is to establish a treatment relationship and to negotiate a treatment contract that is acceptable to both the patient and the therapist. Therapy with the alcoholic is usually a long-term process with multiple treatment contracts that will be redefined and renegotiated as the process evolves. One may have to accept goals such as reduced drinking, elimination of acting-out behavior while drunk, avoidance of missed time at work, etc., as the first step in such a process.

The actual goals are less important than the fact that goals have been negotiated specifically and clearly. Goals can always be changed and renegotiated. Problems are more likely to occur if the goals are nebulous. In such cases, patients and therapists are often left with no way to clearly measure progress (or failure) in therapy or to make adjustments in unrealistic goals.

The therapist's attitude is crucial if successful treatment is to occur. It is extremely important that the therapist convey a strong sense of therapeutic optimism and unconditional positive regard for the patient. The patient must not be made to feel rejected or overly guilty for his behavior, and the therapist must clearly be able to separate his feelings about the patient's behavior from his regard for the patient as a human being. Patients often feel hopeless about their condition and need strong encouragement from the therapist to recognize that alcoholism can be successfully controlled. Regardless of how the patient describes himself, it is safe to assume that he is experiencing considerable guilt, depression, and intense feelings of failure and worthlessness. Strong support is required if the patient is to progress in treatment.

Successful therapists have found that treatment is more productive, particularly in the initial phase, if it focuses on helping the patient gain control over his drinking. Therapists should be acutely aware of the problems that can occur when they deliberately raise topics or engage in therapeutic maneuvers that increase a patient's anxiety during a therapeutic session. While it is often impossible to deal effectively with any patient without generating some anxiety, the degree of anxiety should always be moderated so that it does not overwhelm the patient's defenses. Most patients with serious alcohol problems really have only one functional defense mechanism to deal with anxiety, and that is drinking. As time goes on and therapy helps the patient build new defensive structures, the patient will be better able to tolerate anxiety and may then be able to engage in a more worthwhile exploration of past problems and underlying psychological issues.

In general, alcoholics gain control of their drinking problem not so much by insight into psychodynamic conflicts as by a more transference-oriented "cure" resulting from a positive relationship with a therapist who plays the role of a helpful and advice-giving parent.[65]

In the management of the alcoholic, as with any chronic patient, it is crucial to expect an occasional relapse and to prepare the patient for such a possibility. Chronic patients should always be encouraged to return to treatment whenever it is needed. In such cases, it is imperative for the clinician to understand how to revise treatment contracts and to help the patient set new and more reasonable goals for himself.

Antabuse

Disulfiram (Antabuse) is often a helpful adjunct to treatment. Disulfiram interferes with the action of acetaldehyde dehydrogenase and causes a buildup of acetaldehyde in the patient's blood, should he drink alcohol while taking this medication. Acetaldehyde produces an extremely unpleasant reaction associated with flushing, nausea, vomiting, facial warmth, a sense of suffocation, and difficulty in breathing. In some cases, this reaction can be fatal, particularly if the patient continues to consume alcohol. Nonetheless, disulfiram has been proven to be a safe and effective medication in the vast majority of cases. Exceptions include patients who are psychotic or suicidal or who have extremely poor impulse control. Furthermore, disulfiram is effective only within the context of an ongoing treatment relationship.[66] Patients usually stop taking it unless there are frequent supportive visits with their physician.

In general, patients should be helped to recognize that taking disulfiram is not simply reliance on a chemical crutch, but rather is an active step to assist them in gaining control over their drinking. Treatment should begin with 250 mg P.O. b.i.d. After 10 days, the dose can be reduced to 250 mg daily. Because disulfiram is generally taken early in the day or at a time when the patient is not tempted to drink, the patient may thus resolve the issue of drinking for the next 24 hours. Disulfiram is metabolized slowly and remains in the body for 48 to 72 hours. It is therefore important that the patient be instructed about the risk of starting to drink immediately after he stops taking the medication.

Discharge Planning

In addition to specific after-care plans for any psychiatric problem, a major emphasis must be placed on the patient's need for long-term participation in an alcoholism treatment program.

For many patients, this may simply involve regular attendance at A.A., with family participation in Alanon and/or Alateen. If the patient began active involvement in A.A. while on the inpatient unit, continuation in this program can be easily accomplished.

If the patient is in the very early stages of alcoholism, does not have serious problems with loss of control, and can identify a specific need for psychotherapy, referral can be made to a psychotherapist skilled in work with alcoholics. Psychotherapy should also be considered for more seriously alcoholic patients who have previously failed to achieve sobriety using A.A. alone.

Patients who continue to deny their alcohol problem, or refuse A.A. or psychotherapy, are best referred to a sympathetic internist or family practitioner.

An alcohol clinic staffed by medical professionals and skilled psychotherapists is the best referral for schizophrenic or depressed patients who require ongoing medication as well as alcoholism treatment. An alcohol clinic should also be utilized for persons hostile to A.A. or those psychologically unable or unwilling to participate in group-oriented treatment programs.

If the patient lacks a stable home environment or has a history of repeated failures in outpatient therapy, he should be evaluated for referral to an alcohol halfway house. A structured living situation may be a very helpful transition between the inpatient unit and the community.

COURSE AND PROGNOSIS

There have been no adequate long-term studies on the course of treated and untreated alcoholism. Clinical experience suggests that the long range course of untreated alcoholism is extremely difficult to predict. Some patients stop drinking permanently with no specific therapeutic intervention. Other patients continue drinking and eventually die from this disease, despite numerous efforts at treatment. Still other patients demonstrate repeated cycles of sobriety and drunkenness with an unpredictable outcome.

Given the growing evidence that there is more than one form of alcoholism, it is unlikely that one single treatment approach will ever prove effective for all alcoholics.[28] It is, however, clear that therapeutic intervention has a positive impact on most alcoholics. It is a myth that alcoholism does not respond to treatment, though there is no strong evidence that one therapeutic approach is more effective than any other. Evaluation of a variety of programs funded by the National Institute of Alcohol Abuse and Alcoholism indicated a general improvement rate of approximately 70% of all patients treated, regardless of the therapeutic approach used.[67] Surprisingly, many patients responded with only minimal therapeutic intervention.

Edwards compared an intensive treatment group to an "advise" only group, where married patients were given a stern warning that they were suffering from alcoholism and were advised that they should stop all drinking, continue work or return to work, and work to resolve any marital problems. The patient's spouse was involved in the original evaluation and meeting with the clinic staff and was then interviewed at home on a monthly basis by a social worker who monitored the patient's progress. The results (one third of both groups had only a "slight or no" drinking problem at 12 months follow-up) led Edwards and associates[68] to question the rational and economic justification for more elaborate treatment programs.

In many cases, a positive response to treatment is not correlated with total sobriety. Major gains can be achieved with treatment that focuses on reduced drinking or a greater degree of control over drinking or a greater degree of control over drinking. While sobriety should be recommended for all individuals who have serious drinking problems, no patient should be rejected from treatment because of his difficulty accepting or meeting that goal. Many alcoholics will be unable to accept sobriety until they recognize that controlled drinking is not feasible for them. This recognition may come only after a period of time in treatment.

There has been considerable controversy over whether controlled drinking is possible for alcoholics.[69] There is no question that some individuals, though apparently a relatively small percentage of the total alcoholic population, have been able to achieve a state of controlled, nondestructive drinking. It is unclear, however, which alcoholics can achieve controlled drinking, whether this is permanent or simply a temporary pause in their pattern of drinking, and whether limited drinking should be accepted as a legitimate treatment goal. Many therapists have insisted that these patients will ultimately revert to uncontrolled drinking, though this has not been adequately documented. Unfortunately, there are no guidelines that permit us to reliably identify which alcoholics have a real possibility of achieving controlled drinking. For that reason, complete sobriety should be recommended for all patients.

Inpatient psychiatric units should be encouraged to work with patients with alcohol problems. To do so, it is important that the staff maintain an optimistic and accepting attitude toward these patients and that they be willing to re-admit patients if and when further inpatient treatment becomes necessary.

Therapists will find that work with these patients can be a very challenging and rewarding experience. The therapeutic nihilism associated with this disease is poorly deserved. It hopefully will change as the positive results of current treatment programs become better known.

REFERENCES

1. Vaillant G: *The Natural History of Alcoholism.* Cambridge, Mass., Harvard University Press, 1983.
2. Chafetz ME: Alcoholism and alcoholic psychoses, in Freedman AM, Kaplan HE, Sadock BJ (eds): *Comprehensive Textbook of Psychiatry II,* ed. 2, vol. 2, Baltimore, Williams & Wilkins Co., 1975.
3. Edwards G, Gross MM: Alcohol dependence: Provisional description of a clinical syndrome. Br Med J, *1:* 1058–1061, 1976.
4. Woodruff RA, Guze S, Clayton PJ, Carr D: Alcoholism and depression. Arch Gen Psychiatry, *28:* 97–100, 1973.
5. Cadoret RJ, O'Gorman TW, Troughton E, Heywood E: Alcoholism and antisocial personality. Arch Gen Psychiatry, *42:* 161–167, 1985.
6. Goodwin DW: Alcoholism and genetics. Arch Gen Psychiatry, *42:* 171–174, 1985.
7. Jellinek EM: *The Disease Concept of Alcoholism,* Highland Park, N.J., Hillhouse Press, 1960.
8. The Criteria Committee, National Council on Alcoholism: Criteria for the diagnosis of alcoholism. Am J Psychiatry, *129:* 127–135, 1972.
9. American Psychiatric Association: *Diagnostic and Statistical Manual of Mental Disorders,* ed. 3 (DSM-III). Washington, D.C., American Psychiatric Association, 1980.
10. Young "problem drinkers." *The Boston Globe,* March 20, 1981.
11. DeLuca J (ed): *Fourth Special Report to the U.S. Congress on Alcohol and Health from the Secretary of Health and Human Services January 1981.* Washington, D.C., U.S. Government Printing Office, No. 343-993, 1981.
12. Gallop Poll. *Boston Sunday Globe,* July 2, 1981.
13. Jessor R: Perceived opportunity, alienation, and drinking behavior among Italian and American youth. J Pers Soc Psychol, *15:* 215–222, 1970.
14. Bourne PG, Light E: Alcohol problems in blacks and women, in Mendelson JH, Mello NK (eds): *The Diagnosis and Treatment of Alcoholism,* New York, McGraw-Hill Book Co., 1979.
15. Fox JE: Outpatient alcoholism coverage to be tried. U.S. Medicine, *19:* 24–25, 1983.
16. Winokur G, Reich T, Rimmer J, et al.: Alcoholism. III. Diagnosis and familial psychiatric illness in 259 alcoholic probands. Arch Gen Psychiatry, *23:* 104–111, 1970.
17. Bergman H, Borg S, Hindmarsh T, Idestrom C, Matzell S: Computed tomography of the brain and neuropsychological assessment of male alcoholic patients and a random sample from the general male population, in Beglecter H, Idestrom C, Pankin JG, von Wartburg JP (eds): *Proceedings from the Second Magnus Huss Symposium (1979).* Acta Psychiatr Scand, [Suppl] *286:* 77–88, 1980.
18. Goodwin DW: Is alcoholism hereditary? Arch Gen Psychiatry, *25:* 545–549, 1971.
19. Kaij L: Studies on the etiology and sequels of abuse of alcohol. Thesis, University of Lund (Sweden), 1960.
20. Goodwin DW, Schulsinger F, Hermansen L, et al.: Alcohol problems in adoptees raised apart from alcoholic biological parents. Arch Gen Psychiatry, *28:* 238–243, 1973.
21. Goodwin DW, Schulsinger F, Knop J, Mednick

S, Guze SB: Alcoholism and depression in adopted-out daughters of alcoholics. Arch Gen Psychiatry, *34:* 751–755, 1978.

22. Winokur G, Reich T, Rimmer J, et al.: Alcoholism. III: Diagnosis and familial psychiatric illness in 259 alcoholic probands. Arch Gen Psychiatry, *23:* 104–111, 1970.

23. Goodwin DW: Alcoholism and heredity. Arch Gen Psychiatry, *36:* 57–61, 1979.

24. Cloninger CR, Reich T, Guze SB: The multifactorial model of disease transmission. II: Sex differences in the familial transmission of sociopathy (antisocial personality). Br J Psychiatry, *127:* 11–22, 1975.

25. Crowe R: An adoption study of antisocial personality. Arch Gen Psychiatry, *31:* 785–791, 1974.

26. Cloninger CR, Reich T, Wetzel R: Alcoholism and the affective disorders: Familial associations and genetic models, in Goodwin D, Erikson C (eds): *Alcoholism and the Affective Disorders,* pp. 57–86, New York, Spectrum Publications, 1979.

27. Cloninger CR, Bohman M, Sigvardsson S: Inheritance of alcohol abuse. Arch Gen Psychiatry, *38:* 861–868, 1981.

28. Winokur G, Rimmer J, Reich T: Alcoholism. IV: Is there more than one type of alcoholism? Br J Psychiatry, *118:* 525–31, 1971.

29. Freud S: Three essays on the theory of sexuality (1905), in *Standard Edition,* vol. 7, London, Hogarth Press, 1955.

30. Rado S: The psychoanalysis of pharmacothymia. Psychoanal Q, *2:* 1, 1933.

31. Knight RP: The dynamics and treatment of chronic alcohol addiction. Bull Menninger Clin, *1:* 233–250, 1937.

32. Glover E: On the etiology of drug addiction, in *On the Early Development of Mind,* New York, International Universities Press, 1956.

33. Kernberg OF: *Borderline Conditions and Pathologic Narcissism,* New York, J. Aronson, Inc., 1975.

34. Khantzian EJ: The ego, the self and opiate addiction: Theoretical and treatment considerations. Int Rev Psychoanal, *5:* 189–199, 1978.

35. Tyndel M: Psychiatric study of one thousand alcoholic patients. Can Psychiatr Assoc J, *19:* 21–24, 1974.

36. Cahalan D, Cisin IH, Grossley HM: *American Drinking Practices.* New Brunswick, N.J., Rutgers Center for Alcohol Studies, 1969.

37. Miller PM, Barlow DH: Behavioral approaches to the treatment of alcoholism. J Nerv Ment Dis, *157:* 10–20, 1973.

38. Conger JJ: Reinforcement theory and the dynamics of alcoholism. Q J Stud Alcohol, *17:* 295–305, 1956.

39. Lazare A: Hidden conceptual models in clinical psychiatry. N Engl J Med, *288:* 345–351, 1973.

40. Mayfield D, McLeod G, Hall P: The CAGE questionnaire: Validation of a new alcoholism screening instrument. Am J Psychiatry, *131:* 1121–23, 1974.

41. Hanna E: Towards a conceptual understanding of the development of problem drinking. Paper presented at Workshop in Conceptual and Methodological Aspects of Drinking Contexts, National Institute on Alcohol Abuse and Alcoholism, Washington, D.C., May 3, 1978.

42. Mullin C: *The General Hospital and The Alcoholic,* Boston, Division of Alcoholism, Massachusetts Department of Public Health, 1973.

43. Kaim SC, Klett CJ, Rothfeld B: Treatment of the acute alcohol withdrawal state: A comparison of four drugs. Am J Psychiatry, *125*(12): 54–60, 1969.

44. Greenblatt DJ, Shader RI: Treatment of the alcohol withdrawal syndrome, in Shader RI (ed): *Manual of Psychiatric Therapeutics.* Boston, Little, Brown & Co., 1975.

45. Vaillant GE: Natural history of male psychological health. VIII: Antecedents of alcoholism and "orality." Am J Psychiatry, *137:* 181–186, 1980.

46. Mattein JL: Drug induced attenuation of alcohol consumption. Q J Stud Alcohol, *34:* 444–463, 1973.

47. Viamontes JA: Review of drug effectiveness in the treatment of alcoholism. AM J Psychiatry, *128:* 1570–1571, 1972.

48. Greenblatt DJ, Shader RI: *Benzodiazepines in Clinical Practice,* New York, Raven Press, 1973.

49. Keeler MH, Taylor CI, Miller WC: Are all recently detoxified alcoholics depressed? Am J Psychiatry, *136:* 536–538, 1979.

50. Schucket MA: Alcoholism and affective disorders: Diagnostic confusion, in Goodwin DW, Erickson CK (eds): *Alcoholism and Affective Disorders,* Jamaica, N.Y., Spectrum Publications, 1979.

51. Kline NS, Cooper TB: Lithium therapy in alcoholism, in Goodwin DW, Erickson CK (eds): *Alcoholism and Affective Disorders.* Jamaica, N.Y., Spectrum Publications, 1979.

52. Reynolds GM, Merry J, Coppen A: Prophylactic treatment of alcoholism by lithium carbonate: An initial report, in Goodwin DW, Erickson CK (eds): *Alcoholism and Affective Disorders.* Jamaica, N.Y., Spectrum Publications, 1979.

53. Merry J, Reynolds CM, Bailey J, Coppen A: Prophylactic treatment of alcoholism by lithium carbonate: A controlled study. Lancet, *2*(7984): 481–482, 1976.

54. Judd LL, Huey LY: Lithium antagonizes ethanol intoxication in alcoholics. Am J Psychiatry, *141:* 1517–1521, 1984.

55. Fawcett J, Clark DC, Gibbons RD, et al.: Evaluation of lithium therapy for alcoholism. J Clin Psychiatry, *45:* 494–499, 1984.

56. Quitkin FM, Rifkin A, Kaplan J, Klein DF: Phobic anxiety syndrome complicated by drug dependence and addiction. Arch Gen Psychiatry, *27:* 159–162, 1972.

57. Overall JE, Brown D, Williams JD, Neill LT: Drug treatment of anxiety and depression in detoxified alcoholic patients. Arch Gen Psychiatry, *29:* 218–221, 1973.

58. Jeffreys DB, Flanagan RJ, Volans GU: Letter to the editor. Lancet, *1:* 308, 1980.

59. Issues in alcohol and cocaine abuse, interview

with David E. Smith, M.D. *Alcoholism Update,* 8(2): 1–6, 1885.

60. Ryback R: The continuum and specificity of the effects of alcohol on memory. Q J Stud Alcohol *32:* 995–1016, 1971.

61. Ryan C, Butters N: Further evidence for a continuum of impairment encompassing male alcoholic Korsakoff patients and chronic alcoholic men. Alcoholism: Clin Exp Res, *4:* 190–198, 1980.

62. Stinson DJ, Smith GW, Amidjoya I, Jeffrey MK: Systems of care and treatment questions for alcoholic patients. Arch Gen Psychiatry, *36:* 535–539, 1979.

63. Renner JA: Alcoholism, in Lazare A (ed): *Outpatient Psychiatry Diagnosis and Treatment,* pp. 440–457. Baltimore, Williams & Wilkins, 1979.

64. Whitney A, Grinder N, Sallick RM: A general hospital alcoholism treatment program. Conn Med, *44:* 177–179, 1980.

65. Silber A: Rational for the technique of psychotherapy with alcoholics. Int J Psychoanal Psychother, *3:* 28–47, 1974.

66. Gerrein JR, Rosenberg CM, Manohar V: Disulfiram maintenance in outpatient treatment of alcoholism. Arch Gen Psychiatry, *28:* 798–802, 1973.

67. Chafetz M: Alcoholism. Psychiatr Ann 6(3): 9–93, 1976.

68. Edwards G, Orford J, et al.: Alcoholism: A controlled trial of "treatment" and "advice." Q J Stud Alcohol, *38:* 1004–1031, 1977.

69. McDonald MC: Rand rethinks alcoholism treatment. Psychiatr News, *15:* 1, 1980.

part 2

specific aspects of inpatient psychiatry

chapter 9

the use of the clinical laboratory

A. L. C. Pottash, M.D., Mark S. Gold, M.D., and Irl Extein, M.D.

The importance of the clinical labor- atory in the practice of psychiatry has grown considerably in the last decade. Many of the major trends and develop- ments in modern psychiatry have led to this new emphasis. Progress in neuro- science and neurochemistry research have provided the basic science foundation for which new insights and testing have been built. The growth in the use of psycho- pharmacologic agents ultimately led to the development of methods of therapeutic drug monitoring in psychiatry. Growing concern over the side effects of psycho- tropic medications emphasized the need for treatment with the individualized dos- age regimens which therapeutic drug monitoring allows. In addition, such con- cerns have spurred the search for ad- ditional diagnostic procedures to sup- plement clinical impressions.

The availability of effective and specific psychotropic treatment for major de- pression, manic-depressive illness, and schizophrenia has emphasized the impor- tance of accurate diagnosis. A number of laboratory diagnostic tests have begun to allow physicians greater certainty in their evaluation of need for medications and even in their choice of a particular psycho- pharmacologic agent. As psychiatrists have gained more clinical experience with the use of these medications, the recogni- tion of other side effects has emphasized the need for periodic laboratory as- sessment of basic medical functions, such as tests of renal and thyroid status in pa- tients on lithium. As scientists further

explore brain chemistry, possible clinical applications have been developed, such as measurement of urinary 3-methoxy- 4-hydroxyphenylglycol (MHPG), in order to assess changes in brain norepinephrine metabolism in depression. Advances in immunochemistry led to new and specific measurements of nonendogenous sub- stances relevant to differential diagnosis in clinical psychiatry, such as phencycli- dine (PCP) levels. The drug abuse epi- demic and the development of a new atti- tude about identifying users of illicit drugs have spurred the development and wider use of more specific and accurate tests for such drugs in urine and blood. Increas- ingly aggressive drug testing programs in sports, sensitive industries (such as air traffic controllers), schools, and pre- employment screening are becoming the norm rather than the exception.

Testing to identify medication- responders and "treated" patients at high risk for relapse have been developed, with tests now beginning to be able to separate treatment successes from failure. In ad- dition, as in other branches of medicine, the malpractice crisis which began in the 1970's emphasized the use of laboratory tests in what sometimes approaches a de- fensive strategy. Finally, as psychiatry began to emphasize its place as a branch of medicine, there was renewed interest in differential diagnosis and research in areas of interdisciplinary overlap, such as the relationship of thyroid functions to affective disorders.

All of these trends served to emphasize

the importance of the clinical laboratory in modern psychiatry. The usefulness of the laboratory is not limited to one type of test or procedure and impacts in many areas of diagnosis and treatment. However, it is only recently that psychiatrists have begun to recognize the relatively wide scope of these applications. Many psychiatrists fail to recognize this and become familiar with only one application of the laboratory to inpatient practice, such as the use of therapeutic drug monitoring, or the applications of psychoneuroendocrinology to diagnosis. These are limited viewpoints. When we begin to review the area we see that the clinical laboratory is a major component of the practice of inpatient psychiatry and is indispensable in psychiatric evaluation and psychopharmacologic treatment.

REALISTIC EXPECTATIONS

What has limited the implementation of laboratory advances by psychiatrists? Although some clinicians no doubt view the use of laboratory procedures as incompatible with their own theoretical approach to the patient, other physicians have unrealistic expectations of the infallibility of such testing systems. Psychiatrists argue about which mode of therapy or school of thought should be used in clinical practice, so it is no surprise that unanimity is nowhere to be found regarding the laboratory. Physicians in other branches of medicine have realistic expectations and do not find a laboratory test useless or suspect if it fails to have 100% accuracy. Understanding the limitations of a particular test, they use the results in the context of other signs and symptoms and test results. Some psychiatrists have been slow to remember these basic principles of laboratory medicine and instead espouse a nihilistic view and suggest that lack of sensitivity is proof of the uselessness of a test. In addition, psychiatrists need to remember the concept of interim measures. NASA did not expect to land on the moon before orbiting the earth, and cardiologists would never have defined the uses and limitations of the stress cardiogram unless it was widely used by clinicians. Psychiatrists need ex-

perience with psychiatric laboratory tests to improve their patient evaluation and treatment as well as to impact upon the use and improvement of such procedures. Finally, psychiatrists need to remember that the tradition in medicine is that new tools and techniques developed since residency often necessitate additional postresidency training. Just imagine the consequences of a surgeon not learning the newer techniques of laparoscopy. Some psychiatrists feel that they have learned enough and that nothing "that" important has happened to force them to take an in-depth training program or start to change the way they practice.

Laboratory tests in clinical use vary with regard to both *sensitivity* and *specificity*.[1] The *sensitivity* of a test as we will use the term here describes the ability of the test to correctly identify through an abnormal or positive result a percentage of patients with a given syndrome (true positives). The remaining, unidentified patients are the false negatives. *Specificity* is related to the ability of a test to exclude false positive patients. The sensitivity is defined as the percentage of true negative patients who have a negative test result. The *confidence level* describes the likelihood that an abnormal laboratory result in a given population will identify a true positive patient. For a test to be useful in laboratory medicine, neither 100% sensitivity, 100% specificity, nor 100% confidence level is necessary or even expected. Certain tests, such as the carcinoembryonic antigen (CEA) test in oncology, are most useful in following the course of individual patients and monitoring for relapse, independent of their utility as screening tests. Recent studies suggest that the dexamethasone suppression test (DST) and thyrotropin-releasing hormone (TRH) tests can be applied in psychiatry in this way to monitor biological response to antidepressant treatment and to predict relapse. Of course, it is important to become familiar with the limitations of each particular test. For these and other reasons, laboratory tests can never replace physicians. Diagnosis in laboratory medicine is often based on the review of the results derived from a number of tests, each with a different sensitivity and specificity. The best example of this is the use of the laboratory in the diagnosis of various autoimmune diseases. Some of the commonly used laboratory tests in these medical syndromes have low sensitivities or specificities, although the results of such tests can still contribute to the process of diagnosis.

Psychiatrists in general have had limited exposure to the rapid explosion in the use of diagnostic services experienced in many other branches of medicine as a result of the recent malpractice crisis. However, it is interesting to note that in one review of the malpractice cases involving psychiatrists in California which went on to cash settlement, the largest payment was required in a claim based on "failure to diagnose."[2] The case involved an outpatient diagnosed as a "phobic neurotic" who actually had a vitamin B_{12} deficiency without anemia.

DIAGNOSTIC TESTING

Drugs of Abuse

The ability of clinicians to rapidly and reliably document the abuse of prescription or illicit drugs is critical in accurate diagnosis and development of appropriate treatment plans for psychiatric patients. Using the laboratory, as evidenced by the pathologist's or toxicologist's training, requires a working knowledge of laboratory methodology, pharmacology, and toxicology in order to utilize the proper body fluids for examination and to know the most favorable time of sample collection and the best testing methodology to order. General medical laboratories performing routine "drug screens" frequently generate perplexing results which are difficult for clinicians to understand.[3, 4] For example, urine samples from known abusers and patients maintained on methadone can return with negative results. Important and commonly abused psychoactive compounds such as marijuana, tetrahydrocannabinol (THC), or phencyclidine (PCP, or "Angel Dust") are not tested for in most "drug screens" or else cannot be detected in subtoxic or sublethal doses in the screen. These problems usually are not a result of laboratory error or incompetency but in-

stead reflect limitations of the most commonly used method for drug abuse screening.

Drugs can be detected in human urine by any of several analytical techniques, including colorimetry, gas chromatography, fluorometry, and antibody-based assays. However, the routine "drug screen" performed by most general laboratories uses the rapid, inexpensive, thin layer chromatographic (TLC) technique. This traditional toxicology urine screen is in fact an ideal for what the name implies—rapid determination of toxic levels of drugs in a sample of urine. TLC screens are technically cumbersome and involve highly interpretive methods. When the physician is testing for drugs which TLC methods can identify, when the quantities ingested are large, and when the sample is obtained shortly after the drug abuse event, the TLC tests may be used. However, for identifying the low dose use and abuse, which is the most common type of use seen in the psychiatric patient, antibody-based methods are preferable. We have found antibody methods to give a sensitivity and specificity up to 50 times superior to TLC results for certain drugs of abuse. In addition, antibody-based assays can readily identify marijuana, THC, and PCP. Stronger evidence can be attained by the use of gas chromatography-mass spectroscopy (GC-MS), which analyzes the substance by its fragmentation pattern. Since in various molecules not all bonds are of equal strength, the weak ones are more likely to break under stress. The exact mass of these fragments or breakage products is measured by a mass spectrometer. GC-MS is the most reliable, most definitive, forensic quality procedure, but it is also the most expensive.

Information on the fragmentation pattern is compared to a computer library, listing the mass of the parent compound and its most likely fragments. A perfect match is considered absolute confirmation of the compound. In fact, confirmation by GC-MS is referred to as the "finger printing" of molecules. The use of GC-MS has been out of reach of most laboratories because of cost, the technical expertise needed for operation, and the need for complex sample preparation. However, recent advances in computerization, automated sample preparation, and analytical technology are now placing GC-MS capabilities within the reach of clinical analytical laboratories and clinicians. The sensitivity of GC for most drugs is in the nanogram range but with special detectors for some compounds, *picogram levels* can be measured.

The clinical applications are clear. For example, identifying the psychotic patient who has in fact ingested amphetamine or PCP is of critical importance in the clinical setting. Every psychiatrist recognizes that these drugs are in the differential diagnosis, but only some will vigorously rule it out with a detailed history and the specific laboratory test. With the availability of the clinical laboratory, guesswork and hunch are simply not acceptable when attempting to rule out diagnoses in this area. In one study,[5] 145 consecutive patients seen in the psychiatric emergency services of an urban public hospital were tested specifically for PCP. A surprisingly high 43% of the patients showed positive PCP levels. In other reports, cocaine or cannabis has been shown to produce a clinical picture very similar to that seen in panic states[6] and even schizophrenia.[7] The treatment plan for the depressed patient who by testing is found to be a low dose barbiturate abuser or a person on a self-styled marijuana maintenance program is different from that of the pure endogenously depressed patient, especially if the depression clears once the patient is off drugs of abuse. Inpatient treatment units in hospitals, especially adolescent units, often set limits on acceptable behavior, including prohibiting the bringing of drugs or alcohol onto the unit by patients or visitors, or hiding drugs obtained on passes while out of the hospital. In many hospitals, a common consequence of drug use on the unit is discharge of the patient or transfer to a more restrictive facility. Considering the false positives and negatives of TLC techniques and given the staff response to such drug use by inpatients, perhaps at least antibody-based assays are indicated in such cases to ensure accuracy.

All analytical methods have limitations. Time and dose of the last drug ingestion, as well as drug structure, half-life, and affinity for brain and other lipophilic structures, all affect the length of time the drug can be detected in a sample. False negative results can happen perhaps even easier than false positives, since they are mainly due to the insensitivity of commonly used screening procedures such as TLC (for most drugs equal to 2 μg/ml). Thus, a negative report based alone on TLC may have missed the detection of drugs because the TLC "cut off" between positives and negatives is too high. Another possibility for false negatives is that the sample was taken too long after the exposure, or the wrong biofluid was collected and analyzed for the wrong substance, or the sample was too diluted or too acidic for TLC.

Whatever the case may be, if the suspicion of drug use is strong, inquire at the laboratory for more sensitive screening procedures such as immunoassays, GC and, ultimately, GC-MS and acquire information on the best biofluid and time of collection for the optimum detection of the suspected drug. Collect a first void urine, supervise it, measure the specific gravity, and draw a blood sample to hold if the urine is negative and clinical suspicion remains high. In psychiatry, urinary specific gravity should be measured in all urine drug testing samples to eliminate the possibility that the sample has been tampered with and diluted with tap water.

A comprehensive drug abuse evaluation includes, at a minimum, tests for opiates (morphine equivalents), barbiturates, alcohol, amphetamines, benzodiazepines, methadone, phencyclidine (PCP), cocaine, cannabinoid (marijuana and THC), propoxyphene, and methaqualone. All positive results should be confirmed by the best available technique (e.g., GC-MS). Although a comprehensive antibody-based broad screening drug abuse evaluation including all the common drugs of abuse is indicated in many cases, in some patients with a clear presenting symptom, limited testing may be more cost-effective. For example, evaluation of a newly admitted patient with euphoria should at least include specific testing for amphetamines, cocaine, methadone, opiates, PCP, and alcohol. Psychotic patients should be tested for amphetamines, barbiturates, cocaine, and PCP. A minimum depression drug abuse evaluation should include a screen for benzodiazepines, methaqualone, barbiturates, cocaine, and alcohol. Newly admitted adolescent patients are usually tested for amphetamines, barbiturates, benzodiazepines, cocaine, methaqualone, marijuana/THC, PCP, and alcohol, if a comprehensive drug abuse evaluation is not ordered. Specific drugs, such as PCP, LSD, or cocaine in an acutely psychotic patient, can be assayed in blood in individual cases based on clinical suspicion, or in order to determine which drug(s) the patient was under the influence of at the time of mental status exam or evaluation.

Neuroendocrine Testing

We will be discussing the place of neuroendocrinology in psychiatry primarily in relation to affective disorders. In a typical depressive disorder, patients display both affective and "hypothalamic" symptoms. Affective symptoms may include depressed mood with a loss of interest, motivation, enjoyment, and a prevailing attitude of pessimism, worthlessness, and helplessness and hopelessness. Ruminative thinking, anhedonia, and suicidal thoughts may be present. In addition, somatic symptoms which may be described as hypothalamic may be present, including anorexia, anergia, decreased libido and aggressive drive, insomnia with a sleep continuity disturbance, psychomotor changes (retardation or agitation), and a diurnal variation in symptoms.

Recent studies demonstrating the functional relationships between biogenic amine neurotransmitters and regulation of both limbic and hypothalamic areas of the brain have suggested that studying alterations in secretion of the anterior pituitary hormones in affective disorders may enable us to make inferences about the underlying biochemical abnormalities and differentiate patients on the basis of neurobiologic tests. Discrete neuroendocrine abnormalities in patients with depression have been reported for more than a decade. The working hypothesis is that hypothalamic-pituitary-thyroid axis abnormalities are reliable measures of CNS neurotransmitter dysfunction.

Due to the inherent reserve and compensatory mechanisms of endocrine systems, provocative testing is usually necessary to uncover the abnormalities (Fig. 9.1). The diagnostic tests used in this area were not developed for psychiatrists and in fact have been used for years by physicians evaluating patients with primary endocrinopathies. However, they are of ever-increasing value in inpatient diagnosis in psychiatry. Such tests are especially helpful in the diagnosis of depression and more recently have been applied to evaluation of treatment response in depression. Major depression includes the categories of bipolar and unipolar depressive illness. Major depression of the primary type must be differentiated from secondary depression (depression related to known medical or neurologic illness, or depression in nonaffective psychiatric illness), and nonmajor or "minor," "neurotic," or "reactive" depression. Two categories of tests in endocrinology are particularly helpful, diurnal cortisol and dexamethasone suppression testing, as well as thyrotropin-releasing hormone testing. Due to space limitations, it will not be possible to discuss other diagnostic endocrine tests in psychiatry, such as insulin hypoglycemia[8] and amphetamine growth hormone-cortisol[9] tests or newer acetylcholine receptor, CSF somatostatin, or corticotropin-releasing hormone provocative testing or tests of endorphin function.

Diurnal Cortisol Test (DCT)

The most frequently reported endocrine abnormality in depression is hypersecretion of cortisol. The DCT is a test of the hypothalamic-pituitary-adrenal (HPA) axis which measures cortisol levels and endogenous diurnal rhythm. Normal levels at 8 a.m. range from 10 to 25 µg/100 ml. In normal patients, diurnality is present, and cortisol falls below 14 µg/100 ml by 4 p.m. and is significantly lower by midnight (<6 µg/ml). In the test, the patient goes to bed and arises at his or her regular time. Plasma samples for cortisol by radioimmunoassay (RIA) are taken at 8 a.m., noon, 4 p.m., and midnight. The patient may eat regularly (Fig. 9.2).

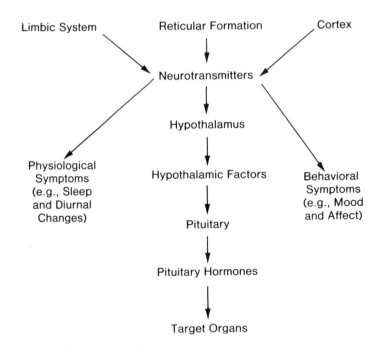

Figure 9.1.   Hypothalamic-pituitary-adrenal axis.

In patients with major depression, there is excessive secretion of cortisol, although sometimes this is seen only in the 4 p.m. or midnight samples. The hypersecretion is not due to stress nor to a change in cortisol metabolism but may be due to Cushing's syndrome. In most cases, although there is hypersecretion of cortisol, diurnality is preserved. Failure to demonstrate diurnality in patients with endogenous depression may be associated with high severity of illness and poor response to treatment.

Adrenal insufficiency is suggested by plasma cortisols persistently below 8 μg/100 ml in the 8 a.m. sample. High or high-normal values in all samples suggest major depression or Cushing's syndrome. Both of these diagnoses have been made "by accident" in patients tested for depression with the DCT.

Cortisol abnormalities are rarely present in schizophrenics or patients with neurotic, reactive, or secondary depression. An abnormal DCT usually disappears on clinical recovery. The DCT can also be done with samples taken every 20 minutes between 1 p.m. and 4 p.m. Twenty-four hour urinary free cortisol can be measured as well. By either method, cortisol production is markedly increased in major depression. The DCT is an independent test which identifies a different patient group than the dexamethasone suppression test (DST).

Dexamethasone Suppression Test (DST)

The DST is another test of the HPA which has been extensively studied in psychiatric patients.[10] The test is widely used in the evaluation of cortisol hypersecretion (e.g., Cushing's Syndrome). The abnormalities seen in patients with affective disorders have been reported and reproduced by researchers all over the world.

Dexamethasone is a synthetic glucocorticoid which acts in the CNS at hypothalamic and limbic sites which regulate corticotropin (ACTH) release. The drug mimics endogenous corticosteroids to inhibit ACTH-cortisol release. The failure of dexamethasone to cause a normal suppression indicates significant limbic-hypothalamic-pituitary system dysfunction, similar to that observed in Cushing's syndrome and certain other specific physical illnesses.

The patient receives 1 mg of dex-

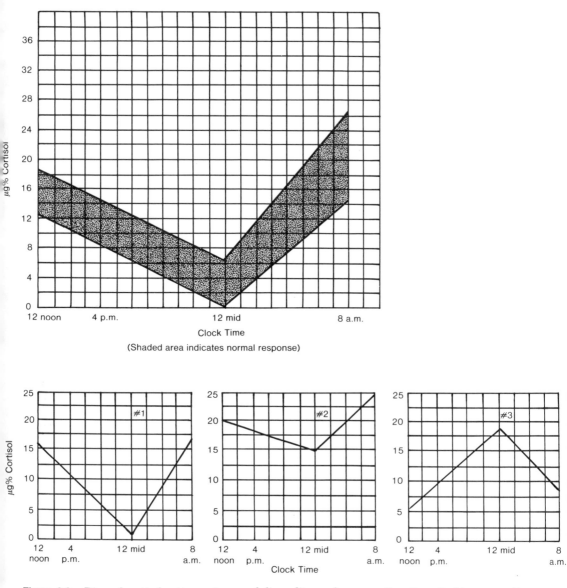

Figure 9.2. Diurnal cortisol patterns. *1,* normal diurnality, no hypersecretion; *2,* cortisol hypersecretion (e.g., primary affective disease, Cushing's disease); *3,* loss of diurnality, cortisol hypersecretion—relative nonresponse to tricyclics.

amethasone orally at midnight. The patient may eat regularly. No subjective effects are reported from the test. Blood is then taken over the next 24 hours (a minimum sampling of 8 a.m., noon, 4 p.m., and midnight) for RIA plasma cortisol determination (Fig. 9.3). Elimination of any of these sample points decreases sensitivity. For example, a 1-time-point DST has a yield of approximately 1 in 3, whereas a 4-point test identifies one of

every two patients with proven major depression.

Normal controls, as well as schizoprenic, manic, detoxified alcoholic, and anxious patients and secondary or nonmajor depressed patients, show suppression of plasma cortisol levels during the DST to values less than 5 μg/100 ml for the following 24 hours. The test is abnormal if cortisol equals or exceeds 5 μg/100 ml at any of the sample points. This failure

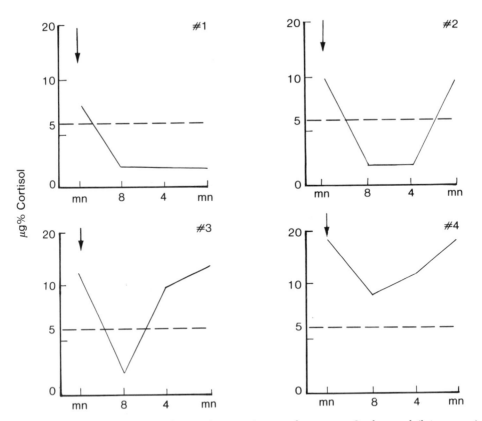

Figure 9.3. Patterns of response to dexamethasone. *1,* normal response; *2,* abnormal (late escape); *3,* abnormal response (inadequate suppression); *4,* abnormal (no suppression), *mn,* midnight.

to suppress is seen in 50% or more of all patients with a clinical diagnosis of major depression and appears to be unrelated to psychosis, anxiety, or stress. There are at least three patterns of abnormal response to dexamethasone: late escape; inadequate suppression; and failure to suppress. An abnormal DST usually reverts to normal upon clinical recovery.

As compared to other laboratory tests in medicine, the DST is a reliable test. The specificity of an abnormal DST in the diagnosis of major depression in most studies is 90–96%, i.e., the failure to suppress on the DST is extremely rare in other psychiatric disorders, with a false positive rate of 5–10%. Though there have been some studies challenging the specificity of an abnormal DST for depression, the DST is a useful test in a properly screened population.[11] The sensitivity in most studies is approximately 50–67%, partially depending on whether 4 or 10 time points are used in the protocol. In summary, a posi-

tive DST (lack of suppression) is of considerable practical usefulness in diagnosis and treatment. It is a test with unusual diagnostic power in that a positive test helps confirm the diagnosis and helps predict treatment and outcome. The DST does not appear to be affected or interfered with by oral contraceptives or the common psychotropic agents, except perhaps by high doses of benzodiazepines. The DST appears to be useful in evaluating depression in alcoholics if utilized at least a week or two after the completion of detoxification. False positives may be caused by pregnancy, high doses of estrogens or caffeine, severe weight loss, uncontrolled diabetes, high fever, dehydration, phenytoin, barbiturates, carbamazepine, meprobamate, methyldopa, and reserpine.

Normalization of the DST after successful treatment has been reported in many studies. Interestingly, depressed patients who show apparent clinical recovery but whose DST remains abnormal are at serious risk for early relapse. In such cases, continued DST abnormalities may indicate the need for alternative antidepressant treatment or electroconvulsive therapy (ECT), or, at the minimum, continued somatic treatment and observation. Some clinicians successfully use normalization of the DST as a guide to when to discontinue treatments in a course of ECT. Other clinicians have suggested that the DST returns to normal before clinical response to antidepressants in patients who are on their way to recovery. DST positive major depressives are poor psychotherapy or placebo responders but good candidates for antidepressant medication or ECT.

In addition to its primary role in identifying patients with major depression, the DST has also been applied in a variety of other ways. It is possible that an abnormal DST will identify patients for whom treatment for depression may be indicated, although they carry other presumptive diagnoses such as schizoaffective depression, borderline personality disorder, dementia, or catatonia. In addition, nonsuppression in depression in children and adolescents may support use of somatic treatments in such cases where clinical presentations are varied and are due to a multitude of factors. Results at the present time regarding the DST's ability to predict response to a particular antidepressant are conflicting. Clinicians using either the DCT or the DST need to be aware of interlaboratory differences in methodologies for cortisol determination. Also, special precision and accuracy are necessary at the lower than usual concentrations used in these tests.[12]

Thyrotropin-Releasing Hormone (TRH) Test

TRH is a tripeptide found in the hypothalamus which, when released, causes secretion of thyroid-stimulating hormone (TSH) from the anterior pituitary gland. TSH then acts directly on the thyroid gland. Endocrinologists have long used the TRH test as a measurement of the responsiveness of this system. Synthetic TRH (500 μg) is administered intravenously to the patient at bedrest after an overnight fast. Samples for TSH are taken at base line, and 15, 30, 60, and 90 minutes after TRH administration via an indwelling venous catheter. TSH is measured by RIA. Delta TSH (ΔTSH) is the maximum TSH response, derived by subtracting the baseline TSH level from the peak. Subjective response to TRH infusion is limited to mild transient autonomic symptoms such as an urge to urinate.

ΔTSH is decreased in patients on corticosteroids, possibly carbamazepine, and certain other drugs, although tricyclics, phenothiazines, and benzodiazepines do not appear to influence the TRH test. ΔTSH is also reduced in cases of hyperthyroidism and alcoholism, as well as in elderly males. In hypothyroidism exaggerated TSH responses to TRH are seen (>25 μIU/ml).

One variation of the TRH test is to measure growth hormone (GH) levels at the same time as the TSH levels. In patients with major depression, as compared to normal controls and patients with other psychiatric diagnoses, a pattern of positive GH response to TRH may be elicited.

Over the last 10 years it has been widely reported by many authors around the world that there is blunted or decreased TSH response to TRH administration in major depression. More recently, several groups have reported a higher TSH response to TRH in bipolar, as compared to unipolar depression, though other groups have failed to replicate this finding. Manic, nondepressed patients often showed a blunted or decreased ΔTSH (<7 μIU/ml).[13] In addition, patients with other psychiatric diagnoses showed a ΔTSH response similar to that seen in normal controls (7-15 μIU/ml). Blunted TSH response is not an inherited marker/risk factor for affective illness.

The results of TRH testing on one group of 147 depressed patients without a history of thyroid disease are presented in Table 9.1. Reviewing the TRH test as a diagnostic test for major unipolar depression in this and some other studies, sensitivity often ranges from 60% to 77% and specificity from 77% to 97%. Similar results, with slightly lower specificity, can be seen when the TRH test is used in the differential diagnosis of mania and schizophrenia.

Table 9.1.
TRH Test Results in 147 Depressed Patients

	Total No. of Patients	No. of Patients with TSH ≤7	No. of Patients with +GH
Group I			
Bipolar, depressed	12	1	6
Unipolar, depressed	44	34	17
Minor depression	10	0	0
Group II			
Schizoaffective, depressed	5	0	2
Opiate addiction	7	0	4
Adjustment/Personality Disorder	7	0	1
Presenile dementia	1	0	0
Group III			
Bipolar, manic	13	6	3
Schizophrenia	14	0	2
Schizoaffective, manic	10	3	2
Anorexia nervosa	5	0	5
Alcoholism	5	3	1
Organic brain syndrome	9	2	2
Miscellaneous	5	0	0
Total	147	49	45

Like the DST and DCT, the utility of the TRH test in inpatient psychiatry is becoming clearer. In addition to its use in identifying patients with early hypothyroidism, its primary use is in the identification of active major depression. In addition, some limited research suggests that unipolar and bipolar patients with similar depressive symptomatology and severity of illness might be separated on the basis of the TRH-induced TSH response. Although fewer manic and schizophrenic patients have been studied, it appears that the TRH test may also be useful in separating from each other clinically similar patients with mania and schizophrenia.

In addition, *changes* in the TSH response to TRH in depressed patients have been used to predict response, in a manner similar to the predictive utility of the DST.[14] In one study,[15] all depressed patients who failed to show a significant increase in ΔTSH after ECT relapsed within 6 months, while the majority of those who showed a change in ΔTSH after ECT remained cured during the same time period. These data have been replicated. An important recent study from Denmark[16] has shown that patients for whom the TRH test predicts likely relapse following an antidepressant response to ECT can have a good prognosis if treated with tricyclics on a prophylactic basis.

Research over the coming years with larger numbers of patients with a wide range of psychiatric diagnoses should further clarify the usefulness of the TRH test in differential diagnosis and evaluation of treatment response.

DST Combined with TRH Test

In many centers, patients receive both the dexamethasone suppression test (DST) and the thyrotropin-releasing hormone (TRH) test. The TRH test is performed 2 or 3 days prior to performing the DST, since corticosteroids affect the TRH results. A few studies have shown that the tests are complementary and that the combination of both tests together leads to increased identification of unipolar depressed patients. Each test identifies a significant proportion of unipolar (major) depressed patients not identified by the other. Since these are patients in whom antidepressant medication is usually indicated and often helpful, these laboratory procedures can aid in clinical decision-making, especially in ambiguous cases. Using both the DST and the TRH test, abnormalities in either can confirm the diagnosis of major depression (and particularly unipolar depression) with high diagnostic confidence and with few false positives, especially when combined with a careful clinical interview (Fig. 9.4). In one study of unipolar patients (excluding alcoholics) (Fig. 9.5), 34% of the patients showed only an abnormal TRH test, and 20% showed only an abnormal DST. In 30% of the cases both cases were abnormal. Any comprehensive evaluation program should use the DCT, DST, and TRH tests to increase identification of true unipolars to 80–90%.

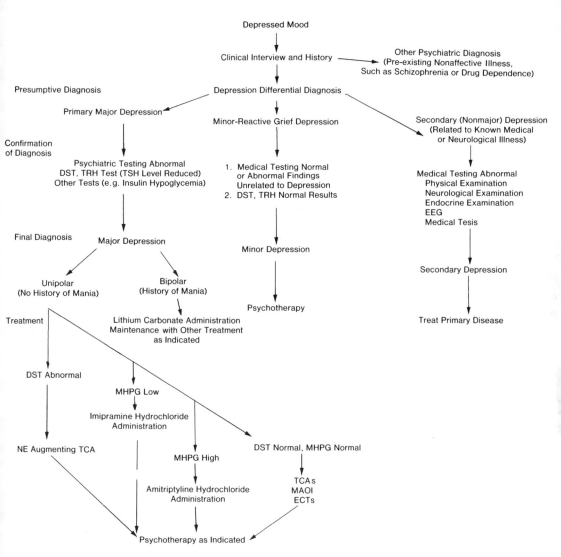

Figure 9.4. Subdivisions and treatment methods for depression, DST indicates dexamethasone suppression test; TRH, thyrotropin-releasing hormone; TSH, thyroid-stimulating hormone; ECT, electroconvulsive therapy; MAOIs, monoamine oxidase inhibitors; TCA, tricyclic antidepressant; NE, norepinephrine; MHPG, 3-methoxy-4-hydroxyphenylglycol. (Reprinted with permission from Gold MS, Pottash ALC, Extein I, Sweeney D: Diagnosis of depression in the 1980's. JAMA, *245:* 1562–1564, April 17, 1981, Copyright 1981, American Medical Association.)

Thyroid Function Tests (TFT's) and Depression

Many of the symptoms of hypothyroidism are similar to the symptoms of depression.[17, 18] In hypothyroidism, depression and/or changes in cognition are common, both of which usually improve with replacement therapy. These observations have led to a great deal of interest in the incidence and coexistence of thyroid disease and depression. Often the covertly hypothyroid patient's first complaint is of depression or lethargy, sometimes leading to a visit to a psychiatrist. Since many psychiatrists merely take the patients' complaints and begin treatment, a number of those patients have been failures in psychiatric therapy and antidepressant treatment. Other physicians order routine thyroid function testing in all newly admitted psychiatric inpatients. Studies on

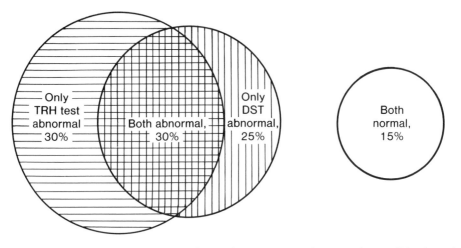

Figure 9.5. Relationship of TRH test and dexamethasone suppression test abnormalities in unipolar depression (n = 55).

such patients showed an incidence of thyroid dysfunction either equal to or greater than that of the general population. However, in most of these studies patients presenting with depression and/or anergia were not separated from patients with other diagnoses. In addition, the diagnostic evaluation only included measurement of peripheral thyroid hormone (TH)—usually thyroxine (T_4) and triiodothyronine (T_3) resin uptake (T_3uptake), and only occasionally measurement of basal thyroid-stimulating hormone (TSH). More recently, however, research has shown that the TRH test is the most useful test in identifying cases of incipient or evolving hypothyroidism.

The most commonly used tests in diagnosing hypothyroidism are T_3uptake and T_4 (by RIA). The T_3uptake is an index of protein binding that allows calculation of the Free Thyroxine Index (FTI). These tests yield a small but significant number of abnormal results when they are used as a screening procedure for hypothyroidism in depression. The addition of a TSH determination significantly increases the sensitivity of the screening battery and is thus recommended. TSH is elevated before T_4 or FTI is decreased.

However, just as the DST is used in both the differential diagnosis of depression and the identification of Cushing's syndrome, the TRH test has also been used to identify cases of hypothyroidism in its ear-

liest stages. The TRH test appears to be the most sensitive measure of thyroid function and is often abnormal (ΔTSH $\geq$ 30 or 35) prior to changes in T_3 uptake, T_4, and TSH.

Endocrinologists have begun to focus on hypothyroidism as an evolving disease entity, rather than as an all-or-none phenomenon. As hypothyroidism develops, all of the laboratory measures of thyroid function become abnormal over time (Table 9.2).

In the earliest phases only the most sensitive measure of thyroid function—the TRH test—is abnormal. This stage may be called "subclinical hypothyroidism" (grade 3). The patient exhibits no clinical signs or symptoms of thyroid disease. In "mild" hypothyroidism (grade 2) there may be isolated clinical signs or symptoms of hypothyroidism, with an abnormal TRH test, elevated baseline TSH, and normal T_3 uptake and T_4. Grade 1 patients show the clinical signs and symptoms of classical "overt" hypothyroidism with abnormal T_3 uptake, T_4, FTI, baseline TSH, and an exaggerated TSH response to TRH. Thyroid hormone administration may be indicated in mild and overt hypothyroidism and possibly in the "subclinical" stage. Patients with ΔTSH $\geq$ 20 and high titers of thyroid autoantibodies are candidates for thyroid hormone.[19, 20]

The results of complete thyroid function testing in 250 depressed and/or anergic

Table 9.2.
Stages of Hypothyroidism [a]

	T_3 Uptake	T_4	TSH	Clinical Symptoms	TRH Test TSH
Overt—Grade 1	↓ and/or normal	↓	↑↑	Many	↑↑↑
Mild—Grade 2	↓ and/or normal	Normal	↑ or normal	Few	↑↑
Subclinical—Grade 3	Normal	Normal	Normal	Few or none	↑↑

[a] ↑ = elevated; ↓ = decreased.

patients are presented in Table 9.3. A significant number of cases showed only augmented TSH response to TRH without abnormalities in T_3, T_4, and baseline TSH. The study also supports the use of baseline TSH determination in the screening battery for hypothyroidism. Only 10% of the hypothyroid patients could have been identified by T_3uptake and T_4 measurements alone. At least 50% of the grade 2 and grade 3 patients have autoimmune thyroiditis as evidenced by antibody testing.

It is possible that previous reports[21] on the antidepressant and antidepressant-potentiating properties of T_3 and TSH in depressed subjects could be attributed to a reversal of early or subclinical hypothyroidism. Research has shown that many patients with subclinical hypothyroidism will require and benefit from T_3 potentiation of tricyclics. It is still open to debate as to whether all patients with depression and/or anergia should be evaluated with TRH testing in addition to T_3uptake, T_4, and TSH determinations, or whether the additional TRH testing should be reserved for treatment failures. Serial thyroid functioning may be useful in some patients to determine whether thyroid tests in the usual normal range represent changes in the hypo- or hyperthyroid direction for an individual which may be related to emergence of symptoms.

Presence of positive items on history or physical strongly increases the possibility of thyroid disease, and a full laboratory workup is mandatory. We feel that all patients presenting with anergia or depression require at least T_4, T_3 RIA, T_3RU, and TSH. This will pick up patients with grade 1 hypothyroidism and will be suggestive in grade 2 disease. Patients suspected of grade 2 or grade 3 hypothyroidism should have the TRH infusion test to confirm the diagnosis and help guide treatment. Patients with an abnormally high ΔTSH $\geq$ 20 should be screened for anti-M and anti-T antibodies.

In one recent study,[22] 20% of depressed patients had detectable titers of antithyroid antibodies. In these patients, T_4, T_3uptake, free thyroxine index, and baseline TSH were all normal. (Unfortunately, TRH testing was not done.)

Lithium-treated bipolar or recurrent unipolar patients present a unique problem.[23, 24] These patients are by definition predisposed to depressive episodes. In addition, they are at risk for lithium-induced hypothyroidism which can cause or increase susceptibility to depression. How

Table 9.3.
Results of Thyroid Function Testing in 250 Depressed Patients

Laboratory Data	No. of Hypothyroid Patients Identified— 250 Consecutive Admissions	Stage of Thyroid Failure
T_3, T_4 decreased and many clinical signs	2 (<1%)	Overt
T_3, T_4 normal but baseline TSH elevated and few or isolated clinical signs	8 (3.2%)	Mild
T_3, T_4 baseline TSH normal but TRH test abnormal (TSH excessive) and isolated clinical signs or asymptomatic	10 (4.0%)	Subclinical
Δ TSH excessive (all above patients)	20 (8%)	Overt, mild, and subclinical

should the psychiatrist work up the bipolar depressed patient who is taking lithium? A TRH infusion test can be of considerable help. Following a ΔTSH in the patient from before treatment to lithium maintenance is of considerable importance in the early identification of lithium-induced grade 3 disease. An increasing ΔTSH should raise the possibility of Grade 2 or 3 hypothyroidism, and thyroid replacement should be considered before starting antidepressants.

Measurement of MHPG

Some clinicians have found measurement of pretreatment urinary 3-methoxy-4-hydroxyphenylglycol (MHPG) to be of assistance in the prediction of a response to specific antidepressant medications. MHPG is the major metabolite of brain norepinephrine. While there has been some disagreement about the use of urinary MHPG as a diagnostic test for depression and some discussion in the basic science community regarding the relative contribution of the brain and periphery to the MHPG measured, most, but not all, studies support the use of the MHPG test to predict response to medication.

Prior to collection of a 24-hour urine, the patient may be on a regular diet but preferably will have been off psychoactive drugs for at least 1 week. Creatinine clearance and total urinary volume are measured at the same time as MHPG to rule out incomplete collection. In patients who are candidates for treatment with antidepressants, low pretreatment MHPG levels ($\leq$1000 μg/24 hours) have predicted favorable response to use of antidepressants such as imipramine and maprotiline, which primarily effect noradrenergic systems.

B$_{12}$ and Folate

Folic acid deficiency has been widely reported in psychiatric patients, alcoholics, drug addicts, epileptics maintained on anticonvulsant medications, women on oral contraceptives, and others (e.g., malnutrition, malabsorption, pregnancy, anemia). However, a firm link between folic acid level and depressive mood has only

recently been made. Some studies have shown an abnormally low folate level in 20–40% of nonanemic depressed patients. Another study showed that folate deficiency is more common in depressed patients, and B$_{12}$ deficiency is more common in psychotic patients. Folate deficiency can impair monoamine (e.g., norepinephrine) synthesis in the brain (folate is the co-enzyme for tyrosine hydroxylase). While folate deficiency is treated with replacement, it is unclear as to whether folate depression exists as a distinct entity or as a life style side effect to depression.

Investigators have also found low B$_{12}$ levels in psychiatric patients. It has been reported that psychiatric symptoms may appear before the development of frank anemia in untreated pernicious anemia. In one California survey,[2] failure to diagnose just such a B$_{12}$ deficiency without anemia led to the largest psychiatric malpractice settlement in 5 years. We suggest folate and B$_{12}$ levels in the context of a comprehensive neuropsychiatric evaluation.[25]

Tryptophan

Tryptophan is the essential amino acid precursor for serotonin. Tryptophan hydroxylase, the rate-limiting enzyme in the conversion of tryptophan to serotonin, is not saturated. Dietary intake is necessary to provide for adequate tryptophan and thus serotonin. Tryptophan is frequently low in depressed, anorexic, drug abusing, and alcoholic patients on the basis of a dietary deficiency. This deficiency may explain sleep and mood changes, aggressiveness, and irritability in these patients. Tryptophan replacement can reverse this dietary deficiency. In addition, lithium may cause a tryptophan deficiency,[26] possibly by accelerating the enzymatic conversion of tryptophan to serotonin. We have theorized that this may explain some postmania depressions in patients on lithium and depressed mood in long-term lithium patients. Tryptophan levels at 8 a.m. (fasting since midnight) on two consecutive days may be indicated in patients who are "pre-lithium" and those who could have a dietary deficiency (e.g., depression, anorexia nervosa, drug abuse, alcoholism), with simple tryptophan replacement if indicated.

Electrolyte Imbalance

Electrolyte imbalance may cause syndromes which could be mistaken as psychiatric problems, such as depression or dementia. On the other hand, patients' psychopathologies may lead to behaviors which cause electrolyte imbalance (e.g., anorexia nervosa or water intoxication in schizophrenia). Both hypokalemia and hypercalcemia are well-known to cause depression or organic brain syndrome. Hyponatremia secondary to excessive water ingestion may produce a clinical picture of lethargy and withdrawal or decreased concentration. Both hypernatremic and hypocalcemic patients often display signs of irritability or impaired cognition. Decreases in magnesium levels may lead to organic brain syndrome or depression, especially in alcoholics. For these reasons, we advocate routine monitoring of serum electrolytes at the time of admission. Sodium, potassium, and calcium are usually included as part of a SMA-22 battery of admission tests. In addition, magnesium levels should be ordered on all patients presenting with impaired cognition, organic brain syndrome, or alcoholism.

THERAPEUTIC DRUG MONITORING

Antidepressant Levels

Laboratory tests to monitor plasma levels of antidepressant drugs have enhanced the physician's ability to use these agents in a more rational manner. While drug concentration is not the sole determinant of clinical response, it is an important refinement of the dose-response curve typical of classic pharmacological studies.

In most patients, physicians expect a normal or negative finding on most medical screening tests, such as a screening electrocardiogram or chest x-ray. In contrast, obtaining a drug plasma level of a well-studied medication always provides useful information. First of all, the test is directed to something that is expected to be there. Some concentration of drug in the blood should be detected and quantifiable because the patient is presumably taking medication. If the drug is nondetectable, either insufficient dosage or a compliance problem is likely. Secondly, a detectable level will be either appropriate or inappropriate. In the latter case, appropriate dosage adjustment would be indicated. Drug plasma monitoring is becoming an integral part of medical practice.

The use of standard dose regimens unrelated to plasma levels has been identified as a major source of antidepressant nonresponse. The reasons for this fact are numerous but include pharmacokinetic, pharmacodynamic, and other factors. For example, liver microsomal enzymes metabolizing antidepressants and converting tertiary tricyclics to secondary may show large intersubject variability (greater than 30-fold). Antidepressant absorption from the gastrointestinal tract is highly variable among patients and in the same patient over time. Absorption may be markedly affected by antacids, sodium bicarbonate, and vitamin C, to name a few substances. Drug interactions may seriously affect blood levels of antidepressants. Antipsychotic medications often increase antidepressant levels, while smoking and prior or current drug abuse will often lower levels. Physicians sometimes forget that poor compliance is a major factor in drug nonresponse even in the most motivated patients. All of these factors explain why routine measurement of antidepressant levels is indicated for patients on these medications, especially for inpatients, many of whom have just started intensive treatment.

There are other reasons which justify the use of such levels. Cardiotoxicity, including prolonged QRS duration and dysrhythmias, has been correlated with high plasma levels. Geriatric patients often show unusual patterns of drug metabolism and often can least tolerate the cardiotoxic effects. On the same dose, elderly patients have higher drug levels than younger patients. In addition, other subjective side effects of antidepressant use may be correlated with plasma concentration.

A significant number of patients who do not respond to antidepressants do not respond because of the use of routine dosages or "drug insert" treatment regimens. Increased response rate is seen when dosages are individually determined by plasma levels. Since this is the case, why have clinicians been slow to uniformly use such tests? We have encountered a number of factors to explain this hesitancy. Some early research showed mixed results with regard to correlation of response to medication level. However, methodology has improved both in the area of technical laboratory performance of the tests and clinical research with regard to precise diagnosis and evaluation of response. The results of new research show a clearer correlation between plasma levels and both response and side effects.

Another reason many clinicians have delayed the use of the plasma levels is because of suggestions in the past that all nonresponders merely require a higher dose of the antidepressant. It was once said that no antidepressant trial in the face of nonresponse is complete without a period on high or very high doses. However, now it is clear that not only is that incorrect but, in fact, the practice is dangerous, since some patients would end up with extremely toxic levels on high dosages. Now clinicians more often say that no antidepressant trial is complete until the patient has achieved therapeutic plasma levels for at least 2–3 weeks. One factor contributing to this change in focus was the discovery that some tricyclic antidepressants have a therapeutic window, so that plasma levels both below and above the range are correlated with poorer response to treatment.

Two other factors which relate to clinicians' delay in full use of plasma levels have been questions of expense and superiority of clinical judgment. Some doctors feel that antidepressant levels add an unnecessary expense for the patient. However, given the much greater expense of a hospital day, any test which could possibly decrease length of stay in an inpatient facility by even one day, and possibly decrease side effects, would appear to be cost-effective. It is clear that there are risks to the patient of being on an antidepressant such as amitriptyline with substandard levels—the risks of not getting better, suicide, and suffering, as well as the medical risks. Finally, psychiatrists' initial response to the development of reliable methodologies for antidepressant level determination has been similar to the initial response of neurologists to the introduction of anticonvulsant levels. Neurologists once felt that clinical judgment was adequate in determining patient medication dosages and felt that anticonvulsant levels were an unnecessary expense. Now, very few neurologists fail to utilize such laboratory tests.

One difficulty many clinicians encounter when they attempt to utilize antidepressant levels is that laboratories vary a great deal with regard to methodology and accuracy of the performance of the tests. Some methods are affected by other psychoactive medications, have low recovery of known standard concentrations, and cannot differentiate between active and inactive metabolites. Measurement of antidepressant levels is a very difficult and sensitive procedure and is not done routinely in many laboratories. When a laboratory does not perform the test in-house, it must send the sample to a reference laboratory, which in many cases increases the length of time it takes for the clinician to receive the results. Clearly, for antidepressant levels to be clinically useful, the results must be returned to the clinician rapidly, to enable the test to be used when making clinical decisions about dosage. It should take a laboratory no more than 24 hours to perform the assay.

During the initial phases of treatment for inpatients we recommend frequent determination of antidepressant level, e.g., at least twice per week. Blood specimens are obtained in the morning, prior to any morning dose, and are collected in Venoject brand tubes or certain Vacutainer brand tubes (but not serum separator and transport tubes (SST) (Table 9.4). With regard to methodology, we feel that the most practical, rapid, and sensitive method of measurement of tricyclic antidepressants is high-performance liquid chromatography (HPLC). Periodically,

Table 9.4.
Antidepressant Levels

Generic	Trade Name	Therapeutic Plasma Levels (ng/ml)
Amitriptyline (AT)	Elavil, Endep	AT + NT (125–250)
Nortriptyline (NT)	Pamelor	50–140
Imipramine (IMP)	Tofranil, SK Pramine	IMP + DES (75–300)
Desipramine (DES)	Pertofrane, Norpramine	150–300
Protriptyline (PRO)	Vivactil	90–170
Doxepin (DX)	Sinequan, Adapin	DX + DDX (75–300)
Clomipramine (CLO)	Anafranil	CLO + DCLO (350–800)
Trimipramine (TRI)	Surmontil	>50
Maprotiline	Ludiomil	180–300
Amoxapine	Asendin	150–450 ng/ml of 8-OH amoxapine

the assay should be cross-validated with a mass spectrophotometric method (Fig. 9.6).

There are essentially four major reasons to monitor.

1. **To Check Compliance.** This issue is important in regard to both initial and maintenance treatment response, especially in depressed patients whose concentration and motivation are impaired.

2. **To Maximize Clinical Response.** Since a relationship between clinical response and drug plasma concentration has been established for certain antipressant medications, plasma monitoring allows the physician to more rationally adjust drug dosage to enhance therapeutic effect.

3. **To Avoid Toxicity.** Since a relationship between drug plasma concentration and drug toxicity has also been demonstrated for some antidepressant agents, drug toxicity can also be minimized by rationally adjusting dosages based on plasma monitoring.

4. **To Help Protect the Physician Legally.** This issue is particularly important in this era of malpractice suits, especially for physicians who

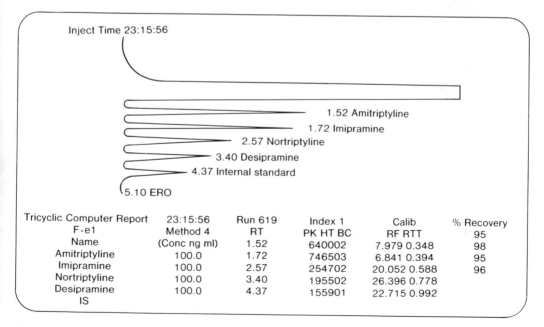

Inject Time 23:15:56

1.52 Amitriptyline
1.72 Imipramine
2.57 Nortriptyline
3.40 Desipramine
4.37 Internal standard
5.10 ERO

Tricyclic Computer Report	23:15:56	Run 619	Index 1	Calib	% Recovery
F·e1	Method 4	RT	PK HT BC	RF RTT	95
Name	(Conc ng ml)	1.52	640002	7.979 0.348	98
Amitriptyline	100.0	1.72	746503	6.841 0.394	95
Imipramine	100.0	2.57	254702	20.052 0.588	96
Nortriptyline	100.0	3.40	195502	26.396 0.778	
Desipramine	100.0	4.37	155901	22.715 0.992	
IS					

Figure 9.6. A tricyclic chromatogram.

give high doses of potent anticholinergic (TCA's).[27]

Recent studies[28, 29] in man clearly demonstrate that the normal bodily metabolism of imipramine, desipramine, amitriptyline, and nortriptyline can result in significant accumulation of hydroxylated metabolites in concentrations equal to or greater than those of the parent compound. Measurement of antidepressant levels should include as many active metabolites as is feasible. Determination of levels of hydroxylated metabolites is now technically possible, although few laboratories perform this procedure as part of their routine measurements of the levels of the parent tricyclic compounds.

Therapeutic plasma level monitoring is useful in helping to define an adequate TCA trial (Table 9.5). In light of the high proportion of treated depressed patients who have inadequate pharmacologic treatment,[30] criteria for adequacy are important. An adequate TCA trial consists of maintaining the patient at a dosage adequate to achieve therapeutic TCA plasma levels for a minimum of 21 days with documented compliance.

Numerous studies support the use of tests of platelet monoamine oxidase inhibitor (MAOI) activity in order to maximize treatment response to MAOI medications.[31] Patients achieving an 80% or greater MAOI inhibition from their own base have higher response rates in MAOI treatment for depression than patients with lower inhibition levels. One study showed a 50% increase in the response rate: those with inhibition over 80% showed a 68% response rate, whereas patients with lower inhibition had only a 44% response rate.

Antiepileptic Medications

Therapeutic plasma concentrations have been defined for most antiepileptic

Table 9.5.
Adequacy of a Tricyclic Antidepressant Trial[a]

1. Dosage
2. Plasma levels
3. Duration
4. Compliance

[a] Minimal trial: 21 days at therapeutic plasma levels.

drugs, so that seizure control can be achieved with little risk or toxicity. The effective plasma level may vary from patient to patient because the severity of seizures may be different, which may explain why seizures in some patients are well controlled at subtherapeutic plasma drug levels.[32] Many clinical studies have confirmed the usefulness of antiepileptic drug monitoring in achieving optimum seizure control.[33–38] Psychiatrists are increasingly interested in the psychotropic effects of some of the anticonvulsants, such as carbamazepine. In addition, many patients seen by psychiatrists have seizure disorders. Methods of monitoring and titrating dose when these medications are used in psychiatry are just as useful. It is important, however, that laboratories offering determination of antiepileptic drugs participate in a quality control program to establish interlaboratory reproducibility and report the method used to determine the blood level. Due to drug interactions, even patients long maintained on a dose of a particular anticonvulsant should be monitored when admitted to an inpatient unit and started on other medications.

Neuroleptic and Other Drug Levels

There is a smaller body of research into clinical use of neuroleptic and antipsychotic levels. However, many of the basic principles of therapeutic drug monitoring discussed above also apply to neuroleptic levels. For example, consistently low levels might indicate noncompliance. Patients with extremely high levels may be considered toxic, may have a high risk of developing tardive dyskinesia, and may require closer observation. Anticholinergic drugs appear to lower plasma concentrations of neuroleptics. In one study[39] levels varied as much as 15-fold in children on the same daily dosage. More recently, research has shown a correlation between neuroleptic plasma level and clinical response.[40] Some studies[41, 42] show the presence of a therapeutic window for plasma levels of haloperidol and possibly thiothixene and fluphenazine.[43, 44] Dopamine receptor binding levels adding all the active metabolites into one blood level-like measurement may be widely utilized over the next 2–5 years.

In addition to antidepressant and neuroleptic levels, psychiatrists need to be familiar with the use of therapeutic drug monitoring of lithium and the all-too-common case of multiple medications prescribed at the same time to the same patient. Simple, reliable, and inexpensive methods of performing such levels make the tests routine in clinical practice. We recommend weekly or at least monthly lithium levels to encourage compliance and reduce relapse rate.

SPECIAL EVALUATIONS

Evaluation of the Drug-Abusing Patient

The current increase in drug abuse in all age groups and increasing awareness of the associated medical complications necessitate a careful and systematic approach to the person who presents to the physician with a history of polydrug abuse.[45, 46] A urine specimen for a comprehensive drug evaluation (described above) should be obtained, under supervision, at the time of admission and periodically during hospitalization, regardless of the history given by the drug-abusing patient. Such patients also should have a thorough evaluation for hepatitis, including hepatitis B surface antigen, B surface antibody, B core antibody, and A antibodies. In addition, a CBC with differential, B_{12}, folate, tryptophan, urinalysis, SMA-22 multitest profile, prothrombin time, partial thromboplastin time, and serology are usually indicated. When inpatient psychiatrists treating patients who abuse drugs do thorough evaluations of such patients they discover a surprisingly large number of medical problems requiring evaluation and treatment.

Evaluation of Impotence

Recent studies have shown that the concept that impotence is almost always psychogenic may not be true. One study[47] showed that 35% of consecutive patients with impotence had previously undiagnosed disorders of the hypothalamic-pituitary-gonadal axis. Impotence is frequently reported in patients with alcohol and drug abuse. At a minimum, serum testosterone levels are indicated in the evaluation of impotence. Further workup may include a penile tumescence-monitored sleep study, measurement of serum luteinizing hormone (LH), prolactin, thyroid functions, and serum LH response to luteinizing hormone-releasing hormone (LHRH test).

Evaluation of the Patient on Lithium Maintenance

The issue of lithium's long-term effects on the kidney has emphasized the need for periodic laboratory evaluation of patients maintained on lithium[23, 24] We recommend measurement of urinary volume and creatinine clearance at least every year, in addition to more frequent measurement of serum creatinine and serum lithium levels.

Lithium significantly interferes with thyroid metabolism and may be an immunostimulant. Five percent or more of patients on lithium become hypothyroid. When patients are started on lithium they should have a baseline TSH, T_4, and T_3 uptake. In addition, some clinicians recommend measurement of thyroid antibodies and a TRH test at the same time.[17, 18] Thereafter, the basic thyroid functions should be repeated a few times during the first year, and then annually (or more often if indicated). It is important not to eliminate the TSH level from the battery.

Medical Evaluations

To uncover a psychiatric disorder caused or precipitated by a prescribed medication, illicit medication, or poison, the psychiatrist must (on the basis of the physical, neurological, and endocrinological examination and review of the history given by the patient and others) generate a formal differential diagnosis and exclude all viable competing diagnoses through testing or other active processes of investigation.

A complete discussion of medical diseases that commonly present to a psychiatrist and imitate naturally occurring psychiatric syndromes are beyond the scope of this chapter but have been discussed elsewhere.[48]

Recognition of these disorders is important because patients may exhibit psychiatric symptoms early, and many of the conditions are treatable and reversible. Psychiatrists have a special role in identifying patients with toxic or medical causes for their psychiatric symptoms. It is incorrect to assume that the consulting internists will be able to thoroughly address this complicated differential diagnosis. As the use of clinical laboratory tests in psychiatry becomes more common, and as the tests become more sophisticated, psychiatrists will increasingly identify patients with toxic and medical syndromes who previously would have been misdiagnosed.[17, 49] The unique role of the psychiatrist will be to attempt to rule out these organic disorders prior to psychiatric treatment, thereby improving the response rate. Increasingly, psychiatrists in clinical practice are willing to accept this responsibility.

REFERENCES

1. Galen RS, Gambino SR: *Beyond Normality: The Predictive Value and Efficacy of Medical Diagnoses,* New York, John Wiley & Sons, Inc. 1975.
2. Slawson PF: Psychiatric malpractice: The California experience. Am J Psychiatry, *136:* 650–654, 1979.
3. Hansen HJ, Caudill SP, Boone DJ: Crisis in drug testing: Results of CDC blind study. JAMA, *253:* 2382–2387, 1985.
4. Schwartz RH, Hawks RL: Laboratory detection of marijuana use. JAMA, *254:* 788–792, 1985.
5. Yago KB, Pitts FN Jr, Burgoyne RW, Aniline O, Yago LS, Pitts AF: The urban epidemic of phencyclidine (PCP) use: Clinical and laboratory evidence from a public psychiatric hospital emergency service. J Clin Psychiatry, *42:* 193–196, 1981.
6. Sweeney DR, Gold MS, Pottash ALC, Davies RK: Neurobiological theories, in Kutash IL, Schlesinger LB (eds): *Handbook on Stress and Anxiety,* pp. 112–122, San Francisco, Jossey-Bass Inc., 1980.
7. Thacore VR, Shukla SRP: Cannabis psychosis and paranoid schizophrenia. Arch Gen Psychiatry, *33:* 383–386, 1976.
8. Gruen PH, Sachar EJ, Altman N, Sassin J: Growth hormone responses to hypoglycemia in postmenopausal depressed women. Arch Gen Psychiatry, *32:* 31–33, 1975.
9. Sachar EJ, Asnis G, Halbreich U, et al.: Dextroamphetamine and cortisol in depression. Arch Gen Psychiatry, *37:* 755–757, 1980.
10. Carroll BJ, Feinberg M, Greden JF, et al.: A specific laboratory test for the diagnosis of melancholia. Arch Gen Psychiatry, *38:* 15–22, 1981.
11. Carroll BJ: Dexamethasone suppression test: A review of contemporary confusion. J Clin Psychiatry, *46:* 13–24, 1985.
12. Ritchie JC, Carroll BJ, Olton PR, et al.: Plasma cortisol determination for the dexamethasone suppression test. Arch Gen Psychiatry, *42:* 493–497, 1985.
13. Extein I, Pottash ALC, Gold MS, et al.: Using the protirelin test to distinguish mania from schizophrenia. Arch Gen Psychiatry, *39:* 77–81,1982.
14. Langer G, Resch F, Aschauer H, et al: TSH-response patterns to TRH stimulation may indicate therapeutic mechanisms of antidepressant and neuroleptic drugs. Neuropsychobiology,*11:* 213–218, 1984.
15. Kirkegaard C, Bjorum N: TSH responses to TRH in endogenous depression. Lancet, *1:* 152, 1980.
16. Krog-Meyer I, Kirkegaard C, Kijne B, et al.: Prediction of relapse with the TRH test and prophylactic amitriptyline in 39 patients with endogenous depression. Am J Psychiatry, *141:* 945–948, 1984.
17. Gold MS, Kronig MH: Comprehensive thyroid evaluation in psychiatric patients, in Hall RCW and Beresford TP (eds): *Handbook of Psychiatric Diagnostic Procedures,* vol. 1, pp. 29–45. New York, Spectrum Publications, 1984.
18. Gold MS, Pearsall HR: Hypothyroidism—Or is it depression? Psychosomatics, *24*(7): 646–657, 1983.
19. Gold MS, Pottash ALC, Extein I: "Symptomless" autoimmune thyroiditis in depression. Psychiatry Res *6:* 261–269, 1982.
20. Sternbach HA, Gold MS, Pottash ALC, Extein I: Thyroid failure and protirelin (thyrotropin-releasing hormone) test abnormalities in depressed outpatients. JAMA, *249*(12): 1618–1620, 1983.
21. Whybrow PC, Prange AJ Jr: A hypothesis of thyroid-catecholamine-receptor interaction. Arch Gen Psychiatry, *38:* 106–114, 1981.
22. Nemeroff CB, Simon JS, Haggerty JJ, et al.: Antithyroid antibodies in depressed patients. Am J Psychiatry, *142*(7): 840–843, 1985.
23. Pottash ALC, Gold MS: Issues in lithium therapy, in Giannini AJ, (ed): *Clinical Foundations of Biological Psychiatry,* pp. 227–234, New Hyde Park, N.Y., Excerpta Medica/Med Exam Publishing, 1986.
24. Pottash ALC: Clinical use of lithium, in Giannini J (ed): *Psychiatric, Psychogenic, and Somatopsychic Disorders Handbook,* pp. 277–280, New York, Medical Examination Publishers, 1978.
25. Goggans FC, Gold MS: Nutritional deficiency syndromes in clinical psychiatry, in Woods S (ed): *Diagnostic and Laboratory Testing in Psychiatry,* pp. 99–106, New York, Plenum Publishing Corp, 1986.
26. Knapp S, Mandell AJ: Conformational influences on brain tryptophan hydroxylase by submicromolar calcium: Opposite effects of equimolar lithium. J Neural Transm, *45:* 1–15, 1979.

27. Preskorn SH, Gold MS, Extein I: Therapeutic drug level monitoring in psychiatry, in Wood S (ed): *Diagnostic and Laboratory Testing in Psychiatry*, pp. 131–154. New York, Plenum Publishing Corp, 1986.
28. DeVane CL, Jusko WJ: Plasma concentration monitoring of hydroxylated metabolites of imipramine and desipramine. Drug Intell Clin Pharm, *15:* 263–266, 1981.
29. Young RC, Alexopoulos GS, Shamoian CA, et al.: Plasma 10-hydroxynortryptiline in elderly depressed patients. Clin Pharmacol Ther *35*(4): 540, 1984.
30. Keller MB, Klevman GL, Lavori PW, et al.: Treatment received by depressed patients. JAMA, *248:* 1848–1855, 1982.
31. Georgotus A, Mann J, Friedman E: Platelet MAO inhibition as a potential indicator of favorable response to MAOI's in geriatric depressions. Biol Psychol, *16:* 997–1001, 1981.
32. Feldman RG, Pippenger CE: The relation of anticonvulsant drug levels to complete seizure control. J Clin Pharmacol, *16:* 51–59, 1976.
33. Cereghino JJ: Serum carbamazepine concentration and clinical control. Adv Neurol, *11:* 309–330, 1975.
34. Eadie MJ: Plasma level monitoring of anticonvulsants. Clin Pharmacokinet, *1:* 52–66, 1976.
35. Kutt H, Penry JK: Usefulness of blood levels of antiepileptic drugs. Arch Neurol, *31:* 283–288, 1974.
36. Kutt H: Diphenylhydantoin. Relation of plasma concentration to seizure control, in Woodbury DM, Penry JK, Pippenger CE (eds): *Antiepileptic Drugs,* ed. 2, New York, Raven Press, 1982.
37. Lascelles PT, Kocen RS, Reynolds EH: The distribution of plasma phenytoin levels in epileptic patients. J Neurol Neurosurg Psychiatry, *33:* 501–505, 1970.
38. Sherwin AL: Ethosuximide: Relation of plasma concentration to seizure control, in Woodbury DM, Penry JK, Pippenger CE (eds): *Antiepileptic Drugs,* ed. 2, New York, Raven Press, 1982.
39. Morselli PL, Bianchetti G, Durand G, Le-Heuzey MF, Zarifian E, Dugas M: Haloperidol plasma level monitoring in pediatric patients. Ther Drug Monit, *1:* 35–46, 1979.
40. Extein I, Augusthy KA, Gold MS, et al.: Plasma haloperidol levels and clinical response in acute schizophrenia. Psychopharmacol Bull, *18:* 156–158, 1982.
41. Magliozzi JR, Hollister LE, Arnold KV, et al.: Relationship of serum haloperidol levels to clinical response in schizophrenic patients. Am J Psychiatry, *138:* 365–367, 1981.
42. Miller DD, Hershey LA, Duffy JP, et al.: Serum haloperidol concentrations and clinical response in acute psychosis. J Clin Psychopharmacol, *6:* 305–310, 1984.
43. Mavroidis ML, Kanter DR, Hirschowitz J, Garver DL: Clinical relevance of thiothixene plasma levels. J Clin Psychopharmacol, *3:* 155–157, 1984.
44. Mavroidis ML, Kanter DR, Hirschowitz J, Garver DL. Fluphenazine plasma levels and clinical response. J Clin Psychiatry, *45:* 370–373,1984.
45. DeMilio L, Gold MS, Martin D: Evaluation of the substance abuser, in Woods S (ed): *Diagnostic and Laboratory Testing in Psychiatry*, pp. 235–247. New York, Plenum Publications, 1986.
46. Gold MS, Estroff TW: The comprehensive evaluation of cocaine and opiate abusers, in Hall RCW, Beresford TP (eds): *Handbook of Psychiatric Diagnostic Procedures*, vol. 2, pp. 213–230, New York, Spectrum Publications, 1985.
47. Spark RF, White RA, Connolly PB: Impotence is not always psychogenic. JAMA, *243:* 750–755, 1980.
48. Estroff TW, Gold MS, Pottash ALC: Psychiatric misdiagnosis, in Gold MS, Lydiand RB, et al. (eds): *Advances in Psychopharmacology: Predicting and Improving Treatment Response.* Boca Raton, Fla., CRC Press, 1984, pp. 33–66.
49. Pottash ALC, Sweeney DR, Gold MS, et al.: The future of private hospitals—Some crucial distinctions. Hosp Community Psychiatry, *33*(9): 735–739, 1982.
50. Gold MS, Pottash ALC, Extein I: Hypothryoidism and depression. JAMA, *145:* 1919–1922, 1981.

SUGGESTED READINGS

Amsterdam J, Brunswick D, Mendels J: The clinical application of tricyclic antidepressant pharmacokinetics and plasma levels. Am J Psychiatry, *137:* 653–662, 1980.

Banki CM, Arato M, Papp Z: Thyroid stimulation test in healthy subjects and psychiatric patients. Acta Psychiatr Scand, *70:* 295–303, 1984.

Bertilsson L, Mellstrom B, Sjoquist F: Pronounced inhibition of noradrenaline uptake by 10-hydroxy-metabolites of nortriptyline. Life Sci, *25:* 1285–1292, 1979.

Brown WA, Shuey I: Response to dexamethasone and subtype of depression. Arch Gen Psychiatry, *37:* 747–751, 1980.

Carroll BJ, Curtis GC, Mendels J: Neuroendocrine regulation in depression. I. Limbic system-adrenocortical dysfunction. Arch Gen Psychiatry, *33:* 1039–1044, 1976.

Carroll BJ, Curtis GC, Mendels J: Neuroendocrine regulation in depression. II. Discrimination of depressed from non-depressed patients. Arch Gen Psychiatry, *33:* 1051–1058, 1976.

Dysken MW, Pandey GN, Chang SS, et al.: Serial postdexamethasone cortisol levels in a patient undergoing ECT. Am J Psychiatry, *136:* 1328–1329, 1979.

Elsborg L, Hansen T, Rafaelsen OJ: Vitamin B12 concentrations in psychiatric patients. Acta Psychiatr Scand, *59:* 145–152, 1979.

Ettigi P, Brown GM: Psychoneuroendocrinology of affective disorders: An overview. Am J Psychiatry, *134:* 493–501, 1977.

Evered DE, Ormston BJ, Smith PA, et al.: Grades of

hypothyroidism. Br Med J, *1:* 657–662, 1973.

Extein I, Pottash ALC, Gold MS, et al.: Differentiating mania from schizophrenia by the TRH test. Am J Psychiatry, *137:* 981–982, 1980.

Extein I, Pottash ALC, Gold MS: Relationship of thyrotropin-releasing hormone test and dexamethasone suppression test abnormalities in unipolar depression. Psychiatry Res, *4:* 49–53, 1981.

Extein I, Pottash ALC, Gold MS: TRH test in depression. N Engl J Med, *302:* 923–924, 1980.

Glassman AH, Schildkraut JJ, Orsulak PF, et al.: Tricyclic antidepressants-blood level measurements and clinical outcome: An APA task force report. Am J Psychiatry, *142:* 155–162, 1985.

Gold MS, Pottash ALC, Davies RK, et al.: Distinguishing unipolar and bipolar depression by thyrotropin release test. Lancet, *2:* 411–413, 1979.

Gold MS, Pottash ALC, Extein I: The psychiatric laboratory, in Bernstein JG (ed): *Clinical Psychopharmacology,* pp. 29–58, John Wright PSG, 1984.

Gold MS, Pottash ALC, Extein I, Sweeney DR: Diagnosis of depression in the 1980's. JAMA, 245: 1562–1564, 1981.

Gold MS, Pottash ALC, Ryan N, et al.: TRH-induced response in unipolar, bipolar, and secondary depressions: Possible utility in clinical assessment and differential diagnosis. Psychoneuroendocrinology, *5:* 147–155, 1980.

Goodwin FK, Cowdry RW, Webster MH: Predictors of drug response in the affective disorders: Toward an integrated approach, in Lipton MA, DiMascio A, Killam KF (eds): *Psychopharmacology: A Generation of Progress,* pp. 1277–1288, New York, Raven Press, 1978.

Greden JF, Albala AA, Haskett RF, et al.: Normalization of dexamethasone suppression test: A laboratory index of recovery from endogenous depression. Biol Psychiatry, *15:* 449–458, 1980.

Greden JF, Carroll BJ: The dexamethasone suppression test as a diagnostic aid in catatonia. Am J Psychiatry, *136:* 1199–1200, 1979.

Kirkegaard C, Norlem N, Lauridsen UB, et al.: Prognostic value of thyrotropin-releasing hormone stimulation test in endogenous depression, abstracted. Acta Psychiatr Scand, *52:* 170–177, 1975.

Lamberg, BA, Gordin A: Abnormalities of thyrotropin secretion and clinical implications of the thyrotropin releasing hormone stimulation test. Ann Clin Res, *10:* 171–183, 1978.

Loo H, Benyacoub AK, Rovei V, et al.: Long-term monitoring of tricyclic antidepressant plasma concentrations. Br J Psychiatry, *137:* 444–451, 1980.

Meyers B, Tune LE, Coyle JT: Clinical response and serum neuroleptic levels in childhood schizophrenia. Am J Psychiatry, *137:* 483–484, 1980.

Pottash ALC, Barker TE, Goggans F, et al.: Dopamine receptor blockade of amoxapine: Comparison of GC 8-OH amoxapine plasma levels and dopamine radioreceptor activity. Soc Neurosci Abstr, No. 155.7, 1982.

Pottash ALC, Black HR, Gold MS: Psychiatric complications of antihypertensive medications. J Nerv Ment Dis, *169:* 430–438, 1981.

Pottash ALC, Extein I, Gold MS: The TRH test in the differential diagnosis of depression. Soc Neurosci Abstr, *6:* 324, 1980.

Pottash ALC, Martin DM, Extein I, et al.: High performance liquid chromatography versus gas chromatography mass spectroscopic analysis of tricyclic antidepressants in human plasma. Soc Neurosci Abstr, 7(213.2):644, 1981.

Pottash ALC, Martin DM, Extein I, et al.: The prediction of therapeutic nortriptyline dosage regimens and related plasma concentrations of hydroxylated metabolites in geriatric depressives. Soc Neurosci Abstr, *9:* 428, 1983.

Prang AJ Jr, Wilson IC, Lara PP, et al.: Effects of thyrotropin-releasing hormone in depression. Lancet, *2:* 999–1002, 1972.

Sachar EJ, Asnis G, Halbreich U, et al.: Recent studies in the neuroendocrinology of major depressive disorders, in Sachar EJ (ed): *Psychiatry Clinics of North America,* vol 3, pp. 313–326, Philadelphia, W.B. Saunders, 1980.

Schlesser M, Winokur G, Sherman BM: Hypothalamic-pituitary-adrenal axis activity in depressive illness. Arch Gen Psychiatry, *37:* 737–743, 1980.

Smith RC, Chojnacki M, Hu R, et al.: Cardiovascular effects of therapeutic doses of tricyclic antidepressants: Importance of blood level monitoring. J Clin Psychiatry, *41:* 57–63, 1980.

Sweeney DR, Maas JW: Specificity of depressive disease. Annu Rev Med, *29:* 219–229, 1978.

Sweeney DR, Maas JW, Heninger GR: State anxiety, physical activity, and urinary 3-methoxy-4-hydroxphenethylene glycol excretion. Arch Gen Psychiatry, *35:* 1418–1423, 1978.

Webb WL, Gehi M: Electrolyte and fluid imbalance: Neuropsychiatric manifestations. Psychosomatics, *22:* 199–203, 1981.

Wenzel KW, Meinhold H, Raffenberg M, et al.: Classification of hypothyroidism in evaluating patients after radioiodine therapy by serum cholesterol, T_3-uptake, total T_4, FT_4-index, total T_3, basal TSH and TRH test. Eur J Clin Invest, *4:* 141–148, 1974.

chapter 10

the therapeutic milieu and its role in clinical management

Cavin P. Leeman, M.D.

HISTORICAL INTRODUCTION

The word "milieu," in the sense of a carefully arranged environment for the treatment of the mentally ill, began appearing in the psychiatric literature during the 1940's. Bruno Bettelheim,[1] in working with children, proposed the creation of a *therapeutic* milieu to reverse the pathogenic effects of the child's earlier, natural milieu. Experiences in military psychiatry during World War II showed that treatment and rehabilitation of psychiatric casualties were often more effective when careful attention was paid to the milieu in which they were carried out. Twentieth century psychiatrists rediscovered what Benjamin Rush had pointed out more than 100 years earlier, that the environment in which treatment occurs can provide additional therapeutic benefit.[2] The work of Rush and other early 19th century humanistic reformers led to the development of moral (psychological) treatment, which has been well reviewed by Bockoven.[3] The principles of moral treatment included the importance of working with mental patients in a kind, nonpunitive way and also of providing a benign physical and interpersonal environment to enhance therapeutic effectiveness. The gains achieved by moral treatment, which contributed to the therapeutic success of American mental hospitals in the first half of the 19th century, were lost in the second half of that century, when overcrowding, understaffing, and a changed social and economic climate turned these same hospitals into custodial warehouses for the insane and the unfortunate.[4, 5]

After World War II, little time was lost in applying the findings of military psychiatry to civilian populations. Thomas Main coined the term "therapeutic community," and applied it to British hospital psychiatry.[6, 7] At almost the same time, Maxwell Jones[8] was developing similar methods. In the therapeutic communities of Main and of Jones, the total structure of the treatment unit was involved in the treatment process. As described by Jones[9]:

It would seem that in some, if not all, psychiatric conditions, there is much to be learned from observing the patient in a relatively ordinary and familiar social environment so that his usual ways of relating to other people . . . can be observed. If at the same time he can be made aware of the motivation underlying his actions, the situation is potentially therapeutic. This we believe to be the distinctive quality of a therapeutic community.

Jones's therapeutic community, described more fully by Rapoport[10] than by Jones himself, was utilized primarily for the treatment of patients with personality disorders. (In the literature of the therapeutic milieu, the term "therapeutic community" has been used both in the narrow sense, in which it is used in this chapter, to refer to the specific form of therapeutic milieu developed by Main and by Jones, and in a broader sense, as a synonym for "therapeutic milieu." The careful reader will not be misled.) Its basis was maximal participation by patients in management of the ward and maximal utilization of the patient community as an agent of change for individual patients. Other workers applied the therapeutic milieu to the treatment of other kinds of patients. The authors who wrote about the therapeutic milieu in the 1950's and 1960's emphasized values, generally humaneness, openness, honesty, trust, democracy, egalitarianism, and permissiveness.[11–13] These writers were not much concerned with specific methods of milieu treatment, and generally did not acknowledge that a milieu approach that was beneficial for some patients might be less beneficial, or even harmful, for others.

Jones's therapeutic community, in which less than 10% of the patients were psychotic, patients considered "too sick" were "as far as possible, screened out prior to admission," and the median length of stay was between 100 and 200 days,[10] had little in common with most psychiatric units of the 1970's and 1980's. Inappropriate application of the original therapeutic community model to very different clinical settings led to a wave of criticism in the 1970's.[14–16] Yet, milieu therapy already included a repertory of methods which, skillfully applied, can make the environment therapeutic for diverse patient groups.[17]

Major trends in psychiatric hospitalization in the 1980's include the admission of ever-increasing proportions of acutely psychotic patients to short-term inpatient psychiatric units, many of them in general hospitals, and increasingly intense pressure to reduce the length of stay on these same units. This pressure comes from a convergence of economic considerations with repeated inability of researchers to demonstrate any clinical superiority of longer stays over shorter stays, for most patients.[18, 19] These trends have necessitated further modification in milieu treatment. Making milieu therapy effective on the acute psychiatric units of today requires clearer role definitions and lines of accountability, as well as focused treatment planning which utilizes the milieu flexibly to meet the needs of each individual patient.[20, 21]

DEFINITION AND MECHANISMS

The essence of inpatient psychiatric treatment, which distinguishes it fundamentally from outpatient treatment, is that it occurs in a controlled milieu. This corresponds to the reason patients are hospitalized, which usually is either the failure of treatment in an uncontrolled outpatient environment or the failure of the patient and his social environment to tolerate one another.[22] The reason for a patient's admission must be addressed promptly and consistently during the hospitalization if the patient is to return safely and expeditiously to the community. This requires evaluating the patient's premorbid environment, and his interaction with that environment. Information-gathering interviews with relatives and other significant figures can be extremely helpful. Within the hospital the patient's behavior should be assessed in varied interpersonal situations, and opportunities should be provided to enhance the patient's responsibility and to restore optimal social functioning.

The general aim of modern milieu therapy is to provide a reasonably stable and coherent social organization which facilitates the development and application of an individual, comprehensive treatment plan, based on realistic and specific therapeutic goals, for each patient. Change should be not only accepted but expected and encouraged. Intact ego functions must be identified and built upon. The environment should be structured yet flexible, within the limits set both by clear, concise general rules and by each patient's individual treatment plan. Appropriate ego-strengthening stimuli as well as exposure and involvement in varied "living-learning" experiences are constantly examined and modified to meet the needs of the individual patient. Initially, some acutely ill patients need marked limitation of exposure to interpersonal stimulation.

The social environment of the milieu allows for experiential and observational learning to occur. Patients are helped to become aware of how they interact in social situations and of the effect their behavior has upon other patients and staff members. This all occurs within the relatively safe context of the ward milieu. Staff members, functioning partly as role models, allow the patient to observe healthier, more effective methods of social interaction.

The autonomy and responsibility of patients are respected and encouraged within the limits determined by each individual's clinical state. This is reassessed frequently, and appropriate changes are made in the treatment plan. As patients improve, they are expected to participate more and more actively in their own treatment. While patients and staff members may participate together in many administrative and therapeutic decisions, final authority on the unit rests with the staff. The degree to which the staff retains responsibility and authority for clinical and administrative decision-making represents a major distinction between the therapeutic milieu of an acute general psychiatric unit and the democratic structure of Jones's therapeutic community. Oldham and Russakoff[23] have delineated how an acute unit can adapt the techniques of a therapeutic community to the needs of a heterogeneous population of acutely disturbed patients and reduced lengths of stay, without turning patients into passive recipients of medically oriented care.

While on the unit, patients are encouraged to maintain as much contact with the outside community as is consistent with their clinical needs and to regain such contact as quickly as possible. Resocialization within the outside community, usually combined with conversion to outpatienthood, and not optimal adjustment to the hospital milieu, is the overall objective.

Abroms[17] has stated that the goals of psychiatric treatment can be reduced to two main ones: setting limits and learning basic psychosocial skills. He lists five types of disturbed behavior which must be controlled or limited for therapy to progress—destructiveness, disorganization, deviancy ("acting out"), dysphoria,

and dependency—and four psychosocial skills which must be learned—orientation (social orientation, not just person, place, and time), assertion, occupation, and recreation. He considers milieu therapy to be "a treatment context," or a "metatherapy," in which the full range of specific treatment techniques available on the unit can be delivered in an individualized, coordinated fashion. Thought of in this way, milieu therapy is "the means of organizing a . . . treatment environment so that every human interaction and every treatment technique (including somatic therapies, individual and group psychotherapy, occupational therapy, etc.) can be systematically utilized to further the patients' aims of controlling symptomatic behaviors and learning appropriate psychosocial skills."

The remainder of this section will consider the mechanisms of the therapeutic milieu. As pointed out by Abroms, they all serve, in various ways, to arrive at and maintain consensus about treatment goals and methods. For a milieu to be therapeutic, clear channels of communication are essential. Attention must be paid to the *entire* network of communication. *Any* information relating to the social and interpersonal processes of the milieu is relevant.

Ward Report

This meeting has the function of sharing initial clinical data about newly admitted patients as well as information about other patients' behavior and the general tone of the milieu during the preceding 24 hours. How it is organized depends on the style of the unit. In a *therapeutic community* patients generally are present and are expected to participate. On a *short-term* unit, both the greater mental disorganization of newly admitted patients and the rapid turnover of patients necessitate that staff members must serve almost unaided as the preservers and transmitters of the unit's culture. In this setting, patients are much less likely to be included in ward report. In a *general hospital,* the psychiatric unit, although typically more egalitarian than other nursing units in the hospital, is likely to preserve much of the traditional medical orientation. A psychiatrist, serving as the director or associate director of the unit, generally chairs report; most of the data are presented by the charge nurse; other staff members of various disciplines contribute additional information and share points of view. Each unit develops its own format. For example, every patient may be reviewed daily, or only newly admitted or problematic patients may be discussed. A feasible compromise is to make report longer (perhaps an hour) on Friday afternoons and on Monday mornings, providing time to discuss every patient and to anticipate and review weekend passes and activities. Shorter (half-hour), selective reports are held on Tuesday, Wednesday, and Thursday mornings. Generally, each day's report should include brief reports on groups which have met the previous day as well as observations on the overall milieu.

Community Meeting (CM)

This is a meeting, typically a half-hour to an hour long, that is usually held several times a week, on a regularly scheduled basis. Additional CM sessions may be held at times of crisis on the unit. At CM practically all of the patients meet together with most of the staff members actively involved on the milieu. CM is the cornerstone of the therapeutic milieu, providing a forum for shared therapeutic work, enhancing the overall therapeutic environment, and helping other forms of therapy to flourish (M. Libbey and G. K. Katz, unpublished observations). Issues related to living and working together on the unit are discussed, including plans for shared tasks and activities and reactions to traumatic events. Sharing information, as well as feelings, about arrivals and departures of patients and staff members in itself can serve a valuable therapeutic function, especially since separation and loss so often are problematic for psychiatric patients.[24] Constructive participation and social assertiveness are encouraged. Communication skills are fostered, and patients are helped to become aware of the transactional impact of their behavior. Staff members support patients' valid perceptions, "teasing" them apart, often with group support, from pathological distortions and socially inappropriate styles of delivery. Community meeting also is used by the staff to facilitate cohesiveness, to assess the state of the milieu and the needs of the community. A particularly important function of CM is the strengthening of the Unit's behavioral norms,[24] which will be discussed later in this chapter, and to influence the tone for the day.

In a *therapeutic community,* CM may be combined with ward report and may be the setting in which passes and changes in privileges are negotiated.

In a *short-term psychiatric unit in a general hospital,* passes and privileges generally are negotiated by patients and doctors individually, and may be reviewed in ward report, without patients being present. In that case, CM is used for discussion of general issues concerning hospitalization. Such discussion helps patients to overcome their sense of shame and unique defectiveness, helps them to observe and to learn from the interpersonal conflicts of others, enhances their self-esteem, and facilitates their learning of interpersonal skills. Generally, all patients are expected to attend CM unless there is a specific clinical contraindication. Exceptions include very actively psychotic or manic patients whose tolerance of interpersonal stimulation is minimal, patients who are so confused that their participation would be disruptive to others and not meaningful to themselves, and patients whose hearing is so impaired as to make their presence a major source of frustration. As emphasized by Russakoff and Oldham, careful attention to making the structure of CM clear and consistent is especially important in a short-term general psychiatry unit.[24]

Ideally, CM is followed immediately by a meeting of its staff member participants alone, without patients, to clarify what the staff has learned from CM, and to review how staff members have worked with one another during CM. Staff members also may identify what information from CM should be shared with leaders of patient activities throughout the day and evening shifts, since themes that emerge in CM tend to persist throughout the day and to come up again and again. The post-CM meeting, or "rehash," is valuable in enhancing the skills of staff members as therapeutic participants in CM, a role which is not without its unique pitfalls.[25-27] Staff members must learn when to participate as members of the community, on a par with patients, expressing feelings and opinions as patients are encouraged to do. They also must learn when and how to utilize their role as facilitators and leaders. When CM seems to have no direction, it is frustrating, particularly if not acknowledged explicitly. When distortions are not challenged, psychopathology tends to be reinforced. When limit-setting is overemphasized by repressive staff members, impaired senses of self continue to languish rather than to recover.

As pointed out by Main, interpretation in large groups such as CM is extremely risky.[28] The author follows Main in recommending "non-interpretive therapeutic interventions," which are "highly personalized statements about one's own sincerely felt position . . . offered only if the declared personal position has been thought out as being revealing also about the situation of others."

While some have recommended a longer post-CM meeting for maximal didactic benefit, even a 15-minute discussion period can be very useful. It has been found helpful for participants to come to this meeting with the following questions in mind: How did it feel to be in community meeting? What would I have liked to happen in community meeting? What could I have done differently (more effectively) in community meeting? (A. Armour and B. Press, unpublished observations)

Patient Discussion and Activity Groups

In addition to CM and formal group psychotherapy (see Chapter 12 for a discussion of inpatient group psychotherapy), a variety of special interest and activity groups can assist patients in identifying problems, sharing thoughts and feelings, developing social skills, promoting mastery, and enhancing self-esteem. Some groups which often are utilized in this way are art therapy group, occupational therapy group, exercise group, cooking group and community lunch, writing group, men's concerns group, women's concerns group, parenting group, work discussion group, alcohol concerns group, current events group, and various games and outings.[29-31] (Also see Chapter 15.) Physical activity is especially important for adolescent patients, as well as for others who have difficulty in discharging tension verbally. Transition group is a special kind of discussion group, attended by selected patients as they approach discharge and then return for a limited number of sessions (for example, three) after they have left the unit. The unique functions of this group are to assist with issues of separation and loss, to ease the transition from the cloistered hospital environment to the community, and to support the reassumption of vocational and familial responsibilities.

Treatment Planning Conferences (TPCs)

As with the meetings already discussed, treatment planning conferences vary in format from one unit to another, depending on the presence or absence on the staff of community-based psychiatrists,* and on other structural variables of the unit. In a general hospital short-term psychiatric unit previously directed by the author (average length of stay 3 weeks, with a range from overnight to about 3 months), in which patients are treated collaboratively by community-based psychiatrists and a hospital-based staff under the direction of a hospital-based psychiatrist. A TPC on each patient is held once a week. The essential participants in each conference are the chairperson (director or associate director of the unit, or other senior clinician), the attending psychiatrist

---

*Some inpatient psychiatric units are staffed entirely by hospital-based personnel. These probably offer the easiest situation in which to provide a stable, cohesive milieu, and the most difficult in which to achieve continuity of care between inpatient and outpatient treatment. The collaborative treatment model, discussed further in the text, probably is the most challenging, but may offer the best combination of a strong, interdisciplinary, therapeutic inpatient milieu and continuity of care. In a third model, in which community-based private practitioners extend their solo practices into the hospital, and the hospital itself serves primarily to contain the patient, efforts to make the milieu therapeutic tend to be fragmented and rudimentary.

(regular attendance is expected, even if he is not salaried by the hospital), a nursing staff representative (preferably the "milieu therapist," the nursing staff member specifically assigned to work most closely with the patient and to coordinate his treatment program), and the social worker assigned to the case. Frequently other members of the staff, such as a clinical psychologist, an occupational therapist, and other members of the nursing staff, also participate. Clinical data presented by each member of the treatment team are reviewed; goals of treatment are agreed upon; and a treatment plan is formulated, with the role of each member specified. Progress is assessed each week, and the treatment plan is modified accordingly. A summary of the TPC is entered into the patient's permanent record, where it becomes a part of the periodic utilization review process (see Appendix 1). On many units, groups of nursing staff members or small interdisciplinary groups may get together between weekly TPC's in order to monitor patients' progress and discuss the details of treatment programs.

When all or almost all of the patients on a unit are treated entirely by hospital-based personnel, the organization of the staff into clinical teams can facilitate efficient collaboration. Team members become accustomed to working with one another, and schedules can be readily coordinated. Team meetings, often held two or three times a week, may serve as TPCs. (When community-based psychiatrists are active on a unit, division into teams is less likely to be practical. Unevenness of admission rates of various psychiatrists makes it difficult to assign each psychiatrist to a particular team. On the other hand, if one psychiatrist is expected to work with more than one team, scheduling can become impossibly complex.)

Discharge Planning Conference

When an inpatient unit is part of a network of mental health services, including partial hospitalization programs, outpatient clinics, community residences, sheltered workshops, and case management services, it may be useful to have regular meetings, twice a month or so, at which representatives of the various programs meet to coordinate services for patients approaching discharge.

Whole Staff Meeting

It is desirable for the entire staff, or as many members as can convene during any one shift, or at change of shift time, to assemble regularly to discuss communication difficulties, conflicts, and other issues that from time to time interfere with working together smoothly. Questions of how authority is exercised, delegated, and shared, and of how decisions are made, are ubiquitous, and are more problematic if not discussed. There need be no pretense of complete equality in decision-making. In fact, honesty as to the loci of power and responsibility is far better than pseudo-egalitarianism. What is most important, however, is that everyone have, and know that he has, the opportunity to be heard. The leader of the whole staff meeting, often but not always the director of the unit, should set a tone for these meetings that avoids superficial triviality on the one hand, and inappropriate interpretation or shifts from the professional context to personal issues on the other. Ineffective leadership, too little structure, or too much emphasis on personal self-disclosure can undermine clinical work.[32] Often these meetings are held weekly for about an hour, although some units have found longer sessions at less frequent intervals more useful. Abroms[17] and others have commented on the immediacy with which the resolution of staff conflicts is translated into therapeutic benefit for patients. The parallelism between themes raised in staff meetings and those brought up by patients in CMs also is a frequent observation. Less often noted is the way that Bion's ideas of group function apply to the staff of a psychiatric unit.[33, 34] The staff is a work group with a work task that is the restoration to health of the patients, but the group also has covert tasks which may subvert the work task, leading to crisis. When that happens, it is important for the staff to work on the issues that have gotten in its way, sometimes in an emergency meeting, and to re-establish the work task.

Administrative or Policy Meetings

It is important for representatives of each professional group on the interdisciplinary staff to meet together regularly, under the chairmanship of the director of the unit, to discuss matters of policy. Guidelines for admission procedures, aspects of the overall program, and recruitment of key staff members are examples of the kinds of issues discussed.

Educational Conferences

An ongoing program of educational conferences provides intellectual stimulation as well as an opportunity for identification with more experienced or gifted clinicians. Often a variety of formats is useful, including didactic presentations, seminars, and also case conferences in which clinical data are presented, a patient is interviewed before the group, and an opportunity is provided for more in-depth discussion than is possible in the more immediately practical TPC's.

FUNCTIONS OF THERAPEUTIC MILIEUS

Gunderson[35] has delineated the following five therapeutic activities which milieus can provide.

Containment

"The function of containment," as defined by Gunderson,[35] "is to sustain the physical well being of patients and to remove the unaccepted burdens of self control or feelings of omnipotence . . . . Containment acts to prevent assaults, homicides, and suicides, and to minimize the chances of physical deterioration or of dangerous accidents in those who lack judgment." Containment is most important for acutely psychotic patients, as well as for the actively assaultive or self-destructive. For patients who do not need it, it may "suppress initiative and hope, and reinforce isolation." Seclusion and restraint are two specific forms of containment which may occasionally be both necessary and therapeutic even on an unlocked unit that admits only voluntary patients. (While many unlocked units do not have seclusion rooms, some do. Restraint, of course, can be used regardless of whether there are seclusion rooms.) Other authors have discussed patterns of use of these interventions, as well as aspects of technique.[36-40] On a unit which strives for an open, therapeutic milieu, every episode of seclusion or restraint has a significant impact on the tone of the milieu and should be reviewed in CM, and possibly in other settings as well.

Support

Gunderson[35] uses the term "support" to refer to "conscious efforts by the social network to make patients feel better and to enhance their self-esteem." A supportive milieu provides nurturance and encourages patients

"to venture into other more specific therapies, such as psychotherapy, rehabilitation, or family therapy. . . . This function is especially important to frightened, depressed, and good-prognosis patients . . . (but) too much emphasis on support can confirm a patient's sense of inadequacy and dependency . . . and be quite toxic to certain borderline or paranoid patients."

Structure

By structure, Gunderson[35] means "all aspects of a milieu which provide a predictable organization of time, place, and person." Structure is emphasized by "fixed role definitions, high order and organization, and hierarchical responsiblity distribution." It is "especially needed by chronic schizophrenics, manic, acting-out, and short-term patients," but "too much structure can . . . leave patients poorly prepared to deal with the less structured world to which they are discharged."

Involvement

"Involvement refers to those processes which cause patients to attend actively to their social environment and interact with it."[35] Specific techniques include "open doors and open rounds, patient-led groups, the identification of shared goals, mandatory participation in milieu groups, community activities, verbalization of problems, and self-assertiveness experiences." The therapeutic communities of Main[6] and Jones[8, 9] are therapeutic milieus which emphasize involvement. Involvement, which particularly addresses patients' passivity, is most important for withdrawn and sociopathic patients, as well as for some schizophrenic patients who are neither acutely psychotic nor flagrantly paranoid. Shershow has commented on the problems associated with overemphasizing this milieu function for patients who cannot make use of it.[15]

Validation

This term refers to "the ward processes which affect a patient's individuality," such as individualized treatment programming; acceptance of privacy and secrets; exploratory one-to-one talks; emphasis on loss; and encouragement to accept challenge, to tolerate uncertainty, and to risk failure.[35] Gunderson feels that "paranoid and borderline patients will profit most from this function," but that very passive, nonverbal, or relentlessly suicidal patients may be hurt by too much emphasis on validation.

General Comments

The astute reader will note some similarity between the milieu functions described by Gunderson and the analysis by Abroms reported earlier.[17] Gunderson's approach seems more readily applicable to characterizing and differentiating various treatment milieus, designed to serve a variety of distinct, and more or less homogeneous, patient populations, with varying clinical needs.† Short-term units with relatively unrestrictive criteria for admission are not free to specialize, however, and do well to strive for an alternative suggested by Gunderson[35]: a "maximally flexible milieu which can provide all therapeutic functions reasonably well, even if it cannot provide any one of them in its optimal form."

There are few conclusive research findings as to which milieu characteristics are

most likely to be therapeutic for various kinds of patients, and space does not permit review of the published studies. The reader is referred to other authors.[45–47]

The importance of adapting the milieu to each patient's individual clinical needs has been emphasized by Leeman and Autio.[20] They called for application of the various modalities of milieu treatment—limit-setting, orientation, nurturance, stimulation, structure, promotion of autonomy and responsibility, and development of insight—skillfully blended in individualized treatment programs to meet specific needs of each patient. Leeman and Autio's seven modalities of milieu therapy correspond approximately to Gunderson's five functions and to Abroms' five types of disturbed behavior and four psychosocial skills (Fig. 10.1). Patients with different problems, or at different phases of their treatment, require emphasis on different modalities of

ABROMS	LEEMAN and AUTIO	GUNDERSON
Setting Limits: destructiveness	Limit Setting	Containment
Setting Limits: deviancy		
Social Skills: orientation	Orientation	Structure
Setting Limits: disorganization	Structure	
Setting Limits: dysphoria	Nurturance	Support
	Stimulation	Involvement
Setting Limits: dependency	Promotion of Autonomy and Responsibility	Validation
Social Skills: assertion		
	Development of insight	
Social Skills: occupation		
Social Skills: recreation		

---

†One aspect of the issue of specificity versus generality is the question of whether voluntary and involuntary patients should be treated on the same unit. Some clinicians have argued that the open therapeutic milieu which is beneficial for most patients is seriously damaged by the locking of doors and the admission of involuntary patients,[41–43] while others feel that voluntary and involuntary patients can be well treated together on a locked unit.[23, 44]

Figure 10.1. Approximate correspondence of functions of therapeutic milieus as analyzed by Abroms, Leeman and Autio, and Gunderson.

treatment, as is discussed in the next section.

INDIVIDUAL TREATMENT PLANNING

Experienced inpatient clinicians have become adept at balancing the general goals of a therapeutic milieu with the individual clinical needs of each patient. Although most psychiatric units still set *some* limits on the range of patients accepted for admission, a heterogeneous patient population is typical, especially in psychiatric units in general hospitals and in general short-term units in psychiatric hospitals. Individual treatment planning is crucial, and Johansen's comment[48] that "Shaping milieu treatment to the individual patient . . . must not be allowed to degenerate into a one-to-one concordance between diagnostic label and treatment approach" is well taken; yet some generalizations appear valid and are summarized in this section. The reader is referred to original sources for more detail.

Limit-Setting for Adolescent Patients

Adolescent patients with character disorders often present unresolved emotional conflicts and antisocial behavior unresponsive to exploratory psychotherapy. For some of these patients, firm, consistent limit-setting by a caring administrator assisted by a ward staff who act as a unified team has proved remarkably effective.[49] (See also Chapter 13.)

Patients with Borderline Personality Disorders

The study of therapeutic failures and special problem patients often has helped to advance medical knowledge. Certainly this has been true in the field of milieu therapy, where first Main, then Burnham, then Pardes and associates, each carefully examined a series of patients who did poorly or were associated with special problems on an intensive, supposedly therapeutic, milieu.[50–52] By today's diagnostic criteria, most or all of these patients would be regarded as suffering from borderline personality disorders. Review of these three classic studies is recommended to inpatient clinicians interested in avoiding the pitfalls for which this diagnostic group has become well known.

Current clinical thinking emphasizes that most of the definitive treatment of patients with borderline personality disorders is accomplished best on an outpatient basis, with brief hospitalizations at times of crisis. Friedman[53] has pointed out the importance of strict limitation of disruptive behavior in order to minimize regression in these patients. Adler[54] has emphasized that the staff must recognize and resist the primitive psychological mechanisms with which borderline patients provoke punishment and incite conflict within the staff. Wishnie[55] has elucidated how these patients can be helped to overcome their magical thinking by reminding them consistently of their autonomy and of the responsibility for their own lives. Structuring the milieu so that most of the patient's work is channeled to a single staff member, and/or close coordination of the various persons working with the patient, can help the patient to synthesize his all good and all bad object images into a more accurate representation of the real persons with whom he is relating.

Peteet and Gutheil[56] have suggested the following themes for the ward management of the borderline patient:

1. The patient is held accountable for his actions; disruptive or self-destructive behavior engenders an administrative response that is individualized and, ideally, negotiated.
2. There is an unrelenting emphasis on the expression of feelings in words rather than actions.
3. An attempt is made to achieve an alliance with the patient around the problems of accountability, verbalization, and controls.

Gunderson[57] has reviewed the literature on hospital care of borderline patients. He finds consensus on the following points:

1. "The general role of the hospital in the overall treatment of borderline patients is that of a backup to outpatient treatment, which provides an essential service during periods of crisis."

2. Hospitalization of borderline patients often involves regression.
3. Ubiquitous staff conflicts, usually "between viewing borderline patients as waifs in need of nurturance or as manipulators in need of limits," complicate the hospital experience.
4. Firm limits should be imposed early and consistently.
5. "Milieu programs must emphasize interpersonal issues."

He suggests that empirical research be undertaken to resolve persistent disagreements concerning the following questions:

1. Does long-term hospitalization enhance the possibilities of psychological growth beyond what is possible in outpatient treatment, or is it contraindicated because of the regressive experiences which it engenders?
2. Is the regression which occurs when a borderline patient is hospitalized inevitable, a reflection of poor management, or related to vicissitudes in the patient's relationships to significant important persons, having little to do with the hospital stay? (The experience of the author, as well as of those workers quoted above, is that regression during acute hospitalization can be markedly reduced by the methods already mentioned.)
3. Are the intrastaff disagreements, so common in the treatment of borderline patients, caused by psychological mechanisms within the patients, the individual psychology of staff members, or diversity of professional experience and roles within the staff? (In any case, the author's experience is that emphasis both on intrastaff communication and on the need to understand, not merely manage, patients, combined with ongoing inservice education, can be quite helpful.)

Some borderline patients may need repeated hospitalization. Once they have become well known to the staff, it may become possible to structure and limit the hospitalization almost from the moment of admission. The following example‡ is illustrative:

The therapist of a middle-aged woman with a borderline personality organization requested that the patient be readmitted following disclosure by the patient that she had stood over her husband's bed the previous night with a knife, thinking of hurting him. On admission, the patient was disheveled, agitated, and apparently helpless. She voiced concern about losing her husband, who had been threatening her with divorce, and expressed little hope for herself. At the end of the initial interview, the patient was told that she could stay on the Unit for 72 hours, with the goals of acknowledging her rage at her husband and of telling her husband about the incident before discharge. This approach was designed to convey recognition of her strengths and responsibilities as a mature adult, and to minimize gratification of her wish to regress and be taken care of. Within the first 24 hours, the patient was no longer agitated, her physical appearance had improved, and she was involved in Unit activities. She talked about her anger toward her husband for threatening to divorce her, but acknowledged that her recent behavior had provoked him. On the third day of hospitalization, the patient arranged a meeting with her husband and calmly discussed the incident and her understanding of what had preceded the events of that night. The following day, the patient was discharged home to continue her outpatient treatment.

Manic Patients

The milieu management of manic patients has been clearly delineated by Gunderson,[58] who has proposed the following principles:

1. Administrative issues should be handled in an authoritarian and non-negotiable manner.
2. Manic patients require firm external controls.
3. While a manic patient is demanding privileges, he needs restrictions.
4. Limits should be enforced consistently and firmly.

Bjork and associates[59] have elaborated further on the usefulness of these prin-

‡The clinical examples in this section were published originally in *Psychotherapy and Psychosomatics,* from which they are reprinted with permission. (Leeman CP, Autio S: Milieu therapy: The need for individualization. Psychother Psychosom, *29:* 84–92, 1978.)

ciples, as well as on the reciprocal influences of the manic patient on the therapeutic milieu, and vice versa. They emphasize that successful hospitalization of manic patients requires that they be given particularly thoughtful consideration, starting even before admission and continuing until discharge. It was from manic patients that Bjork and associates learned the importance of individualizing milieu therapy, as the following quotation makes clear:

In the early therapeutic communities there was a tendency to see and treat all patients more or less alike. That de-emphasized diagnostic differences (an obvious disadvantage for the manic) and focused on a rather homogeneous treatment program in which great importance was placed on active participation by all. For instance, everyone from the most agitated manic to the most withdrawn catatonic was expected to attend community meetings. That proved to be disastrous for one of our first manic patients, who totally dominated and disrupted the community meetings for days, until she succeeded in alienating herself completely from the rest of the community. She became the scapegoat for everything wrong on the ward and soon left and admitted herself to a closed unit. It was then that we modified our philosophy. It has become standard practice to evaluate the manic's ability to tolerate external stimulation and to semi-isolate the patient from the community when necessary. Depending on the degree of excitability of the patient, the isolation can range from complete restriction in a seclusion room to exclusion from large group meetings.

Acutely Schizophrenic Patients

The apparent inability of many acutely schizophrenic patients to select or filter out those stimuli which are relevant to the task at hand has become a commonplace clinical observation. Consistent with this finding is the concept that an active therapeutic milieu may contain an intensity of environmental stimulation that is toxic for some acutely schizophrenic patients. This point of view has contributed to the opposition to milieu therapy already noted.[14] Such opposition has not recognized that a more sophisticated approach requires individualization of each patient's involvement in the therapeutic milieu. The actively psychotic, acutely

schizophrenic patient needs limitation of stimuli and assistance in gradual orientation to the social structure of the unit. The following example illustrates useful techniques:

An 18-year-old man entered the hospital in a frightened, agitated, suspicious, and disorganized state characteristic of an acute schizophrenic episode. The standard admission procedure was deferred. The patient was introduced to the nurse in charge, who showed him to a single room. She reassured the patient that he was among people who wanted to help, and that his behavior was communicating to her his need to be alone. He was restricted to the single room with frequent checks by staff. Following a dose of medication, the patient relaxed and slept. Later, recognizing the patient's difficulty with orientation, the admitting nurse introduced him to the charge nurse for the next shift. This practice continued for several shifts, with only the charge nurse on each shift working with the patient. A daily schedule was established for him. Room restrictions were continued; frequent orientation to time, date and place was instituted; group involvement was restricted; and visitors and phone calls were limited. Nurses whom the patient had come to know ate meals with him in his room. As he improved further, they spent brief periods playing cards with him. Other patients were encouraged to introduce themselves individually to the patient. When he was able to tolerate increased stimulation, he was given a tour of the unit. He was allowed limited periods out of his room in a small lounge. Time for playing pingpong with a staff member was added to his schedule. As his disorganization and confusion dissipated, he was encouraged to attend therapeutic groups and given access to all aspects of the milieu.

Depressed and Withdrawn Patients

Depressed and withdrawn patients may benefit from active encouragement to participate in task-oriented and recreational activities, promoting a sense of accomplishment and mastery, enhancing self-esteem, and facilitating resocialization. A clinical example follows:

A 52-year-old woman was admitted with depression, multiple somatic complaints, and inability to care for herself, culminating in a retreat to bed for the preceding 9 months. On admission, she was tearful, clinging, and insistent that she would be unable to complete even simple tasks. A schedule was established for the patient, including wake-up time, dressing, making her bed, involvement in groups, and rest periods. Gradually, she began to assume increasing responsibility on the Unit and her rest periods decreased. Whenever she was given a new assignment, such as a cooking group, there was a new barrage of somatic complaints. With support and encouragement, she attempted the task and was praised when she succeeded. In time, the focus was shifted to utilization of the patient's skills at home. Passes to go home caused her much anxiety and a return of the somatic complaints, requiring a 'total push' in order to get her to leave the Unit. Staff members worked with the family so that the same kind of program could be continued during the passes, enabling the patient gradually to reassume her responsibilities.

Neurotic Problems

As already noted, "the distinctive quality of a therapeutic community," as envisioned by Jones,[9] is achieved by providing opportunities for the patient to observe both the motivation and the effects of his own behavior. Milieu therapy can facilitate "laboratory" observation of one's own behavior not possible in individual therapy alone. The development of insight often can be combined with other techniques of behavioral change, as shown in the following example:

A 48-year-old woman was admitted for depression. Prominent among her presenting problems was a phobia concerning the handling and preparation of food. This phobia had reached such intense proportions that friends and relatives could no longer be invited to her home. The patient was convinced that those who ate the food she prepared would be poisoned.

The patient initially was restricted from any groups dealing with food and was not allowed to assume any kitchen duties. After forming a working alliance with the patient, her milieu therapist began to deal with the phobia. The therapist's goals were to help the patient to gain a better understanding of the dynamics and to correct the behavior.

The patient viewed her childhood as an unhappy, isolated one and resented her brother for being the favored child. She saw her parents as cold, distant people who stifled any expression of affect. Peer groups were of little interest to the patient, who spent much time with studies in an effort to gain the approval of her perfectionistic father. She felt that he was never satisfied with her performance, and that

she got no support from her hypochondriacal, passive mother, whose main interest was her meticulous housekeeping and preparation of meals. Family meals were unrelieved by conversation, and father often ate apart from the rest of the family. The patient pursued a career as a writer, graduating from college with high honors. Following college, she married her present husband. She felt that their relationship was close and caring at first, but that it had deteriorated over the years to become as cold and distant as her parents' marriage.

With this background in mind, the patient and the milieu therapist came to regard the phobia as a defense against intense rage. The patient feared that expression of her omnipotent rage would be fatal to the persons close to her. Food had become the medium of her rage as a learned response from childhood.

As the patient began to articulate her anger, the therapist began to confront the phobic behavior, beginning by asking the patient to make her a cup of coffee. The patient became increasingly anxious but completed the task. After repeated reassurances that the therapist had suffered no ill effects, the patient was able to repeat the performance with less anxiety. Then she progressed to making lunch for herself and the therapist. At this point the patient was encouraged to join a cooking group composed of patients and staff members, and assumed the responsibility of making coffee for the community. In sessions with her milieu therapist, she continued to learn more about her anger, realizing that often her feelings were justified, and that she was a person of worth. Meetings with her husband and the therapist provided an opportunity for the patient to express her anger directly to him; he responded sympathetically and they developed greater emotional closeness. The patient began to go home on short passes, progressing from simply tolerating her home environment to assisting with a family meal. The phobia remained in check and she began to prepare meals without anxiety. Since the patient's phobia increased whenever there were dinner guests, the milieu therapist arranged with the patient to visit for dinner with the family. Despite the patient's initial anxiety, she was able to prepare the meal. Meanwhile, she had become more articulate in expressing her feelings and needs to her husband, even when they differed from his.

The patient contacted the milieu therapist 6 months after discharge. She no longer was isolating herself, she was entertaining friends and relatives, and she had moved to a larger community where she had assumed a more responsible job. Her phobia and depression had not returned.

THE THERAPEUTIC ALLIANCE, SOCIAL NORMS, AND BEHAVIORAL INCIDENTS

Effective treatment is facilitated by the development of an alliance with the patient. While there is an extensive literature on the therapeutic alliance,[60] little has been written about its unique aspects in relation to hospital settings. Gutheil[61] has emphasized that an important part of the alliance with a hospitalized patient concerns the patient's overt behavior. He suggests that an "administrative alliance exists between therapist and observing part of the patient against maladaptive, self-defeating or self-destructive behaviors as they affect, or appear in, the clinical context." The psychiatrist should strive from his initial contact with the patient to engage with him and to share with him the functions of clinical assessment, decision-making, and behavioral prescription. As Gutheil points out, the degree of participation by the patient may be limited by his capacity, and at times the doctor may have to act in opposition to the patient, but in the patient's interest, for example, denying a pass or insisting on involuntary hospitalization. This, however, should be regarded as a way station on the road to establishment or re-establishment of the alliance.

Johansen and Gossett[62] have expanded on the notion of a dyadic doctor-patient alliance to address concurrent processes within the patient-doctor and patient-hospital relationships. Alliance-formation is influenced by pre-existing needs and expectations of all the participants. As in individual psychotherapy, the alliance may have to be limited at first to a narrow goal, such as the alleviation of a single symptom, to be broadened later, as work proceeds. The inpatient situation, however, is greatly complicated by additional factors involving other members of the treatment team, the hospital community (including other patients), and the patient's family, who may be deeply involved in the patient's admission and perhaps also in treatment decisions. The following example illustrates this point:

A psychotic young man was participating actively in his treatment, including neuroleptic medication. Both he and the staff were pleased with his progress, but his father wanted the treatment changed to megavitamin therapy. On two occasions when his father visited, the patient submitted three-day letters prepared by his father for his signature, requesting discharge. When his father left, the patient retracted the letters, explaining apologetically that, "I can't stand up to my father."

Berger[63] has pointed to the impact on alliance building of the "involuntariness" of many hospital admissions, referring not only to overtly involuntary admissions but also to many overtly voluntary admissions as well. The latter cover a spectrum from those which are arranged under explicit threat of involuntary hospitalization through those in which there is some degree of external coercion from family, friends, or therapists to those in which the only coercion is internal and based on psychic pain, but still subjectively real. It is likely that most patients enter a hospital with feelings of humiliation, failure, shame, and guilt about hospitalization itself, and special attention should be paid to those feelings on admission and thereafter.

There are many ways in which the therapeutic alliance can be fostered from the time of admission. The patient should be approached in a manner that respects his dignity and appeals to the healthier aspects of his functioning, not as a helpless child or as someone whose feelings and needs are unimportant. Admission procedures should be designed to minimize the patient's feeling dehumanized. He should be oriented to the unit in person and also may be given some written material to help him learn what patients and staff can expect from each other. Anxieties about being hospitalized can be acknowlegded openly in community meeting, and emotional support can be provided by other patients as well as by staff members. If the patient is too ill to assimilate information upon admission, it can be introduced when he is ready. Attention should be paid to the process by which the patient came to the hospital and how he feels about it. Acculturation to the unit proceeds gradually and should continue throughout the patient's entire hospitalization.

A depressed woman who had requested hospitalization and was a voluntary patient spoke poignantly in community meeting of the "terrible shame" that she felt, and that "no one of you can begin to understand," at being behind a locked door. The comments of other patients helped her to feel that she was not alone. Her therapist, who was present but had not previously been aware of how his patient felt, brought up the matter again in private sessions, to therapeutic advantage.

The psychiatrist's role in building the alliance is especially important; the prevailing expectations of the doctor's role, as well as the matrix of power, influence, knowledge, and competence of the patient's particular doctor as he functions within a particular psychiatric unit, ensure its importance. To facilitate alliance-building, the psychiatrist should convey to the patient a sense of being acknowledged, respected, and understood. Empathic support must be provided, and appropriate limits set. The relief of suffering as, for example, by the prescription or the administration of medicine, also may strengthen the developing alliance. Other staff-patient interactions may enhance or erode the doctor's efforts, and even patient-patient interactions may exert powerful, and frequently overlooked, influences upon the newly admitted patient. It is not unusual for patients to be extremely helpful in comforting and orienting a new arrival, nor is it rare for newly admitted patients to react with fear or with distancing maneuvers such as "I'm not as bad as that" to the disturbed behavior of other patients, sometimes to the point of deciding almost immediately upon arrival not to stay in the hospital.

A careful diagnostic assessment of a newly admitted patient may permit clinical staff members to anticipate probable management difficulties. This is particularly true in the case of patients who already are known to the staff from prior hospitalizations. Such patients, for example, may have violated the rules against illicit drug use, been noncompliant with medication or with other components of the therapeutic regimen, eloped from the unit, or insisted upon premature discharge against medical advice. An attempt should be made from the beginning, or as soon as the patient's capacities permit, to engage him in an alliance to understand what happened and to avoid recurrence. It often is useful in such cases to set very explicit limits from the moment of admission, sometimes even specifying the sanctions to be imposed for violations of the rules. The use of written contracts, which represents the most formal version of this approach, can be helpful in carefully selected cases.[56] (An example of a written contract is given by Gunderson[57] on p. 183 of his book. Although the example comes from a unit specializing in borderline patients, where it apparently is used with every patient admitted, more heterogeneous units could adopt it selectively.)

Prevailing social norms on the unit must be cultivated and utilized to inhibit violence, the use of illicit drugs, sexual activity between patients, and other forms of behavior that are antitherapeutic either for the individual or for the patient group as a whole. The ward culture must stress individual accountability for one's own behavior, participation in one's own treatment, and the importance of putting feelings into words. For example, "The patient must not run off the ward to show how upset he or she is, but must stay and talk about being upset or at least talk about why he or she wants to run off."[64] Different levels of competence in the relevant skills are acknowledged dependent upon diagnosis, stage of illness, and intellectual and characterological variables, but a shared commitment to these values is expected of all. Generally, it helps to be quite explicit about these matters, in community meeting and in other settings. Knowing that the staff takes norms, expectations, and limits seriously helps the patients to feel safe.

It would be an inappropriate and misguided application of respect for patients' privacy to shy away from openly discussing violations of community norms. Behavior within the hospital setting is community business. This truth becomes obvious when it is realized that patients as a group generally are quite aware of infractions of the rules, although they may not feel free to discuss this behavior with staff members, especially in the face of hesitancy or reluctance. For much of the unit's population, an open discussion, initiated and participated in by staff, provides little new information about patient behavior, while it goes a long way toward re-establishing a stable, caring environment. Russakoff and Oldham[24] have outlined how these issues can be discussed in community meeting. For example, the use of illicit drugs, or sexual activity on the unit, both of which are explicitly proscribed, is brought up either by staff or by patients. Information is collected from the community; hospital policy is reiterated and sometimes briefly explained; and patient distress is acknowledged. The detail in which the staff describes a particular incident depends on their assessment of the amount of information the community needs to know in order to make sense of the situation. Staff members who have not yet heard about the incident can act as monitors; if they are unclear about the situation, they should assume that others are also, and should ask questions. An episode of marijuana-smoking on a psychiatric unit illustrates how this can be handled:

Mr. A, a psychotic patient with a history of episodic substance abuse, told a nurse that he had smoked marijuana on the unit the night before. As part of their one-to-one discussion of the incident, the nurse explained that she could not keep this information confidential but would have to share it with the community. After talking with Mr. A, a staff member on his team brought up the incident in the community meeting the next day, leading to a general discussion of trust and mistrust, and demonstrating to all the patients the staff's concern for maintaining a safe environment. Mr. A's roommate, Mr. B, revealed that he had supplied Mr. A with the marijuana and had used some himself, which helped the staff to understand Mr. B's recent obvious failure to maintain continued improvement. Mr. A, in talking more about the incident, recognized, apparently for the first time, that his use of marijuana was related to his frustration at not being given a pass as soon as he wanted one. This insight proved helpful in his treatment.

Felthous[65] has discussed the importance of a clearly articulated, strongly supported, repeatedly expressed norm against violence. Any violent act must be discussed as a group issue in order to understand what happened and why, and to mobilize community support from patients as well as staff for maintaining a safe, nonviolent environment. Part of the usefulness of clearly expressed norms is the overcoming of patients' unspoken assumptions, such as the ideas that mental illness excuses them from responsibility, that hospitalization protects them from the consequences of misbehavior, and that maintaining control is solely the job of the staff.

The use of the therapeutic alliance and the culture of a therapeutic milieu are powerful but imperfect deterrents to behavioral incidents. The times of greatest vulnerability are early in the hospitalization, before the development of a strong therapeutic alliance, and much later, when the patient may have regressed to a more dependent state. Any incident should be regarded as a form of communication about the state of the alliance, and as a helpful clue to something overlooked (G.A. Clark, unpublished observations). This approach is consistent with the findings of a study by Steinglass and associates[66] on discharges against medical advice (AMA). Based on interviews of patients at admission, the best predictors of discharge AMA within the first week of hospitalization were the expectation by the patient of a short hospital stay ("only a few days") and the expectation that the staff would be of little help. This finding points to the risk of assuming the existence of a therapeutic alliance when in fact none exists. The patients who leave AMA appear to have an interest in temporary hospitalization, whether to appease another person or for some other reason, but not any real interest in receiving either psychological or pharmacological treatment. Steinglass and associates suggest that careful attention to the patient's expectations at the time of admission could provide the opportunity to develop real, although limited, alliances and to tailor brief treatment programs to the needs of these patients, enabling them to leave without the pejorative label "AMA," and perhaps having achieved some modest gains. Conceivably, early recognition of these patients' needs and expectations could lead to therapeutic negotiation which, at least for some, might make effective inpatient treatment possible.

As noted earlier, a second time of vulnerability to incidents occurs late in the course of hospitalization, when the patient's dependancy needs may have come to the fore. Patients with borderline personality disorders are especially likely to react in this way. Staff members must be extremely careful with such patients not to promise, even implicitly, too much comforting and nurturance, and also not to probe into deep intrapsychic conflicts during periods of decompensation. Wishnie's[55] practical emphasis on the here-and-now and on the patient's responsibility for his own life, is extremely useful. Disruptions in the frame of treatment always call for prompt attention, as failure to take up the patient's minor infractions leads almost invariably to escalation to more serious misbehavior. Explicit limit-setting by the staff usually is required, and discussion, clarification, and re-establishment or re-negotiation of the treatment contract are essential.

A corollary of regarding each incident as a form of communication is the idea that the management of incidents is not simply a policing function, but a part of therapeutic work. Ogden[67] has reported on a schizophrenic patient who eloped repeatedly during the first weeks of hospitalization, beginning on the day of admission, as a way of validating his view of the staff as incompetent. Of crucial importance, however, to the understanding of this behavior was the fact that, each time the patient eloped, he returned to the unit on his own, as he had not completely given up on the possibility of being helped. Unfortunately, in the case reported, the staff was hampered by unresolved institutional problems and by increasing feelings of anger and frustration directed at the patient. Thses factors contributed to laxness in elopement precautions and inability to explore with the patient the meaning of his behavior. Thus, a patient whose behavior represented a cry for both control and understanding received neither.

This example is not unusual, in that breakdowns in communication, and other impairments of staff functioning, often interfere with the prevention of behavioral incidents. A familiar problem is posed by the therapist who communicates to other staff members, but not to the patient, his concern about a patient's threatening behavior. It is difficult for other staff members, in working with the patient, to make use of clues that they have not seen themselves; meanwhile, the patient, to whom the therapist has not responded directly, has no way of knowing that the therapist is taking him seriously. The solution, in this situation, is active encouragement to the therapist to explore the issue, first-hand, with his patient. The usual result is the acquisition of more clinical data, and better agreement between the ways in which the patient is perceived by the therapist and by other staff members. Other ways in which staff behavior can contribute to behavioral incidents, for example, by covertly encouraging patients to act upon their own unacknowledged wishes to rebel against authority, are more difficult to discover and to correct.

Elopement

In addition to the general issues already discussed that should be attended to in addressing any kind of untoward behavior, there are specific practical questions about elopement. Should one wait for a patient to return or should somebody look for him? The answer, which depends in part on the clinical assessment of the patient's dangerousness, may not be readily apparent. It can be helpful to telephone a relative. For one thing, this action may determine quickly where the patient is; if not, it can be useful to explore together what the patient is up to and what should be done. Even if the relative doesn't know the patient's whereabouts, he may be able to provide other relevant information about the patient's habits or recent communications. Sometimes the patient may need encouragement to return. At this point, the family's influence on the alliance may be crucial, either in strengthening it or in undermining it, which underscores the importance of good family assessment early in the hospitalization, before incidents occur. Sometimes the patient, although not ready to resume his hospital stay, will agree to return to discuss the possibility of further treatment. This provides another opportunity to explore needs and expectations, correct misunderstandings, and renegotiate a treatment contract. (The term "contract" refers not only to formal written contracts, which are useful, as already mentioned, in exceptional cases but, more generally, to shared commitments to the methods and objectives of treatment.[61]) Administrative flexibility is called for, especially in those instances when the only alternative to compromise is no treatment at all. As in Ogden's example,[67] often the patient returns on his own, communicating something just as important in returning as in the cryptic message of his departure.

Sexual Activity on the Unit

Several unique factors make sexual activity between patients on the unit particularly difficult for staff members to deal with. For one thing, the staff is confronted with the need to deal publicly with behavior that for most people is still a private matter, and with a subject that often makes staff members uncomfortable. For another, unless this issue has been thought through, staff members may feel that they are being inconsistent or hypocritical in forbidding behavior that is regarded, in an appropriate context, as a normal part of mature, healthy functioning. In contrast to most psychiatric units of today, Jones's therapeutic community of 30 years ago was sexually, as well as generally, permissive.[10] But, as Russakoff and Oldham[24] have pointed out, when a couple forms on a unit, the members of the couple usually are either comfortable on the unit and unengaged in treatment, or in the midst of protest. In either situation, their treatment suffers. For disorganized patients who are frightened by sexual urges, frank sexual activity can be terrifying and further disorganizing. Also, like many other kinds of behavior by inpatients, sexual activity between patients often is a form of communication to the staff.

An adolescent boy reported to a nurse that he had "had sex" with a female patient, adding that the staff didn't seem to care about what he did, since he had been in the girl's room for some time with the door closed and no one had noticed. Significantly, this incident occurred immediately after a flurry of episodes in which several other patients had been demanding considerable attention, in community meeting and elsewhere, by means of a series of relatively minor infractions of the rules prohibiting the use of alcohol and of marijuana. In the discussion of those incidents several patients had expressed their doubts as to whether the staff really cared about patients, and whether the staff could and would exert sufficient control to maintain a safe environment.

Refusal to Take Medication

As with other behavioral incidents, refusal to take medication calls for negotiation with the patient, absent a clinical emergency. Some bargaining may be legitimate, perhaps as to dosage form (tablets, concentrate for oral administration, intramuscular injections) or other specifics that are more consequential to the patient's sense of being taken seriously than to the effectiveness of the pharmacotherapy. It is not unusual for a patient to refuse a medication to which he previously experienced an unpleasant or frightening side effect, and to accept a different but pharmacologically similar drug. In this situation, the psychiatrist should be on his mettle to administer the new drug in such a way as to avoid repetition of the same reaction, which almost certainly would further erode the patient's trust. The general goal is to express caring and respect for the patient's autonomy within the frame of basic conditions required for treatment to proceed. In working with a paranoid patient, time may be allowed for alliance-building and for the patient to accept the need for medication. Each case must be individualized, both as to the amount of time allowed and as to whether, in the end, the doctor makes acceptance of medication a mandatory condition of his continuing to be responsible for the patient's treatment. In a true emergency, to control dangerous behavior, a limit to negotiation must be set quickly, and the patient must be medicated, even against his will, if necessary. Whatever is done, however, should be reflected upon later with the patient and should be utilized to clarify and deepen the therapeutic alliance.

SUMMARY

1. Modern milieu therapy, although representing, in part, a rediscovery of the principles of 19th century moral treatment, developed largely from the application of World War II military psychiatry to civilian populations.

2. Jones's therapeutic community, utilized primarily for the lengthy inpatient treatment of patients with personality disorders, emphasized egalitarianism and permissiveness. Its basis was maximal participation by patients in management of the ward and maximal utilization of the patient community as an agent of change for individual patients.

3. Inappropriate and rigid application of the original therapeutic community model led to a wave of criticism; yet, milieu therapy includes a repertory of methods which, skillfully and flexibly applied, can make the hospital environment therapeutic for diverse patient groups. Particular attention to structure, role definitions, and lines of accountability is needed on today's short-term units, which admit a high proportion of psychotic patients.

4. The general aim of milieu therapy is to provide a reasonably stable and coherent social organization which facilitates the development and application of an individual, comprehensive treatment plan for each patient, based on realistic and specific therapeutic goals.

5. The mechanisms of the therapeutic milieu, including a variety of meetings and conferences, serve to facilitate communication and the achievement and maintenance of consensus about treatment goals and methods. Community meeting is the cornerstone of the therapeutic milieu.

6. The functions of therapeutic milieus, as described by Gunderson, include containment, support, structure, involvement, and validation. These correspond approximately to the modalities of milieu therapy defined by Leeman and Autio, as well as to the kinds of disturbed behavior to be limited and the psychosocial skills to be taught by psychiatric treatment, as viewed by Abroms.

7. While milieus on different units can be designed to emphasize different milieu functions, considerable flexibility in applying milieu therapy on any one unit is both possible and desirable. The excellence of milieu therapy, in fact, depends upon the degree to which it is individualized to meet each patient's clinical needs.

8. While every patient is unique, some generalizations as to the needs of various patient groups appear valid and are discussed in this chapter.

9. Effective treatment of any patient is facilitated by the development of an alliance with the patient. In the inpatient situation this process is complicated by additional factors involving other members of the treatment team, the hospital community, and the patient's family, as well as by the "involuntariness" of many hospital admissions, even those which are overtly voluntary.

10. Prevailing social norms on the unit must be cultivated and utilized to inhibit forms of behavior that are antitherapeutic either for the individual or for the patient group as a whole. Clarity of communication and consistency in setting limits are important elements in this approach.

11. Behavioral incidents, such as elopement, sexual activity on the unit, and refusal to take medication, may occur in spite of the use of the therapeutic alliance and the culture of a therapeutic milieu. Any incident should be regarded as a form of communication about the state of the alliance, and its management should be used as a means of strengthening the alliance. Specific issues and techniques which are germane to several particular kinds of incidents are discussed in this chapter.

REFERENCES

1. Bettelheim B, Sylvester E: A therapeutic milieu. Am J Orthopsychiatry, *18:* 191–206, 1948.
2. Daniels RS: The hospital as a therapeutic community, in Freedman AM, Kaplan HI, Sadock BJ (eds): *Comprehensive Textbook of Pyschiatry—II,* vol. 2, ed. 2, pp. 1990–1995, Baltimore, Williams & Wilkins, 1975.
3. Bockoven JS: *Moral Treatment in American Psychiatry.* New York, Springer, 1963.
4. Sederer L: Moral therapy and the problem of morale. Am J Psychiatry, *134:* 267–272, 1977.
5. Morrissey JP, Goldman HH, Klerman LV (eds): *The Enduring Asylum: Cycles of Institutional Reform at Worcester State Hospital,* New York, Grune & Stratton, 1980 (see chaps. 2 and 3).
6. Main TF: The hospital as a therapeutic institution. Bull Menninger Clin, *10:* 66–70, 1946.
7. Goldstein EJ, Goldstein MZ: Cassel—A different kind of hospital. Psychiatric Commun, 6(2): 35–41, 1963.
8. Jones M: *The Therapeutic Community,* New York, Basic Books, 1953.
9. Jones M: Quoted in Wilmer HA: *Social Psychiatry in Action,* Springfield, Ill., Charles C Thomas, 1960.
10. Rapoport RN: *Community as Doctor.* Springfield, Ill., Charles C Thomas, 1960.
11. Schwartz MS: What is a therapeutic milieu?, in Greenblatt M. et al. (eds): *The Patient and the Mental Hospital,* New York, Free Press, 1957.
12. Cumming J, Cumming E: *Ego and Milieu,* New York, Atherton Press, 1962.
13. Edelson M: *Ego Psychology, Group Dynamics, and the Therapeutic Community,* New York, Grune & Stratton, 1964.
14. Van Putten T: Milieu therapy: Contraindications? Arch Gen Psychiatry, *29:* 640–643, 1973.
15. Shershow JC: Disestablishing a therapeutic community. Curr Concepts Psychiatry, *3:* 8–11, 1977.
16. Herz MI: Short-term hospitalization and the medical model. Hosp Community Psychiatry, *30:* 117–121, 1979.
17. Abroms GM: Defining milieu therapy. Arch Gen Psychiatry, *21:* 553–560, 1969.
18. Kirshner LA: Length of stay of psychiatric patients: A critical review and discussion. J Nerv Ment Dis, *170:* 27–33, 1982.
19. Mattes JA: The optimal length of hospitalization for psychiatric patients: A review of the literature. Hosp Community Psychiatry, *33:* 824–828, 1982.
20. Leeman CP, Autio S: Milieu therapy: The need for individualization. Psychother Psychosom, *29:* 84–92, 1978.
21. Kernberg OF: The therapeutic community: A re-evaluation. J Natl Assoc Private Psychiatr Hosp, *12:* 46–55, 1981.
22. Tucker GJ, Maxmen JS: The practice of hospital psychiatry: A formulation. Am J Psychiatry, *130:* 887–891, 1973.
23. Oldham JM, Russakoff LM: The medical-therapeutic community. J Psychiatr Treatment Eval, *4:* 337–343, 1982.
24. Russakoff LM, Oldham JM: The structure and technique of community meetings: The short-term unit. Psychiatry, *45:* 38–44, 1982.
25. Jones M: *Maturation of the Therapeutic Community—An Organic Approach to Health and Mental Health,* New York, Human Sciences Press, 1976.
26. Klein RH: The patient-staff community meeting: A tea party with the mad hatter. Int J Group Psychother, *31:* 205–222, 1981.
27. Goering P, Littman S: Training in large group therapy. Can J Psychiatry, *26:* 53–56, 1981.
28. Main T: Some psychodynamics of large groups, in Kreeger L (ed): *The Large Group: Dynamics and Therapy,* pp. 57–86. Itasca, Ill., FE Peabody, 1975.
29. West WL (ed): *Changing Concepts and Practices in Psychiatric Occupational Therapy,* Dubuque, Iowa, Wm. C. Brown Book Co., 1959.
30. Fidler GS, Fidler JW: *Occupational Therapy: A Communication Process in Psychiatry,* New York, Macmillian, 1963.
31. Wittmann D, Leeman CP: Using Creative writing in an activity therapy group on a short-term unit. Hosp Community Psychiatry, *30:* 307, 311–312, 1979.
32. Abrams RT, Sweeney JA: A critique of the process-oriented approach to ward staff meetings. Am J Psychiatry, *139:* 769–773, 1982.
33. Sacks MH, Carpenter WT, Jr, Scott WH: Crisis and emergency on the psychiatric ward. Compr Psychiatry, *15:* 79–85, 1974.
34. Sacks MH, Carpenter WT: The pseudo-therapeutic community: An examination of antitherapeutic forces on psychiatric units. Hosp Community Psychiatry, *25:* 315–318, 1974.
35. Gunderson JG: Defining the therapeutic processes in psychiatric milieus. Psychiatry, *41:* 327–335, 1978.
36. Gutheil TG: Observations on the theoretical bases for seclusion of the psychiatric inpatient. Am J Psychiatry, *135:* 325–328, 1978.
37. Plutchik R, Karasu TB, Conte HR, Siegel B, Jerrett I: Toward a rationale for the seclusion process. J Nerv Ment Dis, *166:* 571–579, 1978.
38. Hay D, Cromwell R: Reducing the use of full-leather restraints on an acute adult inpatient ward. Hosp Community Psychiatry, *31:* 198–200, 1980.
39. Oldham JM, Russakoff LM, Prusnofsky L: Seclusion: Patterns and milieu. J Nerv Ment Dis, *171:* 645–650, 1983.
40. Tardiff K: *The Psychiatric Uses of Seclusion and Restraint,* Washington, D.C., American Psychiatric Press, 1984.
41. Leeman CP, Berger HS: The Massachusetts Psychiatric Society's position paper on involuntary psychiatric admissions to general hospitals. Hosp Community Psychiatry, *31:* 318–327, 1980.
42. Leeman CP: Involuntary psychiatric admissions to general hospitals: Progress or threat? Hosp Community Psychiatry, *31:* 315–318, 1980.
43. Leeman CP, Sederer LI, Rogoff J, Berger HS, Merrifield J: Should general hospitals accept

involuntary psychiatric patients? A panel discussion. Gen Hosp Psychiatry, *3:* 245–253, 1981.

44. Pinsker H, Raskin M, Winston A: The treatment of involuntary patients in the general hospital psychiatric unit. Gen Hosp Psychiatry, *3:* 301–305, 1981.

45. Kirshner LA, Johnston L: Current status of milieu psychiatry. Gen Hosp Psychiatry, *4:* 75–80, 1982.

46. Gunderson JG, Will OA Jr, Mosher LR (eds): *Principles and Practice of Milieu Therapy,* New York, Jason Aronson, 1983.

47. Vaglum P, Friis S, Karterud S: Why are the results of milieu therapy for schizophrenic patients contradictory? An analysis based on four empirical studies. Yale J Biol Med, *58:* 349–361, 1985.

48. Johansen KH: The impact of patients with chronic character pathology on a hospital inpatient unit. Hosp Community Psychiatry, *34:* 842–846, 1983.

49. Cohen RE, Grinspoon L: Limit setting as a corrective ego experience. Arch Gen Psychiatry, *8:* 74–79, 1963.

50. Main TF: The ailment. Br J Med Psychol, *30:* 129–145, 1957.

51. Burnham DL: The special-problem patient: Victim or agent of splitting? Psychiatry, *29:* 105–122, 1966.

52. Pardes H, Bjork D, Van Putten T, Kaufman M: Failures on a therapeutic milieu. Psychiatr Q, *76:* 29–48, 1972.

53. Friedman HJ: Some problems of inpatient management with borderline patients. Am J Psychiatry, *126:* 299–304, 1969.

54. Adler G: Hospital treatment of borderline patients. Am J Psychiatry, *130:* 32–36, 1973.

55. Wishnie HA: Inpatient therapy with borderline patients, in Mack JE (ed): *Borderline States in Psychiatry,* pp. 41–62, New York, Grune & Stratton, 1975.

56. Peteet JR, Gutheil TG: The hospital and the borderline patient: Management guidelines for the community mental health center. Psychiatr Q, *51:* 106–118, 1979.

57. Gunderson JG: Hospital care of borderline patients, in *Borderline Personality Disorder,* chap. 8, pp. 131–152, Washington, D.C., American Psychiatric Press, 1985.

58. Gunderson JG: Management of manic states: The problem of fire setting. Psychiatry, *37:* 137–146, 1974.

59. Bjork D, Steinberg M, Lindenmayer J, Pardes H: Mania and milieu: Treatment of manics in a therapeutic community. Hosp Community Psychiatry, *28:* 431–436, 1977.

60. Docherty JP (ed): The therapeutic alliance and treatment outcome, in Hales RE, Frances AJ (eds): *Psychiatry Update: The American Psychiatric Association Annual Review, Vol. 4,* Washington, American Psychiatric Press, 1985, pp. 525–637.

61. Gutheil TG: On the therapy in clinical administration. Psychiatric Q, *54:* 3–25, 1982.

62. Johansen KH, Gossett JT: Therapeutic alliance versus "conversion" in hospital psychiatry. J Natl Assoc Private Psychiatr Hosp, *12:* 56–62, 1981.

63. Berger HS: The therapeutic alliance in voluntary and involuntary hospitalization. Arch Gen Hosp Psychiatry, *3:* 249–251, 1981.

64. Tucker GJ: Therapeutic communities, in Gunderson JG, Will OA, Mosher LR (eds): *Principles and Practice of Milieu Therapy,* pp. 35–46, New York, Jason Aronson, 1983.

65. Felthous AR: Preventing assaults on a psychiatric inpatient ward. Hosp Community Psychiatry, *35:* 1223–1226, 1984.

66. Steinglass P, Grantham CE, Hertzman M: Predicting which patients will be discharged against medical advice: A pilot study. Am J Psychiatry, *137:* 1385–1389, 1980.

67. Ogden TH: Psychiatric hospital treatment, in *Projective Identification and Psychotherapeutic Technique,* chap. 6, pp. 111–133, New York, Jason Aronson, 1982.

Appendix 1

FRAMINGHAM UNION HOSPITAL
DEPARTMENT OF PSYCHIATRY
SUMMARY OF TREATMENT
PLANNING CONFERENCE
Date: _____
1. **People participating:** _____

_____

2. **Summary of clinical issues:** (Include relevant description, mental status, problems, precipitants, character and social issues, significant changes since previous conference.)

_____

_____

_____

_____

_____

_____

_____

_____

3. **Diagnosis:** Axis I: _____
   (DSM-III) Axis II: _____
            Axis III: _____

4. **Recommended Treatment Goals** (compare with previous conference):
   a. Hospitalization: _____

_____

   b. Long-term: _____

5. **Recommended Treatment Plan** (include meds, type of Rx and with whom, agencies to be involved, role of O.T. and Social Work):
   a. Before discharge (include usefulness of further hospitalization): _____

_____

_____

_____

   b. Therapeutic Trial Visits: _____
   c. Anticipated length of further stay: _____
   d. After discharge: _____

_____

Signature of Conference Chairman

_____

chapter 11

individual psychotherapy

Jerome Rogoff, M.D.

The only thing we really deal with in our relationships with patients is their actual life experience ... how much of it they integrated and how much of it isn't integrated; how much they can handle and how much they can't handle, but have to postpone or avoid or deny.[1]

Psychotherapy adds insight to injury. Psychic injury may be of any type, may have come in any form, and may be single or multiple, but it has altered the patient's feeling, thinking, behavior, or self-regard in a negative way. Insight may be curative, ameliorative, supportive, merely interesting, or ineffectual, but it is one of the key things psychotherapy has to offer. Psychotherapy offers other things, such as perspective, objectivity, sympathy, empathy, support, and structure. It also offers help in testing reality, bearing ambivalence, containing painful affects, and taking responsibility for one's thoughts, actions, feelings, and fantasies. It offers the opportunity to remember the forgotten, relive the repressed, and relinquish the maladaptive. It can help one mourn the ungrieved, face the feared, or tame or channel aggression.

Whatever psychotherapy does, it does it in the context of a relationship. Psychotherapy is, at its core, the use of a relationship to constructively influence another person's life. Thus, the therapist is himself the instrument of change.

There are many kinds of psychotherapy. Some focus more, others less, on the relationship itself as the means to effect change, but all of them are set immutably in that relationship. In what follows, I will be using as my model what is the most widely practiced form of individual psychotherapy, the psychodynamic model, derived from psychoanalysis but modified in many ways and in many directions. Psychodynamic psychotherapy places major emphasis on the relationship itself between therapist and patient.

The psychotherapy of inpatients is the treatment, by these relational, verbal means, of patients who have been defined, or have defined themselves, as disordered in some major way. They represent the "sicker" end of the spectrum of psychiatric maladies. Such people have had a major breakdown of defenses, coping mechanisms, thought processes, affective tone or response, the will to live, or a combination of these. Treatment is aimed at effecting change, primarily in the patient himself, but often also in the social system (usually the family) from which the patient has come. Change is difficult to measure, and there is no consensus about what should change. Nevertheless, most clinicians seem to agree that there should be some constructive change in the patient's thoughts and feelings about himself and the world around him. Changes in these parameters usually affect behavior. Psychotherapy, then, aims at reducing or eliminating abnormal thoughts, feelings, and behavior, which are what we call symptoms. Psychotherapy also aims at positively influencing underlying conflicts that give rise to the symptoms, contribute to them, or exacerbate them.

What, then, is the role of verbal individual psychotherapy in the treatment of patients, the large majority of whom require and respond to psychotropic medication, the structure of an inpatient milieu, or other therapies, such as ECT or occupational therapy? Researchers have attempted to evaluate the "efficacy" of psychotherapy, especially in relation to drug treatment.[2-5] Psychotherapy, even the shorter-duration variety, requires that a great deal of time be spent by very highly trained specialists, and it is therefore expensive. No one, understandably, wants to pay for something that is not of proven effectiveness, especially if there may be alternatives that are quicker and cheaper. Thus it makes sense to ask about what is known of the effectiveness of psychotherapy. To do so, however, is to enter a labyrinth of ambiguity and uncertainty, for the question makes no sense unless "effectiveness" is defined.[2-6]

Is the measure of effectiveness a reduction of symptoms? Is it a lowering of recidivism? Is it a lessening of fear or pain? Is it an improvement in the lived, experienced quality of an individual's life, an increased ability to cope in the world, or a subjective feeling of mastery, understanding, or well-being? Or is it simply preventing the patient's getting worse? Can one judge from the results of a single hospitalization, or do many patients require a series of them, as would the advanced diabetic or cardiac patient? After all, the vast majority of psychiatric patients are like the majority of medical-surgical patients in that they are chronic and incurable. They require long-term care that aims at amelioration, control, reduction of pain and/or disability, and the prolongation of useful life. With the exception of most infectious diseases (but not herpes, AIDS, or chronic pyelonephritis, to name a few) and a few medically, surgically, or orthopedically treated diseases such as peptic ulcers, appendicitides, pheochromocytoses, or some fractures, the bulk of illnesses that physicians of all specialties treat are not curable. Chronic obstructive pulmonary disease, congestive heart failure, atherosclerosis, diabetes mellitus and other metabolic diseases, most neoplasms, the arthritides, many dermatitides, almost all of the major neurological disorders, renal failure, etc., all demonstrate the truism that the practice of medicine is largely management rather than cure. Psychiatry, as a medical specialty, is no different.

Realistically, then, it makes no more sense to expect psychotherapy—or psychopharmacotherapy—to "cure" mental illness than it would to expect insulin to cure diabetes or digitalis to cure congestive heart failure. Thus the effectiveness, and therefore the role, of psychotherapy has to be understood in terms of its effect on the illness *and* on the total person who harbors or expresses that illness.

In this light, it makes sense to consider the psychotherapy of inpatients from two points of view: its role in the treatment of the *person* afflicted with mental illness, and its role in the treatment of *symptoms* of acute illness. The role of psychotherapy in the treatment of symptoms of acute illness will be described toward the end of this chapter in the sections on the psychotherapy of specific diagnostic entities. Let me begin with the treatment of the person.

THE PSYCHIATRIC PATIENT

The experience of any mental or emotional illness that is severe and disorganizing enough to require hospitalization, is a shattering one for anyone. Try to imagine your very organ of reason, your mind, or your most profound feelings so disrupted that you can no longer function effectively or no longer wish to live. Eugen Bleuler, who coined the word schizophrenia,[7] tried to capture that pain in the term. Schizophrenia does not mean, as it is popularly misconstrued, "split personality." *Schizo,* from the Greek, does indeed mean split or divided, as in the word "schism," derived from the same root. *Phrenos,* also from the Greek, is known to students of anatomy in terms of the phrenic nerve, which innervates the diaphragm; "phrenos" means diaphragm. Split diaphragm? The Greeks were thought to have placed the locus of the soul in this large sheet of muscle that divides the body. Bleuler coined the term to highlight the pain of the subjective experience of having a soul divided against itself.

The same can be said of any major psychiatric illness. One's sense of self, one's identity, one's anchor in at least an approximation of certainty and predictability, one's self-esteem, one's view of others, one's sense of security, one's confidence in the future, and one's trust in one's own powers, to name just the most obvious, are all seriously undermined. (These are all in addition to the social stigma of psychiatric hospitalization: the "loony bin," craziness, dangerousness— the entire gamut of fears and fantasies that the general populace harbors which have consequences that extend to work, family, social circle, and beyond).

Hospitalized mentally ill people, then, are in desperate need of aid, support, and help in reconstructing their lives and picking up the shattered pieces of their self-esteem. There can be no more physicianly endeavor. For this reason psychiatrists have been called "physicians of the soul."

From this vantage point, every psychiatric inpatient requires psychotherapy, at a minimum, of the supportive kind, whatever else in the way of therapy or somatic treatment the patient may require. In this approach to the patient, one is treating not the schizophrenic process, nor the depression, nor yet the character disorder, but the person, in very human terms, who has that illness or malfunction. This form of treatment, founded on empathy, understanding, and a quiet willingness to "sit with," to help bear the pain and make sense out of the experience, goes on quite independently of, and is complementary to, whatever specific therapy, of whatever kind, is indicated. To this end, experience with the natural history of these disorders, coupled with an understanding of one's own feelings and needs, learned, it is to be hoped, in any good training program, is of paramount importance.

One often must deal with a distraught family, whose members need not only realistic explanations and a prognosis, but also help with their own feelings, ranging from fear and guilt to anger and sorrow. Psychotherapy, then, may extend to the family of the patient, for it is often the family from which the patient has come into the hospital, to which the patient will return after the hospitalization, and which constitutes the patient's primary support system. To the extent that the family, as a social system of which the patient is a member, has either contributed to the patient's acute disturbance or has failed to be of effective help in preventing it, or to the extent that the patient has major distortions in his perceptions of the family's role, the family will have to be involved in some psychotherapeutic process, over and above the use of the family for the purpose of gathering data. Family therapy may involve the family members alone or in conjunction with the patient and must be tailored to each patient's and family's individual needs (see Chapter 14).

It is often difficult for students and beginning therapists to comprehend just what goes on in a psychotherapy session because, in part, unlike a surgical or medical procedure, it cannot easily be observed. Psychotherapy depends on privacy. It is always an intimate and quintessentially personal experience for both patient and therapist, and the process can be dampened or destroyed by any direct third party observation.[8] One-way mirrors and video tapes have been employed to try to capture psychotherapy sessions, and they are indeed useful, but it must be remembered that they are limited by both the therapist's and the patient's awareness of their presence, and by the nature of psychotherapy itself, which is an interpersonal *process* over time and not ideally suited for study by temporal cross-sections. Yet, there is nothing arcane or mystical about the process, although it is an art as much as it is a science, is difficult to learn, and has to be experienced to be fully understood.

PSYCHODYNAMIC CONCEPTS

Some terms and assumptions derived from psychoanalysis are helpful in explaining what goes on in psychotherapy.

The Unconscious

The unconscious refers to the memories, thoughts, ideas, feelings (affects), wishes, and fantasies that are in the mind but not readily available to awareness. The contents of the unconscious are quite present, however, and are often powerful, constituting one of the wellsprings of motivation. They quite often underlie symptoms, and may be seen, in disguised form, in dreams. The tasks of psychotherapy include modifying the contents of the unconscious (as when confrontation with reality corrects distorted unconscious memories) or allowing some of the contents of the unconscious sources of pathological behaviors or feelings to emerge gradually and in tolerable doses into consciousness. It is the reliable, continuing, empathic, unfrightened and nonjudgmental therapist, in the context of a trusting relationship, that makes such a process possible. Once made conscious, these formerly unconscious contents can be seen to be less frightening or more bearable than they were believed to be, thus lowering anxiety, and are subject to modification, thus altering their pathogenic quality.

Resistance

Resistance is the operation of forces within the patient that oppose the treatment process, and may oppose getting better itself. It is found in every psychiatric and in many medical (e.g., noncompliance) and surgical treatment situations. The motive for resistance, usually unconscious, is the avoidance of pain. Thus resistance is a species of defense against psychic pain. Many resistances strain the credulity and the patience of the unseasoned caregiver, for their operation serves to keep the patient suffering from the very symptoms and feelings that brought him to the hospital in the first place. Experience teaches, however, that there is in most of us a fear of true psychic change, which is often unconsciously resisted. If the unconscious harbors unacceptable wishes and fantasies, or unbearable feelings, then the dread of change looms even larger.

Regression

Regression is the return to earlier, developmentally less advanced modes of functioning and/or feeling. Distortions in perception, cognition, speech, or mood may occur, and behavior is always affected. The fact of hospitalization, the nature of the therapy situation, the vulnerability of the patient and his dependence on the therapist and staff for help, and the authority of the therapist all conspire to make the patient feel less powerful, less in control, more helpless, and more childlike. The regression can be either a danger or an opportunity in psychotherapy, depending on the patient, the illness, and the therapist's skill and experience. In general, in healthier, psychically resilient patients, the regression made possible by the treatment situation can be tolerated by the patient with the therapist's help, and becomes an opportunity to explore the unconscious. In less stable and more poorly defended patients, which includes most hospitalized patients, the same regression can be dangerous, undermining already compromised defenses and worsening symptoms. An experienced therapist can usually tell the difference and can often modulate the regression, at least somewhat, by properly titrating silence, the emotional availability of the therapist, and the nature of the material pursued in the hour. Structure on the ward provides an antiregressive frame within which the psychotherapy is set. Ongoing supervision by an experienced clinician can enable beginning psychotherapists to learn firsthand how to manage regression.

Transference

Transference is the application in the present of feelings, wishes, or attitudes belonging to the past. These are directed toward a person in the present, but properly should be directed toward another person, usually a parent or sibling, in the past. Transference is usually, if not always, unconscious. The unfolding and then the understanding of transference is the cornerstone of psychoanalysis, but it is less intensely usable as a therapeutic tool in psychotherapy with most short-term inpatients. However, transference remains a very important and useful diagnostic tool, and it is helpful in planning ways of approaching the psychotherapy of the patient. Like regression, transference represents both a possible danger and a possible opportunity. The danger, especially for the kinds of patients who are likely to be hospitalized, lies in the transference becoming a resistance to treatment. A transference relationship with the therapist may take center stage, pushing other meaningful work out of the way. In a so-called psychotic transference, the patient's belief in the truth of his perceptions of the therapist are of delusional proportions, not amenable to reality-testing nor modifiable by empirical means. In such a case the therapeutic relationship becomes the problem, rather than the means to a solution. It represents the latest manifestation of the patient's particular pathology. In most cases the transference is an opportunity, a here-and-now clinical representation of the patient's characteristic ways of relating and of the origins of those ways.

Countertransference

Countertransference is a species of transference. It is the transference of ideas, wishes, feelings, etc., from the therapist to the patient. Strictly speaking, it involves the same misapplication to the patient in the present of mental contents properly directed towards another person from the therapist's past. Countertransference, however, has come to be used widely as a shorthand for all of the therapist's unconscious or exaggerated feelings toward, or thought about, the patient. It should not be used as a synonym for the therapist's conscious, rational feelings, thoughts, and judgments about the patient. There is some true countertransference in every therapeutic relationship, for physicians are only human. It constitutes a problem only when it begins to interfere with the therapist's rational and objective thinking about the patient and to color his interactions, or lack of them, with the patient. The safeguard against such a happening is the acquiring of as much self-knowledge as possible on the part of the therapist, which is why psychotherapy or psychoanalysis for the therapist early in his career can be very helpful. Another safeguard is consultation with other treaters who know both the patient and the therapist. Such consultation is a built-in feature of inpatient work.

Empathy

Empathy is defined by the dictionary as "understanding so intimate that the feelings, thoughts and motives of one are readily comprehended by another." Although there are reams of paper devoted to attempts to define precisely what is meant by the term empathy, this short definition

will do quite well. Empathy is distinguished from sympathy by its profound and intimate quality, in which there is a closer and more immediate affinity between subject and object. If sympathy is, "I understand what you feel," then empathy is, "I feel what you feel, but I recognize the source of that feeling to be within you rather than within me." The capacity for empathy is partly natural, an innate talent, and is partly learned. It is crucial to doing good psychotherapy and may be what separates the ordinary, well-trained therapist from the gifted one.

INITIATING PSYCHOTHERAPY

Although most of the content of what is learned in medical school is directly applicable to the practice of psychiatry, especially with the burgeoning of biological and psychopharmacological knowledge in psychiatry, much of the form, the approach to the patient that is learned in medical school is not useful in doing psychotherapy. In fact, medically trained psychotherapists find that in the early stages of learning how to do psychotherapy they have much to unlearn before they can be free to learn new approaches. For example, the measure of a good reviewer of systems in taking a medical history is the quantity of specific, objective data that can be elicited in the shortest amount of time. The physician asks one question after another designed to elicit short, factual answers, leaving the patient as little scope as possible to wander, to follow his associations, and to talk of feelings and be subjective. Given what we have said about the unconscious and resistance, such a line of questioning yields little psychotherapeutically useful information and could not be better designed to elicit and reinforce the patient's resistance. Like Hamlet, the psychotherapist must "by indirections find directions out."[9] The patient must be given scope and room to digress (but not evasively), to follow his mental associations (but not endlessly), and to express feelings, wishes, and fears (but honestly). Such intimacies are not readily divulged by most people. They require an established relationship, an atmosphere of trust, and time.

A psychiatric history, which is a life history that includes feelings and thoughts as well as facts and events and experiences, is never gleaned at one sitting, but only over time. This is where empathy begins to be crucial. Genuine empathy is a sine qua non of initiating a psychotherapy, which begins, as does any medical treatment, with a careful and thorough history. In psychotherapy, the line between history-taking and therapy is an indistinct one. The therapy begins with the establishment of an atmosphere of empathic listening from the first moments of taking a history. A relationship is begun, signaling the start of psychotherapy. Transferences begin to be mobilized from the start and to develop throughout the relationship.

The student of psychotherapy must first abandon the quest for sharp, well-defined answers and the rapid staccato of a barrage of questions aimed at eliciting measurable or observable data. An attitude of patient, comfortable, curious listening must be cultivated and conveyed; only then can empathy flourish. Measurable data must also be gathered in psychiatry (e.g., a detailed family history of mental illness and/or response to medications or a careful cataloging of symptoms for use in psychotherapy and in the prescription of drugs), but all in good time, emerging naturally and in its place, and never at the expense of empathy.

Another unlearning that has to occur before psychotherapy can be initiated is that of the role of silence and passivity. Doctors are trained to be active, to do something, even if it is initially only to ask questions. Psychotherapy requires expectant listening, tolerating silences, even long ones, without irritation. The therapist's mind remains active, even hyperactive at times, paying simultaneous attention to the patient and the therapist's own responses. Yet, the therapist may do nothing.

Such an attitude of quiet, empathic listening is often in itself therapeutic, over and above what it elicits. Almost any painful feeling can be borne more easily if one does not have to bear it alone. The simple but profound act of sharing one's pain with another, especially an empathic other is, as almost everyone has experienced at one time or another, enormously relieving. I have seen no better description of this than in the short story entitled "Grief," by Anton Chekhov, himself a physician. In this story, Iona, driver of a horse-drawn cab, has just lost his only son. As he picks up each fare, he tries with growing desperation to tell the person or the group of people of the loss of his son. Each time he is either ignored or cursed. He cannot unburden himself, cannot share his pain. He remains alone with his terrible story. Giving up, he returns to the stables. A final attempt to tell his grief to the other cab drivers is also rebuffed.

He puts on his coat, and goes to the stables to his horse; he thinks of the corn, the hay, the weather. When he is alone, he dare not think of his son; he could speak about him to anyone, but to think of him, and picture him to himself, is unbearably painful.

"Are you tucking in?" Iona asks his horse, looking at his bright eyes; "Go on, tuck in, though we've not earned our corn, we can eat hay. Yes! I am too old to drive—my son could have, not I. He was a first-rate cab-driver. If only he had lived!"

Iona is silent for a moment, then continues: "That's how it is, my old horse. There's no more Kuzma Ionitch. He has left us to live, and he went off pop! No let's say, you had a foal, you were that foal's mother, and suddenly, let's say, that foal went off and left you to live after him. It would be sad, wouldn't it?" The little horse munches, listens, and breathes over his master's hand. . . ."

Iona's feelings are too much for him, and he tells the little horse the whole story.[10]

THERAPEUTIC INTERVENTIONS

Empathic listening is not, of course, all there is to psychotherapy. It is, however, the absolutely necessary background to what does go on. The therapist's interventions, in a psychodynamic psychotherapy, in addition to the ordinary necessary communications about time and place of meeting, can be divided into three general classes: confrontation, clarification, and interpretation.

Confrontation is making one or more

comments about what the patient has been saying that draws his attention to something he has not noticed or been aware of. A common example of a confrontation is one with disproportionate affect: Hamlet's mother says of the Queen in the play Hamlet has staged, "The lady doth protest too much, methinks."[11] A confrontation makes the fact of the patient's avoidance clear, makes the matter explicit, and lets the patient know that there is something that needs to be explored further and understood.

Clarification is the process of directing the patient's attention to that exploration. There are several types of clarifications. Examples of some of them follow.

1. Helping the patient to try to understand the sources or reasons for his avoidance (the resistance) by bringing the avoided material to light and defining it accurately. "You have been talking about other people who are ignored, deprived, and abandoned, but you do not mention that today is your birthday and no one has visited you or wished you a happy birthday. Could that be why you feel like crying?"

2. Calling the patient's attention to links between what was said earlier and what has just been said, or to connections between a current event and personal history. "Are you aware that the way you say your boyfriend treats you sounds just like your description last week of how your father treated you when you were little?"

3. Noting feeling states of which the patient is unaware or which are out of proportion to what is being talked about, e.g., rage at a minor slight or giddy elation in response to trivial praise from a person not usually important to the patient.

In this last clarification, the therapist's own feelings, the effect the patient's feelings have on him, are often the means whereby the need for the clarification is discovered. For example, the patient may be talking of enormous sadness about a relationship with say, his sister, but the therapist does not *feel* the sadness; it seems hollow, lacking in genuineness. What the therapist finds himself feeling is impatience, then anger. Scanning himself for countertransference problems and making sure that is not the reason for his anger, he might say to the patient: "I can understand your sorrow about your relationship with your sister, but it seems to me you have other strong feelings about her as well." He might further have to name the feeling. "Are you aware of anger at your sister"?

Interpretation means "to make conscious the unconscious meaning, source, history, mode or course of a given psychiatric event."[12] For example, the therapist might say, "You feel guilty for having survived the accident in which your husband died because you felt relief that you did not die, and momentarily felt, 'better he than I.'"

Needless to say, interpretation of deep unconscious material is a powerful intervention. It must only be used when the therapist is absolutely certain of the accuracy of the interpretation, and when the patient is ready to hear it, which means that the verbal material the patient is presenting shows that the patient is already aware of it just below consciousness. The therapist puts the unspoken into words. However, the therapist must also be certain that the patient can tolerate the emotional impact of the revealed thought or feeling. Correct timing is of the essence in making interpretations. It follows from the above that interpretation is a very rare intervention indeed in a short-term inpatient hospitalization. Most patients are too disturbed to withstand such an onslaught, however gently broached. Moreover, interpretations often promote regression which, for patients who are already too regressed, is counterproductive unless there is an unlimited amount of time to work through the further regression. There are inpatients for whom interpretation is both necessary and effective, especially among the nonpsychotic depressive syndromes, but it must be used cautiously and sparingly, and always under supervision.

In addition, of course, are all the questions a therapist asks that are designed to elicit more material, to help the patient remember and reflect. That is why most questions in psychotherapy are open-ended ones, as distinguished from the specificity of usual medical questions. "Tell me more about that." "What else comes to mind when you think of that?" "Has it always been or felt that way?" "What did or do you feel?" The therapist's first task is to aid the patient's memory and to overcome resistances. Only then does he make connections or try to make the unconscious conscious, and that only with certain well-defined types of patients and never with certain others. (These differences will be discussed in greater detail below, under the headings of the specific diagnoses.) The therapist must avoid thrusting his own associations upon the patient or pushing too early for a closure of the patient's associations by prematurely zeroing in on one aspect of the patient's speech. One such open-ended and effective type of question (the one often parodied in films and on television) repeats a key word in the patient's last sentence:

Patient: "My father is the only other person I ever felt as much hatred toward as I do my boss."

Therapist: "Your father."

The repetition urges the patient to associate while allowing him the freedom to go where he will with it. The use of the patient's own word limits coloration by the therapist. However, the therapist has made a choice, for the simple repetition of a word has not been either random or without purpose. By choosing to repeat "father," he directs the patient's associations, at least initially, to particular historical material, memories, and comparisons. The therapist could have repeated "hatred" (focusing on the affect) or "ever" (focusing on history), or called attention to the extreme nature of the feelings, etc.

THE THERAPIST

The only truth you have is your patient, and the only thing that interferes with that truth is your own perception. You may not be free to observe what there is to be observed, chiefly because it evokes feelings in you that are so troublesome that you quit looking. . . .[13] Perhaps the most difficult, vexing, but crucial core of what must be mastered to perform effective psychotherapy is the management of countertransference. Much of the task of the beginner is to learn to sit, to listen, to be empathic, to bear painful affects and to overcome one's own resistance to them, to learn to be patient and, finally, to learn to use the help of supervision by honestly disclosing one's feelings, one's ignorances, one's bewilderment.

One particular aspect of countertransference to which special attention must be paid by the beginning therapist is that of the rescue fantasy. Doctors are trained to heal, to rescue patients from illness and disease and pain. Yet, nothing could be more inimical to a successful psychotherapy outcome than the therapist's rushing to the patient with a therapeutic zeal meant to satisfy the therapist's inner need to gain quick results in order to feel professionally adequate. Patients' resistances have a field day with such a naive, if understandable, attitude, leaving the bewildered therapist wondering why so genuine a wish to help meets with so little positive response. That is not to say the therapist should appear jaded or blase— far from it—but that he must be patient, respectful, and responsive to the patient's needs, not his own. The therapist cannot rescue the patient; only the patient can do that. The therapist can help the patient to know, contain, and bear his feelings; to know better his thoughts and fantasies; and to learn about his unconscious motivations. Only then can the patient decide whether or not he wants to be rescued and, if so, he can then enlist the therapist's aid in doing it himself.

Similarly, love alone is not enough for these patients. An approach consisting of mostly genuine positive feelings and wishes, will not, by itself, produce much progress, and a therapist using such an approach will often be taken merciless advantage of by many resistant patients. The patient requires treatment, which means emotional containment followed by self-awareness and self-understanding in a supportive context. Treatment is neither pity, sympathy, nor rescue, nor, equally, blame or anger.

Even with a proper therapeutic attitude, true empathy, and what might be called passionate detachment, the therapist may still be pushed away. An accomplished social worker who worked many years with psychiatric inpatients put it this way: "It may be threatening to the patient to have someone interested in him. The patient may push hard to send clinicians running. Don't be fooled—if most people grew up in the families and/or with the genes of these patients, it would be wise for them too to be so guarded about letting someone come close. The patient is trying to survive."[14]

Like the patient, the therapist too must have support in bearing painful affects. The work of psychotherapy may be endlessly interesting and excitingly challenging, but it is surely ineffably lonely. This is all the more so on an inpatient service, where the affects to be borne are primitive, often frightening, and usually bizarre. Moreover, they are right out in the open. A central paradox of the inpatient setting is that while the patients' feelings are all but unknown to them, those feelings assail people around them, particularly when one opens oneself by turning a receptive, nondefensive, empathic self to the patient.

Staff supportive interaction, therefore, must be constant. Inpatients mobilize every resource to aid their resistances, including the exploitation of staff splits and differences of opinion. When these momentarily do not exist, patients will often try to create them. Obviously, coordination of treatment by all members of the staff is of paramount importance. That is one reason why there are so many clinical meetings on psychiatry units. Another is for mutual staff support. Community meetings, staff meetings, team meetings, rounds, staff feelings groups or "didactic" group seminars, impromptu hallway meetings, and seemingly endless supervision all provide places for members of the team to draw from the well of support of one's colleagues.

REQUIREMENTS FOR THE SHORT-TERM

Inpatient Psychotherapy

Though the psychotherapy of inpatients follows general psychotherapy guidelines, it must be modified to fit the usually severe illnesses and particular conditions of hospitalized patients. Short-term intensive psychotherapy as it is commonly practiced on most inpatient units, especially in general hospitals, owes much to the model established by long-term psychotherapy of hospitalized patients (vide infra). The general approach is similar, except that it is meant to be antiregressive rather than regression-promoting, and the goals are more modest. The task of learning to perform the psychotherapy is quite the same.

To begin with, inpatient units are always staffed by a treatment team consisting of some combination of doctors, nurses, social workers, psychologists, occupational therapists, mental health workers (attendants), and sometimes others. The kind of sacrosanct privacy and confidentiality that obtains in outpatient psychotherapy is neither possible nor advisable on an inpatient unit. The patient should be told at the outset that psychotherapy is one of several interwoven hospital treatments and that the entire treatment team will be privy to what develops is the treatment hour. Confidentiality is expanded to include the entire team or staff, but is not compromised one whit beyond that. The psychotherapy hour is still conducted in a private, one-to-one setting. The information gleaned is then shared with the treatment team in order to coordinate all treatment and to allow each member of the staff to be maximally effective in helping the patient to improve or grow. Novice therapists often allow themselves to be put in an untenable position by promising the patient, at the patient's request, exclusive confidentiality, only to be then told of the patient's advanced suicide plans, or plans to run away, or something else that must be shared with the rest of the team.

The milieu aids the psychotherapy as well. Information gleaned by the staff in its all-day observation and interaction with the patient is shared with the therapist. This information can be of inestimable value in making accurate confrontations and clarifications. Psychotherapy in an inpatient setting must always focus on and make use of the patient's behavior, interactions, and relationships on the unit. Material avoided in the intensity of the psychotherapy may emerge more readily in the more casual setting of an occupational therapy group, in a treatment group where the transference to the group therapist is different, or in conversation with a nurse or mental health worker.

The patient's activities on the unit offer reliable feedback to the psychotherapy, giving the therapist a more objective assessment of the patient's progress or lack of it. If a patient fails to make use in the milieu of insights gained in psychotherapy, he is unlikely to be able to make use of them outside the hospital after discharge.

The shortened duration of inpatient treatment dictates that the psychotherapy be not only intensive (three to six meetings per week, depending on the clinical situation) but also more active than in the classical model described below. Supported by the symptom-relieving medications, psychotherapy need not wait for the gradual unfolding of the natural history of the disease process. After gathering the basic history, the therapist should seek to identify the *acute* precipitants of the current illness or decompensation, rather than to focus primarily on past history. All that is learned about the patient's past should, however, be carefully noted and passed on to the long-term outpatient therapist. The therapist should be active in seeking out the underlying conflicts, in searching vigorously through pertinent details of personal and family history, and in pursuing gentle but persistent confrontations and clarifications. Of course, all of this activity must be titrated against the patient's clinical state and vulnerability. The ability to do this comes with time and experience and through careful supervision. As always, however, true interpretation, an ever-powerful tool, must be used sparingly, if at all, and never by one without a great deal of experience in this field. Finally, the therapist should not attempt to remain neutral in relation to the illness: he is an adversary of the disease process and an ally of the patient's restorative, healthier side.[15] This can be made known to the patient in several ways, including support and encouragement for the patient's appropriate behaviors and thoughts, and honest labeling as incorrect or unrealistic those behaviors and thoughts that are inappropriate. Self-revelations on the part of the therapist,

however, are unnecessary and often counterproductive, as they may serve to frighten patients with too much closeness too soon, may be misinterpreted as seductive, or may further blur ego boundaries in patients whose boundaries are already less than clear, thus promoting further regression.

Since both attachments and non-traumatic separation are goals of hospitalization, discharge and follow-up planning should be undertaken, with the understanding and collaboration of the patient, from the very beginning of treatment. If the psychotherapist is not going to be able to continue the therapy after the patient leaves the hospital, this should be made clear at the outset so that the patient does not suddenly find realistic expectations dashed and does not feel rejected. The outpatient therapist should be advised to begin to see the patient before discharge from the hospital in order to facilitate a smooth transition and to take advantage of the knowledge of the staff. The patient may begin to see the outpatient therapist on the unit and then begin to visit him in his office.

For most patients, hospitalization represents, rightly or wrongly, basic disappointments with the primary caregivers in their lives, be they spouse, parents, children, or friends. In the case of patients already in psychotherapy, it always represents some disappointment with the therapist. These disappointments must be broached, explored, reality-tested, and worked through to some resolution. Outside (the service or unit) therapists should be kept advised of this work and involved in it to the extent they can or want to be.

There are patients who do not want to be treated, whose resistance, for whatever mix of conscious and unconscious reasons, will not yield to even the most persistent empathic and interpretative efforts. The wishes of these patients, if they are neither suicidal nor homicidal, nor so disorganized that they cannot care for themselves or be cared for in the community without the likelihood of serious harm befalling them, must be respected, for psychotherapy is a collaborative venture and cannot be forced on anyone. Some of these patients may do well on their own. If not, they will sooner or later seek help, or call attention to themselves so that help is again offered. It may take several professional contacts before these patients realize they do need help.

INPATIENT PSYCHOTHERAPY

The Schizophrenic Patient

In most hospital settings nowadays, especially where Professional Standards Review Organizations (PSRO), Utilization Review Committees, and third-party payers are involved, hospital stays are meant to be relatively brief. When the patient or family is directly paying the expense of a hospital stay, a very costly proposition indeed exists, also militating for as short a hospitalization as possible. Not too many years ago, when the states underwrote most mental hospital care, it was not uncommon to find an average length of stay for a schizophrenic breakdown of a year or more. With that kind of time, a whole experience, and a literature to go with it, developed, based upon the treatment of schizophrenia by psychotherapy alone. After the advent of antipsychotic medication, psychotherapy continued to flourish, either alone or in conjunction with medication.

The rationale for such treatment was the conviction that there were fundamental defects in development and personality (ego defects) that underlay the schizophrenic breakdown. These defects were seen as amenable to change in the context of a long enough, consistent enough, and empathic enough relationship with a therapist who could tolerate the chaos and nerve-wracking affective shifts such a therapy entailed. Such painstaking, patient, thorough, and time-consuming psychotherapy was no less than heroic. In the hands of skilled practitioners it was often very effective. Perhaps the most famous description of such an in-depth treatment was Hannah Green's *I Never Promised You a Rose Garden,*[16] a book and movie which portrayed a fictionalized account of a case conducted by psychiatrist and psychoanalyst Frieda Fromm-Reichmann at the Chestnut Lodge Sanitarium in Rockville, Maryland.

Such therapists as Fromm-Reichmann worked with the conviction that the roots of schizophrenia lay within deeply buried psychic conflicts at a very early or developmentally "primitive" level. Their conviction was derived from their patients' behavior, affects, and cognitions, as well as their histories, and thus was a theoretical viewpoint based on clinical observation and deduction. The idea that psychic conflict is central to schizophrenia remains a bias, as does any other theoretical approach to schizophrenia, since very little is conclusively proven about it.

This kind of therapy of schizophrenia, by relational means alone, began before the advent of antipsychotic medication. However, even after antipsychotic medication became available, because these therapists felt that the efficacy of neuroleptics, when they worked, was transient, and because there was the necessity, often, for lifelong maintenance drug therapy, they continued to aim at bringing about fundamental changes in the patient's character.

These therapists attempted to lessen lifelong fears, to undercut maladaptive defenses, and then, under the aegis of a healing relationship, to help the patient retravel, or in some cases, to travel for the first time, the road of childhood psychic development. Their intent was to build within the patient a more normal ego, free of the crippling defects from which he had suffered so long. When successful, such a psychotherapy could free the patient once and for all from his malady and eliminate the need for ongoing medication. With the knowledge we have now of the deleterious long-term effects of many of our key drugs (such as tardive dyskinesia with the neuroleptics and possible interstitial fibrosis of the kidney with lithium), such an outcome would continue to be much desired. Moreover, the more we learn about the origins of the psychoses, such as schizophrenia and manic-depressive illness, the more plausible, if less single-minded, the underlying assumptions of psychodynamic psychiatry seem to be. For example, it is fairly well established through the study of monozygotic twins and adoptions that there is a definite genetic underpinning to the major psychoses—at least to the more chronic ones. It is equally clear, however, that the concordance between monozygotic twins is far less than 100%, which has led some interpreters of the research data to conclude that the genes provide only a diathesis. It is life experience that determines whether, how, and to what extent genetic diathesis will express itself. It is to that life experience that the long-term psychotherapy of schizophrenia was directed.

Nowadays, such heroic therapies can rarely be undertaken and, from a social and economic viewpoint, even more rarely justified, except perhaps for a privileged few. (This kind of therapy is still practiced in several, mostly private, hospitals.) The more common hospital pattern is for a combination of neuroleptic drug treatment and psychotherapy conducted intensively for anywhere from 2 to 8 weeks. Fortunately, the neuroleptics, despite their dangers and drawbacks, are powerfully and reliably effective, in a reasonably short time, for all but the most chronic of schizophrenics. (Even for these chronic patients, new drug strategies, such as the addition of propanolol to the usual neuroleptics, are providing dramatic results in some cases. It is also to be hoped, even expected, that further research will yield either new antipsychotics without the long-term side effects, or successful treatment for those effects.) The medication usually mitigates the disorganization and fragmentation seen in such acute symptoms as severe withdrawal, hallucinations, and delusions.

In the short-term inpatient treatment of the schizophrenic patient, the psychotherapy goals have to be far more modest, and in crucial ways the very opposite of those described above for the long-term inpatient treatment of those same patients. Regression is to be avoided, as it will prolong the hospitalization and lead to a disruption of the patient's links, however tenuous, to the community to which he will return. Unless long-term treatment can be continued for the time, often years, necessary to bring about permanent change, the worst thing one can do is to embark on such a course with half measures. The mainstays of short-term therapy must be to provide structure in the patient's life, support, clarity, accountability for behavior, and constant help in reality testing, including the reality of the patient's current and possibly long-term limitations of functioning. The patient can be helped to identify and set worthwhile and realistic goals. The family can be helped to understand the patient's limitations and to modify their own unrealistic expectations of him, thus avoiding their disappointment in and anger at him. A realistic modification of the family's expectations can also protect the patient from constant frustration and lowering of self-esteem. Therefore, the focus in a short-term psychotherapy cannot be on the transference, which will invite further regression. The focus should be on the patient's real, present life, and on his coping skills or lack of them. Defenses, even those that in healthier patients would be seen as pathological and explored with a view toward helping the patient replace them with more adaptive ones, should be supported if they help the patient cope or prevent psychotic distortion of reality.

Nevertheless, although medication, structure, and support may lessen the immediate panic, the intolerable affects (such as overwhelming fear, sadness, and a very damaged self-esteem) are still there, as are a sense of loss of control, helplessness, and the severe ego defects that make it difficult for the patient to bear any strong affect. How then, does the therapist approach such a patient in the psychotherapy hour? What does one actually *do* when sitting with a person who is fragmented, frightened, and may be delusional or hallucinating, even if one has the above modest goals well in mind? The therapist attempts to establish a mutual and structured attachment between himself and the patient. From that attachment an integration of the fragmented aspects of the self, the formation of some kind of real relationship with the therapist, and finally separation from the therapist can occur. A fine description of the aims and the process of doing psychotherapy with a schizophrenic patient is offered by Daniel Schwartz, M.D. He is here referring to the more long-term kind of work with schizophrenics, but the principles he outlines in the following paragraph are the same for short-term therapy.

The therapist does things in the early times of therapy. He spends time in the presence of the patient, he tries to appreciate the nature of the patient's dilemma and the patient's activity in relation to that dilemma. He attempts to lend himself to the activity (however dimly perceived) of the patient in dealing with this dilemma. He does this within the limits of his continued survival in the presence of the patient. To these ends he acts and talks in such a way as to favor continuity of himself and continuity of his relatedness to the patient in the face of the patient's attempt to deal with chaotic disorganization of thought, of impulse and of affect. To these ends he provides himself as a rather regular, not easily disorganized human object in the face of the patient's panicky certainty that all human objects (inner and outer) are subject to his destructive rageful activity. He notices and moves toward honest naming of what the patient communicates in words or actions about the patient's state, feeling, observations, and effort—and he does that within his sense of respect for the distance required for safety, and the essentially inviolable privacy of a separate human being. He appreciates the vulnerability of the sense of self to degradation and panic which make withdrawal and disorganization genuine and dangerous. He openly acknowledges the patient's accurate observations about himself or his surroundings, veiled or direct, painful or flattering. And he does this as real in the face of the patient's conviction of the unintegratable nature of accurate perceptions. He notices differences between them. The patient's body and its functions—presenting its refusal to be ignored through anorexia, fecal smearing, sexual gesture, or chill fear—is allowed space and words in the therapy . . . What the patient gets from all of this seems clear: his inundated ego functions find a human being willing to modulate, establish constancy, provide stimulus barriers, apply controls to action in life-threatening situations, focus and name accurately, sequence and remember, distinguish a self from a nonself, a living from a dead, an inside from an outside. That person nevertheless respects the capacity and value of the patient for whom he is providing these partial functions.[17]

The therapist provides the consistent, caring, human environment within which

healing can take place, whether that healing is aided most by medication, by structure provided by the milieu, by psychotherapy itself, or by all three.

THE BORDERLINE PATIENT

The psychotherapy of the hospitalized borderline patient presents a challenge that is in some ways similar to that presented by the schizophrenic patient, and in other ways, very different. The similarities lie in the necessity to consider all aspects of the treatment on the unit in a coordinated fashion, and to understand the nature of the patient's ego defects and limitations. The major differences lie in the degree to which one can hold the patient accountable for his behavior, and in the management of the countertransference—the therapist's own emotional responses to the patient. A small library of volumes on understanding or treating the borderline has been published, partly because the breadth and depth of pathology they evidence makes them a kind of laboratory of pathology, but probably more because they typically arouse such powerful feelings in their treaters that almost everyone who treats them finds himself in need of support, understanding, and help. They invariably have a major impact on psychiatric inpatient units, ranging from nettlesome to disastrous, depending perhaps on the sophistication and awareness of the staff of the unit. (This effect is nowhere better described than in T.M. Main's paper, The Ailment.[18]) Rational short-term treatment of the borderline must be predicated on at least a phenomenological understanding of the pathology of the disorder. (A more complex psychodynamic understanding is required for long-term treatment; see references at the end of this chapter.)

Borderline pathology is character pathology, (which is why it is listed on Axis II of DSM-III), meaning that it is a disorder in the patient's longstanding, habitual patterns of behavior, of thinking, and of feeling. These disordered modes of being are most clearly and importantly seen in the patient's relations with others, and it is in those relationships that the patient characteristically gets into trouble. Although there are many vantage points from which to view the borderline's pathology, I find that the most comprehensive one is that of object hunger as the basic organizing pathology.

Most current thinking about the origin of the borderline's pathology starts with the idea of a developmental arrest somewhere in the second year of life, which means that the ego strengths, the capacities, the coping skills that we all learn at that time are partially or completely lacking in the borderline, or are severely compromised. These ego defects, or missing capacities, are what the borderline patient takes into all subsequent developmental phases, and into adult life. For whatever reason, and many possible reasons have been advanced, such as a constitutional overendowment of aggressive drive that alienates parents and others, inconsistent parenting, neglect and deprivation, or overindulgent parenting, the borderline grows up with an abiding and desperate hunger for love, attention, and reassurance. Moreover, this need is experienced as peremptory, imperative, and essential for psychic survival. The love must be unconditional, the attention constant, and the reassurance unending. This desperate hunger for others in such a way is, of course, unattainable and doomed to failure again and again, which has understandable and predictable consequences for the borderline's behavior.

In the first place, borderlines have to learn very early to control others in order to try to get what they feel they must have from them. Thus they learn, out of survival need, to be exquisitely sensitive to other people's moods, needs, and vulnerabilities. This sensitivity, however, is entirely in the service of the borderline's own needs, and does not in any way take into account the separate, legitimate needs of the other. In common with the other major disorders of character, the borderline lacks true empathic capacity. He uses his sensitivity to try to control others, to manipulate others. Most people do not take kindly to being so controlled and manipulated, which leads the borderline into an endless series of stormy relationships, most of them short-lived. As a consequence, the borderline is left feeling ever

alone. The unsatisfying nature of his relationships, when he has them, only adds to that terrible sense of aloneness.

The desperation with which the borderline seeks to fill his unfillable need makes him exceedingly dependent, with each successive person representing the "last hope" for satisfaction and surcease from longing. It follows that the borderline will be sensitive in the extreme to rejection, either real or fancied. The patient's behavior will, of course, bring about repeated rejection, but even the remotest hint of a slight, or another's merely not anticipating what he wants, will be experienced by the borderline as a rejection. Moreover, the borderline's woes are augmented by what John Murray[19] has termed "narcissistic entitlement," a conviction or feeling that, by virtue of one's past deprivation or suffering, one is absolutely entitled to have whatever one wants or needs. ("I want what I want when I want it!"). The borderline's response to rejection or to a frustration of his narcissistic entitlement is, typically, rage.

The rage of the borderline can be likened to the tantrum of a 2½-year-old: total, disorganizing, and often self-destructive. It is usually filled with hate and destructive impulses, fantasies, and wishes. Because of his abject dependence on the relationship of the moment, rage puts the borderline in a quandary: How can he destroy the person on whom he is dependent for emotional survival? The borderline's solution is to be passive-aggressive, that is, to do aggressive things to himself as a means of "getting to" the other, much as Gandhi got to the British by laying his own life on the line. When carried to the extreme, such behavior gets to be suicidal, although most often the emotional vector of the acts is more homicidal than suicidal. This is the most common meaning of the self-destructive "acting-out" of the borderline, but the picture is enormously complicated by the fact that the aloneness, vulnerability to rejection, fears of imminent abandonment, and concomitant low self-esteem all combine to give the borderline patient a genuine depressive diathesis. For all of the borderline's pseudodepressive symptomatology that is designed to control and manipulate others, he is at the same time susceptible to recurrent bouts of acute depression. Distinguishing between the two is an ongoing major task of the therapist.

Borderlines develop other pathological coping strategies in order to survive. The ambivalence toward people close to them outlined above—murderous rage coupled with abject dependence—is less acutely handled by separating the two feelings absolutely, so that only one of them is felt or allowed into awareness at a time. This way of dealing with ambivalence is called splitting, a term emphasized by Melanie Klein.[20] Splitting becomes a way of life for the borderline, so that people are experienced as either all good or all bad, and the conditions of life come to be experienced in either/or, black-and-white terms. People are idealized, only to be denigrated and devalued at the first whiff of disappointment. (Thomas Sydenham said of these people, in 1682, "All is caprice, they love without measure those whom they will soon hate without reason."[21]

Developmental arrest at such an early point in life leaves the borderline with other ego defects, such as a blurring of ego boundaries, i.e., an uncertainty as to where the self leaves off and the other begins. This, in turn, leads the borderline patient into attributing his own thoughts and feelings to the other, or into taking the other's for his own, and to externalizing responsibility for his actions. When coupled with primitive idealization, it also leads to magical expectations of others.[22] The second year of life is the time children begin to learn to delay gratification, to bear frustration, and to tolerate the anxiety and depression that go with both. It is also the time of learning to control impulses. Whatever the disordered parenting that takes place at that time for the borderline, whether as a response to the child's excessive aggression or as a result of primary flaws in the parents, the future borderline never learns those essential survival skills. These are capacities that are missing in the adult borderline, who thus frequently has an impulse disorder and who reacts with rage to demands to delay gratification or bear frustration.

It should be understood that all borderline patients are not the same, despite sharing several elements of the same pathology. In fact, perhaps depending on how far along the path of ego development the child traveled before he got "stuck," the borderline pathology is a spectrum, with a less ego-developed end, called "primitive," and a more ego-developed end, called "healthier." Patients at the more primitive end of the spectrum are prone to lapses into psychosis under stress. These psychoses may be, acutely, clinically indistinguishable from schizophrenia (in DSM-III terminology, Schizophreniform), but they are unique in other ways. They tend to have a sudden onset and to be short-lived, even if untreated. Nevertheless, they respond very well to neuroleptic medication, which shortens their duration. Furthermore, the level of recovery from psychosis in borderline patients is complete, without residual impairment or sequelae.

One particular kind of psychotic reaction requires special mention, and special warning, viz., psychotic transference. Given the object hunger around which the borderline's life is organized, it is not surprising that the one-to-one psychotherapy relationship will present special problems for the borderline patient, whose characteristic defenses will soon make it a problem shared by the therapist. Whatever the intent of the therapist, and sometimes whatever the therapist says or does, the mere fact of regular, frequent meetings with the patient represents an invitation to the patient to regress. This invitation to regress will be increased to the extent that the therapist becomes overinvolved, loses control of his own responses, or otherwise ignores the warnings to be outlined below. When that happens, the patient will lose the ability to reality test his beliefs about, and his magical expectations of, the therapist. The patient's demands will escalate beyond all bounds and brook no denial of them. At that point, suicidal manipulative behavior and genuine attempts at suicide are likely to occur.

I have found one other observation helpful in trying to understand the borderline, but it is a complex one. Borderlines do not trust the power of words to convey feelings. This is not an alexithymia,[23] in which the patient does not have words for feelings, but a more subtle lack. The second year of life, the age of the hypothesized developmental difficulty or arrest for the borderline, is also the age when language skills are acquired. During that time not only words are learned, but also the value and the use of words are learned. Language is always acquired in an interpersonal context—we learn language from others, primarily parents and siblings, and we use it first to communicate *to* others. Major disturbances in the parent-child field will affect the acquisition of those parts of language skill most dependent on the relationship itself, and on the empathic capacity of the parent. Thus the borderline has all the necessary words for feelings, indeed, often a surfeit of them. What is missing, however, is the sense of trust and confidence in the ability of words to accurately convey one's feelings to another. It is easy to see how this lack contributes centrally to the borderline's sense of isolation and aloneness. Lacking in empathic capacity himself, unable to understand the empathy of others, yet hungering desperately for understanding and involvement with others, the borderline feels condemned to imprisonment in an affectively mute world. Everyone has experienced the relief that talking to someone one trusts can bring when one is troubled, even if such sharing of feeling changes nothing. Any painful feeling state is easier to bear if one does not have to bear it alone. The borderline is convinced that, as far as words are concerned, he has to bear all of his unbearable feelings alone.

However, there is another way to communicate feeling. Bereft of effective words, the borderline can use action. I believe that this mechanism underlies at least some of the "acting out" that is frequently taken for manipulation. It *is* manipulation, not in the service of sadism or hatred, but of communication on the most primitive and essential level. Moreover, borderlines usually take this one step further. The only way they can be sure that their feeling has in fact been understood, since they equally do not trust the therapist's words that he understands how they feel, is to see their own feeling in the therapist. (This process superficially resembles projective identification but is quite different. In projective identification, the patient unconsciously misperceives, in a projective manner, the reality of the other, usually the therapist, who then may or may not "identify" with that misperception. In the process I am describing, the patient is unconsciously trying to communicate affect to the therapist in the only effective way he knows. The patient is not misperceiving the therapist; he is trying to make something happen between them.) Thus, some of the strong feeling that borderlines arouse in the therapist is the result of the borderline's need to communicate, or share, his affect with the therapist. Sometimes this fact can be useful to the therapist, for the feelings he notices arising unbidden in himself, feelings like anger, sadness, helplessness, or sexual arousal, are mirror images of what the patient is feeling at that moment, even if the patient is talking about something else or is unaware of such a feeling. In any case, many borderlines are masters of the ability to make others feel what they feel, and will not rest until they succeed. That also makes them hard to live with.

The role of psychotherapy on an acute inpatient unit, then, has to be based on an understanding of the borderline's needs and limitations. By needs I mean here what the borderline requires in order to grow and to be able to build into his ego the capacities that are lacking, rather than what the borderline experiences as his peremptory needs. Furthermore, given the characterologic, chronic nature of the borderline's pathology, the therapist must realize from the outset that major change is not possible in a short hospitalization, and goals have to be quite modest. In essence, the patient enters the inpatient unit in some kind of crisis, and the immediate task of hospitalization is to contain the crisis, prevent further regression, and return the patient to his usual level of functioning. Perhaps the most common crisis that catapults the borderline patient into the hospital is some sort of rupture of the always tenuous alliance between the patient and his long-term therapist.[24] A necessary feature of any hospitalization of a borderline is a consultation to the outside therapist by the inpatient therapist, with a view toward identifying the nature and source of the impasse between them so that the long-term relationship can resume. Such a consultation has to be conducted with tact, a clear understanding of the borderline's pathology, and a sympathetic knowledge of the powerful ways in which borderlines arouse conscious and unconscious feelings in their therapists.

In a long-term therapy, the borderline will, of course, bring all of his pathological ways of relating into the relationship with the therapist, and will zero in, often with uncanny precision, on bothersome elements of the therapist's own personality. They will also attribute their own often aggressive, occasionally sexual thoughts and feelings to the therapist (projection), while simultaneously using those projections to justify their own aggressive wishes (projective identification). The therapist, in turn, may be unconsciously persuaded that the patient's feelings are his own, and behave accordingly, thereby confirming for the patient his own projections. For example, the patient feels, "I hate you and wish you were dead!" That is untenable because of the patient's total emotional dependence on the therapist, so the patient gets rid of the feeling by attributing it to the therapist. Now it is, "you hate me!" The patient behaves toward the therapist as if the therapist hated him, and before long the unaware therapist starts to feel hatred for the patient, and to express it in subtle ways. The patient picks that up immediately and says, "You see, you do hate me! I knew it, and I am justified in hating you."

If working on these kinds of mechanisms and the origins of the need for them is the central work of long-term therapy, it is *not* the work of a short-term inpatient stay. The patient will bring all of these pathological ways of relating immediately into his relationships with all of the staff and with the inpatient therapist, but the task of the inpatient therapist is to contain affects rather than to explore them and to prevent further regression by stringent limit-setting. This is not the time to "mobilize" the patient's rage. There will be plenty of rage anyway, and encouraging the patient to feel and express his omnipresent rage will only promote regression and needlessly prolong the hospital stay.

More than with any other kind of patient, the inpatient psychotherapy of the borderline cannot be conducted in a vacuum, but must be fully coordinated with all other aspects of treatment and all other kinds of treaters on the unit. The whole staff must know what is being worked on in the psychotherapy, and the therapist must know what the patient is saying and how he is relating to everyone else on the unit. Only in this way will destructive splits be prevented, and frequent meetings of all the primary treaters are essential.

Within the individual therapy hour, the therapist should focus on the patient's behavior on the ward, with current important people in the patient's immediate life, and on the patient's relationship with his long-term therapist. The therapist must be utterly consistent and clear in his role in setting the rules by which the patient must live on the unit. The therapist must also be clear in supporting the limits set by the nursing staff and others on the ward. The therapist can try to help the patient see how his defenses, his ways of relating, are maladaptive for him, and do not succeed in getting him what he wants, but rather, interfere with or prevent his getting what he wants. He can be helped to see how he drives people away rather than engages them. He can be helped to try to make do with what he can get, and to bear the frustration of not having the unhaveable. With a combination of limits and empathy, the therapist can attempt to demonstrate to the patient that he can tolerate what he has been convinced is intolerable, and that he can learn to bear frustrations. The patient can be helped to see the difference between internally experienced needs and realistic external possibilities of gratification. He can be shown the nature of his projections and his projective mechanisms, and how they work against him. To accomplish this the therapist must be utterly honest. (This should not be confused with openness. The therapist should rarely be revealing of personal details of his own life, for this will be an invitation to a psychotic transference for the patient.) The therapist also should not be afraid to set and enforce realistic, nonpunitive, but firm limits. Promises should not be made that cannot be kept, nor should threats of sanctions (discharge, transfer, a loss of ward privileges) be made unless they can be stringently, immediately, and consistently carried out. Finally, responsibility for the patient's behavior must rest with the patient, and only with the patient.

The therapist can use the opportunity of hospitalization to begin to acquaint the borderline patient with his impairment in the use of words. He can be helped to see that he really does not trust the power of words to convey his feelings to another, and that that contributes to his sense of aloneness and isolation. He can be encouraged to begin to try to use words rather than action to bring relief from painful affects. Of course, the therapist should not expect to resolve this problem in one hospitalization, but a beginning can be made and can be carried on by the outside therapist. Finally, the patient can be acquainted with the notion that what he feels to be an issue of survival often is not, and can be dealt with more effectively and more gratifyingly in less desperate ways.

The issue of medications in the treatment of the borderline patient is a particularly thorny one and has to be considered as part and parcel of the psychotherapy, unlike in the treatment of the schizophrenic, in which psychopharmacologic intervention targeted at the psychotic symptoms can be undertaken relatively independently of the psychotherapy. Borderlines, like any other people, may have target symptoms of anxiety or depression for which drug therapy is indicated. However, one must always bear in mind that those symptoms are ensconced in a pathological character structure. Drugs treat symptoms, not character, at least at this point in time. Thus the benefits of medication in the relief of target symptoms must always be weighed against the possible harm they may cause the patient because of the psychotherapeutic context in which they are given. The most obvious example of this is in the potentially suicidal acting-out of the patient. Often that acting-out is in re-

sponse to frustrations necessarily engendered by the psychotherapeutic relationship itself, and in an attempt to manipulate or "emotionally blackmail" the therapist into one course of action or another. When that very therapist—the current focus of all the patient's pathological ways of relating—is the one to prescribe the medication, or when it is a backup physician to whom the patient has been referred by the therapist, the patient frequently finds it irresistible to act out with the medication itself, often endangering his life, and always vastly complicating the therapy.

The prescription of medication always has meanings for any patient and is always to some degree a function of transference and of the relationship with the doctor (which is why drug studies have to be double blind). With the borderline patient those meanings are far more weighty, and more fraught with peril. Borderlines are always looking for magical relief for their emotional pain and are almost always endowing their therapists with magical and omnipotent powers. The last thing most borderlines want to do is to have to take responsibility for their own growth; they would much rather foist that responsibility off onto the therapist. By prescribing medication for the borderline, even for "legitimate" symptoms, and with the best and clearest intentions in the world, the therapist lays himself and the therapeutic relationship open to almost inevitable distortion by the patient. The borderline patient will invariably misinterpret the prescription as an offer of magical cure and will see the therapist as assuming responsibility for the patient's work, growth, and improvement. The issue is *not* what the therapist intends, but what the borderline experiences. Thus the psychotherapeutic and milieu work will be undermined, and regression promoted.

This is not to say that there is never good reason to treat borderlines pharmacologically, but only to be absolutely sure that the reasons are of paramount importance, and that one has carefully weighed the likely benefits of medication against the almost certain psychotherapeutic, management, and safety costs. For example, borderlines do become depressed, and their depressions may be drug responsive. Moreover, if some of the depressive symptoms are relieved, the patient may do better and may even become, at least for a while, less likely to attempt suicide or to engage in self-destructive acts. However, in the long run, the improvement often does not hold and may well dissolve in the next interpersonal crisis. In weighing the use of drugs on the scale of character risks, one often finds that the latter negates the expected benefits to be gained from the former. One therefore often finds oneself in the anomalous position of considering the use of medication that is as likely to hurt as it is to help, *even if it works*. There are times that one will take the risk of trying medication, but only where the expected benefits are clear and overwhelmingly important. In any case, the therapist should disabuse himself of the notion that borderline pathology is simply an affect disorder, or a variant of an affect disorder. It is not, although it may well co-exist with one, be exacerbated by one, or be the cause of one. The same can be said of anxiolytic medication, and it too should be used sparingly if at all, and with the same *caveats*.

There is one clear exception to this pharmacologic humility, that of frank psychosis. Borderlines at the more disturbed end of the spectrum occasionally slip over into psychosis (I am not speaking here of psychotic transference, but of a schizophreniform illness replete with Schneiderian First Rank symptoms). These psychoses must be responded to in the same way as an acute psychosis in any patient: immediate hospitalization with vigorous neuroleptic treatment. However, with the borderline, once the psychotic symptoms have responded adequately to the medication, it can be fairly rapidly tapered off. Long-term maintenance antipsychotic medication is rarely necessary and is often contraindicated.

The definitive treatment of the borderline is of necessity a long-term undertaking. A recent study[25, 26] by McGlashan et al. at Chestnut Lodge demonstrated that borderlines kept in the hospital in an intensive and consistent treatment milieu for an average of 30 months did extremely well when viewed from the perspective of a 10-year follow-up. The cost of such treatment is staggering, and impossible in the usual hospital setting, but it does suggest a strategy and a way of looking at the hospitalization of the borderline. Perhaps we need to view the borderline as needing to do such long-term work on the installment plan, with each successive brief hospitalization a part of a long-range strategy. Viewed in this way, the borderline patient will be seen as someone who will work in long-term outpatient therapy but will need a *series* of brief hospitalizations, preferably in the same setting, all of which are expected parts of the long-range treatment plan and can be anticipated to stretch over years. This is not only a realistic way of viewing the borderline's needs; it can be of enormous help to the morale of the inpatient staff and the long-term therapist, as well as to the patient. Each necessity for brief hospitalization no longer has to be seen as a failure, a defeat, or as recidivism. It is legitimately part of the long-term treatment plan. This in turn allows the staff of the unit to welcome the patient positively rather than with discouragement, and it promotes the willingness of inpatient units to be the consistent, loyal backup to a number of borderline patients.

AFFECTIVELY DISORDERED PATIENTS

Schizophrenia and borderline personality are two of the three most common diagnoses seen on general inpatient units. The third is that of the various major affective disorders, including mania but principally depression, whether of bipolar, unipolar, or endogenous origin, with or without psychosis.

Mania has always been very difficult, if not impossible, to treat by psychotherapy alone. Furthermore, what could be said of the treatment of schizophrenia by psychotherapy does not apply very well to true mania. For one thing, the manic patient rarely sits still, either literally or figuratively, physically or mentally, long enough to engage in any meaningful verbal therapy. Fortunately, pharmacotherapy, in the form of neuroleptics and lithium carbonate, can lyse the manic symptoms entirely so that the underlying characterologic and situational issues can be examined. Once the acute symptoms yield to drug therapy, there is usually plenty to understand in the way of functional pathology. As with the disorders described above, the task of the inpatient therapist is not so much to explore the perhaps etiologically significant historical roots of the patient's pathology, although these may be gainfully delineated, but rather to focus more on the patient's current relationships, including those on the unit and with the outside therapist. A major part of the work will be to help the patient integrate the experience he has just come through, which may be experienced as shattering, or may be mourned as the loss of a treasured euphoria or elation. The manic patient will usually need psychotherapeutic help in learning to accept and live without a "high," and to find gratification in the ordinary feelings and events of life. He will need help in seeing how destructive to his ongoing and valued relationships his manic behavior has been. Without this understanding, it is likely that he will soon fail to comply with his lithium regimen and risk, or even seek, another manic episode. Family work, on the model described above for schizophrenia, will also be necessary and helpful in advancing and maintaining the patient's recovery.

More can be said of the depressions. Here the containment of, and learning to bear, painful affects reaches its apogee. Depression seems to be the most universally human of the major psychiatric disorders. What human life is there without loss and pain? Here, moreover, the countertransference problems are less those of dealing with personal responses to the bizarre, the attacking, and the alien, and more of responses to issues that are much closer to home. If they are threatening, it is because they are so familiar and thus potentially overwhelming.

Freud made the very useful distinction between grief and true depression.[27] The former, it seems, can mimic the latter in every clinical particular, except for duration and one other symptom: a fall in self-esteem. Sooner or later this loss of self-esteem must be the central focus of the psychotherapy of depression.

My own observations[28] lead me to conclude that there are, independent of the final common pathway of the presenting symptomatology, several clinical forms of depression, each primarily involving different major affects, although all depressions have mixed affective pictures. There are depressions whose *primary* disordered affect is *rage*, other depressions whose *primary* affect is *guilt*, and those whose *primary* affect is *shame*. All involve a fall in self-esteem, but each presents a different type of low self-esteem and requires a different slant to the psychotherapeutic approach. The rage-filled depression requires a focus on issues of dependency, deprivation, helplessness, and the fear of abandonment and psychic starvation. The guilt-ridden depression requires a focus on issues of personal badness, unworthiness, aggressiveness and hatred, and problems with authority. The shame-wracked depressive needs to work on issues of adequacy, potency, lovability, attractiveness, competition, fear of success, and high-level narcissism. These clinical distinctions cut across the DSM-III diagnostic categories of depression based on the biological symptom picture that is so useful in planning somatic therapy interventions but is of little help in planning the psychotherapy of depression.

OTHER DIAGNOSTIC CATEGORIES

The role of inpatient psychotherapy in many of the other primary diagnostic categories is often more ancillary than in those discussed above. Some of these other illness do not often appear on inpatient services, and when they do, short-term psychotherapy has little to offer.

Eating Disorders are varied but require either long-term psychotherapy to address underlying chronic issues, or immediate attention to the possibly life-threatening medical complications, such as in the starvation state of anorexia nervosa or electrolyte imbalances of the bulimic or bulimarexic (the eating-disordered patient is not likely to be admitted to the hospital unless the medical condition reaches dangerous proportions). Starvation itself has so many effects, many of which are psychic and emotional, that no effective psychologic or characterologic diagnosis, let alone psychotherapy, can be carried out until the medical crisis has been alleviated. Some of these patients will then be seen to have borderline or psychotic problems, which will be treated as outlined above. Others will respond best, in the short term, to behavioral techniques and/or to medication. The role of the inpatient service is to stabilize these patients medically, set limits, start behavioral and psychopharmacologic regimens, prevent regression, and refer the patient for long-term management and, if indicated, psychotherapy. However, there is one important factor for the psychotherapist to keep in mind in treating the anorexic patient. Many of these patients have, at the very root of their psychopathology, a history of having been responded to by their parents unempathically, as if they were nothing but bodies without any other qualities of self.[29] Thus they may be starving themselves in order to make their bodies go away so that they will finally be responded to in ways that are affirming of aspects of self other than body. Indeed, these patients may be on a desperate search for selfhood, for any sense of self at all. Ironically, but not surprisingly, they have chosen a way that will guarantee that they will be responded to first as bodies, for that is all they have been used to and can neither understand nor trust anyone's responding to them as real people. The therapist cannot change that self-perception in a short-term hospitalization, but he can be sensitive to the fact that everyone is, of necessity, dealing with the patient in physical, medical ways. This manner of caring for the patient is likely to reinforce the patient's distorted and pathologic view of herself, and bolster her determination not to eat, to disappear physically. The therapist must at least try to offset this unwanted effect of the medical treatment by taking pains to relate to the patient empathically around the patient's experience of what is happening, and to quietly insist that the patient is a whole human being with a full range of affects and ideas, however singlemindedly she focuses on body and the avoidance of food. The psychotherapist must also be the one to remind the rest of the staff of the patient's psychological and emotional needs, especially during the times when the patient is most obdurately uncooperative and most in physical danger.

The *psychopathic or sociopathic personality* manipulates therapy as he does everything and everyone else, and rarely truly engages in it. These patients do not often appear on inpatient units, and when they do, they frequently have calculated, ulterior motives, such as hiding from criminal prosecution or building some sort of legal case. The therapist should guard against being "conned" while remaining open to the possibility that the patient may decide to opt for real change. Such patients are best treated in groups, preferably made up of the same kind of patients, so that the disingenuousness is constantly confronted by experts.

The *schizoid character* develops little, if any, usable transference and less real attachment. Moreover, the pathology is so ego syntonic that there is rarely very much motivation to change. These people also rarely end up in inpatient units. When they do, they may be able to use a quiet supportive treatment focused on current, practical issues of daily life.

Substance abusers and addictive personalities often present a blend of oral-dependent and psychopathic issues and may respond, once the addiction is under control and the patient is substance-free, to a psychotherapy that is similar in focus to that of the dependent depressive. Such people, in fact, often do harbor an underlying depression, which may respond to antidepressant medication, but their penchant for substance abuse makes the prescribing of such medication perilous. Psychotherapy before the substance abuse is totally and enduringly under control is practically worthless, as these patients find the work of psychotherapy too arduous in comparison with the immediate, if short-lived, gratifying escape provided by the substance abuse. Moreover, the necessary buildup of affect in the therapy is never allowed to happen, as it is immediately relieved and dissipated by the abuse. For a select few of this category of patients, long-term psychotherapy focused on underlying issues of deprivation, unsatisfiable need, and low self-esteem can prove very effective, but only after the substance abuse has stopped for some time. For the majority, substitutive and behavioral techniques, such as disulfiram or those offered by Alcoholics Anonymous and other specialized treatment groups, are usually far more effective than psychotherapy.

CONCLUSIONS

In psychotherapy, the clinician's instrument to effect change is the clinician himself, his very being, the sum of all that he is: knowledge, memory, experience, character, defenses, defects, talents, and learned skills. One's knowledge of Dostoevsky or Kafka or Conrad is apt to be of as much help with some patients as is one's knowledge of norepinephrine metabolism or of Freud. Whatever is accomplished in psychotherapy happens in the context of, and as a result of, the direct human relationship between therapist and patient. Psychotherapy is usually structured to maximize the flow of information and feeling from patient to therapist, but the therapist calls upon his inner life and self-knowledge as in no other field except, perhaps, artistic creation. In this aspect of psychiatry, the physician embarks on a lifelong voyage of self-discovery, with his patients often his most effective teachers, an education that has no parallel in any other branch of medicine and few parallels, if any, at that intensity, in any other human endeavor. If the outcomes are often no better than those in the rest of medicine, they are, on the whole, no worse, and the process itself offers a challenging and intimate involvement not to be found in any other specialty. For that, one has to sacrifice some of the scientific certainties and clarities, such as they are, of the rest of medicine and some of the comfort of being able to turn to the laboratory or the radiograph for help. The practice of psychotherapy is not for everyone; it is for those temperamentally suited to its demands, and for those who are, by nature, comfortable with and rewarded by intense and sustained human contact.

REFERENCES

1. Semrad E: *The Heart of a Therapist,* p. 103, New York, J. Aronson, 1980.
2. Mintz J: Measuring outcome in psychodynamic psychotherapy. Arch Gen Psychiatry *38:* 503–506, 1981.
3. Smith MC, Glass GV, Miller TI: *The Benefit of Psychotherapy,* Baltimore, Johns Hopkins University Press, 1980.
4. Kazdin AE, Wilson GT: Criteria for evaluating psychotherapy. Arch Gen Psychiatry *35:* 407–416, 1978.
5. Marshall E: Psychotherapy works, but for whom? Science, *251:* 506–508, 1980.
6. Greenspan SI, Sharfstein SS: Efficacy of psychotherapy. Arch Gen Psychiatry, *38:* 1213–1218, 1981.
7. Bleuler E: *Dementia Praecox, or the Group of Schizophrenias,* New York, International Universities Press, 1950.
8. Zinberg N: The private vs. the public psychiatric interview. Am J Psychiatry, *142:* 8, 889–894, 1985.
9. Shakespeare W: *Hamlet,* Act II, scene i.
10. Checkhov A: Grief, in *The Short Stories of Anton Checkhov,* New York, Modern Library, 1932.
11. Shakespeare W: *Hamlet,* Act III, scene ii.
12. Greenson RR: *The Technique and Practice of Psychoanalysis,* vol. I, p. 39, New York, International Universities Press, 1967.
13. Semrad E: *The Heart of a Therapist,* p. 112, New York, J. Aronson, 1980.
14. Taketomo R: Personal communication.
15. Hoffer A: Toward a definition of psychoanalytic neutrality. J Am Psychoanal Assoc, *33*(4): 1985.
16. Green H: *I Never Promised You a Rose Garden,* New York, Holt, Rinehart, & Winston, 1964.
17. Schwartz DP: Quoted in Gunderson J and Mosher L: *Psychotherapy of Schizophrenia,* p. 31, New York, J. Aronson.
18. Main TM: The ailment, Br J Med Psychol *30:* 129–145, 1957.
19. Murray J: Narcissism and the ego ideal, J Am Psychiatr Assoc, *12:* 477–511, 1964.
20. Segal H: *Introduction to the Work of Melanie Klein,* London, Heinemann Medical Books, 1964.
21. Quoted in Groves J: Borderline personality disorder. N Engl J Med, *305*(5): 259, 1981.
22. Modell A: Primitive object relationships and the predisposition to schizophrenia, Int J Psychoanal, *44:* 282–292, 1963.
23. Lesser IM: A review of the alexithymia concept. Psychosom Med, *43:* 531–543, 1981.
24. Jacobs D, Rogoff J, et al.: The neglected alliance: The inpatient unit as a consultant to referring therapists. Hosp Community Psychiatry, *33*(5): 377–381, 1982.
25. McGlashan T: Borderline personality disorder: Part V of Chestnut Lodge followup study, in *The Borderline: Current Empirical Research,* pp. 61–98, Washington, D.C., American Psychiatric Association, 1985.
26. McGlashan TH: The Chestnut Lodge Follow-up Study. III. Long-term outcome of borderline personalities. Arch Gen Psychiatry *43*(1): 20–30, 1986.
27. Freud S: Mourning and melancholia, in *Standard Edition,* London, Hogarth Press, 1971.

28. Rogoff J: Primum non nocere: The inpatient psychotherapy of depression. Presented at the 1985 Annual Meeting of the APA, Dallas, Texas.

29. Rizzuto A, Peterson R, Reed M: The pathological sense of self in anorexia nervosa. Psychiatr Clin North Am, 4(3): 471–487, 1981.

FURTHER READINGS

Adler G, Myerson P: *Confrontation in Psychotherapy,* New York, Science House, 1973.

Anthony EJ, Benedek T: *Depression and Human Existence,* Boston, Little, Brown & Co., 1975.

Arieti S: *Interpretation of Schizophrenia,* New York, Basic Books, 1974.

Basch M: *Doing Psychotherapy,* New York, Basic Books, 1980.

Bernstein S: Some psychoanalytic contributions to the understanding and treatment of patients with primitive personalities, in *Psychoanalysis: Critical Explorations in Contemporary Theory and Practice,* Jacobson A, Parmelee D, New York, Brunner/Mazel, 1982.

Burnham D: The special problem patient: Victim or agent of splitting? Psychiatry, 29: 105–122, 1966.

Chessick R: *Great Ideas in Psychotherapy,* New York, Jason Aronson, 1977,

Drake R, Sederer L: Inpatient psychotherapy of chronic schizophrenia: Avoiding regression. Presented at APA Annual Meeting, Dallas, May 1985.

Gunderson J, Singer M: Defining borderline patients: An overview. Am J Psychiatry, 132(1): 1–9, 1975.

Jacobson E: *Depression,* New York, International Universities Press, 1971.

Kernberg O: Borderline personality organization. J Am Psychoanal, 15(3): 641–685, 1967.

Borderline Conditions and Pathological Narcissism, New York, Jason Aronson, 1975.

Kris A: On wanting too much: The "exceptions" revisited. Int J Psychoanal, 57: 85–95, 1976.

Langs R: *The Bipersonal Field,* New York, Jason Aronson, 1976.

Little M: Transference in borderline states. Int J Psychoanal, 47: 476–485, 1966.

Maltsberger T, Buie D: Countertransference hate in the treatment of suicidal patients. Arch Gen Psychiatry, 30: 625–633, 1974.

Masterson JF: *Psychotherapy of the Borderline Adult,* New York, Brunner/Mazel, 1976.

Olinick S: *The Psychotherapeutic Instrument,* New York, Jason Aronson, 1980.

Pfeiffer E: Borderline states. Dis Nerv Syst: 212–219, 1974.

Schwartz M: What is a therapeutic milieu?, in Greenblatt M, Levinson D, Williams R (eds): *The Patient and the Mental Hospital,* Glenco, Ill., The Free Press of Glencoe, Ill., 1957.

Shapiro E: The psychodynamics and developmental psychology of the borderline patient: A review of the literature. Am J Psychiatry, 135(11): 1305–1315, 1978.

Tarachow S: *An Introduction to Psychotherapy,* New York, International Universities Press, 1970.

Wishnie H: Inpatient therapy with borderline patients, in Mack J (ed): *Borderline States in Psychiatry,* New York, Grune & Stratton, 1975.

chapter 12

group psychotherapy

Irene E. Rutchick, M.S.S.S.

Patients enter the psychiatric hospital in varying states of psychological disorganization and present a wide range of behavioral disturbances, cognitive impairment, and affective symptomatology. They may feel helpless and hopeless, or they may be frightened by an inability to think clearly or by a nightmarish perception of reality. They may be confused and angry because their judgment and behavior are questioned or misunderstood and they are deemed incapable of independent decision-making and functioning. For some, this disorganization may be an acute state in a previously relatively well-functioning individual. For the majority, however, an acute decompensation represents an exacerbation of a chronic or recurrent disorder.

Regardless of presenting symptoms or the acute or chronic nature of the illness, hospitalized patients share a sense of having failed as human beings. The vague, but nonetheless powerful, blows to self-esteem incurred by disturbing thoughts, feelings, and behavior evoke shame and humiliation, which is often concretized and intensified by the act of hospitalization. In addition, patients often feel betrayed by and alienated from the significant people in their lives whom they may perceive as having failed them.

Although many patients experience the hospital as a refuge from overwhelming external pressures and a haven in which frightening impulses can be contained, their personal integrity is threatened in a number of ways.[1-3] The loss of familiar surroundings, meaningful relationships, work, school, or household responsibilities, as well as a change in daily routine, is a demoralizing disruption in a person's life. Sharing living space with others whose pathology is foreign or even a representation of projected self-contempt may prompt the fear and denial seen in the frequently expressed statement, "I'm not that bad. I don't belong here." The many demands for interaction from other patients as well as with staff[4] can be confusing and overwhelming and may replicate internally familiar conflicts.[5] Limited rights of privacy and freedom of movement as well as having most every act open for scrunity may add to the patient's threatened integrity. The type of information elicited to understand and treat the patient's disorder is an act of exposure and is potentially threatening.

At the same time, the hospital provides many sources of dependency gratification that often heighten the patient's yearnings for an all-caring, all-giving authority figure. The inevitable frustration of these yearnings may lead to regression in some patients.[5, 6] For the patient who must protect himself from overwhelming rage evoked by disappointment, regression serves a defensive function, and, if unchecked, the hospital experience may become toxic.

This chapter discusses how the hospital experience is the primary material used in group therapy to treat specific aspects of the patient's acute state and to alter some of the potentially deleterious effects of hospitalization. After a brief history of groups in hospital settings, there is a discussion of the functions of inpatient group therapy and of its specific treatment goals. Next, the technical aspects of group formation and leadership functions will be addressed. Finally, there will be a consideration of countertransference as it relates to inpatient group treatment.

THE HISTORY OF GROUPS IN INPATIENT SETTINGS

The use of groups in hospital settings dates back to the 1920's. In 1921, Lazell lectured to groups of hospitalized schizophrenic patients on the nature of their illness. He reported successful results obtained through universalization, reduced fear of the analyst, and increased social contact.[7] At about the same time, Marsh[8] used a similar format, though his approach was more structured, was broader in scope, and held to the theory that patients could be supportive of one another. In addition to inspirational and formal academic lectures, he instituted art and dance classes for the patient's psychological well-being.

In the 1930's, Wender[9] utilized psychoanalytic concepts in the hospital group treatment of patients we would now call borderline, with the goal of partial personality reorganization. He described the transference as one in which the group symbolized the patient's family. The therapist was seen as the parent and the other group members as siblings.

During World War II the use of groups in military hospitals expanded primarily as a result of economic necessity. It was in such a setting that Bion[10] initiated his study of the conscious and unconscious determinants of group behavior and process.

Following World War II, Standish and Semrad[11] described the technique of "Participation in Casual Conversation" with psychotic patients. Through focusing on the feelings that underlie the manifest symptoms and with the understanding of the therapist, patients were able to express suppressed hostility and to increase social interaction and interpersonal learning.

In the 1950's the growing use of groups in inpatient settings was fostered by an increased understanding of the hospital as a social system and of the psychological impact of hospitalization. There was an attempt to substitute therapeutic groups for the destructive group forces too often seen in an unguided institutional milieu. Frank,[12] in recognizing that hospital patients need to develop a sense of belonging and that psychological illness is often chronic or recurrent, utilized group therapy for the dual purposes of improving communication within the milieu and of increasing the patient's responsibility for himself and others.

As short-term hospitalization for both acute and chronic disorders developed in the 1970's and 1980's, Kibel,[13, 14] Maxmen, et al.,[15–17] and others[18–26] developed conceptual models and modified long-term therapy goals and techniques for their use with the short-term, regressed, hospital patient. Yalom addressed the place for group therapy in today's psychiatric hospital and detailed specific leadership strategies and techniques for interpersonal learning within a single session time frame.[27]

FUNCTIONS OF INPATIENT GROUP THERAPY

Healing

The first and most important task in treating psychiatric patients is to establish a therapeutic alliance in which the therapist and patient work together toward a common goal. For the hospitalized patient, alliance is often a formidable task because of his pervasive feelings of demoralization and heightened yearnings for dependency gratification, which intensify transference and transference-like phenomena.* Group therapy heals by altering feelings of de-

---

*Transference is classically defined as "the unconscious assignment to others of feelings and attitudes that were originally associated with important figures in one's early life."[28] Transference distorts reality. Transference-*like* phenomena occur in the more disturbed patient when distorted perceptions of others result from confusion between self and others and from the need to experience others in a manner that enhances self-esteem.[29] Examples include attributing to others the capacity to gratify a need that is longed for or projecting negative self-images, i.e., unconsciously assigning negative aspects of the self, like hate and sadism, onto others. This chapter expands the classical definition of transference to include distorted perceptions of others that result from transference-like phenomena.

moralization, by enabling patients to contain and tolerate intense transference, and by providing patients an experience which helps them to handle troublesome feelings in an ego-enhancing manner.

Humans are social beings with instinctual desires to belong. Hospitalized patients, experiencing intense feelings of isolation, feel they don't belong anywhere. Isolated and demoralized, these patients frequently perceive their situation to be hopeless, and they feel helpless. They employ defenses such as denial and externalization of problems which impede therapeutic efforts and which may intensify their dilemma.[16, 20]

Group therapy offers an opportunity to mitigate painful feelings of isolation, demoralization, hopelessness, and helplessness. Maxmen[31] specifically refers to four "curative factors," described by Yalom,[27, 30] which have particular relevance for the short-term inpatient:

1. *Universality.* The shared understanding that one's problems and feelings are not unique and that one is not alone.
2. *Altruism.* The opportunity to give to others and to feel needed and useful.
3. *Instillation of hope.* The opportunity to see and hear the progress of others with similar problems.
4. *Group cohesion.* A sense of belonging, which includes trust, acceptance, and support. It is the group equivalent of positive transference.

Furthermore, group therapy helps to diminish helplessness and demoralization as group members experience themselves as therapeutic agents. Patients provide each other support, acceptance, reality confrontation, and feedback. Efforts to help themselves and others enable patients to begin to re-experience their own effectiveness and to increase their self-esteem.[27]

Many hospitalized patients have a primitive character structure or have suffered an intense trauma which renders them vulnerable to intense feelings of helplessness and ineffectualness and which fosters a perception of others, particularly those in authority, as being omniscient and in total control.[5, 13, 32] Although there may be a good deal of comfort and gratification in feeling cared for by an omnipotent figure, these feelings cannot remain constant. First, the personal history of these patients reminds them, consciously and unconsciously, that authority figures are untrustworthy. Second, the therapist, at times, must disappoint and frustrate, which evokes past and present feelings of being uncared for and abandoned. Finally, intense feelings of helplessness give rise to anger with its attendant fear of retaliation. When the omnipotent figure has real control, as with the power to grant passes, determine discharge, etc., the transference reaction becomes even more marked.

Group therapy enables patients to contain and tolerate transference in several specific ways.[12, 14, 30, 33-35] First, a sense of *helplessness* towards authority is diminished significantly when in the company of others. Support for one's point of view, particularly as it relates to the unfairness of authority, provides a source of strength for the patient that is unavailable in one-to-one therapy. Second, it is easier to express *negative feelings* (e.g., hate, aversion, disgust) in a group than it is with an individual therapist. Fears of retaliation are generally reduced in a public forum. The expression of negative feelings is particularly important because they are a frequent source of a treatment impasse which may lead to further regression. Instead of feeling understood and accepted, angry patients are preoccupied by defending against and controlling hostile impulses, leaving them little psychic energy to reality test and to relate to others. Third, seating arrangements in a group promote a certain amount of *safety* by providing distance from the therapist. It is not uncommon, for example, to find the most angry, hostile group member facing the therapist from the far side of the room. Fourth, a therapy group permits the patient to sit back and observe the therapist interact with others. The therapist can emerge more as a real person when the patient is not constantly on the spot and his *anxiety* is diminished. Furthermore, patients experience a sense of caring when the therapist demonstrates concern for others.

Group therapy also heals by providing

patients a "corrective emotional experience," that is, a "reexposure under favorable circumstances to an emotional situation that the patient could not handle in the past."[36] Increased self-esteem and the experience of mastery in a situation that previously evoked feelings of helplessness or anxiety are examples of a corrective emotional experience. The group experience may also be corrective in providing the patient with a human relationship that has been essentially absent in his life. Because many psychiatric patients present with a history bereft of meaningful interpersonal contact, the group may provide a context for the beginning of significant engagement with others.

Traditionally, the concept of the corrective emotional experience includes the integration of both experiential and cognitive factors, though some therapists emphasize one or the other, depending on the type and duration of change expected.[30, 36, 37] In brief therapy, which aims to support ego recompensation, emphasis is placed on experiential factors. Conscious, or cognitive, awareness of the *process* is not required in order for it to be effective. (Awareness of the healing process is distinguished from cognitive activities that are used to promote reality testing.) In fact, attempts to promote cognitive understanding may negate the therapeutic benefit of the experience by undermining defenses.[38] For example, Ms. A. repeatedly used projection in the group (as she did with all relationships), seeing others as angry with her. The group members were able to indicate that, in fact, their distance reflected their own fears and concerns and was not an angry withdrawal. Ms. A. identified with the concerns expressed by others and experienced a rarely felt sense of acceptance in the group which diminished her anger and, thereby, her need for projection. Her use of projection was not interpreted because of her inability to bear her own anger.

Linking: The Individual, The Group, and the Milieu

The small therapy group is a subsystem of the hospital milieu[39–43] and a microcosm of each patient's interpersonal world.[27, 30, 31]

The group reflects all the transactions and tensions of the ward patients and staff[13] and demonstrates each patient's characteristic responses. The therapy group is, therefore, in a position to examine and help correct each patient's maladaptive ways and to ameliorate the destructive tensions which arise on the unit. As milieu events are discussed, distorted perceptions can be clarified and the ego strengthened. Patients can then begin to discern the patterns to their reactions, which serves to diminish feeling sof helplessness and ineffectiveness.

In the same manner that the hospital milieu is reflected in the material of the therapy group, processes in the group may reciprocally have a major therapeutic impact on the milieu.[12, 35] Alterations in the perception of authority, for example, extend beyond the patient's experience within the group and include other staff on the ward. As greater communication is experienced among patients in the group, it extends to the milieu. As patients experience mutual caring and gain greater awareness of the problems of others, feelings of responsibility for the welfare of others are enhanced. Acting out on the ward is thus less likely to be accepted as patients care for and consider others and begin to assume some of the control functions of the staff. Furthermore, because control from peers, unlike staff, is experienced as concern from an equal, it is less likely to result in power struggles.

The therapy group may also stimulate material for the patient's individual therapy. In an atmosphere of diminished defensiveness and with the opportunity to observe others, suppressed feelings and memories often emerge in the group setting. The increased awareness of behavioral and affective response patterns that group treatment provides may also be brought to the individual therapy, where they can be understood more fully.

GOALS OF GROUP THERAPY

The goals of short-term hospitalization include: (1) diagnostic assessment; (2) modification of disabling behavioral, affective, and cognitive symptomatology; (3) ego recompensation to a premorbid baseline level of functioning; (4) modification of environmental stresses which may have precipitated the decompensation; and (5) motivation for outpatient therapy. These goals focus on a return to the premorbid state, not a more fundamental personality change which would require a regressive capacity that decompensated patients cannot tolerate. Although the goals of group therapy are not identical to the goals of the hospitalization, group treatment facilitates the attainment of these goals in the following ways: (1) providing diagnostic data, (2) reality testing, (3) increasing patient responsibility, (4) strengthening self-esteem, and (5) channeling aggression.

Diagnostic Data

A complete diagnostic assessment of the patient requires the integration of material from the patient's individual therapist, the family, and the milieu. The hospital milieu provides patients many opportunities to reenact their world before the hospital and to rediscover their strengths. Because this occurs in the therapy group as well, in a setting that is smaller and more manageable, it is often easier to observe interpersonal behavior and to assess its diagnostic relevance.[27, 35, 44, 45]

The therapy group provides unique opportunities to obtain information about the nature of and the patient's capacity to tolerate and manage pain and conflict. For example, information about what content patients can or cannot hear, which patients are able to relate to others and to whom, which patients develop an aversion to one another, and who identifies with whom emerges in the group setting.

The patient's ego functioning may also be assessed by observing how attentive he is to what is going on. Questions about the quality of the patient's interaction with others; his capacity to listen, support, and empathize with others; and whether he can or can never agree with others can often be answered by observing the patient's behavior in the group.

Finally, group therapy offers an assessment of the patient's capacity to utilize treatment. This, of course, has considerable bearing on discharge planning.

Patients who are unable to tolerate one-to-one therapy may be able to use a group.[46, 47] Examples include patients who experience excessive or unworkable transference problems which are mitigated in group therapy and those patients who cannot acknowledge that they have problems but who may gain sufficient self-esteem from helping others to diminish this defensiveness. The inpatient group may also demonstrate which patients are not appropriate for outpatient group therapy. Patients who are unable to comply with the group rules, who remain silent, or who become excessively anxious when in the company of others are examples.

Reality Testing

Reality testing refers to "the ability to evaluate the external world objectively and to differentiate adequately between it and the internal world."[28] Disturbances in reality testing may be transient, as when the ego is overwhelmed by affects stimulated by a specific situation, or chronic, resulting from faulty identifications and pathological character defenses established by early experiences with significant persons in the individual's life. Brief therapy cannot alter character pathology. However, it can provide an environment for the correction of reality disturbances which are situation specific. Anxiety associated with the feared consequences of projected feelings is thereby diminished, and increased gratification from both interpersonal interactions and productive problem solving is enabled.

The therapy group specifically provides reality assessment when its members provide a variety of perceptions about a single event.[34, 45] This directly and indirectly confronts the individual with the validity of his own perceptions. In addition, the therapist frequently adds his clarification of reality and lessens distortions by helping patients discharge those disturbing feelings which cloud accurate perception.

Increasing Patient Responsibility

As previously noted, hospitalized patients are in an extremely dependent state and experience intense feelings of hopelessness and powerlessness. Unless checked, this situation can promote further regression and render the patient more unable to recognize areas in which his functioning and responsibility remain intact.

Patient responsibility is a sine qua non of group therapy. Group members are therapeutic agents.[15, 30] In the group, patients are expected, by the leader and the other members, to share their concerns, pull their weight, give and take, and work toward group goals. Though they are in the room with a powerful authority figure, patient comments are considered more helpful.[34] This process directly enables patients to experience their own competence and effectiveness.

Group therapy also helps the patient to experience more control by providing him an opportunity to learn about his impact on others and to identify interpersonal problem areas that can be worked on after discharge.[27] Many psychiatric patients are totally unaware that they have an effect on, or are meaningful to, others. Feedback, from peers and the therapist(s), about certain behaviors and attitudes that enhance or block desired interaction with others promotes a beginning capacity for self-reflection which furthers the patient's capacity to assume responsibility for himself and his treatment.

Strengthening Self-Esteem

One aspect of all psychopathology involves maladaptive maneuvers to preserve self-esteem. Severely disturbed and regressed patients devote much of their emotional energy to the maintenance of an inner sense of cohesion and well-being. To accomplish this task they often utilize primitive defenses such as grandiosity, primitive idealization, projective identification, and splitting. Other people are used as objects in the service of meeting individual needs, thereby diminishing the capacity for empathic connection to or, even, an awareness of the needs of others. This narcissistic relationship to others is often a source of conflict and prevents the very need gratification for which these patients are striving.

In group therapy the leader assists the patients to use the leader, other patients, and the setting to enhance self-esteem by fostering relatedness and the adaptive use of defenses.[13, 48] At times this may require the therapist to support defenses that appear maladaptive but are necessary for the patient's psychic survival. The aim becomes making these essential defenses more adaptive.

Mr. B who, prior to hospitalization, experienced a devastating narcissistic assault due to business failures and divorce, preserved his self-esteem on the unit by maintaining an attitude of superiority (grandiosity). Unfortunately, this defense deterred others from engaging with him and exposed him to further rejection. In the group, he raised many issues relating to the trustworthiness of the other members and the leaders. The therapists supported Mr. B.'s "leadership" abilities (narcissism) by valuing his contributions and thereby enabled other group members to share similar concerns. Mr. B. then identified with the other group members and used them to support his grandiosity: "We are more intelligent than the other patients here." His defensive structure remained intact but was more adaptive as he included others in his world.

Channeling Aggression

Aggression is a potent universal drive serving both protective and growth functions. For the severely disturbed and regressed patient whose controls are limited while aggressive impulses are heightened, psychic stability becomes threatened. Many of these patients are overwhelmed by rage, both past and present, while being deficient in the ego development which would permit some neutralization and adaptive use of their aggression.[49, 50]

The combination of pervasive rage, assaults to the individual's integrity imposed by the frustrations of the milieu, and the inability of the patient to adaptively deal with aggressive impulses make it essential that the hospital provide a setting in which the patients are safely enabled to channel their aggression. Group therapy is one place where this can occur.

The group setting can offer neutralization of rageful affect by encouraging problem-solving and ventilation.[11, 14] In addition, because aggressive feelings may lead to disorganization in some patients (e.g., a borderline patient can become psychotic or suicidal) the therapist may need to support defenses like projection and splitting in order to enable patients to externalize their aggression.[13] Group therapy can facilitate this process because the group members provide multiple opportunities for the use of externalizing defenses.

FORMING THE GROUP

The development and provision of group therapy on an inpatient unit requires careful attention to the definition and management of the group's boundaries.[4, 30, 40–42, 51] What care the group intends to provide, for whom, by whom, when, where, and by what methods must all be defined in order for the group to succeed. These organizational and structural boundaries differentiate what is "in" the group from what is "out," thereby providing the patient a sense of safety and control over the extent of his participation in the group.

Milieu Considerations

Earlier in this chapter we considered the impact of the hospital milieu on patients' feelings about themselves and their behavior. In a similar manner, the attitude of the hospital staff toward any therapeutic endeavor has direct implications for the effectiveness of that therapy.[52] If group therapy is a treatment modality valued by the ward staff, patients are more likely to value this form of treatment and to use the group productively. On the other hand, if group therapy is valued only by the group leader(s), with only lip service offered by other staff, patients may devalue the group or act out this staff conflict in much the same manner as the child who becomes symptomatic in response to parental discord. Examples of this are seen when patients schedule individual therapy sessions or obtain off ward passes during group time. It is important, therefore, before starting a group for group leaders to clarify and educate staff about group therapy and to gain administrative and staff support.

Some therapists believe that it is the patients' responsibility to keep track of their therapeutic commitments. If they do not follow through it is seen as a resistance to therapy. However, an active milieu may offer many forms of treatment, thereby placing patients in conflict as to which treatment is important. It is essential that this conflict be recognized and minimized by staff and that staff members, not patients, determine treatment priorities. Whenever possible, group therapy sessions should be scheduled at times that do not conflict with other ward events. Because this may require ward schedule modifications, the entire staff needs to be consulted.

The role of the group therapist(s) in relation to other staff members must be carefully described.[4] Delineating areas of responsibility for decision-making and mechanisms for communication (discussed later in the chapter) must be articulated and agreed upon. The group therapist is seldom the patient's individual therapist or ward administrator. Unless it is clear who determines discharge, medication management, etc., confusion and destructive use of splitting may occur. Who decides what is not as significant as are clear definitions of specific roles and responsibilities for patient care.

Patient Selection

The types of patients usually considered most suitable for traditional group therapy are not the patients seen in the hospital. Outpatient exclusion criteria often include patients who are in acute crisis, actively psychotic or suicidal, nonmotivated, paranoid, schizoid, highly narcissistic, or organically impaired, and those who display high levels of denial or somatization.[30, 44, 46, 53] In the hospital, were these criteria in place, the range of patients would be further reduced by those newly admitted or on the verge of discharge, leaving few patients, if any, who would be suitable candidates.

The rationale and goals for inpatient group therapy allow for quite different inclusion and exclusion criteria.[16, 27] Because hospitalized patients are living together, interacting in gratifying and conflicting ways and sharing many common experiences and feelings, there is a wealth of psychosocial processes that can be harnessed for therapeutic gain. It can be assumed that *all* hospitalized patients can benefit from group therapy, with the following exceptions:

1. Patients who are unable to tolerate moderate external stimulation.
2. Patients whose impulse control is insufficient to offer group members reasonable safety.
3. Patients who are cognitively impaired to the extent that they suffer short-term memory loss and disorientation (e.g., patients who are heavily medicated, delirious, or undergoing electro-convulsive therapy).
4. Patients who are chronically mute.
5. Patients with whom the group therapist feels *excessive* discomfort.

The last criterion requires some elaboration. While the ability of the therapist to tolerate and accept the pathology of the patient always plays a role in the effectiveness of any treatment, the group therapist's attitude toward any one patient affects the treatment of every other group member. In a group, patients identify with one another, and the regressed patient often does not discriminate between himself and others. Therefore, the therapist's attitude toward any one patient will be felt similarly by other patients. For this reason, it is essential that the group therapist have ultimate responsibility for accepting or rejecting potential group members.

Group Composition

Group therapy literature abounds with consideration of what composition groups require for maximal therapeutic benefit.[30, 33, 54-56] The question of whether groups should be homogeneous or heterogenous (referring to diagnostic and psychodynamic homogeneity or heterogeneity, as opposed to such characteristics as age, sex, socioeconomic background, etc.) is dependent upon the goals of treatment, the setting, and often the skill of the therapist. Homogeneous groups primarily offer more rapid identification among members and thus foster a decrease in feelings of alienation and the anxieties of aloneness which facilitate group cohesion.[35] Heterogeneous groups offer the potential for increased interaction and mutual and self-

exploration which are the hallmarks of more intensive psychotherapy.[55]

On an inpatient unit where the number of patients available for group therapy at any given time is limited, it is usually not possible to obtain diagnostic homogeneity. Yet, hospitalized patients, who often have primitive character structure or are severely regressed, demonstrate a certain degree of homogeneity because of their current level of functioning and experience. It is possible to divide hospitalized patients into two groups: (1) patients who have a predominantly psychotic core (i.e., schizophrenic patients), and (2) patients who retain intact areas of functioning despite their decompensation (e.g., borderline patients) or who are expected to recompensate to a nonpsychotic state (e.g., manic-depressive patients). In order to make this division prior to placement in a particular therapy group, a preliminary diagnostic assessment of the patient is made. This will prevent such iatrogenic group problems as the psychotic patient deteriorating further in response to the emergence of intolerable affect and thereby stultifying the group process for healthier patients, or the inability of the healthier patient to "join" because of fears of contagion.

Patient Preparation

If patients are to achieve therapeutic benefit in a brief period of time, a discussion of group goals, roles, and expectations is essential.[4, 15, 27, 30, 53, 57] Patients should be encouraged to think about what they would like to achieve and then helped to translate these thoughts into realizable short-term goals. These goals should reflect current interpersonal difficulties or needs.[20, 21, 27] Goals such as feeling less isolated and alone, learning to communicate with others, or helping another person are common examples.

The curative factors of group therapy which are conscious and understandable (i.e., universality, altruism, instillation of hope, and group cohesiveness) are interpersonal. Furthermore, a focus on current needs and feelings will engage the patients who deny, externalize, or feel hopeless about their situation. With these patients, it may be necessary for the therapist to be firm, saying, for example, "I think the group will help you feel less alone here."

Clarification of the patient's role in the group includes setting expectations for behavior within the group. This is accomplished by a group therapy contract,[4, 40, 44] which informs the patient of the group rules and obtains an agreement to honor them.

A group therapy contract would include:

1. The patient agrees to attend each group meeting and to be on time.
2. The patient agrees to participate in group discussions and to talk about any feelings he may have regarding the group, other patients, staff, or the hospitalization. This includes feelings evoked both within and outside group meetings.
3. The patient agrees to protect the confidentiality of other group members. He will not discuss information revealed by another member during group meetings with patients who are not in the group.
4. The patient agrees to bring to the group any discussion of the group that occurs with other group members between group meetings.
5. The patient agrees to use verbal communication within the group. Touching other patients or the leader(s); either fondly or in anger; hurting one-self; or destroying property are not allowed.

Similarly, the therapist must clarify his role in the group therapy process and make certain commitments to the patients. The therapist's commitments are as follows:

1. The therapist must spell out the structural boundaries of the group, that is, the time, location, length, and frequency of meetings.
2. The therapist will provide a safe atmosphere in which patients can share their concerns freely, and he will intercede if contract violations occur.
3. The therapist will function as a facilitator of group process. He cannot provide "answers" but will help patients talk to and help each other.
4. The therapist acknowledges that material revealed in the group will be shared with staff members outside the group. Staff members will also share information with the group leader which he may raise in the group.
5. The therapist reviews his decision-making authority in the patient's care.
6. The therapist informs the patient if the group is to be observed or recorded.

Location

It is important for patients to have a quiet, consistent meeting place away from the activity of the rest of the unit. Since many regressed patients attach first to surroundings and then to people, the room should be comfortable and sufficiently large to afford spacial distance among members and the leader(s).

Group Size

The optimal size for an impatient therapy group is six to eight members. In groups of less than five, the interaction is insufficient for maximal therapeutic benefit.[30, 58] In addition, the pressure to "produce" and the enforced intimacy may be more than some regressed patients can bear. Larger groups do not afford adequate time for full participation from all members and tend to inhibit quiet members.

Length and Frequency of Meetings

The recommended length for an inpatient therapy group meeting is 45–75 minutes. The upper limit is more productive for nonpsychotic patients who have the capacity for a high degree of interaction. Patients with an agitated depression and those who are acutely psychotic may not tolerate meetings for longer than 45 minutes. Although extra-group patient contact and the discussion of shared milieu events during the session facilitates "re-entry," the ever-changing membership of the group and the ego states of its participants require time before group themes and affects are expressed, even if the group meets daily. Less than 45 minutes is insufficient time for this to occur. The reduced attention span, inability to relate comfortably to others, and low tolerance for affective stimuli make it difficult for many patients to participate effectively for longer than 75 minutes.

The frequency of group meetings is often determined by the constraints of the ward schedule and staff availability. However, given the patients' brief length of stay and the multitude of personal and milieu experiences to be processed, groups should meet ideally four or five times weekly. Frequent group meetings intensify the experience, provide more continuity, and thereby facilitate the emergence of the curative factors.

COMMUNICATION: KEEPING PATIENTS AND STAFF INFORMED

Once the group boundaries (e.g., patient selection, contract, etc.) are established, it is important to formalize methods of communication whereby the boundaries are conveyed and reinforced for both patients and staff. Patients may remain confused about what is expected of them. Staff may not recall which patients belong in group at any given time. It is helpful for patients to have a written schedule of their therapies and activities. It is also helpful to post, for staff and patients, the times and correct membership of the group(s).

A formal structure for providing feedback to the staff is essential. Information regarding both individual patients and general ward issues that become manifest in the group should be communicated to the individual therapist and other primary care-takers directly and to the ward staff through report, rounds, and chart notations.

Acute changes in symptomatology (e.g., suicidality or increased psychotic process) should be communicated directly to the patient's primary caretakers. Diagnostic (see Diagnostic Data) and progress observations about specific individuals are documented in chart notations. For example, "Ms. C. was angry and she distorted supportive comments from others when asked direct questions about her suicide attempt. She was able to identify with another group member's anger, fear and guilt that was evoked by the transfer of

Mr. D. She spontaneously associated to her grandmother's illness, which may be the precipitant for her recent decompensation."

The significance of general ward issues often becomes crystalized in the group. When this happens, this material should be communicated to the ward staff through group report. For example, in one group many patients exhibited increased hopelessness and discussed leaving the hospital against medical advice. Further exploration revealed that patients felt abandoned and out of control in response to staff shortages during a long weekend.

LEADERSHIP TASKS AND TECHNIQUES

Once the group is established, the primary tasks of the group therapist become: (1) reducing anxiety in order to provide a safe atmosphere in which patients can share their concerns; (2) promoting useful interaction among group members; and (3) monitoring the content and process of the group to meet the psychological needs of the individuals within it. Although these tasks are not mutually exclusive, they will be discussed separately for the sake of clarity.

Reducing Anxiety

By nature a group situation is anxiety provoking. There is always some degree of uncertainty as to the behavior of others, some anticipated fear of rejection by others, and the potential for rivalry and aversion toward others.[59] In addition, a group is often a fantasied representation of an individual's family group and can evoke powerful memories and feelings.[55] The group leader must reduce this anxiety to a workable level in order for patients to feel free to share their concerns. This can be accomplished by the clear delineation of the group boundaries and by the consistency and particular attitudes and interventions of the leader.

Consistent group leadership serves important therapeutic functions for the group. In hospital settings, transient group membership exposes the group to continual boundary assaults. Consistent group leadership enables a sense of continuity that changing membership disrupts. Coleaders are often used on inpatient services to provide consistency. If one therapist is sick or on vacation or, on the rare occasion that a patient becomes so agitated that he must be escorted from the room, the remaining therapist is available to ensure continuity and to deal with the feelings of the other group members.

A stable, consistent group leader also provides an opportunity for patients to begin to deal with the anxiety associated with their distorted perceptions of authority.[32] Patients can begin to develop increased reality testing and a sense of security through a process of repeated positive experiences with a consistent authority figure. This security may then be generalized to others in positions of authority. As part of this process, patients must be permitted to express hostility toward the leader either directly or through displacement (i.e., the unconscious transfer of feelings to a less threatening substitute). The leader must tolerate hostility in an empathic, reassuring, and nonretaliatory manner in order for neutralization of the affect and reality testing to occur.[13, 50] If the leader is "attacked" one day and absent the next, this will not be possible.

The *attitude of the leader* is also critical to reducing anxiety. The leader must convey concern, empathy, hope, and nonjudgmental acceptance. This does not mean that all behavior is tolerated. It does mean that all feelings are accepted and that the leader will attempt to help patients to understand their confusion and to control dangerous impulses. The group therapist must be a benevolent authority who will take control when needed, yet remain non-critical, nonpunitive, and nonrejecting.

The leader must be *responsive and active*[12, 20, 21, 27, 60] and demonstrate immediate feedback. Withholding only increases anxiety. The leader must be able to initiate discussion during periods of high anxiety marked by silence. Although silence may be a time for reflection, it generally occurs at the beginning of the session or when aggression has been mobilized.[61] The therapist should help patients to deal with the source of their anxiety rather than suggesting topics that merely fill the gap. For example, a therapist might say, "It is difficult to know where to begin" or "Perhaps, my comments about absences from group were upsetting."

The leader can also demonstrate responsiveness by answering questions directed to him in a brief, matter-of-fact manner and by praising patients for their efforts, regardless of how insignificant these efforts may appear.[20, 48] For example, praise may be given to the silent patient who remains in the room or to the verbally controlling patient who listens to another person.

The leader must be able to *manage intermember conflict* in a manner consonant with the ego capacities of the group members. For severely disturbed patients, conflict resolution will be rather superficial.[20] Direct intervention from the therapist, as when the leader attempts to dilute the one-to-one interaction before it escalates, may be required. At times, it may be necessary for the leader to call a "timeout." More often, techniques like generalization (translating individual conflicts and concerns into group or universal concerns) and the involvement of other group members in the discussion may be used. The therapist should acknowledge the strength it takes to *express differences of opinion* and how differences of opinion are common, and then ask others how they handle such differences. Praise and generalization can diminish the defensiveness of the members in conflict and increase the likelihood that others will express their opinion. Intense feelings may be thereby neutralized by shifting the group focus from the individuals involved to the group, and from affect to cognition.

Healthier patients with better impulse control may tolerate more exploration of their conflict as well as feedback from other group members.[14, 27] Once intense feelings have been neutralized (which may also occur through the group members without direct intervention from the leader) and the patient's self-esteem has been preserved, these patients can use the empathic observations of others to see their role in the conflict and to clarify their patterns of interaction. Although it is not advisable to confront a defense such as projection or to interpret unconscious conflict, patients can understand misinterpreting the intent of others and recognize patterns like the tendency to withdraw or "fight" when hurt.

Scapegoating is a particular form of intermember conflict which requires mention. A scapegoat is a group member who bears the blame for another, often the group leader or others in authority. This form of displacement is dangerous to both the patient being scapegoated and the group members because it gratifies their sadistic impulses.[13] Scapegoating always requires intervention from the leader, who must redirect the anger to himself or other appropriate authority figures.

Promoting Useful Interaction

One should not assume that patients know how to interact or utilize group treatment. Patient's with a history of poor object relations lack the social awareness and ego capacity to interact with others in a mutually helpful manner. The therapist must serve as the connecting link among patients by educating, modeling, and facilitating appropriate interaction.

The *educative process* begins with the explanation of the goals and purpose of the group during both the pregroup preparation and at the beginning of each meeting. Patients are told again and again that they will benefit from sharing their experiences and from listening to and helping one another.[15] This is then highlighted and reinforced during the course of the group by praising efforts to relate, which range from noticing another person to offers of advice and reality clarifications. The leader should first focus on supporting attempts at relatedness and then address content matter. For example, when John tells Carol to stop taking her medication because she is suffering from side effects, the leader might say: "John, I noticed you offered Carol a suggestion. It is good that you were really listening to how distressed she is." In this manner the therapist avoids criticism, enhances self-esteem, and supports an empathic connection between patients. The therapist may then address the content by asking others how they deal with disturbing side effects and how medication can help.

The therapist is also a *role model* in the group.[12, 30] Patients often will imitate the therapist's attitude and manner of relating to others. By observing how the therapist interacts with others, patients see socializing techniques which they can "try out" in the group. The leader may support this by a smile or a nod but should not draw attention to the process verbally because this could engender an inhibiting self-consciousness.

Finally, the therapist functions as a *facilitator of intermember interaction*.[12–15, 20, 21, 27] This can be accomplished by directly asking patients to provide feedback to a given member and to share similar concerns or different perspectives, by redirecting briefly answered leader-directed questions back to the group for comment, and by connecting the themes of seemingly disjointed individual concerns.

For more disturbed patients, the therapist may facilitate by translating primary process thinking (i.e., illogical, unorganized thinking associated with the unconscious) into ordered, rational thought.[60, 62] Psychotic patients who are unable to organize their thoughts feel isolated in part because of an inability to communicate with others. The leader can aid them by making bizarre, frightening primary process or loose statements understandable to others, thereby diminishing anxiety and isolation. For example, the manic patient who is ranting about government injustices might be managed by saying, "You are talking about something important to all of us. Sometimes things happen that feel unfair, especially when someone important leaves. Wasn't the medical student who is leaving today special to you?" For a schizophrenic patient reciting the nursery rhyme, "Here we go round the mulberry bush," the leader might say, "This is your third hospitalization. Do you feel like you are going in circles? Perhaps, you are telling us that you would like some help putting your thoughts in order." Although it is preferable for the therapist to be correct in his interpretation, he need not wait until he is certain what the patient is saying. It is more important to "connect" the verbal but unintelligible patient to others in the room than to be correct. The patient would not be talking if he did not want to communicate.

Monitoring Group Process and Content

Patients can be helped to distinguish internal and external stimuli, to understand the determinants of their feelings, and to clarify distorted perceptions of others through a discussion of "here and now" events. The term "here and now" refers to what is happening in the room at that particular point in time.[30] It refers to observable verbal and nonverbal actions and affect that are available for comment, understanding, and reality testing. "Here and now" is distinguished from people and events outside the purview of those present. On an inpatient unit, the concept of the "here and now" is expanded to include the entire ward, that is, all staff, patients, and ward events because the group members are participants and observers of these events.[13, 15]

A focus on the "here and now" increases group cohesion, decreases isolation, and enables patients to identify interpersonal strengths and problem areas. Patients can also derive more direct gratification from interacting in the present, even if only as observers. In addition, a "here and now" orientation can promote increased ego functioning by strengthening reality testing. For hospitalized patients, intense affect is a source of anxiety and confusion that can disolve ego boundaries and distort reality perceptions. Excessive affect experienced in the group setting is countered by both the variety of perceptions from various group members and the leader's efforts to help patients understand what they are reacting to, validating external experiences (what is outside) and empathizing with the feelings associated with these experiences (what is inside).

Focus on the "here and now" does not mean exclusion of "then and there" material. Patients need to talk about their lives outside the hospital, to provide background material, to discuss passes home and the like. "Then and there" allows for increased understanding and empathy among members, for problem-solving, and for the utilization of externalizing defenses. However, a primary therapeutic focus on understanding the meaning of outside material can be both regressive and demoralizing.[13, 14] Patients are often confused, and their self-esteem has been damaged by what happened "out there." To focus on understanding that material may lead some patients to direct their attention to the negative aspects of themselves which would support a negative self-image.

Interpretation is a technique used to convey to the patient the significance and meaning of his behavior by addressing material that the patient has warded off.[36] Interpretations from the therapist can be received as assaultive because they elicit anxieties associated with parental criticism and intolerable self-consciousness. The therapist may utilize "group as a whole" interpretations (i.e., comments directed to the entire group rather than to an individual) in order to reduce the likelihood of injury and to foster cohesion by bringing together seemingly disconnected individual concerns.[13, 14]

In order to provide "group as a whole" interpretations, the therapist must discern the themes amid the wealth of material presented by patients and then relate these themes to "here and now" feelings, perceptions, and behavior. For example, in a group where one patient was talking about a boss who favored certain employees, another the inconsistency of parents, and a third the injustices of the welfare system, the therapist could hear the theme of unfair authority figures. He could then relate this theme to a current stimulus such as the ward staff members seeming unfair because they transferred a patient to another facility. Patients would thereby be able to gain relief by the expression of intense affect, to understand the source of their current feelings, and would be permitted to question and clarify their concerns about the precipitating event.

There are times when the precipitating event stimulates group affects that are so intolerable that any interpretive attempt will lead to increased defensiveness and isolation among the whole group. Patients may be helped to discharge disturbing feelings, to connect with one another, and to master "here and now" tensions through displaced discussion and concrete problem solving.[38] For example, discussion of the food service, choosing T.V. programs, or sharing the telephone may provide opportunities for active problem solving and enable patients to resolve symbolically tensions that are too disorganizing to deal with directly.

The Leaderless Meeting

The leaderless meeting principally serves two therapeutic purposes. First, it increases group cohesiveness by adding an additional group meeting.[16] A brief hospital stay, coupled with the constraints of staff time, limits the time available for participation in groups. The leaderless meeting affords patients the opportunity to meet together more often, increasing the potential for group camaraderie and cohesion.

The second therapeutic purpose of a leaderless meeting is to foster patient responsibility.[15] In a setting where much of the responsibility for patients' well-being is assumed by the staff, it is important to encourage adult functioning and decision-making whenever possible. Stqff sanction for the leaderless meeting says to the patient, "We believe you are capable, responsible adults." Leaderless meetings promote problem-solving efforts.[52, 63] In addition, some patients are able to talk more freely and to express negative feelings toward the therapist and the institution without the therapist present.[52, 55, 64]

The therapist has the responsibility to organize the leaderless meeting and to expect the patients to attend. In order to foster patient autonomy, the therapist should refrain from asking about the content of the meeting unless it is raised by the patients, or if the meeting was clearly very stressful. If patients do not attend, this should be explored in subsequent leader-led meetings. Absence is usually indicative of lack of trust or feelings of extreme helplessness and passivity among group members. To allow for discussion of the leaderless meeting, when indicated, not more than one leaderless meeting should be held without an intervening leader-led meeting.

The leaderless meeting should not be used with groups exclusively comprised of severely disturbed patients. These patients require the active assistance of the leader to provide control and to safely connect them with others. They are also likely to experience a deep sense of abandonment by the absence of the therapist.

COUNTERTRANSFERENCE

Countertransference refers to the therapist's emotional reactions to the patient. (This chapter extends the classical definition of countertransference to include the therapist's *conscious* as well as unconscious and partly conscious attitudes and feelings towards the patient.) It provides the basis for empathy (i.e., an "emotional knowing" of the patient, resulting from the therapist's partial identification with the patient) and for intervention which is stimulated by the therapist's inner needs rather than the needs of the patient.

Countertransference that relates to the therapist's inner needs may be evoked by the therapist's human needs, his character vulnerabilities, and his reactions to individual group members and to group induced anxiety.[59] The therapist's need to be successful, to overcome feelings of anxiety or inferiority, his desire to be liked by patients, and his competitive feelings toward patients are all examples of countertransference. The therapist may also react emotionally to individual patients because they evoke feelings from his past or because the therapist identifies with the patient's projections. For example, a therapist may feel guilty in response to a patient's complaints about his lack of helpfulness.

Countertransference is more complex in both group situations[55, 59] and inpatient settings[5, 65] than it is in one-to-one or outpatient settings. In group therapy the sources for countertransference are geometrically increased by the number of patients and their interactions with one another and the therapist. Regressed inpatients evoke primitive anxieties which are further complicated by the abundance of projective mechanisms to which the therapist is exposed. These include projections of demoralization, hopelessness, and helplessness. Furthermore, as discussed earlier, the "here and now" of the inpatient group includes all interactions within the hospital milieu. The group therapist who holds additional responsibilities on the unit will therefore bring to the group feelings associated with his extragroup ward activities. These may include feelings evoked by a particular patient(s), by staff conflict, and by general ward tensions.

The therapist's awareness of his feelings towards patients can facilitate treatment, for it provides him clues about the meaning of patients' behavior.[65] For example, the therapist who feels ineffectual may recognize that the patient's provocative struggles with him belie profound feelings of helplessness on the patient's part, which are being passed on by a process of projective identification. (Projective identification is a defense whereby an individual projects a part of himself onto another and then *behaves* in response to this projection.[39]) If the therapist is unaware of his feelings, his interventions will be poorly informed and may create additional patient anxieties and tensions. For example, a therapist who feels guilty in response to the complaints of a patient may be overly solicitous to that patient and neglect the other group members. Or a therapist may be critical of the "resistant" patient, thereby injuring that patient's self-esteem and stimulating other patients' anxiety about who will be the next victim of a punitive, rejecting authority figure.

The therapist's capacity to manage countertransference feelings is dependent upon his self-awareness, his comfort with regressed patients and with his leadership role, and whether he feels supported by the milieu. Personal therapy, ward conferences, and supervision may all be used to help the therapist manage his countertransference. Personal therapy can facilitate the therapist's self-awareness, improve his self-assurance, and begin to work through character vulnerabilities and conflicts which may impede his work. Ward conferences provide an opportunity to share feelings with other staff and to gain greater understanding of a particular patient(s) or ward event(s). Finally, supervision provides the therapist with support through education and problem-solving. It also provides an opportunity to look carefully at how the therapist's feelings affect his responses to individual patients and to group process. Finally, and of particular importance, the supervisor mitigates the inpatient group therapist's susceptibility to overidentification with the patient's feelings of demoralization, hopelessness, and helplessness. By distinguishing reality from the projective mechanisms used by patients and by acknowledging the therapist's leadership accomplishments, the supervisor helps to reduce overidentification and to increase the therapist's empathic capacities and his sense of effectiveness.

SUMMARY

Though hospitalized patients present a wide range of symptomatology, they share many common experiences. These are the basis of and the material for the small therapy group. Feelings of demoralization, isolation, helplessness, and hopelessness, as well as increased dependency yearnings, may interfere with the patient's capacity to form a therapeutic alliance. Group therapy offers a number of "curative" factors which can mitigate these feelings, contain transference, and provide a corrective emotional experience. The goals of group therapy support ego recompensation by reality testing, increasing patient responsibility, strengthening self-esteem, and channeling aggression. The formation of a therapy group requires careful attention to the definition of group boundaries (e.g., patient selection and preparation, group composition, location, length, and frequency of meetings) in order to contain what is "in" the group. This enables the group therapist to utilize techniques that reduce patients' anxiety, promote healing interaction among group members, and facilitate clarification of patient's distorted perceptions and confused experiences. The therapist's awareness of his countertransference facilitates the group process and minimizes his vulnerability to overidentification with the patients' defeatist attitudes.

REFERENCES

1. Goffman E: *Asylums,* New York, Anchor Books, Doubleday & Co., 1961.
2. Rosenberg SD: The disculturation hypothesis and the chronic patient syndrome. Soc Psychiatry, *5:* 155–165, 1970.
3. Almond R: Issues in milieu treatment. Schizophr Bull, *13:* 12–26, 1975.
4. Klein RH: Inpatient group psychotherapy: Practical considerations and special problems. Int J Group Psychother, *27:* 201–213, 1977.
5. Adler G: Hospital treatment of borderline patients. Am J Psychiatry, *130:* 32–36, 1973.
6. Friedman HJ: Some problems of inpatient management with borderline patients. Am J Psychiatry, *126:* 299–304, 1969.
7. Mullan H, Rosenbaum M: *Group Psychotherapy: Theory and Practice,* ed. 2, New York, The Free Press, 1978.
8. Marsh LC: Group treatment of psychosis by the psychological equivalent of the revival. Ment Hyg, *15:* 328–349, 1931.
9. Wender L: The dynamics of group psychotherapy and its application. J Nerv Ment Dis, *84:* 54–60, 1936.
10. Bion WR: *Experiences in Groups,* New York, Basic Books, 1959.
11. Standish CT, Semrad EV: Group psychotherapy with psychotics. J Psychiatr Soc Work, *20:* 143–150, 1951.
12. Frank JD: Group therapy in the mental hospital, in Rosenbaum M, Berger M (eds): *Group Psychotherapy and Group Function,* New York, Basic Books, 1975.
13. Kibel HD: The rationale for the use of group psychotherapy for borderline patients in a short-term unit. Int J Group Psychother, *28:* 339–358, 1978.
14. Kibel HD: A conceptual model for short-term inpatient group psychotherapy. Am J Psychiatry, *138:* 74–80, 1981.
15. Maxmen JS, Tucker GJ, LeBow MD: Group techniques, in *Rational Hospital Psychiatry,* New York, Brunner/Mazel, 1974.
16. Maxmen JS: An educative model for inpatient group therapy. Int J Group Psychother, *28:* 321–338, 1978.
17. Maxmen JS: Helping patients survive theories: The practice of an educative model. Int J Group Psychother, *34:* 355–368, 1984.
18. Druck AB: The role of didactic group psychotherapy in short-term psychiatric settings. Group, *2:* 98–109, 1978.
19. Houlihan JP: Contribution of an intake group to psychiatric inpatient milieu therapy. Int J Group Psychother, *27:* 215–223, 1977.
20. Gruber LN: Group techniques for acutely psychotic inpatients. Group, *2:* 31–39, 1978.
21. Cory TL, Page D: Group techniques for effecting change in the more disturbed patient. Group, *2:* 149–155, 1978.
22. Erikson RC: Small-group psychotherapy with patients on a short stay ward: An opportunity for innovation. Hosp Community Psychiatry, *32:* 269–272, 1981.
23. Oldham JM: The use of silent observers as an adjunct to short-term inpatient group psychotherapy. Int J Group Psychother, *32:* 469–480, 1982.
24. Betcher WR: The treatment of depression in brief inpatient group psychotherapy. Int J Group Psychother, *33:* 365–385, 1983.
25. Russakoff LM, Oldham JM: Group Psychotherapy on a short-term treatment unit: An application of object relations theory. Int J Group Psychother, *34:* 339–354, 1984.
26. Maves PA, Schulz JW: Inpatient group treatment on short-term acute care units. Hosp Community Psychiatry, *36:* 69–73, 1985.
27. Yaloun ID: *Inpatient Group Psychotherapy,* New York, Basic Books, 1983.
28. Werner A, Campbell RJ, Frazier SH, Stone EM: *A Psychiatric Glossary,* ed. 5, Washington, D.C., American Psychiatric Association, 1980.
29. Blanck G, Blanck R: *Ego Psychology: Theory and Practice,* New York, Columbia University Press, 1974.
30. Yalom ID: *The Theory and Practice of Group Psychotherapy,* ed. 2, New York, Basic Books, 1975.
31. Maxmen JS: Group therapy as viewed by hospitalized patients. Arch Gen Psychiatry, *28:* 404–408, 1973.
32. Kibel HD: Group psychotherapy as an adjunct to milieu treatment with chronic schizophrenics. Psychiatr Q, *42:* 339–351, 1968.
33. Slavson SR: *A Textbook in Analytic Group Psychotherapy,* New York, International Universities Press, 1964.
34. Guttmacher JA, Birk L: Group therapy: What specific advantages? Compr Psychiatry, *12:* 546–556, 1971.
35. Battegay R: Group psychotherapy as a method of treatment in a psychiatric hospital, in de Schill S (ed): *The Challenge of Group Psychotherapy, Present and Future,* New York, International Universities Press, 1974.
36. Kaplan HI, Freedman AM, Sadock BJ: *Comprehensive Textbook of Psychiatry,* ed. 2, Baltimore, Williams & Wilkins, 1975.
37. Blanck G, Blanck R: *Ego Psychology II: Psychoanalytic Developmental Psychology,* New York, Columbia Universities Press, 1979.
38. Katz GA: The noninterpretation of metaphors in psychiatric hospital groups. Int J Group Psychother, *33:* 53–68, 1983.
39. Borriello JF: Group psychotherapy in a hospital system, in Wolberg LR, Aronson ML (eds): *Group Therapy: 1976—An Overview,* New York, Stratton Intercontinental Medical Book Corp., 1976.
40. Rice CA, Rutan JS: Boundary maintenance in inpatient therapy groups. Int J Group Psychother, *31:* 297–309, 1981.
41. Astrachan BM: Toward a social systems model of therapeutic groups. Soc Psychiatry, *5:* 110–119, 1970.
42. Klein RH, Kugel B: Inpatient group psychotherapy from a systems perspective: Reflections through a glass darkly. Int J Group Psychother, *31:* 311–328, 1981.

43. Levine H: Milieu biopsy: The place of the therapy group on the inpatient ward. Int J Group Psychother, *30:* 77–93, 1980.

44. Rutan JS, Alonso A: Group psychotherapy, in Lazar A (ed): *Outpatient Psychiatry, Diagnosis and Treatment,* Baltimore, Williams & Wilkins, 1980.

45. Levin S: Some comparative observations of psychoanalytically oriented group and individual psychotherapy. Am J Orthopsychiatry, *33:* 148–160, 1963.

46. Grunbaum H, Kates W: Whom to refer for group psychotherapy. Am J Psychiatry, *143:* 130–133, 1977.

47. Grobman J: The borderline patient in group psychotherapy: A case report. Int J Group Psychother, *31:* 297–309, 1981.

48. Cooper EJ: The pre-group: The narcissistic phase of development with the severely disturbed patient, in Wolberg LR, Aronson ML, Wolberg AR (eds): *Group Therapy 1978: An Overview,* New York, Stratton Medical Book Corp., 1978.

49. Kernberg OF: Borderline personality organization. J Am Psychoanal Assoc, *15:* 641–682, 1967.

50. Slavson SR: Group psychotherapy and the nature of schizophrenia. Int J Group Psychother, *11:* 3–31, 1961.

51. Singer DL, Astrachan BM, Gould LJ, Klein EB: Boundary management in psychological work with groups. J Appl Behav Sci, *11:* 137–176, 1975.

52. Becker RE, Harrow M, Astrachan B: Leadership and content in group psychotherapy. J Nerv Ment Dis, *150:* 316–353, 1970.

53. Bernard HS, Klein RH: Some perspectives on time limited group psychotherapy. Compr Psychiatry, *18:* 579–584, 1977.

54. Samuels AS: Use of group balance as a therapeutic technique. Arch Gen Psychiatry, *11:* 411–420, 1964.

55. Wolf A, Schwartz EK: *Psychoanalysis in Groups,* New York, Grune & Stratton, 1962.

56. Furst W: Homogeneous versus heterogeneous groups, in Rosenbaum M, Berger M (eds): *Group Psychotherapy and Group Function,* New York, Basic Books, 1963.

57. Rabin HM: Preparing patients for group psychotherapy. Int J Group Psychother, *20:* 135–152, 1970.

58. Fulkerson CC, Hawkins DM, Alden AR: Psychotherapy groups of insufficient size. Int J Group Psychother, *31:* 73–81, 1981.

59. Slavson SR: Sources of countertransference and group induced anxiety. Int J Group Psychother, *3:* 373–388, 1953.

60. Horowitz MJ, Weisberg PS: Techniques for the group psychotherapy of acute psychosis. Int J Group Psychother, *16:* 42–50, 1966.

61. Slavson SR: The phenomenology and dynamics of silence. Int J Group Psychother, *16:* 395–404, 1966.

62. Cutler MO: Symbolism and imagery in a group of chronic schizophrenics. Int J Group Psychother, *28:* 73–80, 1978.

63. Astrachan BM, Harrow M, Becker RE, Schwartz AH, Miller JC: The unled patient group as a therapeutic tool. Int J Group Psychother, *17:* 178–191, 1967.

64. Gould E, Garrigues CS, Scheikowitz K: Interaction in hospitalized patient-led and staff-led groups. Am J Psychother, *29:* 383–390, 1975.

65. Hannah S: Countertransference in in-patient group psychotherapy: Implications for technique. Int J Group Psychother, *34:* 257–272, 1984.

chapter 13

the adolescent and the young adult

Dean X. Parmelee, M.D.

The psychiatric hospitalization of an adolescent or young adult represents a crisis for the individual, his family, school, and community. A psychiatric unit has special tasks in the evaluation and treatment of this age group: (1) to stabilize the charged situation surrounding the crisis, (2) to assess developmental strengths and weaknesses of the patient and parents, and (3) to initiate a treatment plan and follow-up care which actively involves the patient and his family as well as his school and other community resources. This chapter summarizes the emotional development of the adolescent and the related parental responses during this phase, discusses the diagnostic approaches useful for the evaluation of the adolescent, describes the special philosophy and treatment techniques which an inpatient service must have to effectively treat this age group, discusses common management problems inherent in such a service, and reviews therapeutic modalities which are particularly useful in an inpatient setting.

THE DEVELOPMENTAL PROCESS OF ADOLESCENCE

As in other developmental stages, the passage through the years of adolescence and on into early adulthood (13–20 years of age) is difficult. However, the often held view that all adolescents have a tumultuous time has not held up to rigorous investigation.[1] Whether or not an individual will go through the adolescent years with the behavioral turmoil and disruptiveness towards self or others that requires psy-

chiatric intervention depends upon many factors: genetic constitution; resolution of earlier conflicts from the oral, anal, and Oedipal stages; parental support for growing independence and autonomy; and a community sensitive to the importance of providing a structured yet adaptable school system and sufficient jobs and activities to maximize channels for socialization, career choice, and nonregressive roles in the peer group.

The onset of puberty initiates a multitude of changes in an individual's biology and personality functioning. Biological changes, which give the hallmark and thrust to adolescence, usually surprise and often frighten the budding adolescent even if there has been much intellectual preparation through school, father-to-son or mother-to-daughter "talks," and peer group (street) initiation. Sexual feelings, fantasies, and activities add a dimension to life which, for varying periods of time, totally absorb the adolescent. Sexuality also prompts relationships (real or imaginary) which can be remembered for a lifetime and sets the groundwork for either a rich, fulfilling adulthood or one fraught with frustration, a sense of inadequacy, and emotional aloneness. From puberty and extending to early adulthood there occurs a maturation of cognitive functioning with its ability to conceptualize and organize experience[2, 3] and a growing sense of morality and one's place in the world.[4] Social maturation, representing the coalescence of development in the entire "biopsychosocial"[5] sphere, enables the adolescent to begin to control the biological impulses coming from within, to use them creatively through sublimation and relatedness to others, to remember and to integrate the affects and experiences from the past in planning the future, and to maintain an ethical and moral value system which adds integrity to a developing identity.

Parents experience the adolescent years and the entry into adulthood of their children with a variety of internal and external responses. For much of the period, there unfolds a series of realizations which push the parent through a developmental process of his or her own. Memories, attitudes, fears, and wishes from the parent's own adolescence, which may have been buried during earlier child-rearing times, surface and reverberate with the observations of and interactions with the growing adolescent child. The expectations which a parent held for a particular child at birth are brought more to the focus as the "final product" nears completion. Inevitably there is a mixture of disappointment and pride and, most adaptively, a parent will not look for or expect some outpouring of gratitude from his youth for his devotion, will not be too shocked or too hurt if there is bitter criticism for failings and deficiencies, and will realize that his son or daughter is increasingly responsible for the shape and course for his or her own life.

DEVELOPMENTAL TASKS OF THE ADOLESCENT AND YOUNG ADULT

Separation-Individuation

The biological growth of puberty and its attendant emotional changes rekindles for the adolescent and his parents remnants of a phase and possible crisis which took place between the ages of 18 and 36 months, namely, separation-individuation.[6, 7] For the toddler, rapid motility, a heightened curiosity about everything in sight, and a quest to do more without help leads to a period of testing-out what can or cannot be done alone while simultaneously learning how parents feel about increasing independence. For some parents, this period is traumatic for it signifies a loss of the child's close dependence on

them. If their own self-esteem is based upon being the "needed ones," they may be unable to genuinely feel parental pride in their youngster's progress. Parental withdrawal from actively encouraging independence and even support of regression may then occur. When this happens the child is left feeling that to grow, to become and feel more competent, and to explore the world will increase the hazard of upsetting mother and father and possibly losing their love and affection.

The dilemma for the adolescent is similar. To be more independent of parents and to behave, appear, and feel different and separate from parents causes one to run the risk of having parents feel hurt, become angry, or not give continued and necessary support. The adolescent "tests this out" frequently throughout the whole period of adolescence and even into young adulthood. Consider these three examples of adolescents of different ages who are expressing their dependency needs while trying to establish independence:

Thirteen-year-old Billy, now called "Slick" by his buddies, has just finished an evening of bowling and pizza. He wipes the cheese and tomato sauce spill from his black leather jacket, lights up his 20th cigarette for the day, and struts over to the pay phone. "Mom, it's almost eleven, come and get me."

Mr. and Mrs. N. are puzzled and somewhat annoyed with their 15-year-old, Jack. He has said months earlier that he wanted to get his Social Security number and work papers for a summer job. It is now May and he has done nothing about it, despite offers to help fill out the Social Security form. Prodding brought only a "Later." Finally, when the gentle prodding moved into nagging, he burst out, "You want me to get a job so you don't have to give me any allowance, and if I do something you don't like, you can throw me out."

Nineteen-year-old Michelle had not surprised her parents by wanting to go out of state for college. She had always been what they described as the "independent type." However, after her first year they were surprised to add up collect calls and travel expenses for coming home on every vacation and many long weekends. When her father asked her why she always brought home a bag or two of laundry for her mother to do, she laughed and said, "I guess I have to know if you still care about me."

IDENTITY

The solidification of an "identity"[8] is a second developmental task for adolescents. Though the foundations for identity are laid during earlier years, it is during the teenage years and into early adulthood that there occurs an integration of past experiences, identifications with important others, and opportunities in new social roles. Usually a "career" is chosen and, when done without undue pressure from others, it catalyzes a sense of meaning to life, one's meaning to others, and a capacity to realistically plan a future. Two examples demonstrate how two young persons from very different backgrounds struggle with this in the process of finding out what they want to do in life.

Danny, age 16, though quite bright, was too restless in a classroom setting to do well, especially after his father, a blue collar worker, died. He dropped out of school and worked as a janitor for a department store for 2 years. When not working, he often retreated to his garage room "out back" and did pencil, ink, or charcoal sketches. After a year or so, he paid for some art courses at the museum and at age 19 he decided he wanted to be an artist. It took another 2 years to save enough money to go to art school full-time; and when he landed a commercial artist's job after another year, he commented that dropping out of school and cleaning floors for several years gave him "time to think" and "growing room" to decide who he was.

Born to a couple of academic physicians, Margaret had been accustomed to the idea that she would be one too. Straight A's throughout high school and 2 years of college left her feeling pleased but somehow unsure of her future. She joined the Peace Corps for 2 years in Boliva and wrote her parents prior to returning to college, "I had to do the unexpected to find out how strong I really am. Being a wiz in school has always been easy. Living here so much on my own has brought out more of me than I knew was there. I'm ready to go on to medical school because it will now mean something to me."

MUTUALITY

A third important task for the adolescent and young adult involves the development of mutuality. This implies the capacity to deal with others in a nonmanipulative, cooperative, and respectful fashion and to be able to sustain a sense of intimacy with and commitment to significant others, i.e., girlfriend, boyfriend, friends. A more mature sexuality unfolds. "Sex" is no longer a simple act of discharging tension or "proving" one's adequacy to self or others. Sexual behavior becomes an expression of mutual caring and shared excitement and pleasure between two partners. Parents, although probably still viewed as old fashioned and unchangeable, are considered to be helpful rather than just occasionally useful and are seen as potential allies for the child-rearing years ahead. Others in school or work who were once feared or regularly challenged as authority figures come to be seen as being more benign and possibly less exacting. As mutuality becomes more evident in their son or daughter, parents experience relief, for there is no longer a sense of struggle in interaction, a need to set "limits," or a worry about "what will become of" their child.

PSYCHIATRIC HOSPITALIZATION OF AN ADOLESCENT OR YOUNG ADULT

Having reviewed the emotional and developmental tasks of the "normal" adolescent and young adult, we will now turn to a description of the reasons for and process of a psychiatric hospitalization. With the growing number of adolescents and young adults taking up hospital beds in the United States,[9] we must keep in mind that there are a variety of hospital settings for this age group: state hospitals, general hospital psychiatric wards for adults and adolescents, private hospitals either with all adolescent wards or mixed adult/adolescent, and pediatric wards in general or children's hospitals with some beds specified for psychiatric cases. Wards can be described as "locked" and "unlocked" or "secure" and "least restrictive." The clinician working with adolescents and young adults must know what facilities in the community are appropriate for which psychiatric disorders. He must also know the treatment philosophies of the hospital programs, for some may be regressive and foster dependency while others may expect "too much" maturity and be unable to promote increasing levels of responsibility.

When Should a Youth be Hospitalized?

This is a controversial subject. The Joint Commission on Accreditation of Hospitals,[10] The American Medical Association,[11] and the American Psychiatric Association[12] have all attempted to establish hospitalization criteria, of which clinicians need to be aware. In general, hospitalization is indicated if:

1. The young person's behavior or threatened behavior indicates that his life or someone else's is in danger and that the family or other support system cannot provide safety. This may include episodes of drug abuse, often hallucinogens, amphetamines, and cocaine, in which the level of unpredictability creates potential for life-threatening behavior. It also includes psychotic states in which there may be eminent danger.

2. A young person has had a prolonged period of disturbing and disruptive behavior for which outpatient intervention has been unsuccessful or refused. Such behaviors include: physical or intense verbal fights with family and peers, truancy, school failure when grade placement has been appropriate, drug and alcohol abuse, running away, promiscuity, and increasing isolative or withdrawn behavior. Often these behaviors occur in the context of considerable family turmoil, and the only way to find out "what's going on" is to hospitalize one or more of the members of the family. In such a situation, it's important to clarify from the start that there is a family problem as well as the problems of the identified parent.

3. The young person and the family have been in outpatient treatment for some time with either no progress or persistent resistance to change. The clinician may then elect the more intense and exploratory therapeutic environment of a hospital as necessary to elicit hidden data and to design a new therapeutic strategy.

4. The youth has been requested or required to enter a hospital by the court for a formal psychiatric evaluation. Issues may involve custody, questions of competence (if over 16), criminal responsibility, and presence or absence of significant psychiatric illness prior to sentencing or as part of pretrial hearing.

ADMISSION TO THE PSYCHIATRIC HOSPITAL

Once the decision to hospitalize an adolescent or young adult is made, the clinician begins a methodical diagnostic and treatment evaluation and a formulation of the goals for the hospitalization. The attending clinician must be active with the patient and family in letting them know:

1. What kind of hospital has been chosen—private, locked or unlocked.
2. What tests will be performed—laboratory, psychological, EEG, and other neuropsychiatric evaluations.
3. What types of therapy are offered—psychopharmacology, electroconvulsive therapy, individual, group, family, behavioral, psychotherapy.
4. What are the requirements of hospitalization in terms of cost and level of family participation.
5. How long it will take to have sufficient information to plan treatment and to establish a discharge date.

Many inpatient programs which serve adolescents and adults insist on the family's active participation from the beginning. This is essential in diffusing scapegoating of the patient and giving the message to the patient that the hospital should not be seen as a "new, better home with more understanding parents." No admission should be scheduled, except in life-threatening emergencies, without there being a clear understanding between the parents and the clinician that their active participation throughout hospitalization is mandatory. Their responsibilities as parents do not end with the admission papers; rather they can expect to learn how to be more effective and help their youngster grow up. Parents who express great relief with the admission will be difficult to engage in a meaningful process of change. Most therapy appointments are held during "working" hours, and parents need to make arrangements to attend. The clinician may want to offer a letter to the parents' employers requesting flexibility of working time for "medical reasons."

Nursing staff play a central role at the time of admission, and they should participate in the initial family and individual interviews, be introduced as integral members of the evaluation and treatment process, and orient a new patient and family to all aspects of the hospital environment. Information about the new environment should include:

1. Rules about use of foul language and threats of or use of violence.
2. Regulations as to remaining on or leaving the unit and grounds.
3. Hours for bedtime, visiting, and timed therapeutic absences.
4. Expectations for tidy bedroom, appropriate dress, and respectful manner in communicating with peers, adults, and family.
5. Times and locations for all required meetings.

The Diagnostic Process

The diagnostic process for the hospitalized adolescent or young adult requires a multifaceted approach, of which the descriptive psychiatric assessment is only a part. Along with a thorough medical and neurological evaluation, the thrust of the diagnostic process should be along developmental lines. The data is obtained from interviews with the patient, parents, family, and teachers; observations by the nursing staff; and psychological and educational testing.

The diagnostic process should attempt to answer the following questions: (1) What is the level of psychosocial development? (2) How far along is the movement for separation and individuation with parents and family? (3) What is the quality of relationships with peers and authority figures? (4) Is the level of school performance parallel to intellectual and social capacities? (5) Is serious psychopathology present, as evidenced by antisocial acts, firesetting, bizarre and idiosyncratic thinking, and persistent suicidal preoccupation? (6) Given that various psychotherapeutic approaches are avail-

able, what approaches are going to work best during and after the hospitalization?

Mental Status Examination

The formal mental status examination with an adolescent is often regarded as a chore to be avoided. Antagonism, negativism, and hostility can make for a most difficult and embarrassing encounter. Often the adolescent is written off as "too uncooperative to be formally interviewed." Nevertheless, a premium must be placed on finding some way to talk with or otherwise interact nonverbally with the adolescent in order to obtain data for the mental status examination. For example:

Joseph, age 17, was admitted because he had been caught stealing and then wearing women's clothes. The psychiatric resident responsible for the intake interview could not elicit even nods to yes or no questions of the mental status examination. He did learn afterwards from the parents that Joseph had grown up on a dairy farm and was generally very active physically. Before leaving for the day, the resident asked Joe to play ping pong. The invitation was accepted and the resident learned how a dairy farm is managed, how cows are milked, how milk goes to market, and even how prices are set. The lad's speech, memory, and cognitive processes were intact; there was also no indication of delusional thinking or other evidence of formal thought disorder. The following day's ping pong game allowed for further nonintrusive questioning as well as some spontaneous talk about the "problem."

As with adult patients, questions about suicidal thinking and behavior should not be shunned. The incidence of suicide by adolescents has increased dramatically, as has the increased use of guns for suicide.[15] Ask about plans, impulsive ideas, the presence of a gun in the parents' or neighbor's home, dreams about killing oneself. "Accidental" behaviors should never be overlooked and passed off as "accidents" by the examiner.

Sixteen-year-old Karen was admitted following an overdose of 100 aspirins. During an initial interview, in inquiring about the history of feelings to kill herself, the examiner asked about "accidents" over the past year. She laughed and told how a month earlier she was accidentally "shocked" by her curling iron in the bathroom. It was on the sink, she was washing her hair, and father had always told her never to have it near water. Further discussion revealed that she had recently stopped wearing seat belts in the car and was always wishing for "some accident to end it all."

Interview with Parents

Much information must be obtained from the parents of the hospitalized adolescent or young adult. As with establishing rapport with any patient, trust and a working relationship with the parents is essential for the diagnostic evaluation. When a youth has been hospitalized, the parents frequently feel at fault or are angry. They are sometimes relieved. The clinician must be cautious not to be or appear judgmental, especially when the history reveals episodes of abuse, neglect, or incest. Conducting the interview with an attitude of neutrality, searching for clues as to why the current crises occurred, and offering oneself as a "consultant" to the parents as to how to best meet the needs rather than wants of their son or daughter will elicit considerably more data than a simple checklist of questions. One must review with the parents, either together or separately, the following alerts and should elicit their questions about diagnosis and prognosis.

1. The history of events leading to the hospitalization and "the last straw."
2. Past history including major life changes such as moves and separations; the early developmental data, such as birth history, seizure history, surgeries, medications, and school performance.
3. Family history. In addition to medical illnesses in family members, has there been a psychiatric hospitalization, alcoholism, or trouble with the law? Did any relative ever commit suicide or disappear?
4. Marital history. How did the parents meet? Was the child wanted? How did they share parenting, if at all? What have been the marital issues since the patient entered adolescence? How are they coping with their son or daughter's being hospitalized?

Many clinicians find it difficult to separately interview the adolescent and the parents because of some "potential" break of trust or confidentiality. In these cases, another person is appointed to gather the history from parents. Sometimes this interview of the parents and the subsequent working with them is not felt to be as important as the "therapy" with the adolescent or young adult. I do not hold to this division of therapeutic labor because it can lead to, if not further, the young person's idea that his problems stem from his "awful" parents. This division may also give the therapist a false sense of relationship and promote "saving" the patient. Furthermore, parents must feel accepted and supported directly by the clinician in order to be able to risk making some changes in their attitudes towards and behaviors with their son or daughter.

Educational History and Psychoeducational Testing

Even though they occur over a period of several years, school and college years are the closest events to a pubertal rite which our society offers. High school or college for the adolescent and young adult is a major arena for the demonstration of competencies in several areas of development: cognitive, interactional, and physical. The young person admitted to an inpatient psychiatric service will usually have a history of attendance, learning, or conduct problems in school. If he has begun college, the downfall is often described as "too much pressure." Exploring the patient's feelings about school and obtaining information on attendance, grades, and conduct can begin a process of calling to task what the young person is doing with his own life. This exploration can enforce one message which an inpatient experience should give: "You are not powerless and it is time to take responsibility for your life." Furthermore, the objective assessment of the school performance and school program can lead to the design of a more effective special needs education plan, if indicated.

Seventeen-year-old Bobby was hospitalized after 3 years of family turmoil, truancy, school failure, and minor run-ins with the law. In an early therapy appointment he said he saw no reason to learn algebra, earth science, or any of those "useless things." His therapist simply asked why not drop out of school.

B: "What would I do? Nobody would hire me."

T: "They're not going to hire you in 3 more years anyway. You're not going to graduate."

B: "Well, I want to pass those dumb courses but I never can concentrate. I want things right away, I hate to wait. Besides, it's my mother and jerks like you who want me to go to school."

T: "Then don't. Why waste your time? You're over 16, your mother has given up trying to control you anyway. It's all yours now, you can't blame her."

B: "Well, maybe I should learn how to put up with stuff and people I hate. Other kids do it. I think they kiss everybody's ass, but they'll stay out of jail."

This interchange initiated meetings with the guidance counselor, and a program of work study was started before leaving the hospital. This patient might have started a year or two earlier with such an individualized program, but he was always absent and unwilling to explore alternatives. The school officials had long since given up on him. The role of the clinican in such a case is paramount. School officials feel relieved him. The role of the clinican in such a case is paramount. School officials feel relieved that someone else may help them and that the patient

can re-enter the school system with a program more suitable to his needs. Likewise, for the young adult in college, there needs to be communication between the hospital clinician, the school dean, and the health service of the college.

In most cases the administration of a full battery of psychological and educational tests is indicated. Most commonly, the tests selected are those described in Table 13.1. An experienced tester can elicit considerable data towards a more accurate psychiatric diagnosis as well as provide objective information on intellectual and academic levels of achievement, which school and college personnel especially appreciate.

ADOLESCENT INPATIENT TREATMENT SERVICE

Design of the Therapeutic Milieu

When the administration of a hospital has decided that the psychiatric program will accept and treat adolescents and young adults, it must be prepared for changes throughout the institution.[13] The psychiatric unit, whether it will be for adults and adolescents or exclusively for adolescents, must carefully assess

Table 13.1.
Psychological and Educational Tests Useful in Evaluating Adolescents and Young Adults

Test	Format and Features for Age Group
Wechsler Adult Intelligence Scale (WAIS)	Eleven subtests, ages 16 and above, taps various aspects of intellectual functioning. Verbal and performance IQ's and full scale IQ based on age levels.
Wide Range Achievement Test	Subtests for academic and grade level screening.
Bender (Visual Motor)-Gestalt Test	Patient asked to copy geometric designs. Totally nonverbal. Yields information about perceptual-motor maturity, impulse control, motility management. May be correlated with brain damage.
Benton Revised Visual Retential Test	Geometric designs to copy. Nonverbal. More objective than Bender for measuring possible brain damage.
Rorschach Technique	Ten inkblots for eliciting verbal associations. Projective, lack of structure in contrast to Wechsler Intelligence School for Children (WISC), Bender, Benton, Achievement tests. Valuable for assessment of personality structure.
Thematic Apperception Test (TAT)	Projective. Pictures are stimuli for making up a story. Useful for revealing personality structure, interpersonal perceptions and conflicts.
Sentence Completion Text (SCT)	Incomplete sentences eliciting responses which may be used to tap conflict areas and level of ego development.
Draw A Person-Family Test	Graphomotor projective. Patient draws a person, then one of the opposite sex. Assesses body image, self-concept, attitudes toward sexual development and acceptance of sex role.

strengths, weaknesses, and priorities, and it must be clear to staff, patients, and the hospital what the treatment philosophy is for this unit and its patient population. This written philosophy, drawn up by the staff of a unit, can also provide guidelines for the more practical management of the unit. Unit rules and regulations, admissions policies, staffing patterns, and clear role definitions and responsibilities for both staff and patients will clarify philosophy and articulate management guidelines.

As was mentioned earlier, there are several types of inpatient services for adolescents and young adults. To be maximally effective, treatment must grow out of a philosophy which will promote a young person's acceptance of fuller responsibility for all of his actions, thoughts, and feelings, and which will assist his parents in moving away from infantilizing struggles and attitudes. All in all, no matter what diagnostic grouping an inpatient service treats, the goal is to provide an environment, a "therapeutic milieu,"[14] in which "growing up" can take place for the young person and his family. The following four points are useful in drawing up a statement of treatment philosophy.

1. Expectations for the patient's proper hospital behavior are parallel to those in society. The unit is prosocial, that is, one learns to be respectful to peers, staff, and family at all times.

2. A patient cannot stay in the hospital forever. The amount of time necessary is the time needed to be able to use outpatient treatment resources. The baseline assumption is that there will be a return to home and school with new strengths.

3. Parents are not to be blamed. They are to be helped in becoming more effective parents.

4. Psychotherapy does not occur only in the therapist's office. Nursing staff are not "babysitters" and the only "limit setters." All personnel, from the housekeeper to the director, share the responsibility of confronting immature behavior and serving as models for "growing up."

Common Management Issues

The following management issues arise frequently in the inpatient treatment of adolescents and young adults.

Profanity, Aggression, and Violence

The disturbed adolescent struggles to maintain control over his aggressive impulses. His peer group may or may not help channel these impulses constructively. The frequent and abusive use of profanity represents a loss of control for which the adolescent is asking for external controls. The use of profanity should be forbidden on the unit. However, the consequences for its use should depend on the treatment plan of the individual patient. Consider these examples:

Laurie, age 16, was a tyrant at home. The slightest frustration or limits set on her behavior resulted in intense rage expressed by rapid fire vulgarities. Her parents became so afraid of provoking her that they increased the free rein she already had. Once on the unit, she started immediately with her choicest four-letter epithets. The nursing staff and other patients quickly let her know that she had to find better ways of communicating her fury because she would be ostracized and would be spending most of the time in her room until she could be more respectful of others. A month later, after finally settling down, she told everyone in a group meeting she felt "more in control" of herself and better about herself because "people wouldn't let themselves be treated badly by me."

Tom, a 20-year-old schizophrenic, was slowly recuperating from his second psychosis. A major dynamic issue for him was learning how to deal with his domineering mother. In family meetings he was encouraged to speak up to her. She herself asked him to help "control" her. The nursing staff worked on this issue with him because he was equally passive with everyone on the ward, sometimes appearing catatonic. One day, surprising all, he screamed at a nurse when she politely asked him to pick up his room, "You do it, you f--bitch!" Tom immediately became terrified at his loss of control and the potential for revenge from the nurse. He ran out of the room. The nurse caught up to him, reassured him he was not going to be physically punished and let him know that he could say "No" to her without the swearing and that she would still like him. The next day in psychodrama he was able to practice "with feeling" how he would set his mother straight in the next family meeting.

Threats and acts of violence towards others or property are also forbidden. They are forbidden in society, and in this regard, as well as in others, the psychiatric ward is no different. One cannot hide behind "mental illness" or have license to be violent. Whenever there is a threat or act of destructiveness towards property or person, it should be addressed quickly with everyone on the unit. Adolescents and young adults who have a history of such behavior have to be told from the start of the hospitalization that the hospital units is not a jail, that such acts may result in transfer to a locked unit, and that the hospitalization may be the last chance to get control of these destructive impulses before the penal system is involved. Acutely psychotic individuals, driven by internal aggressive stimuli as they often are, settle down more quickly when they perceive that the milieu maintains a strict attitude of safety for persons and property.

All members of the milieu staff have to be consistently watchful for small signs that the patient may be losing his sense of respect for others and for their safety. Usually escalation of acting-out behavior occurs when there is a staff failure to observe this breakdown early and to intervene quickly. Many psychiatric units serving adolescents have closed their adolescent service following episodes of dangerous, out of control group behavior. Cameron,[16] in his review of the beginnings of the adolescent unit at Bellevue Hospital, demonstrated that such episodes usually represent the end product of a series of interactions between staff and patients. The starting point is often as simple as a statement to a staff member as "go to hell." If the staff member is feeling even slightly intimidated by the youth and does not wish to "cause more trouble" he will try to appear indifferent to such a comment. Invariably, however, there will be further comments and actions by this patient or other patients, all increasingly provocative. Consider this vignette showing how chaos developed when the early signs of deterioration in a milieu's equanimity were neglected.

At morning report, staff were aghast at the descriptions of the previous night. Two runaways, several holes kicked in walls, one staff member injured by a flying object, four patients (adolescents) restrained because of assault or threatened assault. Over the next 2 days the following sequence of events was pieced together and reviewed. Earlier in that day, one of the more angry adolescents had stormed into her room after bolting from a family meeting and then refused to talk. She taped a sign on her door: "Stay out—enter at your own risk." The sign was still on the door the next morning for no one wanted to "upset her more" by insisting that she remove it. She continued to be defiant and uncontrollable the next day and incited the rest of the kids to defend her because the "bad" staff was "abusing" her. By bedtime it was "staff against patients."

The use of restraints and seclusion is a controversial subject both therapeutically and legally. For adolescents and young adults the use of restraints and seclusion on a psychiatric unit runs counter to a growth-promoting treatment philosophy. Restraints and seclusion represent the ultimate in external control, and the use of them generally discourages the patient's wish to gain fuller control of himself. With nonpsychotic, character-disordered, male adolescents in particular, there is often an attitude of "machismo" about getting into a big enough struggle to end up in restraints or seclusion or both. Furthermore, the entire process of placing someone who is "out of control" into restraints or seclusion is usually viewed by patients as a "violent and scary act," regardless of the situation or the individual involved. When restraint or seclusion is absolutely necessary, as with an acutely psychotic patient, it is paramount that the staff involved immediately clarify to other patients why this was necessary and convey the expectation that everyone be in control of his impulses.

Elopement

Eloping or "running away" from a psychiatric unit is a multidetermined phenomenon for the adolescent or young adult. The therapeutic approach to elopement should begin at the time of admission. The young person should be informed that he cannot run from problems by "taking off," for they go with him. This may sound simplistic, but it gives a message that will be repeated throughout the patient's entire psychotherapeutic experience, whether inpatient or outpatient. If a patient elopes, upon his return, in addition to standard consequences (punishment) for the runaway behavior, such as floor restriction, the young person must be required to explain his action in terms other than, "I felt like it," or "I don't know." As with all other acting out behaviors, it is essential to stress that action needs to be replaced with words and that the feelings which occur before the action, e.g., "I was bored; I was too depressed to stay around," have to be tolerated.

Psychotic adolescents, or those seriously suicidal, will "run" from a unit when they feel unsafe. Clues to an impending "take-off" commonly occur and should be watched for from the psychotically ill or suicidal young person. Appropriate measures in response to such clues include one-to-one nursing observation, restriction to common areas, or even "locking" the unit. Nonpsychotic "runners" do so to be "caught" and to come back to tell of their exciting adventures. It is remarkable how the ambivalence of the independence-dependency struggle is played out with "running away":

John C., age 18, saw no reason to be in the hospital. To his mind, his parents should have been hospitalized. One night he kicked open an alarmed fire escape door and ran off (the unit was not locked). He hitched to a neighboring town and became "suspicious" that a police officer was watching him. He went over to the police officer and said, "I know you're looking for me, aren't you?"

The chronic "runner," usually female, is often struggling with the issue of closeness. The chronic "runner" tests the milieu from the first day of hospitalization by behaviorally saying, "If you really want to help me, find me." As staff and milieu members readily demonstrate their care and interest, they then begin to find out that the patient feels "you are getting too close."

If the clinician can continue to clarify and confront the patient for several ep-

isodes without becoming too angry and discouraged and help the staff deal with their despair so they don't "drive away the patient," there will be a decrease in the frequency of elopement and an increase in the verbalization of affect. Simultaneously, the parents of a runaway, who have probably been suffering with the problem for years, can be helped to understand this dynamic and to move beyond their constant state of anger and worry.

Drugs and Alcohol

It is rare for an adolescent or young adult to enter a psychiatric hospital and not have had more than a passing experience with drugs and alcohol. The experimentation with and abuse of various mood and mind-modifying substances can be of epidemic proportions in some communities. The psychiatric hospitalization of an adolescent or young adult can be the first opportunity for the clinician to see the patient "drug free" and to begin to make drug-taking behaviors dystonic. Many will enter the hospital boasting "everybody does it." Yes, many do, unfortunately, and "They may or may not end up here. You are here and have a problem." The group process of the milieu can be the most effective tool in changing the view that "doing drugs (alcohol) is fun." This attitudinal change starts with the entire staff insisting on a drug-free environment and recognizing that a young hospitalized person has the kinds of problems that require a drug-free life style.

After his weekend pass home, Leon brought a decorative plastic mirror made by one of the more popular liquor brands. He hung it up over his bed along with the basketball star poster. During a staff meeting later in the week, the discussion focused on several episodes of patients talking about planning to get "plastered" when they went home on pass. There was also an incident of an empty liquor bottle found in a trash barrel. The staff member who had checked Leon in upon return that past weekend had not confronted him about the mirror because "all normal kids have them on their walls."

In the course of a careful diagnostic evaluation of a young person and family, it is often found that parents have serious drug and alcohol problems. The hospitalization of the "identified patient" can serve as a way to open up the parents or other family members' drinking/drug problem and to initiate therapeutic interventions.

Peter, age 19, entered the hospital at the recommendation of his college dean because of repeated episodes of drunkenness. His parents, well-to-do and seen as pillars of society, were shocked. For several weeks Peter persisted in saying that his "getting a buzz on" was no problem. Finally, he blew up at his parents in a family therapy session. "Who are you to tell me I have a problem? Both of you drink like skunks every night after work. Dad, you even passed out driving—that's how you wrecked your car last year." Peter began to work on his own problem when his parents sought treatment for themselves.

Timed Therapeutic Absence

The timed therapeutic absence (TTA) is integral to that nonregressive milieu philosophy of expecting the patient's return to home, family, and school (college). At the admission interviews it is wise to inform the adolescent and his parents that, at first, day passes, then weekend passes, are started as soon as family meetings have started and that a major goal of the treatment plan is to teach them how they might get along better when together. There is often much resistance to the ideal of early, regular, and frequent passes home. Resistance can take the form of the young person dreaming of a home away from home and having more understanding parents; of parents who are too relieved to have their disturbed and disturbing teenager someplace "safe"; of staff members feeling that the patient is "not ready" and that they are better parents; and, worst of all, nowadays, third party payers who see such passes as meaning that the patient does not need to be in the hospital if he can go out on pass! For the psychotic or suicidal young person, passes should be part of the treatment plan as soon as the danger period has passed.

The young adult needs TTA's as much as an adolescent, even when the treatment plan may be "to get him out of the home." The design of the TTA can include time at home in decreasing amounts, time looking for alternative living, and actual staying at alternative living situations such as a halfway house. If the patient has finished high school and is unemployed, then time must be arranged and built-in for job counseling, training, and hunting. Starting back to work or college before discharge from the hospital ensures more vigorous testing of the gains made during the hospitalization.

THERAPEUTIC MODALITIES

Individual Psychotherapy

Individual psychotherapy during a psychiatric hospitalization occurs in a variety of situations and times as the patient's needs mandate. The routine activities of the day, visits home, "doing nothing," are all grist for the mill of psychotherapy. Most adolescents and many young adults will begin individual psychotherapy with much skepticism, often making for a trying experience for patient and psychotherapist alike. With the exception of individuals with sociopathic-antisocial character disorders, individual psychotherapy is highly recommended for adolescents and young adults whose problems are severe enough to require hospitalization.

The standard, 50-minute, sit-down, patient-does-all-the-talking session is frequently unrealistic at the start. The therapist must be prepared to have brief, 15–20 minute daily sessions with the acutely psychotic patient, be very quick witted and limit-setting with the hostile and cantankerous, and energetic enough to play ball or draw pictures with the nonverbal. Over a period of a couple of weeks with a persistent therapist and a supportive milieu, most older adolescents and younger adults will settle in and use the session time to talk and even reflect. Younger adolescents need more time to develop some capacity to observe themselves and verbalize affect. The more distrustful adolescent or young adult also needs more time to make sure that the therapist will survive the patient's anger without retaliating.

As soon as dialogue has begun between therapist and patient, goals for individual psychotherapy should be articulated. This is usually reassuring to the adolescent because psychotherapy can seem so nebulous and open-ended. Goals, when kept small and within reach, create a sense of order to psychotherapy and keep the regressive pull of transference needs at a controllable and nonthreatening range. Typical goals are:

Being able to spend time with parents without full-blown arguments or fights.

Being able to concentrate on school work for 1 full hour per day.

Being able to tell boys "no" and not fear rejection.

Being able to stay for a full therapy session.

Being able to "talk-out" self-destructive feelings instead of cutting wrists.

Not "running" for 2 days in a row.

When small goals are achieved, there develops a healthy and firm alliance between patient and therapist. "Therapeutic alliance" means much more than a sense of "liking" in the relationship. Alliance develops over time as the patient realizes the therapist is not going "to save" him or "give in" to childish demands and that the therapist is an "ally" in being able to change immature and self-defeating ways of living. I do not support the older model of therapeutic orientation in which a therapist/administrator split is created on the unit. Many a therapist welcome this older model because it takes him away from having to "struggle" with the adolescent patient, thereby keeping their "therapeutic alliance." This is nonsense. Struggles and limit-setting provide the real substance for a therapeutic alliance. The therapist who is afraid to engage with the adolescent to prevent regressive behavior is not going to be helpful. I know that there is trouble in a therapy if I hear an adolescent say that his therapist wants him to ask someone else "for permission" to do something or to be given a discharge date, or whatever.

Family Therapy

Over the past 30 years, family therapy has developed into a major and effective treatment modality for disturbed adolescents and young adults.[17] In large part this has occurred because the adolescent and young adult years are characteristically unsettled and far more subject to the family context. Therapeutic interventions made with everyone, or more than one, in a family can yield more effective and lasting results. Many young persons correctly perceive that the situation will be hard for them to change, if not impossible, if their parents and others in the family will not try to do so as well. The crisis created by hospitalization can usually allow the clinician to get all members of a family, including grandparents, involved in treatment.

There are many models and theories of family therapy, all of which have merit, and the clinician is encouraged to be familiar with the practice of each.[18-22] No one approach is perfect for every case. The intensive diagnostic evaluation process which a hospital setting provides yields a great deal of information on how the entire family system operates and on the problems of its particular members. The clinician must use this data to design a family therapy program suited to the needs and dynamics of the case, not according to one or another family therapy school.

The first family therapy meeting is best scheduled on the day of admission or within a short time thereafter. At this meeting, the clinician asks each member to state his views of the family's problems, which allows him to challenge the assumption that all problems stem from the identified patient. Ground rules for subsequent meetings are also set at this meeting and include frequency (usually once per week), who should attend, what topics are for the family meetings, and what topics are for individual therapy or parent-marital guidance therapy.

Lisa, age 18, entered the hospital following a suicide attempt with her mother's sleeping pills. There was a several year history of intense family fighting. The first family meeting predictably started off stormy, with yelling, screaming, and threats of violence between members. The parents became engaged in a screaming fit between themselves about their nonexistent sex lives with each other and accusations about outside affairs. Lisa smiled with her parents' increasing hostility towards each other and denied having done so when confronted. The clinician forcefully established some rules for the remainder of the meeting and subsequent meetings: (1) no threats of violence; (2) one person talking at a time; (3) parents' more personal, marital issues to be dealt with separately, away from the children; and (4) a trial use of videotape for members to learn more about their nonverbal behaviors with each other.

The problems of Lisa and her family typify some of the family problems seen in and treated effectively in the inpatient setting. The hospital environment serves as a safe container for the family's intense feelings for one another, while helping them to begin to observe rather than always react. Needed boundaries between family members can also be set. By looking at such a family developmentally, goals and strategies can be determined to assist growth of individual members as well as improve the family unit's overall functioning.

Group Psychotherapy

Group psychotherapy offers the adolescent and young adult an experience which can greatly supplement the work of individual and family therapy. For individuals with sociopathic antisocial personalities, the group psychotherapy setting can provide some of the socialization processes which never occurred in their families and probably will never occur elsewhere. Unfortunately, more than one or two persons with this diagnosis in a therapy group of 8–10 leads to destruction to the group. It is important to compose a group with persons of varied levels of psychopathology and at different stages of hospitalization. Psychotic young persons often need time to recompensate before they can tolerate some "heavy talk" about sex, families, and each other's relationships. When they do seem ready to join, the therapist must be alert to providing additional structure and concrete goals so that they are not overwhelmed by the freer affect of the others.

For the first 2 months, Ken, age 17, a psychotic, refused to join the family therapy meetings. In individual therapy he spoke little and only about how his parents were determined to "destroy" him. In the adolescent group, which met four times per week, he observed how others were struggling with their families, usually in a more healthy fashion. He became able to tolerate confrontation about his delusions. A big project then developed in the group: getting Ken to communicate with his parents. First, the group members helped him write a letter to them, then they helped him play-act the first phone call, then finally they spent several sessions role playing members of his family and the "first" family therapy session. After this first session he was able to go with his parents out to dinner and continued to make progress.

Parents and Multifamily Groups

Most parents whose son or daughter has been admitted to a psychiatric unit are bewildered and respond very positively to the opportunity to tell their tale of woe to other parents in a parents group. Initially, such a group is "support" in orientation. As members return weekly they begin to give each other advice on how to handle similar situations that they have been through. The therapist for the group needs to be active in providing information about (1) the treatment philosophy of the unit; (2) what is normal and abnormal behavior for an adolescent and young adult; and (3) how to set realistic limits and to compromise. The work of the parents group allows many parents to move out of their overwhelmed and angry positions and to feel that they are not the only parents who have problem kids. Many parents are finally able to set limits and yet give empathically to their children when they are prodded and supported in doing so by other parents rather than by "professionals." Furthermore, parents whose marriages have faltered with difficulties in parenting an adolescent can learn from other parents how some adolescents do indeed split parents apart and how they have to find ways to work together for the sake of the child and their marriage.

Complementing a parents group and the frequently held adolescent group should be a weekly multifamily group. A workable number of families is four, and initially the leader has to be active in "joining" the various elements such as "mothers who never get any help, fathers who feel left out." Hot issues like a family's planning an AMA discharge at the insistence of the adolescent are best handled in this kind of setting.

The Point System

A great many adolescents and young adults, as well as older adults, enter the hospital with behaviors which are considered "regressed," "inappropriate," "immature," or "self or other destructive." Sometimes the patient himself can state that he would like to change these behaviors but "can't." Frequently the behaviors are not recognized by the patient or are seen as "no problem for me." The Point System is a therapeutic modality designed to foster and reward behavior which is "grown up" and to encourage the exercise of independent, responsible thinking and acting. It works best when seen by the clinician and nursing staff as integral to the functioning of the other therapeutic modalities and not as a "behavior control" device of the milieu.

Basic to the initiation of a point system is the understanding of a "Contract."[23] Earlier we discussed the development of mutuality in adolescence, particularly in late adolescence and on into early adulthood. Negotiating a point system through the contractural process is an exercise of mutuality between two parties and serves as a template for further interactions. A contract is negotiable, involves both sides, and is specific in its writing. The following are the steps involved in the process of contracting.

Pinpointing

Pinpointing is a listing by patient, parents, clinician, and nursing staff of the behaviors which are seen as preventing the patient from living more independently and appropriately for his age. Examples include refusing to attend family therapy meetings, verbal abuse, running away, and staying in bed until noon. For the actual contract, it is best to list behaviors as *positive* behaviors, i.e., a point given for getting up at 8:00 a.m. rather than a point lost if he sleeps past 9:00 a.m.

Negotiation and Writing of the Contract

After behaviors have been identified and listed in *positive* terms and points assigned, staff and patient determine, through negotiation, what rewards are given for the earning of points (see Table 13.2). As much as possible, specifics should be written so that manipulations, loopholes, distortions, etc., are kept at a minimum. Parents should be involved in the negotiations so that they also learn how to negotiate and follow through consistently, thereby enabling them to carry on with the program during passes and after hospitalization.

Using the Contract

Nursing staff (parents during TTA's) are responsible for the charting of the points. This is best done soon after the desired behavior and when the patient knows what a point has been given for. Verbal encouragement along with point assignment is helpful. It is not helpful for a parent of staff to become angry when a desired behavior does not occur. It is more important to reward it when it does. Points have to be given consistently and should not be taken away for undesirable behaviors.

Changes and Termination of Contract

Because of the negotiation process, contracts are flexible. During the hospitalization it is usually a good sign if the point system contract undergoes changes. Certainly, as there are more TTA's and the problems at home become more crystallized, the contract changes to more of what it will be like after discharge. Once patient and parents can state that communication is more mutually respectful and the other therapeutic modalities are working well, then there can be a trial period (also negotiated) for "being off" the point system.

SUMMARY

Psychiatric hospitalization of an adolescent or young adult should be a thoughtful and carefully considered process. Central to the process is a thorough working knowledge of adolescent development and family process from which a diagnostic assessment and a treatment plan can be made. The psychiatric unit which is designed to be nonregressive, and only a temporary place-away-from-home,

Table 13.2.
Adolescent Program Point System

NAME: _____   DATES: START: _____
                                                          ADD UP _____

DAY		EVENING		RESPONSIBILITIES
Max	Earned	Max	Earned	
1				1. Attend group (or additional activity on nongroup days)
1		1		2. Attend activities (scheduled)
1		1		3. Attend tutoring (or additional activity on nontutoring days)
		1		4. Attend community meeting
1				5. Rounds (dressed and bed made)
1				6. Attend module meeting
3		3		7. Trustworthy behavior
3		3		8. Expressing feelings in helpful ways
3		3		9. Dealing with authority figures

PRIVILEGES

25 points/day maximum

23–25 =
22 =
21 =
20 = (can begin to earn offgrounds trips)
19 = (can begin to earn all meals in cafeteria)
18 = (can begin to earn some meals in cafeteria)
16–17 = (minimum)
15 or below = floor or room restriction

Points begin *(time)* on day 1 and are added up at *(time)* on day 2. Privileges begin *(time)* on day 2 until *(time)* day 3.

COMMENTS:

can bring together multiple therapeutic modalities, no one of which would be a sufficient treatment choice on an outpatient basis. An overriding goal of the hospitalization is to coalesce the strengths of the young person and his family so that outpatient treatment can begin or continue with a firm foundation.

In this chapter, I have highlighted those developmental tasks of adolescence which have particular bearing on setting up a therapeutic milieu for disturbed adolescents and engaging them and their families in a psychotherapy experience which is more than "Band-Aid" crisis intervention. Using the treatment principles and details set forth, I have found very few adolescents or young adults who require lengthy (more than 3 months) hospitalization or subsequent referral to a residential school.

REFERENCES

1. Offer D, Offer JB: *From Teenage to Young Manhood: A Psychological Study,* New York, Basic Books, 1975.
2. Elkind D: Recent research on cognitive development in adolescence, in Dragastin SE, Elder GH (eds): *Adolescence in the Life Cycle,* pp. 49–62, New York, John Wiley, 1975.
3. Neimark ED: Intellectual development during adolescence. Rev Child Dev Res, *4:*541–594, 1975.
4. Kohlberg L, Gilligan C: The adolescent as a philosopher: A discovery of the self in a postconventional world. Daedalus, *100:* 1051–1086, 1971.
5. Engel G: Clinical application of biopsychosocial model. Am J Psychiatry, *137:* 535–544, 1980.
6. Mahler MS: *On Human Symbiosis and the Vicissitudes of Individuation, Infantile Psychosis,* New York, Interntional University Press, 1968.
7. Mahler MS: A study of the separation-individuation process and its possible application to borderline phenomena in the psychoanalytic situation. *Psychoanalytic Study of the Child, 26:* 403–424, 1971.
8. Erikson E: *Childhood and Society,* New York, W.W. Norton and Co., Inc., 1950.
9. Schonfeld WA: Comprehensive community programs for the investigation and treatment of adolescents, in Howells JG (ed): *Modern Perspectives in Adolescent Psychiatry,* pp. 483–511, New York, Brunner/Mazel, 1971.
10. Joint Commission on Accreditation of Hospitals: *Accreditation Manual for Psychiatric Facilities Serving Children and Adolescents,* Chicago, 1974.

11. American Medical Association: *Peer Review Manuals I and II*, Chicago, 1972.
12. American Psychiatric Association: *Manual of Psychiatric Peer Review,* Washington, D.C., 1976.
13. Ricci R, Pravder M, Parmelee D, LaBran E: A comprehensive short-term inpatient treatment program for adolescents. Presented at Annual Meeting of the American Psychological Association, Montreal, September, in press, 1980.
14. Bettelheim B: A therapeutic milieu. Am J Orthopsychiatry, *18:* 191–206, 1948.
15. Albin RS: Suicide rates increasing among adolescents. Psychiat News, *XVI*(9): 26–31, 1981.
16. Cameron K: Group approach to inpatient adolescents. Am J Psychiatry, *109:* 236–240, 1953.
17. Wells RA, Dilkes TC, Trivelli NC: The results of family therapy: A critical review of the literature. Fam Process, *11:* 189–207, 1972.
18. Ackerman NW: Family psychotherapy and psychoanalysis: The implications of difference. Fam. Process, *9:* 5–18, 1970.
19. Boszormenyi-Nagy I, Framo JL: *Intensive Family Therapy,* New York, Harper & Row, 1965.
20. Bowen M: Family therapy and family group therapy, in Kaplan HI, Sadock BJ (eds): *Comprehensive Group Psychotherapy,* pp. 384–421, Baltimore, Williams & Wilkins, 1971.
21. Haley J: Family therapy. Int J Psychiatry, *9:* 233–242, 1970.
22. Satir V: *Cojoint Family Therapy: A Guide,* Science and Behavior Books, Palo Alto, Calif. 1964.
23. Lazare A, Eisenthal S, Wasserman L: The customer approach to patienthood: Attending to patient requests in a walk-in clinic. Arch Gen Psychiatry, *32:* 553–558, 1975.

the family

Ira D. Glick, M.D., and John F. Clarkin, Ph.D.

THE FAMILY MODEL OF INTERVENTION

Family work on an inpatient unit has gone on, or not gone on, as the case may be, throughout the history of inpatient work. The regard and help given families has reflected prevailing theories of individual patient psychopathology as well as the capacity of hospitals to "adopt" patients. Shorter lengths of stay[1] and a now-developed literature on *hospital* and *family* theory and practice, have combined to inform us of: (1) the limits of hospital practice; and (2) the importance of including and allying with families for the effective short *and* long-term care of the hospitalized psychiatric patient.

This chapter (adopted, in part, from Glick, I.D., Kessler DR: *Marital and Family Therapy,* ed. 2, chap. 16, pp. 220–231, New York, Grune & Stratton, 1980) will focus on the new model (or orientation) of the evaluation and treatment of families on a short-term (weeks, not months or years) psychiatric unit.[2] Models of approach will be empirically, rather than theoretically, based. General guidelines for inpatient family work will be provided, and specific approaches for specific diagnostic disorders elaborated. Table 14.1 contrasts the individually-oriented model with the family-oriented model as they are utilized in a hospital setting.[3]

Background

Psychiatric residents, psychology interns, and social work students currently in training may not realize it, but not that many years ago the family with a member in a psychiatric hospital was seen as, at best, purveyors of hospital information to the social worker and as payers of the bills. At worst, they were seen as malignant, pathogenic individuals who had played a major role in causing the patient's symptoms and who tended to make nuisances of themselves by interfering with the patient's treatment by the hospital staff.

The staff acted *in loco parentis* and often inappropriately blamed the family for the patient's symptoms. The family was frequently not allowed to visit during the early part of the hospitalization. The psychiatric hospital, in turn, was associated with much fear and stigma and, in many cases, families were only too happy to stay away. Prior to the availability of effective somatic treatments, hospital stays were much longer, and already fragile family ties were broken. At the time of discharge, the hospital staff members would tend to remove the patient from the family setting, because they viewed the family as an adversary.

In other cultures, families are sometimes considered a vital part of the psychiatric hospitalization of any of their members.[4] Because of a scarcity of trained professionals, families are needed in the hospital to care for the needs of the identified patient. They, in fact, often stay with the patient in or near the hospital. The assumption in other cultures is that the patient is an integral part of the family network, and it is unthinkable that the patient would return anywhere else but to the family.[5]

Over the last 15 years, there has been an increasing use of family intervention in inpatient settings,[6] but not without problems. In an article published in 1977, An-

Table 14.1.
Family Therapy in Individually Oriented Hospitals and Family-Oriented Treatment in the Hospital: A Comparison

Issue	Individually Oriented Hospitals	Family-Oriented Hospitals
Locus of pathology	In the neurobiological system or psycho-dynamics of the individual	Dysfunctional individual behavior related to dysfunction in family interactions as well as individual neurobiological and psychodynamic factors—a biopsycho-social model
Locus of change and healing	In the biosystem or the intrapsychic system of the individual	In the individual within the family as a significant piece of the individual's ecology
Diagnosis	DSM-III, axes I, II, III	DSM-III, axes IV and V, and charac-terization of family interactions in re-lation to the symptoms or complaints
Role of the staff	To care for and to provide therapy for the patient	To facilitate changes in the family through family interaction or through planned interactions with patient
Visits	During visiting hours, informal	Visits are a part of the treatment. Those people who visit are a part of the treat-ment plan
Role of family therapy	A modality to work on those aspects of the patient's problem which seem to be re-lated to family functioning	The orienting therapy of the overall treat-ment program
Discharge planning	Related to the condition of the individual and his/her ability to function outside the hospital	Related to the condition of the family and its ability to provide safety and continued growth for members

derson[7] outlined some of the difficulties, many of which still remain to some degree:

Regrettably, however, the family therapy literature is not particularly helpful to those working on inpatient units; such concepts as "defining the family as the patient" tend to alienate both the medical staff of an institution and the already overwhelmingly guilt-ridden families. The polarized approaches of family therapists, who generally operate on a "system" model, which overemphasizes interactional variables, and of psychiatrists, who generally operate on a "medical" model, which overemphasizes individual variables, disregard the complex and complementary interplay of biological, psychodynamic, and interactional factors . . . . A collaborative relationship between families and the hospital staff could be developed by the establishment of treatment contacts and by combining these two models, thus accepting the patient's illness as the focus *while* recognizing the importance of family variables.

This quote states extremely well the problem of integrating theories of etiology and pathogenesis. This is a problem shared alike by patient, family, and hos-pital staff. Some advances have been made since 1977. The research on expressed emotion in the family environments of schizophrenics has put biological and environmental influences into perspective, thus focusing treatment strategies.[8, 9] In addition, research designs that include pharmacotherapy in various doses plus family intervention[10] recognize and provide data on the importance of therapeutic attack on biological and social fronts simultaneously.

Function of the Psychiatric Hospital Vis-À-Vis the Family

Brief psychiatric hospitalization, which is the norm in this country, serves the function of providing a safe and controlled environment in which to treat acute symptoms of depression, suicidal ideation, alcoholism, severe personality disorder, and psychotic thought and behavior.[2] In addition, the hospitalization serves major functions for the family of the patient. By hospitalization the identified patient is temporarily removed from the family environment when it seems no longer able to contain the patient. In acute family crises, hospitalization may be a means of decreasing behavioral eruptions and thereby may offer substantial relief to a desperate family that is headed for serious deterioration. This enforced separation is undertaken with the goal of evaluating and changing the domestic conditions so as to improve the family's patterns of interaction.[11]

Hospitalization can also serve the function of dramatically symbolizing the problems of both patient and family and bringing them to a point that calls out for attention and resolution. Hospitalization permits observation, evaluation, and discussion of family interaction patterns around the patient and permits the establishment of motivation for seeking marital and family treatment after the patient's return to a better functioning family setting. Hospitalization may also set the stage for overt (as opposed to previous covert) consideration of separation in deadlocked marital or parent-child interactions.

Family Influences on the Hospitalization Process

While not trying to imply that the family interactions are a major, or sole, cause of the serious individual symptoms, it seems clear that the hospitalization of the family member can serve important functions for a disturbed family system.

1. The family is in a crisis, and the hospitalization can be an attempt to solve the crisis.[12–14] For example, some dysfunctional couples have described the outcome of a psychotic episode and their attempts to cope with it as a strongly positive experience for them.[15]

2. The family extrudes the identified patient from the family in an attempt to solve a crisis.

The M family consisted of mother, boyfriend, and two teenage daughters. The eldest daughter had anorexia nervosa. The other sibling was functioning well in high school. The mother had longstanding chronic paranoid schizophrenia and was extremely dependent on her own mother. The mother had been divorced about 10 years previously and had finally found a boyfriend.

After the mother formed a relationship with her boyfriend and was seriously considering marriage, she began to argue with the elder daughter more frequently. The daughter began eating less and became paranoid. The mother then contacted a pediatrician, stating that the daughter was seriously ill and needed hospitalization. The mother confided to the family therapist she was unable to take care of the identified patient's demands because she was fearful of losing her boyfriend *since caring for her daughter would prevent her from spending time with her boyfriend*. The pediatrician hospitalized the daughter.

This case illustrates how one family member can extrude another member from the family in order to take care of his or her own needs. The mother was afraid of losing her boyfriend and therefore restructured the family by having the identified patient hospitalized.

3. The family uses the hospital to get treatment for a member other than the identified patient. The hospitalized member is not necessarily the only "sick" one (or at times, not even the "sickest" one) in the family.[16] A family approach allows for the observation and evaluation of all significant others, with appropriate treatment (including medication) for the group and for the nonpatient individuals who may require it. Therapists concentrating on the treatment of one individual may entirely overlook even gross, florid psychological disturbance in a close relative. When therapists view their role as that of therapist to a family unit, this sort of blind spot is less likely to occur.

4. The family uses the hospital as a resource to regain a "lost" member. For example, a father who drinks and is never home is finally convinced to go into a hospital because of his drinking. The family's motivation is to have him back as a functioning father and spouse, but the family may also need to keep him "sick" for its own needs and homeostasis.

5. The hospital is used as a neutral arena to change longstanding maladaptive patterns of family functioning. An example is the family with an alcoholic member. For such a family, hospitalization of the identified patient will sometimes allow for change of an underlying family pattern. Of course, for this to happen, the hospital staff must plan the appropriate family interventions; simply separating the iden-

tified patient and the family is necessary but often not suficient for change.

6. If the identified patient has a chronic progressive or deteriorating condition like, for example, childhood schizophrenia, then the family may use the hospital as a respite to relieve family burdens.

If these assumptions about the needs of the family around the hospitalization are correct, then it follows *that in such cases the treatment program is inadequate unless it includes the family*.

The Process of Family Treatment by the Hospital Team

The process of family intervention by the hospital team involves steps similar to those of outpatient family treatment: involving the family, assessment, defining the problem, setting goals, treatment, and referral for assistance following discharge. However, the context of hospitalization is unusual in the extent of pathology of one member, the seriousness of the event, and the crisis for the family, all of which require special mention and attention. Treatment, of course, should be individualized and fit to the needs of the particular family.

Although all the necessary research has not yet been done, preliminary work suggests that there are different interview techniques for different types of families. As a rule of thumb, psychoeducational techniques are most indicated for families in which one member has a schizophrenic disorder or affective disorder, and psychodynamic techniques are more indicated for patients with personality disorder.

Involving the Family

Contact with the family should start very early, *preferably prior to hospitalization,* when the family is trying to arrange admission, or certainly by the time of the actual admission. Many hospital personnel have had the experience of beginning discharge planning late in the course of hospitalization, only to discover at that time that the family, implicitly or explicitly, resists having the patient at home. It usually has to be pointed out to the family that hospital treatment of the identified patient involves (or requires) treatment of all family members. This also

may be made a condition of admission. A family representative may be appointed to be the central communicating link with the primary therapist in the hospital.

Evaluating the Family

Evaluation of the family should involve the presence of the identified patient unless he is so psychotic that this is impossible or too disturbing to the patient. The evaluation will follow the usual outline for hospital work, with construction of a family genogram and with particular emphasis on the immediate events, including family interactions and changes, leading up to the hospitalization. The evaluation should be constructed in such a way as to provide information as to whether further family intervention is needed during hospitalization and, if so, what would be the potential focus of that intervention.

Negotiating Goals of Family Intervention

Keeping in mind that the hospitalization is brief, the therapist must quickly focus on the general goals of family intervention and those most specific to the individual family at hand. Negotiation of these goals with the family should be accomplished by the end of the evaluation session or in the next session. This negotiation with the family must be done with confidence, delicacy, firmness, and empathy. Families are frequently upset about the condition of their loved one; may see no need for the hospitalization; may see no need for their participation in therapy, as the patient is the only sick one; or may be hostile to the hospital for not quickly "curing" their family member.

Education about the illness in order to reduce family guilt over creating the condition, information about the length of hospitalization, and expectation for change will reduce anxiety and allow realistic focus on the future. Realistic expectations for change may reduce unrealistic expectation of cure and subsequent disappointment and devaluing of the hospital and its staff. Education about needed family assistance will help in discharge and posthospital treatment compliance. Sessions can vary in length from 30 minutes to 1 hour and can be scheduled on a daily, biweekly, or weekly basis, depending upon need and/or anticipated discharge date.

Common Goals and Techniques of Inpatient Family Intervention

There are six overriding goals that dictate the focus of family intervention when one family member is an inpatient. These goals set the course of the work with each family so that the aim and thrust of the intervention are clearly defined from the beginning of the hospitalization. While our own inpatient family intervention research[17] has been with two major diagnostic groups (schizophrenic spectrum patients and major affective disorders) these goals are not so specific to diagnostic groups as they are specific to the serious problems presented to the family by a member in crisis who is hospitalized for major pathology.

Such a family, whatever the diagnosis, is presented with multiple *tasks:* (1) forming a conceptual understanding of the patient's illness; (2) deciding about the family's responsibility for the illness; (3) making some alliance with hospital treatment staff while trying to ascertain whether the staff blame them for the condition of their family member; (4) beginning to conceptualize the possible future course of the illness, and adjusting any previous images and expectations of the ill member in light of the nature of the illness; (5) deciding on what postdischarge treatment will be needed for the patient; and (6) making some decisions as to what living arrangements will be most beneficial for the family member once discharged. These tasks faced by the family are enormous, especially on first hospitalization of the patient. Without specific, organized attention from the therapeutic staff, these decisions are often faced without professional help despite the fact that the patient (family) is paying enormous fees for the hospitalization.

The six goals of inpatient family intervention are designed to meet the needs of the family as delineated above in a systematic fashion. It is our hypothesis that, if these family needs are addressed, the family can be a major asset in the recovery of the identified patient. If these needs of

the family are not met, the family may react with hostility and chaos, and may become an irritant to the patient, possibly leading to future exacerbation of symptoms, rather than becoming an asset to the patient in the crucial posthospitalization phase. The six *family treatment goals,* with their corresponding treatment strategies and techniques, are as follows.

Goal 1: Acceptance of the Reality of the Illness and Understanding of the Current Episode

This goal, while so obvious, is the cornerstone of the other goals. Unless the family achieves some acceptance and understanding of the seriousness of the episode that caused the hospitalization, their conception of the patient in terms of setting future goals, and their acceptance of needed future treatment following hospitalization, will be compromised.

The family therapist can choose from a number of techniques to accomplish this goal. He can actively engage the family and patient and form a working alliance by recognizing and expressing the burden of stress experienced by the whole family. He can explore each family member's perception and articulation of the illness. While the therapist may not agree with the family member's understanding of the illness, he can identify with and emphathize with the family's previous attempts to deal with the illness. In order to reduce inordinant feelings of responsibility for the illness, the therapist can provide the family with factual information about the illness, and (in the case of schizophrenia and major affective illness) articulate the biological, genetic causes of the illness as seen today. Once the family has some trust in the therapist and realizes that he is not attempting to blame the family for the current episode, the therapist can begin to explore with the family the emergence and development of the current symptomatic episode, so as to begin to identify stresses both external and internal to the family.

The therapist can also educate the family about the course of the disorder, including likely early signs, progression, and future recurrences.

Goal 2: Identification of Precipitating Stresses to the Current Episode

Once the family has in some fashion, even tentatively, accepted the reality of the illness, the next step is to identify (while still fresh in the family's mind) precipitating stressors to the present episode. By so doing, the abstract notion that stress can influence a patient vulnerable to psychiatric illness becomes a concrete reality in the family's daily life. Only when this link between theory and reality is made will progress be likely to occur.

Strategies and techniques to achieve this goal are mainly educative, cognitive, and problem solving in nature. The therapist can encourage the family to think about the recent stresses, both in and outside the family, that may have contributed to the patient's regression. In addition, the therapist and family can rank the stresses in order to clarify their importance and thus prioritize the brief interventions. In the best of situations, the family comes to a consensus about the most important recent stresses and their role in the patient's illness.

Goal 3: Identification of Likely Future Stressors, Both Within and Outside the Family, That Will Impinge on the Identified Patient

Goals 1 and 2 are concerned in great detail with the immediate and remote past: the recognition of illness and the stressors that might have contributed to its eruption. Once these goals have been partly accomplished, there is a natural pull on the part of the family and therapist to consider the immediate future. In fact, in some cases the pull to focus on the future (e.g., discharge) comes too early in the hospitalization; this generally signals defensive derial that must be met with refocusing on goals 1 and 2 before proceeding to goals 3 and 6.

Goal 4: Elucidation of the Family Interaction Sequences That Stress the Identified Patient

Telling the family that they probably put stress on the family is accepted intellectually and vaguely at best. When, however, in the immediacy of the moment the family is shown that what they are doing is leading to the patient's upset (e.g., talking crazy or getting up to pace about the room), learning can take place.

While the goals[1-3] are approached by cognitive and educative strategies, the attempt to demonstrate how current family interaction stresses the patient more closely approximates systems or traditional family therapy. After pointing out when such an interaction occurs in the session (e.g., "Every time you criticize him, as you did just now, he puts his head down and murmurs something that sounds like nonsense under his breath"), the family's perception of being blamed, and responding with resistance and hostility, can be softened by doing one of several things. The therapist can educate the family members about the fact that current family interaction does *not cause* the disorder but is likely to *trigger* current symptoms. In addition, the therapist can emphathize with the family regarding their feelings of frustration and anger toward the patient's behavior which leads them to criticize him. They can then be told that they need to find (with your help) better ways to try to influence the patient.

Goal 5: Planning Strategies for Managing and/or Minimizing Future Stresses

By the middle or toward the end of hospitalization there is often some belief in family members that the past is over. However, the therapist must remind them that what happened in the past could happen in the future and that planning is needed to ensure that history does not repeat itself.

The therapist can invite and initiate discussion of a possible return of symptoms and how the family means to cope with them. There must be discussion about the family's expectations of the patient's future level of functioning, with realistic lowering of expectations in some cases and, for some families, stimulating hope. The therapist can also help the family anticipate any potential stress related to the patient's re-entry into the community, including re-entry into employment, education, job, etc.

Goal 6: Acceptance of the Need for Continued Treatment following Discharge from the Hospital

This goal, which is central to preventing relapse and rehospitalization, comes full circle to goal 1 (reducing denial of the illness). For families who have seen a patient go through numerous hospitalizations there is no problem in anticipating the future possibility of rehospitalization. However, these families may be so discouraged and burdened that they need support and encouragement. For families going through a first hospitalization there is more danger of denial of future episodes and thus more chance of denying the need for aftercare.

The therapist can use a family technique of visualizing possible replays in the future of what just led to the present hospitalization. How would they perform differently the next time? What are the early signs that something is going wrong? Who would they contact? Additional education about typical courses of the condition may further emphasize the need for aftercare.

Not every family will need work on all goals. Some families will be so damaged and defective that only a few basic goals can be approached. However, in our experience most cases can fit into this general schema.

Particular Decisions in Hospital Family Intervention

Timing

Contact with the family should start during the *decision-making process* leading to hospitalization (e.g., the emergency room). Family therapists disagree about when in the psychotic process to begin famly sessions with the patient present. Some believe that family therapy with the patient present should begin only when the active symptoms begin to diminish.[18] This seems reasonable, although it is our experience that this can be used as a rationalization to put off family treatment, and that many patients, even in some psychotic state, become *more* coherent during family sessions that are well-planned and focused by the therapist.

Staffing

Who should do the family therapy? In our opinion, the primary hospital therapist is the one in the best position to do the family therapy because he has the best overall grasp of the case. The advantages of one therapist doing both the individual and the family therapy, in our opinion, far outweigh the disadvantages. Time constraints may not always make this possible, however, and alternative solutions may have to be devised.

Family therapy has been carried out by all members of the hospital treatment team. Nurses, at visiting or other scheduled times, can meet with the patient and family. Occupational and recreational therapists can provide family treatment. They can prescribe activities for the family, such as preparing a meal together or going on a picnic together. Professional staff of every discipline can have crucial roles in changing longstanding behavior patterns in the family system.

The hospital milieu is especially advantageous for observing and pointing out family interaction patterns. For example, if an adolescent child is paranoid about the nursing staff, it can be demonstrated to him that this is similar to the way he reacts to his mother. Furthermore, accurate, on-the-spot observation of the family may reveal that the patient has good reasons for his symptoms.

How can the need for maximal communication among staff members be reconciled with the need for confidentiality of the patient and the therapist? Communication between staff is crucial for effective treatment. The family should be told that the therapist will use all the material that is available from both the individual and family contacts to help the family function better.

How about a cotherapist? Some therapists believe that family therapy in a hospital setting is the most difficult kind of psychotherapy. They recommend that every family therapist have a cotherapist to share the emotional strains of family therapy. Cotherapy in a hospital setting may be more practical than in a private office practice.

There should be one member of the family designated as the *family representative*. One member of the ward staff can be assigned as liaison to the family and should be available to the family at times that are mutually convenient, such as on nights and weekends. These role assignments are crucial in situations in which there are "factions at war" within the family.

Family Techniques and Their Hospital Utilization

A variety of family therapy techniques are now available and are virtually mandatory for use in the modern hospital setting. These include:

1. Individual family therapy
2. Multiple family-group therapy and conjoint couples group[19]
3. Family psychoeducational workshops (also known as family survival skills workshops or family support groups)[20]
4. Family psychodrama and family sculpture are nonverbal techniques that are often more helpful than cognitive techniques when treating a hospitalized (especially nonverbal) sample of patients.

It is rare for family treatment to be the primary therapy for hospitalized patients. Usually for psychotic patients it is prescribed along with medication and other rehabilitative therapies. For nonpsychotic patients it is usually part of a treatment package consisting of individual therapy, rehabilitation therapy, and other interventions.

Case Example. A 17-year-old boy was admitted after having been extremely agitated and disoriented at home, refusing to eat or sleep. The working diagnosis was of a schizophrenic disorder. In the hospital he continued to be wary, eating only when his mother ate with him and avoiding participation in activities involving other patients. The staff had decided to administer neuroleptic medication. They sat down with the boy and his mother and explained their observations and concerns. They then described the drug and the effects they hoped it would have. They also discussed side effects and remedies for these and focused specifically on how the boy and his mother would be able to evaluate the effectiveness of the drug. Specifically, if the boy were to find out that he could think more clearly and under-

stand what is going on around him, then the medicine would be working. He could also help the staff decide what will be the best dose.

The boy hesitated and his mother had some questions. Finally, however, she told the boy that she thought he should try it, and he agreed. Two days later he said that he felt better and wanted to stop the medication. The staff told him that there had not really been enough time to evaluate it. They spoke again with him and his mother. Agains she told the boy that she wanted him to take the medication. Again he agreed to do so. A week later he said he felt better but wondered if an increased dose would help him sleep better; in another conference with him and his mother a new dosage schedule was arranged.

The medication discussions provided the boy and his mother with a different kind of relationship. His mother had been consulted as a parent, and her competence to evaluate and help her son was underscored. The boy, on the other hand, had a new experience of negotiating with his mother. Decisions were not made for him; instead, he was included with his mother in an active decision-making process. As the hospitalization progressed he felt freer to ask questions of both his mother and the staff, and the answers he received helped to clarify the confusion of his psychotic state. The neuroleptic and the contextual experiences described may have worked synergistically.

It is important to note that family intervention in a hospital setting is hard work. The resistant behavior emanating from the family is often intense, while the benefits are often not seen until well after the patient is discharged. Family therapy also requires good communication, socialization, and control skills by the family therapist and, to boot, is very time consuming.

A Working Model of Inpatient Family Intervention

The GAP Committee on the Family has summarized very succinctly the new family model:

Hospitalization should be viewed in most cases as an event in the history of the family, an event that can be devastating or valuable depending upon the skills and orientation of the therapeutic team. When hospitalization is viewed in this way, it becomes central to understand the role of the patient in the family system and to support the family as well as the patient. The hospital becomes an important therapeutic adjunct not only for severely dysfunctional individuals and their families, but also for families who are stuck in modes of relating that appear to interfere with the development and movement of individual members. For these families, hospitalization aims to disrupt the family set; this disruption can be used to help the family system to change in more functional ways.

Family-oriented programs can be implemented within existing hospital resources, though there is a general trend toward adapting and revising hospital environments to include family members in patient care. (This trend is also noted in other specialties, such as "rooming in" in obstetric and pediatric units.) Effective programs involve the staff, from admission clerks on up, in building an alliance with the family. Stewart describes this as 'the engagement of the family with the institution in a relationship that achieves mutual understanding and support and establishes clarity, acceptance, and commitment to mutually agreed upon goals for the treatment of the hospitalized patient.'[21] This active reaching out is different from a commitment to change-oriented family treatment. Involvement of the family (as we are describing) makes possible the avoidance of staff overidentification with the patient against the family, as well as reducing the stigma of psychiatric hospitalization and increasing system-wide motivation for aftercare.

Many different types of staff/family interaction are possible and helpful. One may separate the tasks of alliance building, formal family therapy sessions geared to change, and staff and family interaction around medications, visits, and so forth which can also have a therapeutic function.[22]

An example of an innovative, well-functioning family-oriented approach in an inpatient setting can be found in Table 14.2.

Guidelines for Recommending Family Therapy in a Hospital Setting

The guidelines for recommending family therapy in a hospital setting are similar to those for outpatient settings. Moreover, if the family is present and available it is more efficacious to utilize family evaluation and often some form of family intervention than to withhold it.[23]

A careful distinction has to be made between evaluation and family treatment, given the brief length of stay for most hospitals in the world. As a rule of thumb, every family should be evaluated, then

educated about family treatment. Treatment, when indicated, should, whenever possible, be started in the hospital, though most goals will be accomplished after discharge.

Prototypic situations that call for some form of family intervention during hospitalization include the following:

A suicidal and depressed adolescent living in the parental home is hospitalized following a car accident. There is some suspicion that the father is alcoholic and that the parents are not aware of the adolescent's depression, nor the adolescent's day-to-day functioning.

A 22-year-old male college student is hospitalized following an acute psychotic episode in the fall of his first year away from home. Family sessions are indicated with the parents to educate them about the unexpected illness, to help them and the patient evaluate their mutual expectations for his performance, and to encourage follow-up psychiatric care which the son has never before needed.

A 39-year-old divorced woman living with her two children, ages 11 and 13, is hospitalized following a paranoid psychotic break in which she stabbed herself in the abdomen in the presence of the children. Family sessions with the children are needed to assist the mother, now in a denial phase, to communicate with the children about her illness episode and to talk about the future.

A 23-year-old female who lives with her parents is hospitalized following an exacerbation of schizophrenic symptoms occasioned by her younger sisters leaving for college. The patient also had gone off her medication. The parents are suspected of high "expressed emotion" (they are critical of their daughter and mother is constantly with her day and night). Family treatment is started during the hospitalization to promote proper after-care, including medication and family therapy.

The indications for family therapy can be seen as coming from the patient, from the family, and from the interaction between the family and the patient's illness. Patient-related criteria would include current living conditions (e.g., living with spouse or family of origin) and life cycle issues (e.g., patient is a young adult trying to separate or an older adult living with and very dependent upon the family of origin). Family criteria include family

Table 14.2.
Inpatient Family Intervention[21, a]

Definition: Inpatient family intervention (IFI) is work with the patient and his or her family together in one or more family sessions. It is aimed at favorably affecting the *patient's* course of illness and course of treatment through increased understanding of the illness and decreased stress on the patient. It has been carried out by inpatient social workers, first year psychiatry residents, or both together as co-therapists.

Description:

I. *Assumptions*
  1. IFI does *not* assume that the etiology of the major psychotic disorders lies in family functioning or communication.
  2. It *does* assume that the *present-day* functioning of a family with which the patient is living or is in frequent contact with can be a major source of stress or support.

II. *Aims*
  1. IFI aims to help the family to understand, live with and deal with the patient and his or her illness; to develop the most appropriate possible ways of addressing the problems presented by the illness and its effects on the patient; to understand and support both the necessary hospital treatment and long-range treatment plans.
  2. It aims to help the patient to understand his family's actions and reactions and to develop the most appropriate possible intrafamily behavior on his part, in order to decrease his vulnerability to family stress and decrease the likelihood that his behavior will provoke it.

III. *Strategy and Techniques*
  A. *Evaluation*
  1. Evaluation is accomplished in one or more initial sessions with the family, with the patient present when conditions permit. Information gained from other sources is also used.
  2. The patient's illness and its potential course are evaluated.
  3. The present effect and the possible future effect on the family are determined.
  4. The family's effect on the patient is evaluated, with particular reference to the stress caused by expressed emotion and criticism (EE).
  5. Family structure and interaction and the present point in the family life cycle are evaluated in order to determine whether particular aspects of the patient's role in the family are contributing to exacerbations of illness or to the maintenance of illness and/or impairment.
  B. *Techniques*
  1. The family and patient are usually seen together.
  2. Early in the hospitalization an attempt is made to form an alliance with the family that gives them a sense of support and understanding.
  3. *Psychoeducation:* (a) The family is provided with information about the illness, its likely course, and its treatment; questions are answered. (b) The idea that stress from and in the family can cause exacerbation of the illness is discussed. (c) The ways in which conflicts and stress arise within each family are discussed, and a problem-solving approach is taken in planning ways to decrease such stress in the future. (d) The ways in which the illness and the patient's impaired functioning have burdened the family are discussed and plans made to decrease such burden.
  4. In some cases, the initial evaluation of subsequent sessions suggest that there are particular resistances due to aspects of family structure or family dynamics that interfere with the accomplishment of (2) and (3) above. If it is judged necessary and possible, there may be attempts in one or a series of family sessions to explore such resistances and make changes in family dynamics. Such attempts may use some traditional family therapy techniques. Such families may be encouraged to seek family therapy after the patient's discharge.

[a]The material in this table has been taken in part from a study, *Inpatient Family Intervention: A Controlled Study*, funded in part by an NIMH Grant (MH 34466), and was drafted by Drs. J. Spencer and I. Glick.

conflict which appears to contribute to the patient's difficulties or significant psychiatric illness in one or more other members of the family. Criteria related to the interaction of family and the patient's illness are exemplified by deficit behavior around the illness (e.g., family denial of illness, family not supporting the vulnerable pa-tient, family not supportive of treatment for the patient's illness, and danger that the patient will harm a family member).

As to contraindications, it should be noted that even though family intervention may be indicated during the hospitalization, there are many situations in which that does not seem to be needed, nor is it the treatment of choice upon discharge from the hospital. When the patient is living alone but needs the family support during hospitalization, individual treatment will often be recommended upon discharge. When the individual patient is striving with some success for independence from parents, individual treatment may be best. If the parents are severely in conflict (with this coming to the fore as the patient individuates) marital treatment may be recommended for them.

Results

The only controlled study of family intervention in an inpatient setting is by Glick and associates in which inpatient family intervention (with a heavy family psychoeducational component) is compared to hospitalization without family intervention for patients with schizophrenic disorders and affective disorders.[17] The sample includes 130 patients and their families for whom family intervention was indicated and who were randomized into one of the two treatment conditions, which were guided by treatment manuals. Assessments were made at admission, discharge, and 6 and 18 months postadmission, using patient and family measures from the vantage points of patient, family, and independent assessors.

Preliminary results from global outcome data obtained at discharge and at 6 months from the first three-quarters of the sample suggest that, for all groups combined, family intervention was more efficacious than the comparison treatment. Family intervention was more efficacious for schizophrenics with good prehospital functioning and for patients with affective disorders (especially females). Family intervention did not seem efficacious for chronic schizophrenics, although it was helpful for their families. Our clinical experience suggests that the specific interventions of psychoeducational groups can help the often demoralized family of the chronic patient to reestablish itself as a viable unit and to lessen their burden of shame, guilt, despair, and isolation.[24]

Other Types of Family Involvement as an Alternative to Psychiatric Hospitalization

At times of family crisis, psychiatric hospitalization of a family member is one solution. With the gradual shift of psychiatric services out of the hospital and into the community, other alternatives have emerged. Schizophrenic patients, in some cases, can be kept out of hospitals by sending the treatment team to see them in their homes.[25, 26] Day hospitalization with a focus on family treatment is another alternative to psychiatric hospital admission.[27] Day hospitals also have moved toward utilizing family therapy as a primary method of treatment because their population is chronic, and difficulties with family relationships are common.

Case Example. In the L family there were two brothers, A and M. The father had died, and the mother was the grieving widow. One son, A, lived by himself, managing marginally, while M, the other son, came to a day hospital for management of his schizophrenia.

Treatment at the day hospital was oriented around helping M to obtain volunteer work. Whenever the volunteer counselor and his therapist at the day hospital came close to finding a job placement for him, they noticed that the patient would start screaming, become paranoid, and collapse on the street. Further investigation of these symptoms revealed that on the nights before the patient was to go to his appointments, his mother would, in painstakingly minute detail, describe her anxiety about not knowing his whereabouts and how her heart would not pump as a result. She told him that she would not want to stop him from work but that she needed to know that he was safe in the day hospital, rather than at some volunteer job where she could not call him.

This case is typical of many chronic patients whose level of function is marginal. Any change in that level is often perceived as a threat by the family.

Often a change in the balance of family forces precipitates the request for hospitalization. Understanding the shift can thereby result in strategies to prevent extrusion of the identified patient. Although hospitalization may be avoided, continued family work is needed to change behavior patterns that exacerbate the identified patient's condition.

Reading for the Family

Over the past decade, a number of excellent books have been written for families with a mentally ill member. They include books by Wasow[28] and Bernheim et al.[29] The recent book by Korpell[30] uses a more traditional, individual-oriented model and is therefore not recommended by us.

REFERENCES

1. Glick ID, Hargreaves WA: *Psychiatric Hospital Treatment for the 1980s: A Controlled Study of Short Versus Long Hospitalization.* Lexington, Mass., Lexington Press, 1979.
2. Glick ID, Klar HM, Braff DL: Guidelines for hospitalization of chronic psychiatric patient. Hosp Community Psychiatry, *35:* 934–936, 1984.
3. Group for the Advancement of Psychiatry: *The Family, the Patient, and the Psychiatric Hospital: Toward a New Model,* p. 24. New York, Brunner/Mazel, 1985.
4. Bell J, Bell E: Family participation in hospital care for children. Children, *17:* 154–157, 1970.
5. Bhatti RS, Janakiramaiah N, Channabasavanna SM: Family psychiatric ward treatment in India. Fam Process *19:* 193–200, 1980.
6. Harbin HT: Families and hospitals: Collusion or cooperation? *Am J Psychiatry 135:* 1496–1499, 1978.
7. Anderson CM: Family intervention with severely disturbed inpatients. Arch Gen Psychiatry, *34:* 697–702, 1977.
8. Falloon IRH, Boyd J, McGill, C, Strang JS, Moss HB: Family management training in the community care of schizophrenia, in Goldstein MJ (ed): *New Developments in Interventions with Families of Schizophrenics,* San Francisco, Jossey-Bass, 1981.
9. Falloon IRH: Communication and problem solving skills training with relapsing schizophrenics and their families, in Lansky MR (ed): *Family Therapy and Major Psychopathology,* New York, Grune & Stratton, 1981.
10. Goldstein MJ, Rodnick EH, Evans JR, May RA, Steinberg MR: Drug and family therapy in the aftercare of acute schizophrenics. Arch Gen Psychiatry, *35:* 1169–1177, 1978.
11. Rabiner E, Malminski H, Gralnick A: Conjoint family therapy in the inpatient setting, in Gralnick A (ed): *The Psychiatric Hospital as a Therapeutic Instrument,* pp. 160–177, New York, Brunner/Mazel, 1969.
12. Sampson H, Messinger S, Towne RD: Family processes and becoming a mental patient. Am J Sociol, *68:* 88–96, 1962.
13. Sampson H, Messinger S, Towne RD: The mental hospital and family adaptations. Psychiatr Q, *36:* 704–719, 1962.
14. Langlsey D, Kaplan D: *The Treatment of Families in Crisis,* New York, Grune & Stratton, 1968.
15. Dupont R, Ryder R, Grunebaum H: Unexpected results of psychosis in marriage. Am J Psychiatry, *128:* 735–739, 1971.
16. Bursten B: Family dynamics, the sick role, and medical hospital admissions. Fam Process, *4:* 206–216, 1965.
17. Glick ID, Clarkin JF, Spencer JH, Haas G, Lewis A, Peyser J, DeMane N, Good-Ellis M, Harris E, Lestelle V: Inpatient family intervention. A controlled evaluation of practice: Preliminary results of the six-months followup. Arch Gen Psychiatry, *42:* 882–886, 1985.
18. Guttman H: A contraindication for family therapy: The prepsychotic or postpsychotic young adult and his parents. Arch Gen Psychiatry, *29:* 352–355, 1973.
19. Davenport YB: Treatment of the married bipolar patient in conjoint couples psychotherapy groups, in Lansky MR (ed): *Family Therapy and Major Psychopathology,* New York, Grune & Stratton, 1981.
20. Anderson CM, Hogarty GE, Reiss DJ: Family treatment of adult schizophrenic patients: A psychoeducational approach. Schizophr Bull *6:* 490–505, 1980.
21. Stewart RP: Building an alliance between the families of patients and the hospital: Model and process. Natl Assoc Private Psychiatr Hosp J, *12:* 63–68, 1982.
22. Group for the Advancement of Psychiatry: *The Family, the Patient, and the Psychiatric Hospital: Toward a New Model,* New York, Brunner/Mazel, 1985, pp. 27–29.
23. Gould E, Glick ID: The effects of family presence and family therapy on outcome of hospitalized schizophrenic patients. Fam Process, *16:* 503–510, 1977.
24. McLean C, Grunebaum H: Parent's response to chronically psychotic children. Paper presented at the American Psychiatric Association Annual Meeting, Toronto, 1982.
25. Pasamanick B, Scarpitti F, Dinitz S: *Schizophrenics in the Community,* New York, Appleton-Century-Crofts, 1967.
26. Davis A, Dinitz S, Pasamanick B: The prevention of hospitalization in schizophrenia: Five years after an experimental program. Am J Orthopsychiatry, *42:* 375–388, 1972.
27. Zwerling I, Mendelsohn M: Initial family reactions to day hospitalization. Fam Process, *4:* 50–63, 1965.
28. Wasow M: *Coping with Schizophrenia: A Survival Manual for Patients, Relatives and Friends,* Palo Alto, Calif., Science and Behavior Books, 1982.
29. Bernheim K, Lewine R, Beale C: *The Caring Family: Living with Chronic Mental Illness,* New York, Random House, 1982.
30. Korpell H: *How You Can Help: A Guide for Families of Psychiatric Hospital Patients,* Washington, D.C., American Psychiatric Press, 1984.

chapter 15

occupational therapy

Sharan L. Schwartzberg, Ed.D., O.T.R., and Janet Abeles, M.Ed., O.T.R.

The clinical picture of a mental disorder is always associated with an impaired pattern of social or occupational functioning. Patients often present complaints about a loss of interest or pleasure in daily activities and difficulties in occupational performance. For the staff, these complaints and the evidence of a diminished ability to function are in part the foundation of a diagnosis and treatment plan. At the same time, as a result of admission to a psychiatric inpatient unit, patients' usual routines of homemaking, self-care, work, and leisure activities are also disrupted.

This chapter will describe a therapy explicitly designed to focus on problems in occupational performance and daily living skills—namely, occupational therapy. First, occupational therapy is defined and then described within the framework of an historical overview and theoretical analysis of various conceptual models used in psychiatric inpatient settings. The assumptions of these psychiatric models and corresponding occupational therapy models are explained. Next, a biopsychosocial approach to inpatient occupational therapy is proposed. Through a program example, the purpose, methods, and value of such an occupational therapy program are detailed and illustrated. Finally, contemporary problems in occupational therapy are discussed, and some concluding remarks are made in regards to the future of occupational therapy and inpatient psychiatry.

DEFINITION

Occupational therapy is the art and science of using purposeful activities to minimize pathology, to facilitate learning of performance component skills necessary for occupational performance and role adaptation, to maintain or enhance function, and to promote health.[1-3] Thus purposeful activities are goal-oriented doing processes, involving interaction with both the human and nonhuman environments.[4] The performance component skills are the sensorimotor, cognitive, psychological, and social skills needed for occupational performance. Such performance involves life task activities of self-care, work, and play or leisure necessary for the satisfaction of personal needs and social roles.[5] In particular, psychiatric occupational therapy in the acute inpatient setting focuses on: functional evaluation, symptom reduction, supporting function or the maintenance of abilities to relate to the human and nonhuman environments, mobilization for rapid return to the community, and discharge planning.[2, 3]

HISTORICAL OVERVIEW

Although the former contemporary definition of occupational therapy helps to explain current practice, it is interesting to note that occupations or activities have been used as a form of treatment for the physically and mentally ill throughout recorded history.[6] However, the value of activities therapy is not as well understood as the more widely accepted methods of verbal group therapy,[7] individual psychotherapy, and psychopharmacologic treatment. Nevertheless, it was in the first decades of the 20th century that individuals wishing to re-establish mid-18th century moral treatment principles labeled these "second moral treatment" programs occupational therapy—an alternative for physicians who were dissatisfied with the prevailing medical model view of mental illness as an incurable disease of the brain.[8] Over the years, various forces acted to change the face of occupational therapy. These changes have broadened the theoretical frames of reference in occupational therapy practice. An examination of psychiatric models and their parallels in occupational therapy lead to an examination of the assumptions underlying various schools of thought.

Assumptions

Given the historically close alliance between occupational therapy and medicine, it is no surprise that there are similarities in the conceptual models of these professions in the specialty area of mental health. Close examination of these models can clarify the relationship between occupational therapy and inpatient psychiatry.

Psychiatric Models

Lazare[9] outlines four conceptual models of clinical psychiatry: the medical model, the psychologic model, the behavioral model, and the social model. As this discussion is concerned with modern day inpatient practice, we would add a fifth model—the biopsychosocial model. Using this configuration of clinical psychiatry, we can make several assumptions regarding occupational therapists' primary concern: occupational performance, that is, depending upon one's conceptual bias, the perceived relationship between mental illness and dysfunction in occupational performance varies (see Table 15.1).

As Lazare[9] points out, the ideology of the psychiatrist is one factor that implicitly determines which model is selected for patient evaluation and treatment. A similar case could be made in regard to the occupational therapist; however, an additional variable exists within the hierarchy of hospital practice. That is to say, it is more likely that occupational therapists are conceptually bound by both their professional ideology and the orientation of the psychiatrist in charge of the inpatient unit. As a result, we see similarities in the clinical models of occupational therapists and psychiatrists.

Occupational Therapy Models for Psychiatric Inpatient Settings

As was discussed earlier, there is a relationship between assumptions about mental illness and occupational performance dysfunction. A closer inspection of models in psychiatry and occupational therapy also reveals parallels (Table 15.2). Six occupational therapy models for inpatient psychiatry are presented since they appear most broadly representative of actual practice. Each will be briefly illustrated and explained. The biopsychosocial model is illustrated and elaborated upon in the discussion of our occupational therapy program model. We wish to emphasize that our intent is not to compare the empirical validity of the models or to imply that they are superior to other models. Other than some emphasis given to their suitability for short-term care, our purpose is to simply describe commonly reported theoretical models for short and long-term inpatient settings.

1. Neurobehavioral Model. Case Example. In the first occupational therapy session, Mr. T., age 43, with a diagnosis of schizophrenia, was unable to copy a simple mosaic tile design or catch a large beach ball. He appeared to have a limited attention span (15 minutes), an inability to think abstractly, was easily distracted, and demonstrated abnormal posture, poor balance, and a pattern of restricted movement. Furthermore, he did not interact with the therapist unless asked a specific question and his affect remained flat throughout the evaluation.

The occupational therapy inpatient treatment goals established were to begin a program to (a) increase range of motion, (b) increase spontaneous movement, and (c) improve posture. Treatment involved a daily 15–30 minute, developmentally sequenced program of sensory input through individual and group gross motor activities. The activities were structured by the therapist, involved repetitive pleasurable action and limited choice and distractions, and were physically demonstrated with repeated, simple verbal directions—continuously refocusing Mr. T.'s attention on the activity outcome. Activities used were primarily games involving a beach ball, balloon, parachute, jump rope, and beanbag chair. After several weeks of treatment, Mr. T. appear to be

Table 15.1
Assumptions about Mental Illness and Occupational Performance

Psychiatric Model	Assumptions
Medical Model[9]	Mental illness is a physical disease due to some defect in the nervous system or biochemical mechanism of genetically predisposed individuals. Disturbances in motor behavior are primary symptoms of neurophysiological defects, and disturbances in work, play, and self-care are secondary psychological symptoms.[10, 11]
Psychologic Model[9]	Impaired development of early relationships and resultant unconscious conflicts confound the ability to care for self and to derive gratification from or sublimate aggressive impulses in socially acceptable work and play activities.[12–15]
Behavioral Model[9]	Abnormal work, play, or self-care behaviors are a result of inadequate learning of performance components or the cognitive, sensorimotor, psychological, and social skills necessary for occupational performance.[16]
Social Model[9]	Disordered work and play environments foster mental illness and contribute to deteriorated habits of living—the absence of a pleasurable and balanced routine of work, play, rest, and sleep.[17]
Biopsychosocial Model	Occupational performance problems are the sequelae of the dynamic interaction between biological, psychological, and social components of a mental disorder.[18] Psychogenic and sociogenic factors involved in occupational performance, such as stress, loss, or sudden change in activity level or stimuli, can trigger and hence precipitate an episode of mental illness in genetically predisposed individuals.[10]

more active and socially responsive. He was referred to an occupational therapist in the day hospital for continued neurobehavioral treatment.

As demonstrated in the case example, this model is concerned with the relationship between biological functions and task performance.[2] According to Clark,[19] "the theoretical premise is that normalization of sensory and motor patterns, and their integration for interaction with the environment, will promote adaptive development of conceptualization, manipulative, and social skills." Function or dysfunction is viewed as the ability or inability to process information from the environment in order to act.[19] Task performance evaluations are used to evaluate perceptual-motor and sensory-integrative functions affected by the central nervous system.[20] In treatment, developmentally sequenced sensorimotor activities are used to nor-

malize the nervous system.[19, 21-24] It is of interest to mention that Kaplan[20] observes that "although some acutely ill inpatients demonstrate neurological deficits, short-term treatment is generally incompatible with neurologic reintegrative approaches".

2. Psychodynamic Model. Case Example. Seven patients are seated around a table about to share free associations to their freely created clay objects. The occupational therapist asks the patients to say whatever comes to their minds and to talk about what their clay object looks like and what it makes them think of or what it reminds them of.

The major theoretical premise of the psychodynamic model is that activities can provide insight and opportunities for need expression and sublimation, thereby fostering personality change and symptom abatement.[25-27] Measures of function and dysfunction are the ability or inability to seek and obtain gratification of needs

Table 15.2.
Occupational Therapy and Psychiatric Models

Psychiatry	Occupational Therapy
Medical Model[9]	Neurobehavioral Model
Psychologic Model[9]	Psychodynamic Model
Behavioral Model[9]	Behavioral/Educational Model
	Developmental Model
Social Model[9]	Occupational Behavior Model
Biopsychosocial Model	Biopsychosocial Model

and self-satisfaction.[28] As the case example illustrates, projective activities are used for the purpose of uncovering unconscious processes.[25, 29] However, Kaplan[20] maintains that projective evaluation techniques are suitable for initial evaluation of the longer-term psychiatric patient and do not appear suitable for a short-term evaluation concerning adjustment to community living. Treatment programs include short-term group and individual activities that provide an opportunity for aggressive impulses to be expressed appropriately and directly, to engage in conflict-free activity,[30] and for the testing of living skills in an environment of thinking, feeling, and action.[26]

3. Behavioral/Educational Model. Case Example. An occupational therapist is reviewing situations patients may encounter as they return to former jobs after hospitalization. Two patients have just volunteered to role play "the first day back on the job." One will be the recently discharged patient and the other the patient's job supervisor. All the patients have just seen a videotape depicting a former psychiatric patient successfully overcoming barriers toward her reemployment.

In this model the theoretical premise is that behavior is learned—additionally, that more adaptive occupational behaviors can be taught and learned through here and now activities and the practice of isolated behavioral skills. Adaptive behavior is the presence of knowledge, skills, and values needed for living in the community, and maladaptive behavior presents the absence of such knowledge, skills, and values.[31] Performance evaluations are used to assess functional behavior in work, leisure, or self-care.[20, 29, 31] Activities therapy treatment[31] focuses on increasing knowledge, skills, and values needed for future living. As demonstrated in the case example, the methods employed include learning through doing, the immediate here and now human and nonhuman environment, and the teaching-learning process.[31] The short-term setting can provide an opportunity for learning behaviors necessary for immediate adjustment to community living; however, a short length of stay does not allow for much repetition or range in the learning process.

4. Developmental Model. Case Example. The occupational therapy department at "General Hospital" offers two levels of inpatient group treatment. The lower level task groups are composed of patients who have difficulty concentrating and are unable to make decisions, share materials, and offer support to other group members, or are involved in group activities requiring problem-solving and co-operation. The occupational therapist selects and sets up activity projects that have simple and familiar procedures, which easily result in successful end products. The activities demand little concentration, can be completed in one session, and do not require group interaction. The therapist also attempts to fulfill members' emotional and social needs. The higher level task groups involve patients in cooperative activities. Members are expected to give and receive feedback, arrive at a consensus about the group project, and be able to share group leadership, membership, and task roles. The therapist serves as a role model, teacher, and activity resource consultant.

In the developmental model, it is assumed that performance component skills are multidimensional and learned in a stage-specific developmental progression that can be simulated through developmentally sequenced purposeful activities.[32-34] Function or dysfunction is seen as the presence or absence of age- or stage-appropriate adaptive skills or behaviors.[28]

According to Kaplan,[20] "in the short-term setting, the appreciation of developmental factors is critical in correctly understanding an individual's current situations. However, decisions need to be made about which abilities are most crucial to evaluate for a given individual because of time factors." Treatment programs simulate a developmental progression of purposeful activities in adaptive skill areas, and behavioral methods of teaching-learning are applied.[33, 34] As the case example demonstrates, in acute care, such progressions are of value for activity analysis and adaptation. However, the major contribution of the developmental model appears in psychiatric rehabilitation programs where one is more likely to find a longer length of stay and larger homogeneous developmental subgroups of patients.

5. Occupational Behavior Model. Case Example. Mrs. B., a 65-year-old mother of three independent children, was admitted to the hospital a month after her husband's death. She complained of loss of interest in her usual homemaking activities, had difficulty making simple decisions, was hardly eating or sleeping, felt isolated and depressed, and had suicidal thoughts. In an interview the occupational therapist learned that Mrs. B. had won several baking contests. She gently urges Mrs. B. to stop by the kitchen at 2 p.m. that afternoon. A group of patients were planning to bake pies and had expressed concerns about the best way to proceed.

Proponents of this model have assumed that life roles organize behavior and that individuals are curious and intrinsically motivated to explore their environment. It is also believed that patients can learn necessary habits and skills through exploration and practice with occupational tools, behaviors, and environments.[35–37]

Function consists of temporal[38] and occupational adaptation in the performance of life roles that are satisfying to self and others. Dysfunction constitutes unsatisfactory social roles, skill and habit deficits, and an imbalanced use of time—a daily life routine that is disorganized or lacking in pleasure.[17] Evaluation usually consists of history-taking in regards to: habit patterns; occupational role solidification and performance in the past and present; and past, current, and future interests, values, and goals.[20, 39–43] The history is aimed at identifying target problems, in the environment and in an individual's performance, that contribute to role dysfunction. Treatment programs provide learning experiences that encourage temporal and occupational exploration and adaptation. They aim to develop competency in the performance of work, play, and self-care activities through experience in such a balance of activities in the hospital milieu.[17, 36, 37, 44, 45]

The occupational behavior model is generally incompatible with a medical orientation and thus presents many communication problems for occupational therapists working in general hospital psychiatric inpatient units. It does, however, provide a means by which to begin an analysis of the relationship between an individual's mental disorder and occupational performance deficits, and as the case example implies, acknowledges a patient's assets and the necessary ingredients of a hospital milieu that maintains and promotes health.

6. Biopsychosocial Model. In this model it is assumed that individuals are dynamic and open biopsychosocial systems intrinsically motivated to do and have an effect on the environment. It is also believed that a health-satisfying environment of purposeful activities in conjunction with an opportunity to learn adaptive skills for doing can help an individual reconstitute to an adaptive level of behavior.[8, 16, 18, 46–50]

Function is viewed as the ability to adapt to the sequela of a mental disorder or one's biopsychosocial configuration—hence, to be able to participate in community life or environmental systems and achieve personal and social goals. Dysfunction is the inability to engage in satisfactory roles and occupational performance as a dynamic result of the interaction between biological, psychological, and socioenvironmental circumstances. Likewise, the physical disease process itself can be triggered by psychogenic and sociogenic factors related to occupational performance dysfunction.

In evaluations, therapists analyze the interactions between internal (biological-psychological) and external (social) mechanisms by assessing both the strengths and weaknesses in an individual's past and present occupational performance, life roles and skills, interests, goals, and available human and nonhuman resources. Usual evaluation methods include history-taking[31, 41–43] and observation of patient performance[31] in occupational therapy and unstructured and semistructured unit activities. Treatment methods include the use of purposeful activities in individual treatment and in open and closed functional task groups,[51, 52] the therapeutic relationship, activity analysis, and activity adaptation in the form of graded structured activities and graded structured relationships. These methods and their therapeutic rationale are further explained in the following section, which illustrates our program model.

PROGRAM MODEL

The occupational therapy program to be described represents a case example of the biopsychosocial model for inpatient occupational therapy. It illustrates the Mount Auburn Hospital occupational therapy program on the psychiatric unit, Wyman II. Mount Auburn Hospital is a nonprofit, 305-bed community/teaching hospital located in Cambridge, Mass. Wyman II is a 16-bed voluntary short-term unit which offers an integrated biopsychosocial approach to the evaluation and treatment of psychiatric disorders. A structured program, implemented by a multidisciplinary team, includes occupational therapy, psychiatric evaluation, medication evaluation and treatment, individual and group therapies, family meetings, and psychological evaluation. The staff consists of occupational therapists, psychiatrists, psychiatric nurses and counselors, psychiatric social workers, and psychiatry and psychology interns.

There are two full-time occupational therapists who engage fully in implementing the occupational therapy program, contributing to treatment planning meetings, and participating in community meetings and activities of the Wyman II milieu. The occupational therapists on Wyman II also maintain an active relationship with the consultation and liaison team as well as with other medical/surgical occupational therapists in the hospital. They provide consultation on relevant psychiatric concerns as well as participate in business and inservice education meetings with the occupational therapy department.

Wyman II provides treatment for patients 16 years of age and older. Upon special consideration and permission of the unit director, patients between the ages of 14 and 16 may be admitted. The average length of stay is 21 days. The Wyman II patient population typically includes a broad range of diagnostic groups: personality disorders, affective disorders, anxiety disorders, schizophrenic disorders, eating disorders, and psychotic disorders.

Purpose

The following section will identify and explain what our biopsychosocial model of occupational therapy entails. Specifically, this section will detail our program model by explaining the purpose of occupational therapy in terms of evaluation, treatment, and health needs for the activity milieu and discharge planning.

Evaluation

The occupational therapy evaluation begins with a systematic process of data collection. Initial data is gathered by chart review, interview, and observation of patient performance in occupational therapy and in unstructured and semi-structured unit activities.

Chart Review. The first step of data collection is carried out prior to the initial meeting of patient and therapist. By reading the admission summary and staff notes, the therapist collects information to structure the initial patient-therapist interaction. More specifically, the therapist determines whether the standard evaluation method can be carried out or whether it will need to be adapted to meet the patient's particular needs.

Interview. In most cases, the second step is an interview. A general written questionnaire (Fig. 15.1) and goals sheet (Fig. 15.2) is given to each patient when he or she is first introduced to the occupational therapy program in the initial interview. The general questionnaire is designed to collect historical data about the patient's prehospitalization, adaptive and maladaptive patterns of occupational behavior, and interpersonal and community relationships. The specific activities of daily living required by the patient's occupational roles and given environment and the patient's perceptions of his or her effectiveness and satisfaction in the performance of these life tasks and leisure interests are also noted. Additional questionnaires for specific major life roles (worker, student, homemaker, retiree) are given, as appropriate, to each patient to elicit further data. For example, the worker questionnaire asks for data related to the patient's educational and work histories; present and prior use of vocational resources; specific job tasks required in the daily work routine; perceptions of which tasks are liked and performed well, not liked and not performed well, liked and not performed well, and not liked and performed well; perceptions of the quality of interactions with both co-workers and supervisors; and perceptions of factors influencing occupational choice.

The goals sheet is given to each patient along with the questionnaire(s). It is a checklist of possible goals that the patient can choose to focus on in occupational therapy treatment. The goals are directed

Figure 15.1. Mount Auburn Hospital Occupational Therapy General Questionnaire

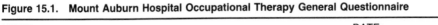

NAME: _____ DATE: _____

1. Which of the following household chores do you have responsibility for:

_____ Cooking   _____ Laundry   _____ House Cleaning

_____ Shopping   _____ Budgeting

   Which one(s) do you have difficulty with?
2. Where do you live? Do you live with others, alone, in a boarding house, etc.?
3. What do you use for transportation?
4. Do you have any fun?
5. What is fun to you?
6. Are there things you would like to do in your spare time that you don't do now? What are they?
7. Do you have any habits which interfere with your daily life?
8. Are there any physical activities you particularly enjoy doing?
9. What kinds of things do you and your family do together?
10. Do you have relatives you get together with fairly often?
11. Do you have any especially good friends you see often? How often? How did you meet them? How do you enjoy spending your time with them?
12. Do you enjoy reading? What?
13. How much time do you spend watching TV?
14. Do you have hobbies or other special interests?
15. Do you belong to any clubs or organizations?
16. How do you spend your weekends?
17. How would you describe yourself to others?
18. What outlets do you use for dealing with feelings?
19. What is your philosophy of life?
20. What do you hope to accomplish by this hospitalization?

towards improving performance skills in the areas of socialization, work, leisure, self-maintenance, activities of daily living, and the balance among these. Specific goals include: to feel more comfortable in groups, to explore and evaluate life-style and the role of leisure and recreation, and to express feelings more directly.

The completion of the questionnaire and goals sheet is followed by a semistructured interview in which further history-taking and data clarification occur. The interview provides the foundation for the developing therapist-patient relationship and provides rich material related to the individual's occupational performance requirements, skills, and perceptions.

The use of a questionnaire and goals sheet, as components of the interview and evaluation process, provides several advantages:

1. The organization of data collection under a conceptual framework that guides interpretation of the data and its translation into a treatment plan.
2. The participation of the patient in the identification of strengths and

weaknesses in performance areas, and subsequent involvement in mutual goal-setting to the degree of the individual's readiness and capability.

3. The opportunity to assess the patient's task and social skills in structured and semistructured activities.

There are clinical situations in which the use of the questionnaire and goals sheet is not appropriate, and data must be elicited by alternate means. Possible reasons for adapting the evaluation process include language barriers, illiteracy, blindness, and physical disability. The individual's mental status at the time of evaluation is also considered. The grossly psychotic or organically impaired patient may not be able to engage in the process of filling out the occupational therapy questionnaire. As the therapist's ultimate aim is to involve the patient in the evaluation process, external and environmental demands and prerequisite psychological, cognitive, sensorimotor, and social skills are considered in the decision to use or not use the questionnaire and goals sheet.

Figure 15.2. Mount Auburn Hospital Occupational Therapy Goals Sheet

In light of your answers on the questionnaire, which of the following goals do you feel the greatest need to work toward in occupational therapy?

_____ To feel more comfortable in groups
_____ To learn to talk more easily with people
_____ To learn to ask for help
_____ To explore the role of social and recreational activities in my life
_____ To do something fun
_____ To learn to structure my time more effectively to include:
_____ Grooming   _____ Social Activities
_____ Household Chores   _____ Recreation
_____ To learn to manage money better
_____ To find an apartment or other living arrangement
_____ To successfully complete a craft project
_____ To learn better skills to organize and complete a task
_____ To clarify career interests
_____ To identify strengths and weaknesses in work skills
_____ To define and assess difficulties in my job
_____ To learn to apply and interview for a job
_____ To look for a job
_____ To learn some ways to relax more
_____ To learn to deal with my feelings more directly and appropriately
_____ To find outlets for angry feelings
_____ To learn to recognize my needs and get them met
_____ To learn more about who I am and what is important to me
_____ To build my self-confidence

Observation of Task Performance. This occurs through observation of patient performance in a combination of formal structured occupational therapy activities, such as participation in a cooking group, unstructured use of time, and semi-structured unit activities such as tending to self-care and operating the unit's laundry facilities. The assessment tasks are selected for their ability to elicit performance component skill data in the biological, psychological, and social domains. The biological component is concerned with the integrating function of the nervous system. For example, for the patient undergoing biological treatment, e.g., medication, tasks yield data about the side effects such as incoordination, blurred vision, and drowsiness. The psychological component refers to how the individual experiences, organizes, and responds to the human and nonhuman environment. In this area, tasks evaluate such concerns as the patient's concept of self and others, his capacity for reality testing, and the coping strategies employed in a variety of situations. The social component focuses on interpersonal interactions as well as environmental and cultural circumstances. The tasks yield data such as the patient's readiness to use available supports and the nature of his or her value system as it relates to personal time management. Finally, it is the dynamic result of the interaction between these components—the actual performance in work, play, and self-care, and the patient's perceptions and wishes about the use of time—that lead to an understanding of the individual's occupational functioning.

The occupational therapy evaluation on this short-term unit provides a basis from which to plan treatment. It provides a base line from which to re-evaluate change during the course of hospitalization. The evaluation serves as a systematic screening of functional skills and limitations. When specific problem areas are identified, a further in-depth evaluation may be conducted. In such instances, occupational therapy evaluation tools used include standardized tests, activity histories and configurations, interest checklists, projective activities, activities of daily living performance checklists, and individual or group tasks.

Treatment

Occupational therapy treatment is broadly designed to correspond with a short-term hospitalization's overall goals of diagnostic assessment, symptom reduction, and rapid reintegration into the community. The occupational therapy treatment goals are coordinated with and reinforce the treatment team's goals for the patient's hospitalization. The patient collaborates in treatment planning as fully as possible.

Symptom Reduction. One of the objectives of occupational therapy treatment with the acutely ill patient is symptom reduction. In our model the problem-oriented intervention for reducing acute symptomatology is applied to restore performance component skills. While in the acute care setting symptom reduction is a realistic and attainable short-term goal, we also find that it is essential to identify longer-term remedial goals that extend beyond the course of hospitalization.

According to Fidler, in short-term acute settings, activity selection for symptom reduction is "based on those experiences that may be expected, for a given patient, to reduce anxiety, diminish hyperactivity, stimulate response and psychomotor activity, reduce confusion and alert or focus attention".[3] For example, a concrete, success-oriented task may be chosen for the depressed patient because of its tendency to interfere with pathological ruminations and to reduce a sense of worthlessness, both of which are symptoms that can accompany a clinical depression. For the acutely disorganized psychotic patient, an activity may be used to relieve anxiety. Thus the activity serves as an anxiety-relieving agent and is selected because its properties inherently facilitate integrative action which has a positive effect on the overwhelmed person.

Skill Development. A second treatment objective is performance skill development. Activities are chosen to facilitate development or learning of skills and attitudes in the areas which will enable the patient to function more effectively in work, leisure, self-care, and socialization. This aspect of treatment involves the patient in a problem-solving process that includes problem identification, goal-setting, planning, and resolution. Depending upon the length of stay, the complexity of patient needs, and the extent of psychopathology manifested, the problem-solving process may reach only the initial phases of implementation in the short-term hospital stay. Carry-over of performance skill development occurs through recommendations for continued outpatient treatment in the community.

While development of major skills can be an unrealistic expectation of a short-term crisis intervention program, increasing the patient's awareness of effective alternatives to a specific and immediate problem may be possible. Treatment may include teaching compensatory techniques or strategies for accomplishing a task. In certain cases, as with patients who have a deteriorating dementia, treatment may be more concerned with both providing education and counseling for the patient's family and environmental manipulation.

Maintenance of Intact Skills. In addition to restoring and developing skills, occupational therapy is directed at maintaining function and preventing further disability. Intact performance skills are maintained through engagement in activities that provide practice in the skills and reinforce success. Fine notes that "in such instances, the primary concern is for the provision of activities that make it possible for the individual to use existing skills and interests, experience intrinsic gratification and meet basic needs for acceptance, achievement, creativity, autonomy and social interaction.".[2]

Life-Style Awareness and Development. Another treatment objective is to increase the patient's awareness of how he or she occupied time prior to hospitalization, as well as increase knowledge of more satisfactory alternatives. An integral aspect of this objective involves teaching, through discussion and experience, the elements and potential value of a balanced routine of work, leisure, self-care, and socialization. Kielhofner states that "balance refers to more than just so much work, play, and rest. Rather, balance recognizes an interdependence of these life spaces and their relationship to both internal values, interests, and goals, and external demands of the environment."[38]

Health Needs—The Activity Milieu

By including a variety of activities, the occupational therapy program reinforces the value of a balanced routine or life-style (Fig. 15.3). For example, the occupational therapy groups and group schedule were designed to fulfill the ordinary human biological need for movement, the psychological need for a product, and the social need for interaction. The patient's daily routine also includes verbal psychotherapy groups balanced with the nonverbal occupational therapy formats such as movement and task-oriented activity groups.

Given our biopsychosocial orientation to occupational therapy, the program offered is based on the assumption that problems in doing may arise from a lack of doing. For this reason the activity groups are so designed to first meet healthy needs for movement, action, and productivity. Thus adaptive patterns of behavior are supported and integrated through experiential involvement in the groups.

In several ways the occupational therapy program and its specific groups support an active therapeutic milieu. One way is by building cohesiveness within the patient community in order to facilitate work in the milieu and in the verbal insight-oriented groups. The other is by helping to structure the milieu to meet the patients' health needs. A balanced routine, offering a variety of treatment modalities, fosters active patient participation rather than regression and dependency.

Discharge Planning

Discharge planning is recognized as an important objective in a short-term hospitalization. It is essential for maintaining a continuous treatment process from the hospital into the community. Discharge planning involves identification of treatment needs and requires a knowledge of community resources. It is concerned with planning a course of action that recognizes the therapeutic process initiated on the inpatient unit and addresses treatment alternatives to be continued or started postdischarge.

Discharge planning begins when the patient is admitted to the hospital. It may involve evaluating the patient's occupational performance and responsiveness to various occupational therapy formats so that recommendations and referrals can be made for appropriate outpatient care. For example, a socially isolated patient who gradually became less withdrawn through active participation in a structured socialization group may derive similar benefits from an outpatient socialization group. Another aspect of discharge planning may revolve around family education to prepare the family for the patient's re-entry into the home activity environment.

Community re-entry may involve directing the patient to a community resource. In establishing treatment services aimed at furthering rehabilitation goals, the occupational therapist often acts as a liaison between the hospital and the community. Long-term treatment needs concerning issues of vocational performance, basic life skills, or socialization may require referrals to such institutional resources as partial hospitalization programs and vocational adjustment programs or noninstitutional community resources such as adult education programs.

Methods

Purposeful Activity

Occupational therapy's emphasis on the meanings and uses of actual engagement in purposeful activity distinguishes it from other psychiatric therapies. Purposeful activity is a goal-directed doing process. The Fidlers note that "*doing* is a process of investigating . . . responding, managing, creating and controlling. It is through such action with feedback from both nonhuman and human objects that an individual comes to know the potential and limitations of self and the environment and achieves a sense of competence and intrinsic worth."[53] The value of the purposeful activity is based upon the social, cultural, and personal meaning, both real and symbolic, and relevance to the individual.

Figure 15.3. Occupational Therapy Program Schedule

MONDAY

11:00–12:00 a.m.
Open Occupational Therapy

Individual activities are performed in a parallel task group setting for a variety of therapeutic purposes.

2:00–3:00 p.m.
Movement Group

Physical exercises and recreational activities are performed to encourage self-awareness, discharge tension, and reinforce the importance of regular movement in a balanced life routine.

TUESDAY

11:00–12:00 a.m.
Self-Expression Group

A task incorporating verbal and nonverbal expression is performed and followed by processing of feelings and experiences.

1:00–2:00 p.m.

Patients are selected for these concurrent groups on the basis of need:

Work Group

A group task is performed or a discussion is conducted that focuses on vocational issues in work or school.

Cooking Group

A group task is carried out, involving shared selection, preparation, and consumption of food for the development of self-care and social skills.

WEDNESDAY

11:00–12:00 a.m.
Movement Group
or
Task Group

Depending upon the need, one of three task groups is conducted:
Quick Crafts—Individual completion of a simple, structured, short-term task; designed to provide a success experience and immediate gratification.
Current Events—Newspaper and news magazine articles are read and discussed by group members.
Garden Group—A seasonal vegetable and flower garden is planted and maintained through both individual and cooperative efforts.

3:00–4:00 p.m.
Open Occupational Therapy

THURSDAY

11:00–12:00 a.m.
Self-Expression Group

1:00–2:00 p.m.
Goals Group

A structured problem-solving group designed to assist patients in identifying realistic short-term goals for the hospitalization.

FRIDAY

11:00–12:00 a.m.
Life Skills Group

Practical skills and techniques for time and stress management, relaxation, avocations, assertiveness, and socialization are explored and practiced.

Unit Responsibilities

Weekly tasks are assigned to encourage a shared commitment for both the upkeep of the unit's common areas and the carry through of planned social activities.

2:00–3:00 p.m.
Open Occupational Therapy

We suggest that a wide range of purposeful activities be offered in the acute care hospital and that attempts be made to include many of those activities with which people fill the majority of their time. The general activity categories include: (a) work and prevocational tasks, (b) activities of daily living, (c) arts and crafts, (d) self-expressive or creative tasks, and (e) avocational pursuits.

The Nonhuman Environment

The nonhuman environment, an essential element in the occupational therapy doing process, refers to all aspects of the external environment that are not human. The nonhuman environment connotes the physical space and the objects, both natural and man-made. On the inpatient unit, it refers to the occupational therapy room, its arrangement of tables and chairs, and the equipment and materials used in the room. It also includes the community environment outside the hospital that the patient will be interacting with after discharge.

Searles[54] examines the relationship children have with their nonhuman worlds as they grow and develop. He explains the role of nonhuman object relationships: they increase awareness of the capacity for feeling, help to safely express feelings and absorb conflicts, facilitate awareness of physical-cognitive abilities and limitations, and serve as a place to practice developing interpersonal skills. These potential meanings are also found in the purposeful activities, and are thereby utilized to accomplish therapeutic aims.

The nonhuman environment can serve as both the means and the end in the occupational therapy treatment process. First, it can be viewed as an entity to be manipulated and mastered. In this instance, the treatment emphasis would be on helping the individual to use the nonhuman environment to learn specific performance skills or social roles, i.e., filling out a job application or learning to cook as part of an individual's move towards separation and more independence. The nonhuman environment can also be viewed as a vehicle or bridge for helping individuals to acquire greater self-understanding and more satisfying interpersonal relationships. Thus, it is used as a means for learning something else. For example, a creative writing exercise may be used to help the individual identify his feelings, or engaging in a group task may help the individual to recognize how he works with others.

Therapeutic Relationship—The Human Environment

The human environment refers to the interactions, both verbal and nonverbal, between the therapist and the patient. The therapeutic relationship is built upon the therapist's use of self. According to Tiffany, "in the occupational therapy process, the therapist's 'use of self' means bringing together knowledge, skills, caring and basic personality strengths to help the client overcome difficulties and maximize abilities."[55] In this acute care setting, the psychoanalytic concept of transference is not utilized. Rather, each therapist establishes and maintains his own identity as a helper. The occupational therapist assumes a variety of roles, including that of teacher, facilitator, counselor, coach, advocate, and supervisor. For example, our experience indicates that for the patient with a borderline personality a consistent approach and clear definition of rules and expectations elicits the most adaptive functioning. For the depressed patient, a supportive and accepting approach is used.

Activity Analysis

Activity analysis, in a biopsychosocial model, is concerned primarily with the biological, psychological, and sociocultural characteristics of the elements of an activity—the materials, process, and product. The analysis has two major purposes: to identify the capabilities required to engage in an activity and to identify components of the activity that may be emphasized or adapted in promoting development or restoration of function.

Nonhuman Environment—Materials, Process, and Product. In analyzing the biological dimension of an activity, we look at the kind and level of sensory-integrative, motor, and cognitive behaviors and actions required for successful completion. Materials are described by such aspects as their sensory input. An analysis of activity process may include identifying levels of thinking (abstract versus concrete) required and the motoric actions (gross or fine movements, repetitions, coordination) involved. The product may be analyzed in terms of its adaptive or survival value to a human organism.

Psychological processes of an acivity are analyzed along such lines as the potential for self-expression, originality, and creativity; the required ego skills; the affective feeling states potentially generated; and the symbolic and unconscious feelings, needs, and drives associated or gratified by the activity. Materials are described by such properties as resistiveness, pliability, controllability, and symbolic potential for sexual identification and reality testing. In our psychological analysis we are also concerned with identifying potential meanings, both real and symbolic, of the self-created product.

The acquired sociocultural properties of an activity reflect the values and beliefs of individuals and groups of people. Thus the various elements of an activity are analyzed for their symbolic meanings or inferences to gender, religion, age, ethnicity, and socioeconomic status.

Human Environment—Patient and Therapist Relationship. In addition to the nonhuman environment, in an activity analysis we also examine the inherent social and interpersonal processes or demands of an activity. In the analysis we ask: How much and what type of relatedness and communication are necessary to successfully complete the activity? Activities may require the involvement of other patients or the therapist, or may be best suited as solitary occupations.

Activity Adaptation

Activity adaptation refers to the strategic process of grading an activity along a planned continuum. This process is developmentally and sequentially operationalized to facilitate restoration and maintenance of functioning, as well as to promote new learning and more adaptive behaviors and attitudes. Based on the activity analysis, we now ask: are the properties of the activity meaningful and the processes and product relevant to the patient's life situation, occupational roles, and performance needs, or should they be modified in some way to better suit the patient's needs?

Graded Structured Activities— Individual and Group. The following are some general principles we observe in grading activities:

1. The steps of an activity and the requirements for action should proceed from *simple to more complex.*
2. The activity should be initially presented at a level at which the patient can *succeed.*
3. The demands of the activity should increase as the performance skills of the patient increase.
4. The patient should be led away from *inactive behavior towards more active and productive behavior.*

In grading structured activities for the individual, we consider the variability of symptomatology. For example, the depressed patient with an impaired attention span would be more assured of success if he or she were engaged in a short-term task or one that could be operationalized into smaller achievable steps. For the schizophrenic patient who has difficulty with informational processing and abstract concepts, an environment with limited stimuli and a visual sample of an end product would be beneficial for prompting success.

Group activities, including both modality and content, are graded according to the needs of the group members and the hospital setting in which the treatment takes place. On the short-term unit, where there is rapid patient turnover and patients display a wide range of individual pathology and occupational performance dysfunction, the group program is graded in the areas of activity process and program content. While the heterogeneous groups reflect diverse needs for activities and are graded to be meaningful and to accomodate both the higher and lower level functioning patients, the homogeneous groups are developed to address common areas of need.

Graded Structured Relationships— Individual and Group. In the biopsychosocial model, it is believed that the relationship between therapist and patient is dynamically influenced by the needs and behaviors of the patient and the subsequent response of the therapist. Interpersonal issues such as dependency, hostility, passivity, and need for control are emphasized and dealt with to an extent that is determined on an individual basis.

For the patient who experiences poor vocational adjustment and dysfunctional co-worker and supervisory relationships, for example, tasks may be structured to place the therapist in the role of authority figure and supervisor and the patient in the role of co-worker with another patient. In such a situation the therapist may model appropriate worker behaviors, give the patient feedback and suggest alternative behaviors, and reality test as needed. If the patient's primary treatment goal is to develop specific occupational performance skills, interpersonal issues would be named and identified as they occur but would not be a major focus of interaction. Rather, the therapist would structure the relationship to focus on the role of the therapist as facilitator or educator and the role of the patient as learner.

Finally, depending on the individual's treatment plan, the therapeutic relationship can be structured to emphasize the ego building and supportive value of individual or group activities rather than their uncovering aspects. The therapist may choose to gently instruct a patient on the processes of a particular activity, or may decide to devise a plan whereby the patient needs little or no instruction and can instead use written instructional aids such as those given in prefabricated embroidery or window-staining kits.

The choice of activity and its adaptability are finally determined by the constraints imposed by a particular setting. On the short-term unit, one must consider whether it is feasible to adapt an activity or whether it is more economical to select an alternate task. In making such a program decision, we find it necessary to consider the time factor for both preparation and completion of an activity, the cost of materials, the amount of space required, and the staffing demands, needs, and resources.

Our purpose in this section was to describe a model for occupational therapy on a psychiatric inpatient unit. As was just mentioned, therapists face some complex decisions in their daily practice. The following concluding remarks aim to outline some of these problems and point us to occupational therapy in the future.

CONTEMPORARY PROBLEMS IN OCCUPATIONAL THERAPY

As a profession, occupational therapy has always been concerned with the disabled individual's rights to a meaningful and productive existence. Grounded in our humanistic and existential philosophy has been the general belief that purposeful activities serve to prevent disease, promote health, and facilitate learning or desired change.

Current "bottom-line health care" management[56] and payment systems based on diagnostically related groups demand efficiency and cost control. Internally, occupational therapists have been debating the relative merits of our various conceptual models, and several have called for a unified theoretical base or paradigm for practice, education, and research. Basing her work on recent advances in neurosciences, Allen[57] convincingly questions and challenges the validity of our basic assumption that activities can prevent or change a psychiatric disease process caused by a biologic abnormality. She suggests that given the rapid effectiveness of psychotropic medication, the occupational therapist should focus treatment on the cognitive disability by changing the task rather than attempting to change the patient. Allen calls for a radical shift in acute care: from believing we can treat the cause of a disease to providing programs that detect changes in task performance and compensate for learning and memory aftereffects or disabilities.

In addition to these problems, hospital administrators and other disciplines often lack an understanding of the educational preparation, role, and value of the occupational therapist. Thereby psychiatric patients need rehabilitation programs which may be considered too costly, especially since the mentally ill are not viewed as a profitable market.

CONCLUSION

The various approaches and model for inpatient occupational therapy outlined in this chapter are based on our best knowledge of theory, research, and practice. As evidence about psychiatric disorders changes, one can expect modifications in the theory and practice of occupational therapy.

It is therefore imperative that a coherent model of occupational therapy be communicated, understood, and valued. This emphasizes the need for occupational therapists to make informed clinical and administrative decisions on the basis of empirical data, hence, the need for more research on both the cost-benefit and cost-effectiveness of occupational therapy and its qualitative value to the individual suffering from an acute psychiatric illness or chronic mental disability, on the well person, and on the individual at risk for a psychiatric condition.

Based on predicted shortened lengths of hospitalization we also suspect there will be a need for the development of structured, standardized functional evaluations. To assist in discharge and treatment planning, these tools must rapidly produce objective data about what the patient will be able to do or not do in community environments. Occupational therapy programs will emphasize symptom reduction and after-care planning. It is likely that occupational therapy program resources will shift, in part, to community programs and outpatient practice. Finally, we will see the role of occupational therapy in general hospital liaison psychiatry flourish as the biopsychosocial and occupational nature of individuals is better understood.

REFERENCES

1. Occupational therapy: Its definition and functions. Am J Occup Ther, 26: 204–205, 1972.
2. Fine SB: Occupational therapy: The role of rehabilitation and purposeful activity in mental health practice. Rockville, Md., American Occupational Therapy Association White Paper, 1983.
3. American Occupational Therapy Task Group of the APA Psychiatric Therapies, Fidler GS, Chair: Overview of occupational therapy in mental health, pp. 9 and 10, Rockville, Md., American Occupational Therapy Association White Paper, 1981.
4. Mosey AC: *Occupational Therapy Configuration of a Profession,* New York, Raven Press, 1981.
5. American Occupational Therapy Association: Standards of practice for occupational therapy. Am J Occup Ther, 37: 802–804, 1983.
6. Kielhofner G, Burke JP: Occupational therapy after 60 years: An account of changing identity and knowledge. Am J Occup Ther, 31: 674–689, 1977.
7. DeCarlo JJ, Mann WC: The effectiveness of verbal versus activity groups in improving self-perceptions of interpersonal communication skills. Am J Occup Ther, 39: 20–27, 1985.
8. Barris R, Kielhofner G, Watts JH: *Psychosocial Occupational Therapy Practice in a Pluralistic Arena,* Laurel, Md., RAMSCO, 1983.
9. Lazare A: Hidden conceptual models in clinical psychiatry. N Engl J Med, 288: 345–351, 1973.
10. Kaplan HI, Sadock BJ: *Modern Synopsis of Psychiatry/IV,* ed. 4, Baltimore, Williams & Wilkins, 1985.
11. King LJ: Occupational therapy research in psychiatry: A perspective. Am J Occup Ther, 32: 15–18, 1978.
12. Menninger KA: Work as a sublimation, in Sze WC (ed): *Human Life Cycle,* pp. 413–425, New York, Jason Aronson, 1975.
13. Neff W: Psychoanalytic conceptions of the meaning of work. Psychiatry, 28: 324–333, 1965.
14. Reisman D: The themes of work and play in the structure of Freud's thought. Psychiatry, 13: 1–7, 1950.
15. Walder R: Psychoanalytic theory of play, in Schaefer CE (ed): *Therapeutic Use of Child's Play,* pp. 79–93, New York, Jason Aronson, 1976.
16. Mosey AC: A model for occupational therapy. Occup Ther Ment Health, 1: 11–31, 1980.
17. Meyer A: The philosophy of occupational therapy, Arch Occup Ther, 1: 1–10, 1922.
18. Mosey AC: An alternative: The biopsychosocial model. Am J Occup Ther, 28: 137–140, 1974.
19. Clark PN: Human development through occupation: Theoretical frameworks in contemporary occupational therapy practice, Part 1. Am J Occup Ther, 33: 505–514, 1979.
20. Kaplan K: Short-term assessment: The need and a response. Occup Ther Ment Health, 4: 29–45, 1984.
21. King LJ: A sensory-integrative approach to schizophrenia. Am J Occup Ther, 28: 529–536, 1974.
22. King LJ: 1978 Eleanor Clarke Slagle lecture toward a science of adaptive responses. Am J Occup Ther, 32: 429–437, 1978.
23. Vander Roest LL, Clements ST: *Sensory In-*

tegration: Rationale and Treatment Activities for Groups, Grand Rapids, Mich., South Kent Mental Health Services, Inc., 1983.

24. Ross M, Burdick D: *A Sensory Integration Training Manual for Regressed and Geriatric Patients,* Middletown, Conn., Connecticut Valley Hospital, 1978.

25. Azima H, Azima FJ: Outline of a dynamic theory of occupational therapy. Am J Occup Ther, *13:* 215–221, 1959.

26. Fidler GS, Fidler JW: *Occupational Therapy: A Communication Process in Psychiatry,* New York, Macmillan, 1963.

27. Holmes C, Bauer W: Establishing an occupational therapy department in a community hospital. Am J Occup Ther, *24:* 219–221, 1970.

28. Briggs AK, Duncombe LW, Howe MC, Schwartzberg SL: *Case Simulations in Psychosocial Occupational Therapy,* Philadelphia, F. A. Davis, 1979.

29. Hemphill BJ (ed): *The Evaluative Process in Psychiatric Occupational Therapy,* Thorofare, N.J., Charles B. Slack, 1982.

30. Hyman M, Metzker JR: Occupational therapy in an emergency psychiatric setting. Am J Occup Ther, *24:* 280–283, 1970.

31. Mosey AC: *Activities Therapy,* New York, Raven Press, 1973.

32. Llorens LA: *Application of a Developmental Theory for Health and Rehabilitation,* Rockville, Md., American Occupational Therapy Association, 1976.

33. Mosey AC: Recapitulation of ontogenesis: A theory for practice of occupational therapy. Am J Occup Ther, *22:* 426–432, 1968.

34. Mosey AC: The concept and use of developmental groups. Am J Occup Ther, *24:* 272–275, 1970.

35. Florey LL: Intrinsic motivation: The dynamics of occupational therapy theory. Am J Occup Ther, *23:* 319–322, 1969.

36. Reilly M: A psychiatric occupational therapy program as a teaching model. Am J Occup Ther, *20:* 61–67, 1966.

37. Reilly M: The education process. Am J Occup Ther, *23:* 299–307, 1969.

38. Kielhofner G: Temporal adaptation: A conceptual framework for occupational therapy. Am J Occup Ther, *31:* 235–242, 1977.

39. Black MM: Adolescent role assessment. Am J Occup Ther, *30:* 73–79, 1976.

40. Florey LL, Michelman SM: Occupational role history: A screening tool for psychiatric occu-

pational therapy. Am J Occup Ther, *36:* 301–308, 1982.

41. Henry A, Kielhofner G, et al.: *The Occupational Performance History Interview Preliminary Version,* Rockville, Md., American Occupational Therapy Association, 1985.

42. Matsutsuyu JS: The interest checklist. Am J Occup Ther, *23:* 323–328, 1969.

43. Moorhead L: The occupational history. Am J Occup Ther, *23:* 329–334, 1969.

44. Neville A: Temporal adaptation: Application with short-term psychiatric patients. Am J Occup Ther, *34:* 328–331, 1980.

45. Shannon PD: The work-play model: A basis for occupational therapy programming in psychiatry. Am J Occup Ther, *24:* 215–218, 1970.

46. Howe MC, Briggs AK: Ecological systems model for occupational therapy. Am J Occup Ther, *36:* 322–327, 1982.

47. Kielhofner G (ed): *Health through Occupation Theory and Practice in Occupational Therapy,* Philadelphia, F. A. Davis, 1983.

48. Mosey AC: Meeting health needs. Am J Occup Ther, *27:* 14–17, 1973.

49. Reed KL, Sanderson SR: *Concepts of Occupational Therapy,* ed. 2, Baltimore, Williams & Wilkins, 1983.

50. Reed KL: *Models of Practice in Occupational Therapy,* Baltimore, Williams & Wilkins, 1984.

51. Fidler GS: The task-oriented group as a context for treatment. Am J Occup Ther, *23:* 43–48, 1969.

52. Howe MC, Schwartzberg SL: *A Functional Approach to Group Work in Occupational Therapy,* Philadelphia, J.B. Lippincott, 1986.

53. Fidler GS, Fidler JW: Doing and becoming: Purposeful action and self-actualization. Am J Occup Ther, *32:* 305–310, 1978.

54. Searles HF: *The Nonhuman Environment in Normal Development and in Schizophrenia,* New York, International Universities Press, 1960.

55. Tiffany EG: Psychiatry and mental health, in Hopkins HL, Smith HD (eds): *Willard and Spackman's Occupational Therapy,* ed. 6, p. 295, Philadelphia, J.B. Lippincott, 1983.

56. Levey S, Hesse DD: Sounding board: Bottomline health care? N Engl J Med, *312:* 644–646, 1985.

57. Allen CK: *Occupational Therapy for Psychiatric Diseases: Measurement and Management of Cognitive Disabilities,* Boston, Little, Brown & Co., 1985.

psychological testing

Gerald P. Borofsky, Ph.D.

Most inpatient psychiatric units regularly use psychological testing for diagnostic, prognostic, and treatment planning purposes. On the inpatient psychiatric unit, testing is usually done by a clinical psychologist who is a member of the unit's staff or a member of the hospital's psychology service. On smaller inpatient units an outside consultant is sometimes used to provide psychological testing. At teaching hospitals, pyschological assessments are also done by predoctoral interns or postdoctoral fellows in clinical psychology. In the same manner as residents, these interns and fellows are supervised by a senior member of the psychology staff.

The clinical psychologist typically holds a Ph.D. in clinical psychology and is licensed as a psychologist in the state where he practices. Along with his other clinical skills, the clinical psychologist has extensive experience in the administration, scoring, and interpretation of psychological tests.

On many inpatient units close collaborative relationships develop between clinicians and psychologists. Under optimal conditions, these relationships are based upon mutual respect. In such cases the resulting teamwork leads to the highest quality of patient care. Clinicians usually find that their work with clinical psychologists is most productive when they understand the concepts, methods, and tests used by the psychologist. Accordingly, this chapter attempts to assist the reader in obtaining an understanding of how the clinical psychologist uses psychological tests on an inpatient psychiatric unit.

WHAT ARE PSYCHOLOGICAL TESTS?

The clinical psychologist uses tests to *systematically sample* a patient's psychological functioning on a wide range of psychological tasks and under a variety of different psychological conditions. Some tests evoke strong emotional responses and therefore sample how a person copes under conditions of emotional arousal. Other tests are unstructured and therefore sample how a person copes with unstructured situations.

Psychological tests such as the Wechsler Adult Intelligence Scale-Revised (WAIS-R) sample a person's cognitive functioning on a standardized set of structured intellectual tasks. Other tests, such as the Rorschach Inkblot Test (Rorschach) and the Thematic Apperception Test (TAT) sample how a person functions when he is emotionally aroused in an unstructured situation. Yet other tests such as the Halstead-Reitan Neuropsychological Examination (Reitan) and the Luria-Nebraska Neuropsychological Examination (Luria) sample the general effectiveness of a patient's higher cortical functions as well as the adequacy of specific cortical functions. Still other tests such as the Wide Range Achievement Test (WRAT) sample a person's level fo skill, aptitude, and achievement.

The choice of what tests to use for a particular patient is largely determined by the specific questions the clinician raises in the referral. For this reason (as is discussed later) it is very important for the psychologist and clinician to discuss the specific referral questions *prior* to testing. This procedure allows the psychologist to fully understand the specific diagnostic, prognostic, and treatment planning questions the clinician wishes addressed. Such discussions also allow the clinician and psychologist to clarify any questions they may have.

On the inpatient psychiatric unit most referral questions are complex ones—requiring data from a wide range of psychological tasks and under a variety of different psychological conditions. For this reason the psychologist uses a *battery* of tests rather than a single test. Based upon his discussions with the referring clinician, the psychologist will put together a battery of tests which will enable him to broadly assess a person's strengths, vulnerabilities, and capacities as well as to systematically sample those psychological functions bearing on the specific referral questions.

RELIABILITY AND VALIDITY

Reliability and validity are two terms that psychologists commonly use when discussing psychological tests. If there is a low degree of reliability and validity, then the test results cannot be considered to be very accurate. On the other hand, if there is a high degree of reliability and validity, then the test results can be considered to have a high degree of accuracy.

Reliability

Psychologists use the term reliability in referring to: (1) a specific test and (2) the test findings. Most concisely put, reliability means *consistency*. If a test is said to be reliable, this means that if the test is given to a person on Monday morning and again on Tuesday morning, the results from both tests will be more or less the same (barring any major changes in the person's life or clinical circumstances during the interim). When a test is said to produce reliable *findings,* this means that if a person is tested by psychologist A on Monday morning and by psychologist B on Tuesday morning, the conclusions reached by both psychologists will be more or less the same.

Validity

Psychologists use the term validity in referring to (1) a specific test and (2) the

test findings. When we ask if a test is valid, we are simply asking if the test measures what it purports to measure. In most cases the validity of a specific test is established through a process of empirical research. People with similar scores on test "X" are compared with each other. Using psychological constructs researchers determine what these individuals have in common with each other as well as what differentiates them from other groups of individuals who have different scores on test "X".

A determination of the validity of test findings enables the psychologist to separate subjective intuitions and fantasies from empirically validated fact. In clinical practice the validity of a psychologist's findings is established by ensuring that he always systematically scores the test data, using one or more of the accepted techniques which have been developed for this purpose. Once the data are scored, an individual patient's scores on a test are then compared with the scores obtained on that test by various comparison groups (e.g., borderline personality disorders, schizophrenic disorders, etc.).

It can be seen that the concepts of reliability and validity are central to the enterprise of psychological testing. If a psychologist uses unreliable and invalid tests and proceeds to interpret them in an unreliable and invalid (i.e., subjective or "intuitive") manner, the clinical value of the tests is clearly minimal. On the other hand, when a psychologist uses reliable and valid tests and interprets them in a reliable and valid manner, the clincal value of psychological tests is considerable.

SOME CHARACTERISTICS OF PSYCHOLOGICAL TEST DATA

In order to maximize reliability and validity, the psychologist draws upon certain methodological principles inherent in the scientific method when collecting and interpreting test data. Some of these principles, as they relate to psychological testing, include: (1) standardized methods of administering tests and recording data; (2) standardized methods of categorizing (scoring) clinical data; (3) use of comparison or control groups when interpreting data; and (4) use of empirically validated hypotheses when interpreting data.

Standardized Methods of Administering Tests and Recording Data

As discussed earlier, an important principle of the scientific method is that information gathered by a clinician should be more or less the same regardless of the clinician's transient moods, personality organization, or degree of clinical experience. Psychological testing embodies this principle by *standardizing* the method of data collection. In order to maximize reliability, test manuals specify the exact manner in which the test should be administered. For this reason, a Rorschach given by an enthusiastic, 30-year-old psychologist in Berne, Switzerland, will be administered in exactly the same way as a Rorschach given by a grouchy, 50-year-old psychologist in Boston, Mass. The Wechsler Adult Intelligence Scales-Revised (WAIS-R) are administered in an identical manner whether they are given in San Francisco or Baltimore.

Standardized Methods of Categorizing (Scoring) Clinical Data

In order to maximize reliability, test manuals provide explicit and precise directions as to how a patient's test responses should be scored. On the WAIS-R, for example, specific instructions tell the psychologist how to score each answer given by a patient. Likewise, there are comprehensive and standardized systems for scoring Rohrschach responses.[1-5] For example, if a person sees "two angels carrying a woman to heaven" on Card I of the Rorschach, this will be scored the same way (for all practical purposes) by any psychologist who examines the data, regardless of what his theoretical orientation may be or what graduate school he attended.

Use of Comparison or Control Groups When Interpreting Data

When interpreting or reaching conclusions about the "meaning" of a patient's test responses, the psychologist makes *explicit* comparisons with scores obtained by other groups. In order to speak of the adequacy or inadequacy of a person's ego functioning or to speak of a person's rigid or flexible methods for testing reality, the psychologist compares the data obtained from an individual patient with data obtained from appropriate comparison groups. By comparing data obtained from an individual patient with normative data obtained from comparison groups (e.g., a group of patients independently diagnosed as having a borderline personality disorder) the psychologist is, for example, able to determine the degree to which a given patient has flexible or rigid methods of testing reality. By comparing an individual's scores on the Rorschach to the normative scores obtained by various comparison groups, the psychologist is able, for example, to conclude whether or not a person is likely to regress to a psychotic level of functioning when confronted with unanticipated emotional stress.

Use of Empirically Validated Hypotheses When Interpreting Data

Since most *clinical* hypotheses (in psychiatry and psychology) are conceptually derived from one or more theoretical perspectives (as opposed to being derived from a set of empirical facts),[6] it is necessary to distinguish the fanciful projections of a clinician's inner psychological world from empirically validated facts.

For this reason, the interpretation of test data relies heavily upon research findings which have correlated specific test findings with specific levels of psychological functioning. One brief example would be of a Rorschach record that might have a number of responses containing the word "blood." In the absence of empirical fact one psychologist might interpret these responses as "meaning" the patient is potentially violent while another psychologist might interpret these responses as "meaning" that the person is masochistic and sees himself as the victim of others' aggression. The only way to determine which (if either) interpretation is correct is by a process of empirical validation (in the case of "blood" responses there has been no correlation between this response and any clinically significant variable, with the exception of persons told to fake mental illness on the Rorschach who give larger numbers of "blood" responses.)

To minimize such "wild" speculation, the psychologist follows certain rules in interpreting the test data. If a psychologist is to interpret a particular score as a manifestation of mental illness, for example, then the psychologist first ensures: (1) that such a score is in fact obtained by individuals who have been independently diagnosed as being mentally ill; and (2) that such a score is not obtained by members of a "normal" comparison group. Through the application of these rules, the psychologist is able to *validly 0interpret the test data.*

GENERAL TYPES OF PSYCHOLOGICAL TESTS

There are several categories of psychological tests from which the psychologist draws when he puts together a battery of tests. These general categories of tests are: (1) tests of *intellectual functioning;* (2) *projective* personality tests; (3) *nonprojective* personality tests; (4) *neuropsychological* tests; and (5) tests of specific *skills, aptitudes,* and *achievements.*

Tests of Intellectual Functioning

These types of tests measure a person's current level of intellectual functioning as well as his intellectual capacity. Commonly known as IQ tests, the more reliable and valid "intelligence" tests assess a person's intellectual performance by comparing the individual's test scores to various sets of norms.

In addition to providing general measures of intellectual functioning and ability, these tests enable the psychologist to assess a number of component aspects of general intelligence. Some of these component aspects include a person's general fund of information; his awareness of what is called for in social situations; the capacity for understanding and communicating the abstract and metaphorical expressions of ideas; the capacity to comprehend relationships between objects, events, and ideas; the adequacy of the person's ability to concentrate and attend to

what is happening around him; the ability to understand cause and effect relationships, etc.

The most reliable, best validated, and most clinically useful tests of intellectual functioning are the Wechsler Tests: Wechsler Intelligence Scales for Children-Revised (WISC-R) for school age children up to middle adolescence and the Wechsler Adult Intelligence Scale-Revised (WAIS-R) for older adolescents and adults. Another widely used but clinically less useful intelligence test is the Stanford-Binet Intelligence Scale.

Projective Personality Tests

Projective personality tests systematically measure a person's psychological strengths and vulnerabilities by assessing how well the person copes when emotionally aroused. The requirements of a projective test are quite different from those of other psychological tests. The person taking the test is asked to respond to ambiguous and vague materials such as inkblots or pictures. In some projective tests, the person is asked to describe what he sees in these ambiguous inkblots or pictures and to describe the reasoning process by which he reached his conclusions (e.g., Rorschach Inkblot Test). In other tests of this type the person is asked to make up a story about what he thinks is going on in a particular picture (e.g., the Thematic Apperception Test).

Why are these tests called "projective"? Because the inkblots and pictures are unstructured and ambiguous and therefore allow for many different interpretations. Different individuals see different things in the same inkblot, just as different individuals tell different stories for the same picture. The ambiguity of the inkblots and pictures allows a person to "project" his own personality into his responses. It is for this reason that those tests are called projective.

For reasons that have to do with basic brain functioning,[7] a person confronted with ambiguous and unstructured situations becomes emotionally aroused and begins to feel anxious and/or depressed. Some people manage to cope quite effectively with these dysphoric affects when they are aroused, while others fare less well (e.g., make suicide attempts, act in antisocial ways to gain attention, take drugs to avoid feeling depressed or anxious, act violently, become psychotic, etc.). By using reliable and well-validated projective tests such as the Rorschach Inkblot Test and the Thematic Apperception Test, the psychologist is able to gain considerable insight as to how an individual functions in unstructured situations when he is experiencing dysphoric affects. For all of us, coping is more difficult under such conditions. Whether a person's functioning remains adequate or whether there is a regression in functioning under such conditions can be systematically, reliably, and validly measured by projective tests, as long as the test results are systematically analyzed and scored in a reliable manner.

Some of the most reliable and best-validated projective tests are the Rorschach Inkblot Test, the Sentence Completion Test, the Tasks of Emotional Development Test (TED), and the Thematic Apperception Test (TAT).

There are a number of projective personality tests which are frequently used on an inpatient psychiatric unit even though there is minimal evidence that they are reliable or valid for assessing psychological functioning. These are drawing tests such as the Human Figure Drawing Test (HFD), the House, Tree, Person Test (HTP), and the Kinetic Family Drawing Test (KFD). While these tests may be a potentially rich source of data for generating clinically interesting hypotheses, the low reliability and validity of these tests make their use in reaching important clinical decisions inadvisable.

Nonprojective Personality Tests

Nonprojective personality tests usually consist of a large number of declarative statements (e.g., "I often black out and forget where I am"; "I very often think that there is something seriously wrong with my body"; etc.) which the person answers "true," "false," or "I can't say." A person's answers to individual questions are grouped together in various systematic ways, and the answers are scored in a reliable manner. The patterns of scores for a given person are compared with the patterns of scores for various groups (e.g., patients with major affective disorders, patients with schizophrenic disorders, etc.). Based on the similarities and differences which result from these comparisons, the psychologist reaches specific conclusions about the psychological functioning of the person taking the test. (These tests are somewhat speciously called "objective" tests by their advocates in an effort to compare them favorably to projective personality tests. In point of fact, if *any* psychological test is scored in a reliable manner and is interpreted validly, then it is an *objective* psychological test. If any test is not scored and interpreted in this manner, then it is a *subjective* psychological test.)

In contrast to the conclusions reached on the basis of projective test results, nonprojective tests give an indication of how the person himself rates the day to day adequacy of his psychological functioning.

Nonprojective tests do not give an objective measure of how well a person functions when he is emotionally aroused. In general, nonprojective personality tests are less effective in providing an in-depth understanding of how well a person copes when he is under stress.

The most commonly used nonprojective personality test is the Minnesota Multiphasic Personality Inventory (MMPI). This test consists of 566 declarative statements which the person answers "true," "false," or "I can't say." This test is frequently used on inpatient psychiatric settings. By itself the MMPI can only serve as a screening test, that is, a test which generates specific hypotheses for the psychologist to follow up with more comprehensive methods of testing, such as projective personality testing. However, when it comprises one element of an overall battery of tests, the MMPI can be helpful in providing reliable, valid, and clinically useful information.

Neuropsychological Tests

In recent years there has been a growing awareness of the widespread and previously undiagnosed presence of impaired higher cortical functioning among individuals who are suffering from apparently psychogenic disorders. Various studies[8] have estimated that some 20% of individuals diagnosed as having a psychogenic disorder are also suffering from some type of organic brain syndrome. (Given the artificiality of the mind-body dualism, which seems to hinder progress in our fields, such a finding is not at all surprising.) For this reason, neuropsychological tests have assumed an increasingly greater role as part of the psychological testing battery.

Neuropsychological tests systematically measure a range of brain functions which influence and regulate behavior (so-called brain-behavior relationships). Some of the brain-behavior relationships assessed by neuropsychological tests include: (1) the capacity for learning new skills and ideas; (2) the capacity for complex conceptual tracking without being distracted; (3) the capacity to make fine sensory discriminations; (4) the capacity for fine motor speed and fine motor coordination; (5) the adequacy of perception and perceptual reasoning; (6) the adequacy of perceptual-motor functions; (7) the adequacy of constructional skills; (8) the adequacy of short-term memory; (9) the capacity to persist in difficult tasks without distraction; (10) the capacity to flexibly shift expectations and effort as environmental conditions change; (11) the adequacy of language-related functions; and (12) the capacity to inhibit impulses when under stress. In contrast to advanced methods of radiological diagnosing, such as the CT scanner, a battery of neuropsychological tests enables the psychologist to document the *functional* brain behavior relationships which have been impaired by a brain syndrome.

Typically, several neuropsychological *screening* tests are included in the battery of tests constructed by the psychologist. If the findings from the screening tests are suggestive of an organic brain syndrome, then a *comprehensive battery* of neuropsychological tests is indicated in order to both confirm the diagnosis and to document the specific functional systems in the brain that are impaired. For this reason, a single test such as the Bender-Gestalt Test or the Benton Visual Retention Test is, *by*

itself, not an adequate method for assessing the functional status of a person's higher cortical functioning. Some comprehensive batteries of neuropsychological tests are the Halstead-Reitan Neuropsychological Examination, the Luria-Nebraska Neuropsychological Examination, and the Boston Veterans Administrative Neuropsychological Examination.

Tests of Specific Skills, Aptitudes, and Achievement

Although this category of tests is less frequently used on an inpatient unit, there are, nonetheless, some situations where tests of skills, aptitudes, and achievement may have a useful role to play. These kinds of tests are used to compare an individual's level of skill, aptitude, and achievement against specific sets of norms. For example, the Wide Range Achievement Test (WRAT) is a commonly used test which assesses the grade level of a person's reading, spelling, and arithmetic skills. The Iowa Test of Basic Skills and the Stanford Achievement Tests are also commonly used test batteries which assess a student's level of skill and achievement in a wide range of areas related to school performance.

These tests might be used by a psychologist when questions arise as to whether or not a person is functioning at a level commensurate with his age, present grade, and/or highest grade attended in school. These tests form a part of the battery when questions of learning disability are raised. These tests can also be used to assess whether or not a person has the basic aptitudes and skills necessary for success in a specific type of occupation.

WHAT IS MEASURED BY PSYCHOLOGICAL TESTS?

As noted earlier, psychological tests systematically sample a person's psychological functioning on a wide range of psychological tasks and under a variety of psychological conditions. For this reason, the data obtained by psychological tests can be helpful in addressing questions related to diagnosis, treatment planning, and prognosis.

Diagnosis

Data from psychological tests can be used to address several issues.

Differential Diagnosis Using the DSM-III Multiaxial Evaluation System

Data from psychological tests can be used to establish differential diagnoses on Axis I and Axis II. (Axis I of the DSM-III evaluation system addresses itself to the presence or absence of clinical syndromes. Axis II addresses itself to the presence or absence of personality disorders and specific developmental disorders.) Specific issues which can be effectively addressed using psychological test data include:

1. The establishment of a differential diagnosis on Axis I. For example, by assessing the degree of disruption in a patient's thought processes, the data from psychological tests can be used to make the differential diagnosis between a schizophrenic disorder and an affective disorder. The data may also be used to articulate the underlying factors that go into the differential diagnosis.
2. The establishment of a differential diagnosis on Axis II. For example, by assessing the stability of a patient's reality testing under unstructured conditions of emotional arousal, the psychological test data can be used to make the sometimes difficult differential diagnosis between a borderline personality disorder and a narcissistic personality disorder.
3. A specification of how the Axis I and Axis II diagnoses interact in a given patient. All Axis I diagnoses exist within the context of an individual patient's personality organization. The Axis I diagnosis expresses itself in somewhat different ways depending on the patient's particular personality organization. For example, the clinical expression of a major depressive episode in an histrionic personality will be different from the clinical expression of a major depressive episode in a paranoid personality. By assessing the underlying psychological functions

in a patient's personality structure, the data from psychological tests can be used to articulate the interweaving of a patient's personality structure of the Axi I disorder.

Assessment of Ego Strengths and Ego Vulnerabilities

Because psychological tests *systematically* assess a patient's psychological functioning, the test data are particularly useful in assessing a patient's functioning with regard to his overall ego *strengths* and ego *vulnerabilities*.

Psychological tests can assess a patient's ego functioning under a variety of different psychological conditions (e.g., under structured and unstructured conditions, under conditions of emotional arousal or emotional neutrality). The same type of assessment can be made with regard to *specific* ego functions. The test data can also be used to assess the *developmental level* at which specific ego functions operate in a given patient. That is, a given patient can be assessed as to the degree of differentiation, integration, flexibility, stability, and modulation represented in his overall ego functioning. The types of ego functions that can be assessed by psychological testing include:

1. Reality testing
2. Judgment
   a. Social awareness
   b. Anticipatory functions
3. Sense of reality (e.g., vulnerability to depersonalization and/or derealization)
4. Methods of regulating drives (Libido and Aggression)
5. Methods of regulating dysphoric affects (Anxiety and Depression)
6. Adequacy of attention, concentration, and memory
7. Thought processes (Information Processing)
   a. Congtive capacities (e.g., IQ)
   b. Cognitive style
   c. Capacity for self-crucial, reflective thought
   d. Capacity for understanding and communicating the abstract-metaphorical expression of ideas
   e. Method of regulating primary pro-

cess thought (e.g., rigidly vs. flexibility)

   f. Degree of awareness and understanding of cause and effect relationships

   g. Methods of reasoning (e.g., logical vs. disordered)

   h. Thought content (e.g., richness vs. impoverishment, complexity vs. simplicity)

   i. Capacity to use thought as a mediator of drives and affects

8. Level of moral development and degree of superego development

9. Adequacy of analytic functions (e.g., the capacity to make conceptual and affective discriminations)

10. Adequacy of synthetic functions (e.g., the capacity to comprehend relationships among objects, events, and ideas)

11. Perception of the self

   a. Self perception—Degree of differentiation and integration

   b. General affective tone with regard to the self

   c. Degree of stability of self-esteem (e.g., stable vs. labile, rigid vs. flexible)

   d. Methods of regulating self-esteem (e.g., projection vs. introjection)

   e. Body image representation

Assessment of Specific Diagnostic Questions

Data from psychological tests can also be used to address specific diagnostic questions about an individual's personality organization. Questions which can be addressed include:

1. Assessment of interpersonal relationships

   a. In *developmental* terms (e.g., symbiotic, part-object, etc.)

   b. In *drive* terms (e.g., oral, anal, phallic, etc.)

   c. In *psychosocial* terms (e.g., trust vs. mistrust, identity vs. role diffusion; etc.)

2. Articulating areas or themes of conflict which are adaptively and/or maladaptively managed by the person (e.g., situations which evoke dependence, situations which arouse

sexual feelings or feelings of aggression, etc.)

3. Assessment of specific traits (e.g., impulsiveness, homicidality, suicidality, vulnerability to psychotic regression, etc.)

Differential Diagnosis of Higher Cortical Functions

Neuropsychological assessment procedures provide clinically useful information regarding the diagnosis of cortical dysfunction and the description of specific behavioral effects resulting from brain lesions. They also provide clinically useful information regarding the prognosis and management of individuals with brain syndromes. Such neuropsychological data provides a rational basis for deciding whether or not to order more extensive and more expensive neurodiagnostic procedures.

More specifically, data from neuropsychological tests can:

1. Provide early diagnostic information as to the presence or absence of cortical dysfunction.

2. Provide early differential diagnosis of primary organic or functional disorders and the relative impact of each. For example, this can be particularly valuable in clarifying the difficult diagnostic problem of differentiating early dementia from depression.

3. Determine whether cortical dysfunction is diffuse or focal and provide data on lateralization and localization.

4. Describe the specific effects of a brain lesion on a person's behavior, cognitive functioning, emotional functioning, and social adjustment.

5. Estimate the person's premorbid level of functioning and make an accurate assessment of any deterioration in cortical functioning.

6. Determine the presence and differential contribution of both organic and psychological factors in individuals with learning disabilities, behavior disorders, or hyperactivity.

7. Provide objective data for those

cases of trauma and/or suspected cortical dysfunction in which litigation is involved.

Treatment Planning

Data from psychological tests can also be used to address questions related to treatment planning.

Type of Treatment(s) Indicated

Based upon assessment of an individual's ego functioning and/or higher cortical functioning, a recommendation for the indicated *type* of treatment may be possible.

1. Somatic Therapies. For example, the test data can be used to address questions such as, "Is the patient suffering from a brief reactive psychosis or is he suffering from a chronic bipolar affective disorder?"

2. Environmental (Milieu) Therapies. The test data can also be used to assess whether the person can tolerate the high levels of emotional arousal and the unstructured setting which characterize psychodynamic psychotherapy without experiencing a psychotic regression, or whether the patient must limit his experiencing of emotional stimulation solely to structured situations such as a milieu group in order to avoid such a regression.

3. Psychotherapy. If the test data reveal that a patient can tolerate the emotional stimulation and relative lack of structure which characterizes this form of treatment without experiencing psychotic regression, then a recommendation for a specific form of psychotherapy can be made. Such recommendations are typically based on an assessment of the specific areas of conflict which are maladaptively managed by the patient, e.g., if a person has specific difficulties in the management of dysphoric affects (anxiety, depression) and/or drives (libido, aggression), then a recommendation for individual therapy would most probably be made. If, in addition, the test data revealed that interpersonal relations and social interactions had been maladaptively managed by the patient, then a recommendation of group therapy as well as individual therapy might be made. If

the test data revealed themes of maladaptively managed conflict in the areas of marriage and family, then a recommendation for marital or family therapy might well be in order.

Specific Treatment Considerations

By providing a comprehensive overview of a patient's deficits and residual abilities, an individualized treatment plan can be developed. The development of such a treatment plan would consider factors such as the following.

1. Structured versus Unstructured Treatment. Essentially all forms of psychological treatment require the patient to experience some degree of emotional arousal. The state of the patient's ego functioning determines whether he can tolerate such emotional stimulation under the relatively unstructured conditions of psychodynamic psychotherapy or whether he requires the structure of a milieu group or "supportive" psychotherapy in order to avoid a psychotic regression when emotionally aroused. Naturally, there is an hierarchical gradient between these two extremes of structured and unstructured. The test data can enable the psychologist to make a recommendation as to the optimal balance of structure and lack of structure, based upon the state of the patient's ego functioning.

2. Emotionally Stimulating versus Emotionally Suppressing Treatment. The degree of emotional stimulation a patient can tolerate (independent of the degree of structure) without a psychotic regression varies depending on his ability to cope adaptively with dysphoric affects and drives. For example, if the test data show a serious weakness in the patient's capacity to resist psychotic regression when stimulated by drives and/or affects, then a recommendation is made that psychotherapy should be less emotionally expressive and more "supportive." If, on the other hand, the test data reveal that the patient does possess adequate ego resources to effectively resist psychotic regression when he experiences dysphoric affects and drives, then a recommendation for a more expressive and exploratory form of psychotherapy will be made.

3. Specific Areas of Vulnerability to Maladaptive Forms of Regression. The nature of psychological test data is such that the psychologist can describe the specific thematic areas of a patient's life which are maladaptively managed or which represent a potential for maladaptive or psychotic forms of regression. For example, for some patients the characterological tendency to deny or repress conflicts involving dependency leaves them vulnerable to psychotic forms of regression when they become lonely. Other patients are unable to adequately differentiate sex and aggression in close interpersonal relationships, thus leaving them vulnerable to pathological forms of regression when sexually aroused. The test data allow the psychologist to note such areas of vulnerability and to assess the degree of vulnerability to regression that a specific patient may have.

4. Recommendation for Specific Foci of Treatment. In detailing a patient's specific areas of ego vulnerability, the psychologist alerts the clinician to specific aspects of the patient's psychological functioning which may require special attention during treatment. For example, if the test data reveal that a patient is vulnerable to reacting to situations of potential dependence by avoidance and flight, the psychologist can alert the clinician that the inevitable evocation of dependency which accompanies most forms of psychotherapy may be accompanied by heightened efforts by the patient to leave treatment. Being thus forewarned, the clinician can typically take effective action to minimize the untoward aspects of this tendency in the patient.

Anticipated Resistances to Treatment

The test data can be used, for example, to assess whether a patient will threaten to leave treatment if the therapist attempts to have him focus upon the emotional rather than the intellectual aspects of his experience.

Anticipated Transference Reactions

For example, the test data can be used to assess whether the patient will attempt to idealize the therapist for defensive purposes and will resist seeing the therapist as a "real" person. However, positive idealizations are likely to shift rapidly to negative ones if the patient's expectations are not met.

Probable Countertransference Reactions in Working with the Patient

For example, the test data might be used to anticipate that a patient's tendency to overintellectualize and the instability of the patient's idealizing tendencies may be a potential source of frustration to the therapist.

Prognosis

Baseline data obtained from psychological testing can be used to address issues of prognosis. For example, the test data can be used for: (1) setting realistic treatment goals; (2) specifying factors that may limit treatment outcome; and (3) monitoring therapeutic progress.

Setting Realistic Treatment Goals

For example, the test data might be used to anticipate that with intensive individual psychotherapy the patient should make a full recovery in the area of work. However, in the area of interpersonal relationships the prognosis is less positive.

Specifying Factors That May Limit Treatment Outcome

For example, the test data might indicate that a patient's lack of sensitivity to nuances of emotion in interpersonal relationships augurs poorly for the future possibility of an intimate relationship.

Monitoring Therapeutic Progress

For example, the test data might indicate the advisability of reassessment of a person's functioning after a period of treatment and comparison of the results with his baseline level of functioning obtained from the initial testing or of assessment of a patient on readmission and comparison of those data with his baseline level of functioning at the time of a previous admission or discharge.

REPORT OF TEST FINDINGS

When the psychologist finishes testing a patient, he scores the patient's responses and interprets the test data. These findings are then integrated into a written report which addressed the clinician's specific referral questions. The written report becomes a permanent part of the patient's record.

INDICATIONS FOR PSYCHOLOGICAL TESTING

Although it is difficult to articulate all possible indications for psychological testing, there are a few general guidelines which may assist the clinician in deciding whether or not to order psychological tests. Psychological testing should be ordered:

1. On a patient's first admission to an inpatient psychiatric unit. First admissions typically require a comprehensive workup including the systematic gathering of baseline data. Psychological testing is *always* indicated on a first admission in order to obtain diagnostic, prognostic, and treatment planning information as well as baseline data against which subsequent changes can be measured.

2. When there appear to be changes in the patient's status during hospitalization. Clinically observed changes in a patient's status can be systematically confirmed and documented with the data from psychological tests.

3. On a readmission to the unit or on a readmission from some other inpatient psychiatric unit. When a former patient is readmitted, psychological testing data can be used to assess the patient's current status as well as any changes since the last admission. When a current patient on the unit was previously a patient on some other psychiatric inpatient unit, a request should *always* be made to the other unit for a copy of the *actual test data* as well as a copy of the written report of findings. After reviewing these materials with the unit psychologist, the

clinician may have certain specific questions which he wants addressed. On the other hand, the clinician may decide after consultation with the unit psychologist that a more comprehensive psychological assessment is warranted.

4. Whenever the clinician has specific questions related to diagnosis, treatment planning and/or prognosis. If the clinician wishes to specifically address any of the types of issues discussed in the previous section, then psychological testing should be ordered.

If the clinician decides to order psychological testing, then the question arises as to when during a patient's hospitalization the testing should be done. The answer to this question is highly dependent on the patient's clinical status. To *maximize* the reliability and validity of the test findings as well as the amount of diagnostic, prognostic, and treatment planning information, it is best not to order testing at the height of a florid psychosis or at the nadir of a psychotic depression. At these times ego functioning is so severely disrupted that it is difficult to assess the subtle interplay between a patient's ego strengths and his ego weaknesses. The clinically obvious statement that a patient's ego functioning is massively disrupted can, of course, be confirmed. However, an assessment of the more subtle interactions of ego functions for diagnostic, prognostic, and treatment planning purposes is best made when there is at least some stability in a patient's overall ego functioning. For this reason, it is probably best to wait and order testing once the most acute phase of a patient's disturbance has somewhat abated.

PSYCHOLOGICAL TESTING COSTS

The cost of psychological testing varies depending on the referral questions involved and the types of tests administered. In all cases, an estimate of the costs can be obtained from the psychologist prior to testing. Where cost becomes a deciding factor in ordering testing, the clinician should consult with the psychologist to discuss the situation. In most cases some form of workable resolution is easily achieved.

In most states psychological testing on an inpatient psychiatric unit is fully covered by Blue Cross and other private insurance carriers. Testing is also covered by Federal Employee's Health Insurance, CHAMPUS, Medicare, and Medicaid.

REFERRAL PROCEDURES

Once the clinician decides that the psychological testing is indicated, he orders the testing, and an appointment is scheduled. This is usually done by the clinician notifying the unit secretary or by calling the psychology office directly. Referral information usually includes the patient's name, his hospital number, and location of the patient in the hospital, as well as the referring clinician's name and phone number. When possible, it is helpful to have a rough estimate of the time frame within which the results of the testing are required. Usually the testing is done and a verbal report of findings is available within several days to a week of the time of the referral. When there is a need for a more rapid reporting of test findings, the clinician should be sure to indicate that when making the referral.

Before the patient is tested it is extremely important that the clinician and psychologist discuss the case with each other. Ideally this is done face to face *if at all possible*. Given the practical realities of a busy inpatient unit, however, a 5- to 10-minute phone conversation can often suffice—particularly when the clinician and psychologist have developed a close and effective working relationship in which there is free and open communication.

The purpose of this meeting is to ensure that the psychologist fully understands what the clinician wants from the testing. For a psychologist to satisfactorily address a clinician's referral questions he must fully understand the specific details of those questions as well as the specific information in which the clinician is interested.

PREPARING THE PATIENT

Before the patient is tested it is also extremely important for the clinician to meet with the patient. The purpose of this meeting is to inform the patient that he has been referred for psychological testing, and to prepare the patient for testing by:

1. Explaining the clinician's reasons for ordering testing and explaining the importance of the tests (e.g., "I feel that since the tests measure how people cope with different types of situations, the tests will enable me to more fully understand you as a person and therefore put me in the best position to be of help to you.")

2. Explaining what is involved in the testing procedure (e.g., "The psychologist will ask you a variety of questions, many of which involve the kinds of things you already know about. On other tests he will ask you to use your imagination in answering the questions.") It is usually advisable to ask the patient if he has taken psychological tests before. If the answer is "yes," the patient can be assured that the upcoming tests are identical or quite similar to the tests he has taken in the past. If the answer is "no," the patient can be assured that these tests are somewhat similar to other types of tests he may have taken in the past at school or at work.

3. Explaining how long the testing takes. The length of time will depend on the number of tests administered, the clinical status of the patient, and the degree of cooperation and effort which the patient exerts. More comprehensive referral questions usually involve longer periods of time. If desired, the clinician can get an estimate of the time involved from the psychologist. The patient should be given this estimate with the caveat that it is a rough approximation.

4. Answering any questions the patient may have about the testing. The clinician should directly ask the patient if he has any questions about the testing. Most questions from patients are quite straightforward and are generally motivated by a desire for factual infor-

mation and/or a desire to allay anxiety. If the clinician is unsure how to answer a patient's question he should consult with the psychologist and then get back to the patient with the answer.

5. Arranging an appointment with the patient to provide him with feedback about the test results. Because patients know that the testing is important to their care they are generally interested in knowing the psychologist's findings. Communicating the test findings to the patient can be done by either the clinician or the psychologist. In either case, however, an appointment should be set up with the patient prior to testing. The clinician may feel that he is not sufficiently knowledgeable to explain the intricate details of the test findings and that the psychologist may be better suited for the job. There are several points to keep in mind in this regard. First, the clinician usually has an ongoing relationship with his patient, and therefore the patient is usually more comfortable in discussing these matters with the clinician. Second, the patient is rarely, if ever, interested in the technical details of the report. He usually wants to know just the main points and what the general diagnostic, prognostic, and treatment planning implications are. A "plain English" discussion of these implications by the clinician is all that the patient desires in the way of substantive information and emotional reassurance.

Since the goal of psychological testing is to obtain a comprehensive view of the patient's psychological functioning, it is important to maximize the patient's cooperation and effort during the testing. While a patient's full cooperation is not essential, it does enable the psychologist to assess the patient at his best level of functioning. By meeting with the patient prior to testing, the clinician can uncover and hopefully allay any anxieties the patient may have about the testing, while at the same time encouraging the patient to do his best.

After the psychologist completes the testing and before the data are formally scored and interpreted, the psychologist usually writes a brief note in the chart listing the date and time testing was completed, a preliminary diagnostic impression, and preliminary answers to the specific referral questions. The psychologist will also contact the clinician by phone to give a brief impression and to arrange a time for discussing the full findings once the data are scored and interpreted.

Given the administrative realities of a busy inpatient psychiatric unit it may take up to a week from the time of testing before a written report of findings is placed in the patient's record. Oftentimes this is too slow a pace for the clinician who requires information more rapidly. For this reason, it is especially important that the clinician arrange to meet with the psychologist, on a more immediate basis, to discuss the test findings. This discussion allows the clinician to raise questions, to clarify points that may seem ambiguous, and to gather more detailed information where necessary. When the clinician and the psychologist have a close effective working relationship in which there is free and open communication, this phase of the process usually takes 10–15 minutes and can, if absolutely necessary, be done over the phone.

It is often tempting for the busy clinician to bypass one(or more of these steps. However, when a clinician follows each of the steps outlined above, he is most likely to obtain the maximum amount of clinically useful data from psychological testing.

REFERENCES

1. Beck S, Beck A, Levitt E, Molish H: *Rorschach's Test. I. Basic Processes,* ed. 3, New York, Grune & Stratton, 1961.
2. Exner JE: *The Rorschach: A Comprehensive System,* New York, John Wiley, 1974.

3. Klopfer B, Ainsworth MD, Klopfer WG, Holt RR: *Developments in the Rorschach Technique,* vol. I, New York, Harcourt, Brace & World, 1954.
4. Piotrowski Z: *Perceptanalysis,* New York, Macmillan, 1957.
5. Rickers-Osviankina M (ed): *Rorschach Psychology,* ed. 2, Huntington, NY, Krieger, 1977.
6. Lazare A: Hidden conceptual models in clinical psychiatry. N Engl J Med, *288:* 345–351, 1973.
7. Sokolov EN: Neuronal models and the orienting reflex, in Brazier MA (ed): *The Central Nervous System and Behavior: Transactions of the Third Conference,* New York, Josiah Macy Jr. Foundation, 1960.
8. Strub RL, Black FW: *The Mental Status Examination in Neurology,* Philadelphia, F. A. Davis Co., 1977.

SUGGESTED READINGS

Golden CJ: *Diagnosis and Rehabilitation in Clinical Neuropsychology,* Springfield, Ill., Charles C Thomas, 1978.
Golden CJ: *Clinical Interpretation of Objective Psychological Tests,* New York, Grune & Stratton, 1979.
Henry WE: *The Analysis of Fantasy,* Huntington, N.Y., Krieger, 1973.
Rabin AT (ed): *Projective Techniques in Personality Assessment,* New York, Springer, 1968.
Rapaport D, Gill MD, Schafer R: *Diagnostic Psychological Testing,* rev. ed., New York, International Universities Press, 1968.
Schafer R: *Psychoanalytic Interpretation in Rorschach Testing,* New York, Grune & Stratton, 1954.

chapter 17

legal issues in inpatient psychiatry

Harold Bursztajn, M.D., Thomas G. Gutheil, M.D., and Bonnie Cummins

INTRODUCTION

Any contemporary textbook on inpatient psychiatry would be incomplete without a substantial section devoted to the legal issues which impact on inpatient clinicians. The past 20 years have spawned a changing but increasingly expanding body of legislation and case law regarding the rights, care, and treatment of the mentally ill. One result of this growth has been an expansion of the contact points between psychiatry and the law, especially in the areas of criminal, victim compensation, and family law. Since numerous books have been written on these classical contact points, we will focus on those emerging areas of contact where the inpatient psychiatrist's understanding of medicolegal issues is critical to the care of *any* hospitalized patient. In particular, the exercise of good judgment and careful understanding of today's most pressing legal issues regarding informed consent, liability, and patient rights are a must if the quality of hospitalized patients' care is to be enhanced rather than compromised by these developments. The focus of this chapter therefore will be on an integration of emerging legal requirements into the clinical process. Matters of documentation, an essential aspect of all medicolegal activity, are addressed in the next chapter.

INFORMED CONSENT

Informed Consent: From Pro Forma to Process

When informed consent is approached as a form to be signed by the patient in order to meet legal requirements, it is experienced by both the clinician and patient as little more than a manipulation: clinical utility is absent, and its legal value is dubious. On the other hand, when the criteria for informed consent are understood as gaining their meaning from a two-person process, the criteria can serve to build the doctor-patient relationship and alliance.

Quality care and the informed consent process are the wheel and axle of the vehicle of psychiatric inpatient diagnosis and treatment. The inpatient psychiatrist is legally mandated to obtain and document informed consent prior to the administration of all diagnostic and treatment interventions. The doctrine of informed consent stipulates that the patient must consent to the procedure(s) before it is performed and that this consent is predicated on *voluntary* acceptance and *competence* in understanding reasonable *information* about the procedure or treatment. Failure to obtain patient consent may be legally deemed as battery. Failure to meet the criteria for informed consent may constitute negligence. The criteria for informed consent can be satisfied by determining the patient's voluntariness of consent and capacity to take part in the informed consent procedure.

Voluntariness

Voluntariness, in relation to informed consent, most simply means that the patient's choice was made in the absence of coercion. Some would argue that institutionalized individuals cannot "voluntarily" choose since their present needs and future wishes are tied to their caretakers' recommendations. Acceptance of this premise would deny institutionalized individuals the right to make any important decisions and seriously compromise the promotion of individual autonomy that informed consent seeks to achieve. Voluntariness of consent should be understood, therefore, as free patient choice in the absence of coercion or undue influence. This applies equally to voluntarily or involuntarily hospitalized patients.

To some extent many psychiatric patients are either "unduly influenceable" or "uninfluenceable." An example of undue influenceability is the overly dependent patient who, although over 18, is symbiotically tied to a parental figure and cannot distinguish his own wishes from those of the parent. The psychiatrist must consider whether he has become such a figure for his patient, via the process of transference. On the other end of the spectrum is the overwhelmingly counterdependent and uninfluenceable patient who remains aloof and excludes dialogue.

At times a patient may be *both* overly influenceable and uninfluenceable. This can occur when a patient is so tied to a real or imagined parental figure that he is unable to exercise a will of his own sufficient to engage in dialogue. Such a patient may present as counterdependent to the examiner ("I won't listen to anything you have to say"), while experiencing himself as powerless, weak-willed, and dependent for his survival on an all-powerful parental figure. Exploring with the patient his experienced vulnerability to domination or

abandonment is critical to moving beyond such a clinical stalemate. It is also critical to undertake such an exploration in order to safeguard against the legal proceedings that the patient may focus on as a substitute for working through clinical conflict.

Capacity (Competence)

"The ability to understand rationally"—i.e., competence—is a legal concept, determined by the court.[1] Competence most often refers to the capacity to understand the nature and consequences of one's actions or decisions. Some individuals are recognized as generally incompetent, others as showing specific incompetence. In the latter group, the individual may be competent to arrive at personal decisions but not treatment decisions. The general rule today is that involuntary commitment does not presume incompetence. In fact, a committed mentally ill person is presumed competent unless legally adjudicated otherwise.

It is neither possible (because of limited resources) nor desirable to legally determine competence for each patient prior to the delivery of clinical services. The process of deciding to obtain a judicial competence evaluation is therefore integrated into the work of the inpatient unit.

Several tests for determining competency to consent to treatment have been used both by psychiatrists and the courts. Certain populations appear at risk for incompetency: acutely psychotic patients who might exhibit delirium; chronic (long-term) institutionalized patients who may have lost critical reasoning capacity; organically impaired patients; elderly senile patients; depressed patients who may be generally hopeless about the future; and retarded patients.[2] These groups should be assessed by psychiatrists if competency to consent to treatment is at all in question. To be judged psychologically competent, an individual should: (1) show an awareness of his current situation (living circumstances, relationships, health status, etc.); (2) possess a factual understanding of his issues (exhibit a clear and realistic comprehension of the facts which bear upon decision making); and (3) show the capacity to manipulate data rationally for decision making. These criteria should be applied to both general and specific competency assessments.

Implicit in the above criteria is that the patient demonstrate these capacities in the presence of another person, namely, the psychiatrist. As such, competence can be most properly considered in a two-person context. The willingness of the examiner to provide the experience of safety and to engage in alliance building and the patient's ability to take advantage of help by engaging in a dialogue regarding the decisions in question are critical elements in any competency assessment. We may call this element of competency "interpersonal competency" or competency to engage in a therapeutic alliance.[3] Keeping in mind that dialogue is a two-person process will give the benefit of the doubt to, for example, the foreign-speaking patient by placing the onus for achieving a dialogue on the clinician, who may have to seek a bilingual examiner or interpreter. On the other hand, the competence of a paranoid, aloof patient who, while able to recite "facts" refuses to engage in a dialogue regarding risks and benefits, even with an empathic examiner, becomes far more questionable under this criterion.

A primary concern to psychiatrists regarding competence of patients in an inpatient setting is *consent or refusal of treatment*. Since precise competency standards for the treatment decision do not exist, examinations on questionably incompetent patients should be performed and findings documented. One approach is to use a consent form which has a written information component and an oral dialogue questions component to assess level of patient understanding of information. The dialogue exemplifies the next component of informed consent—that is, the clinician's provision of reasonable information about the procedure or treatment.

Information

Adequate consent, as we have discussed, entails *voluntary* behavior, the *capacity* to participate rationally in the process, and must also include reasonable and appropriate *information* conveyed to the patient. The current standard as to what kind and how much information is reasonable is that the physician should disclose all information that a reasonable person might want in deciding to accept or reject treatment: what the treatment consists of, benefits and risks; alternatives, with their benefits and risks; and no treatment, with its benefits and risks. Since an exhaustive list of risks and alternatives is by no means practical or even possible in all cases, the clinician may wish to use a modified decision analytic sliding scale approach in determining how to engage the patient in the informed consent process. Stated more simply, the greater the probability of an outcome, or the greater the magnitude of the gain or loss associated with the outcome, the more incumbent it is upon the physician to enter it into the dialogue.

Special Situations

The requirements of informed consent do not apply to all situations. Emergency, therapeutic privilege, waiver, and incompetency involve special legal and clinical consideration.

Emergencies

In medical emergencies, physicians may render medical services in the absence of a formal consent, if taking the time to secure consent (from the patient or substitute consent for patient) would pose a life-threatening delay of needed treatment. In psychiatry, treatment may be given in the absence of consent when a patient becomes violent or self-mutilating and requires intervention to prevent immediate harm to himself or others. Unfortunately, the law to date does not generally recognize a broader sense of emergency, which would include depressed patients in severe distress or even psychotic patients in overwhelming psychological pain (if they are nonviolent or not actively suicidal).

Therapeutic Privilege

Another exception to informed consent is that of therapeutic privilege. If the information about the nature of the patient's condition and treatment might be *directly* damaging to the patient, it can be withheld. Such information, however, cannot be withheld if the damage would be mediated solely by the decision of an adequately informed patient to refuse treatment. For example, the clinician's concern that a psychotic patient may refuse neuroleptics when informed of the risk of tardive dyskinesia is not sufficient grounds for withholding that information. In such a case, where the damage of a continuing untreated psychotic state is at issue, a careful competency assessment needs to be undertaken rather than invoking therapeutic privilege.

Waiver

The right of informed consent can be waived by the patient. The patient may say "Tell me what to do, I don't want to know." This waiver should be respectfully explored by the clinician in order to assess the meaning of the patient's wish *not* to know, which may involve a degree of denial ranging from the healthy to the psychotic. Only such an exploration will suffice to document the patient's competence to waive informed consent. Blind compliance, as much as blind refusal, should alert the physician to potential pathology that may need to be addressed in the course of inpatient treatment.

Incompetency

Patients who have been already judged by a court to be incompetent cannot then give informed consent. A court-appointed monitor or substitute decision maker must then be obtained for purposes of informed consent.

Summary

In approaching informed consent as a two-person process we seek to turn legal constraint to clinical advantage through the clinical dialogue. In doing so, the therapeutic alliance can be strengthened to withstand the uncertainty which characterizes inpatient treatment of high-risk populations. In sharing uncertainty throughout the decision-making process, one may preserve realistic hopes in the patient without fostering magical wishes for omnipotence. The disappointment of magical wishes by tragic outcomes forms the basis of many a malpractice suit.

MALPRACTICE

Defining Malpractice

Malpractice law is a subcategory of tort law, that branch of civil law concerned with providing of redress for damages suffered as a consequence of a breach of duty. Malpractice is negligent or substandard practice by a professional, or a failure to perform a duty that results in an injury to patient or client. Psychiatrists are liable for malpractice, though the claims against psychiatrists are fewer than those against other medical specialties. The action taken in a tort is a demand for compensation for damages to the injured party. Four conditions must be met to have a malpractice claim.

Duty to Care

In order for a patient to allege that a physician's negligence caused him damage he must first prove that the physician assumed a "duty to care" or a treatment relationship with him. Once a duty to care has been established, the physician is responsible for nonnegligent care. Duty to care can be terminated if the patient is medically discharged or transferred to another facility or physician.

Negligence

The physician who takes on the duty to care for a specific patient also takes on the duty to care in a nonnegligent manner. The level of care is generally assessed against what other members of the medical specialty (with similar training and therapeutic orientation) would customarily do in a similar situation, that is, community standards.[4, 5] In some jurisdictions, however, the care given has been assessed as negligent in comparison with what a hypothetical "reasonable and prudent" practitioner might do, or against an even more abstract risk-benefit standard for care.

Harm

A physician is liable for damages only in the event that the breach of duty to care directly caused harm of a physical and/or emotional nature.

Causation

A physician who has established the duty to care for a patient in a nonnegligent way and has breached this duty is still liable *only* if the alleged harm can be found to have been the direct or "proximate" consequence of this act.

In summary, any patient suing a physician for malpractice must prove these four elements to be true by a preponderance of the evidence.

Historically, psychiatrists have been sued less frequently than other physicians. Among psychiatrists, in recent years, the most frequent causes for action alleged in malpractice suits have been for psychiatric negligence leading to patient suicide.

In a recent panel on psychiatric malpractice, the insurers of American Psychiatric Association members presented data of complaint frequency for the most recent 1250 claims.[6] Their data were as follows:

Suicide	219
Improper diagnosis	102
Sexual misconduct	86
Breach of confidentiality	59
Death	58
Fracture	52
Attempted suicide	42
Legal process	41
Missed diagnosis	39
General Liability	33
Homicide	32

Malpractice Risk Management

Suicide

As is evidenced by the aforementioned list of psychiatric malpractice claims, suicide poses, by far, the greatest malpractice threat to psychiatrists. The cases cited point to suicide as accounting for close to 20% of all malpractice suits. The percentage increases when we include injury from a suicide attempt. A relatively high number of suicides occur among individuals who have seen a therapist in the previous year.

When there is a risk of suicide, as in the chronically suicidal borderline patient, then benefits of less restrictive care (e.g., unlocked units or outpatient care) need to be weighed against the risks of being unable to prevent acting out of acute exacerbations of suicidality (e.g., overdose). In such a case, it is useful to engage the patient himself—and, where appropriate, the family—in the informed consent process. Planned transitions to less restrictive environments, e.g., transfer from closed to open units, provide an opportunity to assess and to enhance the patient's capacity for engaging in dialogue and sharing responsibility—a capacity which is at the heart of therapeutic alliance building and the maturational process. For example, the hypomanic patient needs to be asked what he understands the risks and benefits of any planned transition to be. The clinician needs to monitor how character and psychopathology may shape or distort individual understanding and to confront hypomanic denial of difficulties and risks.

The informed consent process in this way supports the most mature side of the patient's self. By helping patients engage in a dialogue where they are supported in remembering, observing, and anticipating, the therapeutic goals of enhancing these capacities and recruiting them to serve the patients' best interests are advanced. With the understanding of these capacities the patient becomes less vulnerable to being overwhelmed by affect and the acting out of suicidal impulses.[4, 5, 7]

The inpatient psychiatrist will more frequently be the target of malpractice action because of treating a select population of more disturbed patients who are at greatest risk for tragic outcomes. By the same token, in treating a population where patient competence and ability to take responsibility are more often at issue, the inpatient psychiatrist needs to repeatedly engage the hospitalized patient in a process of assessment of the patient's ability to assume responsibility for his own actions. In the absence of such review, the psychiatrist is vulnerable to the assumption that inpatients are less able to take responsibility for themselves than outpatients, and thus an inpatient psychiatrist should be held to a necessarily higher standard of care.[8, 9] This blanket assumption ignores the fact that many inpatients, during the course of their hospitalization, regain their ability to assume responsibility and that inpatient treatment can include an unlocked environment and leaves of absence. By carefully engaging the patient in a dialogue-based, informed consent process when, for example, leaves of absence are being considered, the inpatient psychiatrist gains both a valuable and responsible ally in his patient. This also decreases the likelihood that the hospitalized patient's responsibility for any tragic outcome will, in a jury's hindsight, be automatically discounted, consequently holding the psychiatrist to a higher standard of care than warranted.

Inpatients and outpatient psychiatric populations present different legal dilemmas. With outpatients, a malpractice suit is usually based on the allegation that the treating psychiatrist was negligent for not hospitalizing the patient or negligent in prematurely releasing the patient. These cases are less often successful, as courts do recognize the difficulty in predicting suicide.

For inpatients, documentation of the clinical evaluation and decision to *discharge* is one protection against suit for the suicide of a recently discharged inpatient. When the patient is being discharged against medical advice and the risk of suicide is felt to be of a chronic nature but the patient is not felt to be committable, this reasoning should be shared with the patient and, when possible, with the family. Documentation of the decision-making process, the consultation obtained, and the participation of patient and family are critical.

Inpatients thought to be at *high risk* of suicide constitute another medicolegal problem. Hospital procedures, be they close observation, one-to-one supervision, or some other intervention, should be openly reviewed. The inpatient environment itself should be as free as possible of opportunities for suicide, including, for example, insecure windows or access to sharp objects. A shared understanding by staff, patient, and family as to what is being done and why in the context of an overall treatment plan is the best protection.[9]

Suicide litigation involves two main issues: (1) whether the psychiatrist should have predicted that a patient was likely to harm himself, and (2) if the risk was apparent, whether the psychiatrist took adequate precautions to protect the patient from self-harm. If a psychiatrist did not conclude that a hospitalized patient was in danger of self-harm and so did not take adequate precautions, the court will ask whether a reasonable and prudent psychiatrist would have predicted the risk. Courts do acknowledge the uncertainty of prediction in this area and will usually not hold liable a physician who exercised reasonable care. When the risk was apparent but the psychiatrist did not prevent the suicide, the courts question the adequacy of precautionary measures taken. The determination of adequacy is difficult for courts and juries acting in hindsight in that measures seen as deterrents to suicide (such as close observation, seclusion, etc.) may, in fact, prove antitherapeutic in the long run, even though they impede immediate self-harm.

Determining the risk of suicide in a given patient is an uncertain matter. Psychiatrists can reduce liability by documenting the decision-making process and the provision of reasonable care, the following of customary procedures in assessment of risk, and noting, when obtained, consultation with colleagues (in difficult cases).[4, 5]

Bearing Tragic Outcomes

"Outreach" by the hospital treatment team to families of a patient who commits suicide or homicide[2] is an important clinical practice. Though clinicians are barraged by their own feelings of failure, anger, and sadness in the face of such clinical tragedies, to whatever extent possible the clinician can and should try to put these feelings temporarily aside and offer support to the family. Attending funeral services for a patient who has committed suicide is appropriate and is usually appreciated by the family. Most importantly, this practice is good, humane care. It is also legally sound behavior. This supportive family "postvention" decreases the likelihood that the grieving family will act out its guilt, will displace the anger directed at the deceased onto the psychiatrist and treatment team, and then sue for malpractice.

Homicide perpetrators pose different types of problems. The inpatient staff will need to face fears for their own safety in order to provide quality clinical care. Anger aroused by the crime (in the treatment team) must never be translated into less-than-appropriate treatment. Outreach with the family (who may be related to the victim) again is both a humane act and a form of malpractice prevention.[2] By the same token, the perpetrator's family may also be in need of support.

Medication Side Effects

Informed consent as an ongoing process[10] is particularly critical in an area that is as anxiety-provoking to patients as are medication side effects. We shall focus on how the process of informed consent can be applied to prescribing antipsychotic medication and its possible side effect of tardive dyskinesia. The discussion that follows is, however, generalizable to any medication that has potentially serious side effects (e.g., antidepressants and cardiac toxicity, antianxiety agents and addiction, and lithium and renal toxicity). The process of informed consent allows the clinician the opportunity to turn legal constraints into clinical advantage.[11]

Tardive dyskinesia (movement disorders of face, tongue, and extremity muscles) is now an established side-effect of antipsychotic medication. The development of tardive dyskinesia (TD) does not reflect negligence in administration of antipsychotic drugs, for it can occur under optimal neuroleptic drug regimes. However, failure to warn patients of the risk of TD (as of any major side-effect likely to occur) has in the recent past led to huge out-of-court settlements and in-court awards.[12, 13] Clinical case and malpractice liability concerns, therefore, insist that psychiatrists fully inform patients of this side-effect, obviously in an unthreatening and supportive fashion. Some researchers (recognizing the potential for malpractice suits in this area) suggest that written rather than oral informed consent be used with patients who are at high risk of TD.[14] However, progress notes which document an ongoing process of review may be more clinically sound and no less a safeguard against suit.

Consent and liability issues with neuroleptics are of major import.[15–17] The timing of consent is critical. If a patient is, by reason of psychosis, acutely incompetent and in need of emergency treatment, and if treatment results in a restoration of competency, informed consent should await recompensation and should then be obtained if and when further neuroleptic treatment is indicated.[18] In addition to a legal necessity, a doctor-patient dialogue regarding the risks and benefits of acute and chronic neuroleptic treatment can engage the patient in an educational process that is itself alliance-building and potentially restorative of self-esteem. Ego capacities of remembering, observing, and anticipating are also exercised by the consent process. The patient can learn to report any change which might indicate the reappearance of psychosis or the emergence of the earliest symptoms of tardive dyskinesia and thus provide an "early warning" system for re-evaluation of neuroleptic therapy. Moreover, the extent to which the patient can improve his ego capacities in the course of treatment is itself a useful indicator of the ongoing process of recovery. In fact, improvement in the capacity to participate in the informed consent process may be an indicator that the neuroleptic dose can, *ceteris paribus*, begin to be tapered. If the patient remains chronically unable to engage in such a dialogue, the clinician may have to take sole charge of monitoring, which can entail supplementing the clinical examination for tardive dyskinesia with periodic formal tests, e.g., the AIMS test (an abnormal involuntary movement scale).

Our empirical research, at the Program in Psychiatry and the Law at the Massachusetts Mental Health Center, has demonstrated that psychiatrists' willingness to prescribe neuroleptics varied depending on whether they were asked to "risk" or to "accept" a particular probability of side-effects.[19] Moreover, court judges grossly overestimated the probability of occurrence of tardive dyskinesia as a side-effect. Obviously, the clinician must pay careful attention to the language in which he engages in the informed consent dialogue. Furthermore, psychiatrists face the major task of educating the legal profession regarding the actual balance of benefits and side-effects of neuroleptics.

Review of the emerging case law with high awards may be instructive. In what is becoming a landmark case, *Clites v. Iowa*,[20] the Iowa court of appeals awarded $760,000 to a mentally retarded man who had been treated with neuroleptics for his aggressive behavior. The plaintiff alleged that the physicians had both used the drugs negligently (lack of patient monitoring, absence of drug holidays, neuroleptics used as tranquilizers to control behavior) and had not secured informed consent.

A second case, *Faigenbaum v. Cohen*,[21] involved the failure to warn about and the failure to diagnose tardive dyskinesia. In this case, tardive dyskinesia was misdiagnosed as Huntington's chorea. The plaintiff sued the hospitals, drug companies, and physicians. The original verdict awarded $1.5 million to the plaintiff. (The current appeal is based on the state's claim of immunity from suit for its hospitals and physicians.) The drug companies and private practice physicians have already settled.

A third case, *Hedin v. U.S.*,[22] awarded $2.1 million to a veteran and an additional amount to his wife (for loss of companionship) on the basis of negligent prescription of neuroleptics by Veterans Administration physicians.

Two of these three cases found for the plaintiff partly on the basis of inadequately obtained informed consent or lack of any informed consent. The message to inpatient psychiatrists should be clear: always obtain informed consent prior to continued treatment with neuroleptics.

Chronic patients needing high doses of neuroleptics constitute a population at high risk for tardive dyskinesia. General counsel for the APA urges reobtaining informed consent every 6 months for those patients on high doses of antipsychotic drugs. Only in an emergency should these drugs be used without consent. Therapeutic privilege, which holds that informed consent can be withheld if the physician believes that knowledge of risks would be directly detrimental to the patient, is another exception. However, most courts accept only extremely narrow instances of therapeutic privilege.

As a rule, substitute consent from a legal guardian should be obtained instead of using therapeutic privilege.

Psychiatrists are also well advised to follow the APA guidelines on tardive dyskinesia.[17] These guidelines include (1) using the lowest effective dose of neuroleptics for a given patient, and (2) examination for early signs of tardive dyskinesia every 3 to 6 months; if signs of tardive dyskinesia appear, a review should be held to consider whether lowering the dosage, changing to a more benign drug, or stopping treatment is contraindicated. Tardive dyskinesia litigation in the future may shift from a community standard of care to a standard of strict liability.[13] Such a shift would at the very least mean that the burden of proof would be on the physician to prove that he did not act negligently rather than on the plaintiff to prove that the physician did. In a more extreme form, the treating psychiatrist may be held responsible for the patient suffering tardive dyskinesia irrespective of any proof of nonnegligent prescribing.

Improper Diagnosis

Malpractice claims that involve improper diagnosis occur only second in frequency to suicide claims. This category deserves explanation, for we are all aware that clinical diagnostic errors and ambiguities are inevitable. Malpractice involving improper diagnosis, however, does not pertain to human error in judgment. Rather, it applies to negligence, as in failing to use the diagnostic procedures and equipment that a prudent, competent psychiatrist would use to reach a diagnosis. An example of diagnostic negligence would be to treat as a psychiatric disorder an organic disorder that should have been suspected, and an internal medicine consult obtained.

Homicide and the Problem of Confidentiality

Although cases in which a psychiatric patient commits a violent act against a third party do not occur frequently, they may result in large financial awards. The parallel to suicide cases is apparent: both involve the uncertainty which surrounds the accurate prediction of violence. Furthermore, cases of violence raise questions about whether and how prophylactic measures were taken by the psychiatrist to prevent a potentially violent patient from doing harm. Courts have been less sympathetic towards psychiatrists' difficulties in predicting dangerousness towards others than they have in cases involving violence towards the self (suicide).

There have been a number of cases involving identifiable victims and the *duty to protect or to warn*. These cases involve both outpatients and recently released inpatients. The outcome of most of these cases has held the psychiatrist liable for injuries to the victim when (1) he knew or should have known that a patient was likely to harm a specific individual and (2) he failed to warn or otherwise protect that individual. An often-quoted case that held a therapist liable for failing to prevent a violent act towards a patient's victim was *Tarasoff v. Regents of the University of California*.[23] In this case, a former student contacted a school psychologist for therapy. The psychologist tried to initiate civil commitment of the young man based on the supposition that this patient might harm his ex-girlfriend, Tatiana Tarasoff. The university police who subsequently interviewed the young man decided that he should not be committed. He murdered Tatiana Tarasoff shortly thereafter. The family sued the university and the involved clinicians on the basis that they should have done more to protect the young woman. The California Supreme Court held that once a therapist does in fact determine, or under applicable professional standards reasonably should have determined, that a patient poses a serious danger of violence to others, he bears a duty to exercise reasonable care to protect the foreseeable victim of that danger. The duty to warn or protect exists in many states, when specific threats are made against specific victims. Some states go even further than the Tarasoff decision, holding that psychiatrists may be liable even if their patients harm persons not specified in advance.[24]

The court creation of a therapist's duty to protect third parties was anticipated by some psychiatrists to harm the therapeutic alliance needed to treat patients by negating the confidentiality of the patient-therapist relationship. The courts were accused of creating a situation whereby either the patient leaves treatment (and may then be more likely to continue to act out violent impulses) or more patients are civilly committed.[25] We have elsewhere attempted to show how the effects of the Tarasoff decision on the care of a potentially violent patient can be turned to clinical advantage. In selected cases it has been possible to foster the therapeutic alliance by engaging the patient in a process similar to informed consent and thus enabling him to explore his ambivalence about the destructive act.[11]

While the courts have often found the clinician liable in cases in which (from hindsight) the violation of confidentiality would have resulted in saving the life of a third party, an opposing trend is also noted. Recently both Massachusetts and New Hampshire courts indicated that in nonemergency cases, the clinician may be found liable for breaking confidentiality[26, 27]! In view of these opposing trends, the clinician can avoid court-created paralysis by carefully documenting his reasoning and, when in doubt, seeking consultation.

Sexual Misconduct and Other Boundary Violations

On an inpatient unit the intensity of affect and the states of regression of many patients often favor various boundary violations. These include inappropriate socialization with patients, fraternization by staff, exchange of gifts and money, special favors, and the entire spectrum of sexual misconduct. While most of these are problems in therapy and administration, the last has an additional weight.

While charges of sexual misconduct have been brought against physicians in various specialties, a psychiatrist who engages in sexual contact with a patient is clearly betraying the patient's trust. The rule clearly stated by the American Psychiatric Association (APA) code of ethics is that any sexual activity between patient and therapist represents improper behavior on the therapist's part.[2] In addition, there may be both civil and criminal prosecution for battery when such misconduct, however rationalized, occurs. It should be noted that the current malpractice insurance policy offered to APA members specifically excludes coverage for liability incurred on the basis of sexual misconduct.

Inpatient clinicians should be particularly sensitive to the vulnerability of hospitalized patients and staff to respond to feelings of frustration, hopelessness, and helplessness by a flight toward sexualization. The clinician should be aware that under the doctrine of *respondeat superior*, he may be held liable for sexual acting out with patients by staff members under his direct supervision.

Inpatient units treating populations at high risk for sexual exploitation (e.g., adolescents or substance abusers) can meet the standard of care only if they provide adequate psychiatric supervision of clinical staff. Staff should be supported in understanding sexually provocative patient behavior and their own fantasies and feelings as transference and countertransference reactions to be clinically addressed.

Malpractice Prevention

While the delivery of quality care, documentation, and consultation are critical avenues of malpractice prevention, they are not the limits of preventive approaches. Physician sharing of the uncertainty of diagnosis, treatment, and outcome with patients is yet another malpractice prevention strategy.[10] Malpractice suits in medicine often result from patient and family disappointment and helplessness in the face of tragic outcomes, rather than negligence. Informed consent, when practiced *pro forma*, often carries the suggestion of a guarantee and leads to unrealistic hopes. Instead, we recommend that informed consent be used as a starting point in the establishment of a true therapeutic alliance. Uncertainty is then mutually acknowledged, and clinical decision making becomes a dialogue which is characteristic of the psychiatrist-patient relationship at its best. Such a dialogue is particularly critical in those areas where paradoxical legal trends have dramatized the conflict between societal needs, such as the need for protection of third parties (illustrated above) and of individuals' rights, such as the right to protection of confidentiality.[11]

PATIENT RIGHTS

When beginning treatment, or when therapeutic impasse has been reached, or even when the patient has made genuine progress, the clinician may hear the patient speak the language of "rights": "I signed myself into the hospital so I have a right to sign myself out." Perhaps the most important reason for the inpatient clinician to understand the legal context of patient rights is to diminish the anxiety engendered by such assertions so as to allow for clinical exploration of their meaning. It is useful for the clinician to remember that while the legal model invokes the adversarial posture of "your rights versus my rights," the same position in psychiatric treatment is diagnostic of a narcissistic lesion in the doctor-patient alliance which needs to be explored. In the course of such an exploration one may often find the patient harboring the fear that the doctor-patient relationship will reproduce past relationships in which the only protection against domination and exploitation was to act oppositionally. Here again patient rights can be best protected if they are integrated into the informed consent process. By this process the patient comes truly to understand the risks and benefits of exercising their rights. Informed consent can only proceed if the clinician is guided by the psychodynamic model of man in conflict with himself, rather than the legal model of defendant versus plaintiff rights. A clinical alliance rather than a legal adversary process must always be the goal of treatment.

Admission to the Hospital

Voluntary Admission

Voluntary admission is defined by statute. Statutory law often explicitly prescribes conduct. Examples of statutory law are the setting of speed limits and the rules of civil commitment. In general, statutes are enacted at the state level. Medicine has recently come to be increasingly regulated by statutory law.

The majority of hospitalized psychiatric patients have voluntarily signed themselves into the hospital. Even incompetent patients can be "voluntarily" admitted by their guardians. Some patients voluntarily request hospitalization, knowing that commitment procedures will be started if they refuse voluntary admission. In this context critics have questioned the meaning of "voluntary" in the face of impending commitment proceedings. Most states do not require legal competence for voluntary admission. While voluntary admission is permitted, leaving the hospital at will is not. In some states voluntarily admitted psychiatric patients, upon entering the hospital, must sign a form acknowledging that they may be detained (for a period of time that differs state by state, e.g., New Hampshire, 24 hours) beyond the request for discharge. Involuntary commitment procedures may be initiated during this time, if necessary.

Voluntary admission is favored by many mental health professionals in that it usually indicates that patients recognize that they need care and that the institution is capable of delivering treatment. However, voluntary patients should understand that in most jurisdictions they cannot impulsively leave the hospital at any time. The staff should inform all voluntary admittees, upon admission, about procedures required if they then wish to leave against medical advice and about what restraints may be placed upon their leaving under those circumstances. Failure to do so would represent breach of informed consent.[28] The clinician who is unaware of the statutes governing voluntary admission and the nature of the admission process is at risk of running afoul of the law. More importantly, however, from a clinical perspective such knowledge is critical in understanding the patient's expectations upon entering the hospital.[29]

The inpatient clinician must know what information the patient has been given in order to evaluate the patient for the presence of distortions of reality (such as denial) and to alert the clinician of potential pitfalls in other emotionally charged areas. Referring to the initial understanding can also be an aid in maintaining a doctor-patient alliance on what has been termed a situational basis, e.g., "Here are the rules that you and I have to live by."[30] Such a clinico-legal situational alliance can serve as a safe haven to return to when navigating through the storms of transference and countertransference that buffet psychiatric treatment.

Involuntary Admission

In the past 15 years the standards by which a noncriminal person can be involuntarily hospitalized have been significantly altered. Traditionally, the state's power to commit a mentally ill person was based on two principles—*parens patriae* (e.g., unable to care for self) or the police power doctrine (e.g., dangerous to others).[31] Civil commitment statutes in most states now require dangerousness, either to self or others, coupled with mental illness, as the basis for the restriction of liberty that hospitalization is argued to represent. In those states where the courts changed the civil commitment standard to that of dangerousness, many psychiatrists have regarded this change as a devaluation of the traditional medical concept of illness and need for treatment.[31]

Involuntary commitment standards vary from state to state and are constantly changing among the states. Every inpatient clinician (states also vary as to who can commit e.g., physicians, psychologists, judges) should keep abreast of the recent statutes in his state. A general summary follows.

Most states have provisions that allow for short-term emergency hospitalization until a court hearing is held. In most states at least one physician must sign the commitment certificate. Some states allow the police or courts to sign in the absence of a physician. The criteria for emergency commitment are the same as those for court-ordered commitment. All states have stringent time limits for the emergency commitment, but sometimes the bureaucratic lag between emergency commitment and mandatory court review practically extends this limit.[32]

At the end of the emergency commitment period, commitment can only continue upon a petition to the court. Most states currently require a judicial hearing for nonemergency commitments, and patients considered for civil commitment may be represented by attorneys. The psychiatrist's role is one of initiating a petition for commitment or assisting the court in the commitment process. It is the court that decides the commitment question.

Admission and the Incompetent Patient

Committability and incompetency are no longer legally synonymous. Mental patients are presumed legally competent unless adjudicated otherwise. Some states, however, are beginning to require psychiatric competency evaluations performed on new admittees and guardianship petitions filed on those suspected of incompetency.

Treatment

Medications

Patients, both voluntary and involuntary, under the doctrine of informed consent must be given a reasonable explanation of the treatment which the psychiatrist proposes. Informed consent must include risks, benefits, and side-effects of the treatment; other treatment options; and the probable course of the disorder without treatment. In many jurisdictions, since commitment no longer presupposes incompetence, both voluntary and involuntary patients, upon receipt of this information, have the right to accept or refuse the proposed treatment. The right to refuse treatment is waived only if: (1) a narrowly defined emergency exists such that failure to treat the patient would result in a substantial likelihood of physical harm to the patient or others or (2) the patient has been adjudicated incompetent.

If the patient refuses treatment and is thought to be incompetent, the process of finding a legal guardian should be started. In *Rogers v. Commissioner*, the now famous Massachusetts right-to-refuse-treatment case, a mental patient may refuse treatment until and unless adjudicated incompetent by a judge.[33] If the patient is found incompetent, the judge (*not the psychiatrist, not the guardian*) decides for the patient whether the patient, if competent, would have consented to be

treated by antipsychotic drugs (this is termed a substituted judgment standard). This ruling is an example of the increased judicialization of patient care. Fortunately, other jurisdictions have relied more heavily on clinical judgment for patient treatment determinations when incompetence has been established.[34]

ECT, Psychosurgery, and Other Modalities

Today most psychiatrists are exceptionally careful about informed consent when proposing electroconvulsive therapy (ECT). This caution was prompted by suits for failure to obtain informed consent and liability for injury. Despite the fact that ECT is safer today and much less likely to cause injury (injury is a precondition for negligence and liability), documented ECT abuse (overreliance on ECT and inappropriate usage of ECT) has led several states to design regulatory controls on its use.[35] However, before a general right to refuse treatment was recognized, the statutory right to refuse certain kinds of treatment such as ECT, psychosurgery, and aversive conditioning was protected by law. In effect, even if patients do consent to one of these treatments, statutes closely guard their usage.

Seclusion and Restraint

Seclusion and restraint represent the maximum restriction on space and movement for inpatients. Seclusion as a treatment technique provides protection to a seriously ill acting out patient who may harm himself or others. By minimizing sensory stimuli, seclusion can allow the patient an opportunity to regain self-control in the absence of other people. Seclusion and restraint (like ECT and psychosurgery) have court-ordered restrictions on their use.[36] Familiarity with the restrictions in your state is essential.

Before utilizing seclusion or restraint, the clinician must consider and document trials of less restrictive alternatives such as medications and voluntary space restrictions (e.g., an open "quiet room" to decrease stimulation). It is essential to carefully monitor any patient in seclusion or in restraint. Monitoring should be both medical (e.g., "periodic checks of vital signs") as well as behavioral (e.g., "observation checks"). When a patient is being removed from a restricted environment (e.g., by increasing periods of time out of seclusion), monitoring should also include examination for any evidence of a recurrence of the behavior that necessitated the original seclusion. All restrictions must be time-limited and subject to periodic review at times which are often specified by statute. Periodic review is not only legally necessary but also clinically essential. The milieu staff who are involved in restricting the patient and helping to wean the patient from such restrictions must have clear written guidelines for these procedures. Documentation of the reasoning involved in both initiating and weaning the patient from such restricted environments is an essential legal and clinical communication tool.

Discharge from Hospital

A critical treatment period for inpatient hospitalization is the time around discharge, be it planned or unplanned. "Pure" voluntary admittees (check your state definition) can leave the hospital when they wish, limited only by reasonable hours. "Conditional" voluntary patients (again, check local statutes for precise terms) usually must give anywhere from 24 hours to several days notice of their desire to leave; time is allotted for staff to conduct an evaluation of commitability and to initiate commitment procedures if indicated.[37] If a patient desires discharge and is *not* commitable but staff feel it is inadvisable for the patient to leave, the best medicolegal protection is to have the patient sign a form acknowledging his awareness of the physician's opposition to discharge. A leave against medical advice form (AMA) offers some modest protection to physicians in the event that a discharged patient unpredictably proceeds to harm either himself or a third party. In cases where there is a high degree of uncertainty as to whether the physician should petition for commitment or release the patient AMA, a second opinion from a colleague or, if available, a forensically trained psychiatrist, is warranted.

Involuntary patients (civilly committed, emergency committed, or criminally committed) may attempt to obtain a writ of habeas corpus for discharge. The patient appears in court (immediately), and the state must find that the criteria for commitment continue to be met.

An *involuntary discharge* occurs when a patient wishes to remain in the hospital and the physician recommends discharge. It is important to document the *clinical indications* for discharge in this situation, as it may mobilize narcissistic rage and threats to sue on the part of the patient and family.

An example of an indication for involuntary discharge is offered by a borderline patient for whom uncontrollable regression on an inpatient basis may be of higher risk than the benefit of continuing hospitalization and who is not judged to be acutely harmful to self or others.[38] Occasionally the narcissistic rage mobilized in such patients by the discharge may be of sufficient intensity that plans may need to be changed and the patient transferred on an involuntary commitment to a state facility. If the patient has an involved family, they should be contacted with the patient's permission and educated as to the reasons for discharge and informed of alternative sources of emergency care and any conditions that might need to be met for readmission. The sobering alternative of hospitalization in a state facility may be a regression-limiting and, at times, even a lifesaving alternative for the patient who has previously exploited the private or general hospital as a "hotel."

SPECIAL PATIENT POPULATIONS

There are several special patient populations that add unusual circumstances and concerns to established medicolegal constraints. In defining these groups and elucidating certain general considerations, we seek to aid the clinician in turning these constraints to clinical advantage.

Alcohol Abusers

The alcohol abuser or alcohol-dependent patient presents special medicolegal concerns. These individuals suffer social, fa-

milial, occupational, and/or behavioral/
legal (driving while intoxicated (DWI),
violence while intoxicated) complications
of alcoholism. Of special note to inpatient
clinicians is a recent Florida case which
found a cause of action against the hospital and physician for damages incurred
by an inpatient receiving treatment for
alcoholism, who, when on leave of absence
from the hospital, was involved in an
automobile accident while driving intoxicated.[39]

Clearly, any patient with a recent history of driving while intoxicated should be
carefully evaluated for risk when granted
a hospital leave. One possible safeguard
for patients with a history of DWI is to
make leaves contingent on not driving
while on leave. Another is to have the
patient's initial leave be followed by a
drug and alcohol screen. When in the
course of the patient's treatment sufficient
progress has occurred so that driving
while on leave comes to be indicated as
part of the patient's rehabilitation, permission to drive must be preceded by careful clinical evaluation. It should also be
noted that alcohol and other substance
abusers represent a population particularly vulnerable to affective and other psychiatric disorders. Failure to accompany
detoxification with proper psychiatric
evaluation is clearly substandard care. In
the case of a tragic outcome, it may lead to
a cause for malpractice action.

Substance Abusers

Substance abusers comprise another
special inpatient population. While the
term substance abuse in an umbrella for
dependence on opiates, nonnarcotic
agents, and alcohol, we will discuss primarily the opioid abuser. Of import to
inpatient clinicians is the need to carefully
monitor (using physiological criteria) patients for whom methadone is prescribed
for heroin withdrawal, because that drug
can also be abused. One safeguard is to
give each patient the prescribed dose at
regular intervals supervised by staff.

Another problem is with confidentiality. The substance abuser may
report a variety of illegal drug use prior to
hospitalization. Here, as with all patients,

the clinician is under obligation to maintain the standards of confidentiality, unless there is an ongoing direct threat to a
third party.[23, 26]

Substance abuse patients may also enter the hospital with criminal charges
against them. Because of the frequency of
this problem, it is important to ascertain
both their current legal status and their
motivation for seeking treatment. These
patients may have transiently impaired
judgment during the detoxification period
which may affect informed consent. The
clinician must evaluate each patient to
determine whether the patient has sufficient judgment to grant informed consent or whether the situation can be
equated with an emergency. In the latter
case, once the acute crisis has passed, patient competency must be reassessed and
consent reinstated. For some of these patients competency may not exist because
they have permanently impaired judgment due to chronic organic brain
syndromes.

Sociopaths

The hallmarks of sociopathy include:
apparent inability to experience depression, lack of motivation for change,
and absence of anxiety.[40] The psychiatric
examination of sociopathy must include
their medicolegal history. Though these
patients may present themselves as victims of family, parents, the law, and previous physicians,[41] the clinician should
still ask what charges are pending against
the patient and who the patient has sued
or is currently suing.

More sophisticated sociopaths may view
admission to a hospital as an invitation to
reach into the physician's or hospital's
malpractice insurance "deep pocket."
When such an attitude exists it must be
confronted. Staff may need to be supported
by the unit leadership when they become
the subject of repeated malpractice
threats.

Classical sociopaths are most often
found in public hospitals, have long criminal records, and may wish to use the hospital to avoid jail or even to continue their
criminal activities (e.g., drug dealing).
Private hospital settings may discover

what Dr. Leston Havens has described as a "white collar" sociopath.[42] This sociopath wishes to take advantage of what he perceives as vulnerability of inpatient settings to "legal blackmail": "If you discharge me, I'll speak to my lawyer." Whenever a patient is hospitalized under legal coercion, it is critical to clarify the patient's motivation for admission and treatment. In working with sociopaths, inform them, from the start, that you will contact their probation officer, lawyer, etc. Inform them of your responsibility to both them and the referring agency (e.g., the court). In cases in which you believe that your responsibility to the referring agency would preclude sufficient confidentiality to proceed with treatment, you can refer the patient to a colleague who can serve as the treating psychiatrist.

Borderline Patients

Borderline patients demonstrate extreme impulsivity, intense anger, unstable relationships and moods, and the inclination towards suicidal behavior. Clinicolegal problems go hand in hand with these symptoms.[38] Intense countertransference reactions such as abandonment are common and can lead to frank professional negligence. Furthermore, the impulsivity and suicidality characteristic of this patient group increases the liability risk for their caretakers. Medical decisions with this patient population should involve the patient in sharing the uncertainty. Borderline patients must be encouraged wherever possible to assume responsibility for their behavior and treatment.

Organically Impaired Patients

Organically impaired patients are those whose brain dysfunction results in impaired judgment, intellectual ability, orientation, and memory. Two steps should be taken whenever an organically impaired patient is admitted to an inpatient unit. First, the competency status of the patient must be established. Second, if the patient has been legally adjudicated incompetent, ascertain whether prior guardianship has been obtained. If guardianship should be obtained, make that a

recommendation to the family. It is important to differentiate for the family those conditions which are reversible and require only temporary guardians, versus those conditions which are irreversible and require permanent guardianship.

Elderly Patients

Not every elderly patient who appears incompetent is incompetent. In cases where incompetence does exist it may be a treatable organic problem or a depressive pseudodementia. Organic problems are not necessarily irreversible. In order to guard against a premature declaration of incompetency in clinical cases such as these, and against the hopelessness that accompanies such a ruling, the clinician should initially petition for temporary guardianship and then reevaluate at a later point in the hospitalization.

Elderly patients represent a population particularly vulnerable to victimization. In some cases they may have suffered abuse or neglect by their family or other caretakers. The regularity of this problem in elderly paranoid patients calls for inquiry into victimization as a part of the full psychiatric assessment. One must differentiate such cases from cases in which, although victimization is alleged, the claim of victimization turns out on closer examination to be an appeal for help with the loneliness and grief that can accompany illness and aging.

Patients in Overcrowded Facilities

Discharge or transfer of patients under conditions of overcrowding deserve special attention. Under these circumstances inpatients may need to be discharged or transferred. Though it may not be the optimal time for discharge for some patients, more seriously ill patients need the space and staff resources. The inpatient clinician may thus be forced into a process of decision making closely resembling the triage of the wounded that is practiced in wartime on the battlefield.

A charge of abandonment may be precipatated by a discharge under such circumstances. One must be mindful of countertransference issues and make sure that when a patient is chosen to be discharged he indeed has a good chance of functioning in an outpatient setting. Inpatient staff must be explicit with the patient as to reasons for discharge and must monitor for his reactions, which can include hopelessness and rage around experienced abandonment. The rationale for discharge should be thoroughly documented in the chart. Whenever possible, discharge resulting from overcrowding should be addressed in the milieu and with the patient's family. Alternatives (e.g., transfer), must be carefully explored prior to discharge. When adequate clinical exploration accompanies such discharges, the patient may experience the accompanying difficulties as surmountable and even growth promoting.

The Poorly Insured Patient

The poorly insured patient may not be able to afford an optimal stay in a private inpatient setting (this includes private psychiatric as well as general hospitals). In order to avoid abandonment, all decisions regarding transfer to a public facility should be explained, and the patient and family, when possible, should be included in the decision-making process. Provision of adequate follow-up is, as with all patients, critical.

The EAP-referred Patient

Patients often are referred by an Employee Assistance Program (EAP) when their work performance becomes impaired by intercurrent psychiatric illness.[43] EAPs which specialize in helping employees with drug and alcohol problems may also refer for admission. In either case, on an inpatient setting, the psychiatrist's first responsibility must be to diagnose and treat the patient, without regard to whether the patient's illness falls within the purview of the referring EAP. For example, a patient referred for admission as a drug abuser must also be evaluated for an underlying depression or some other treatable psychiatric disorder. This must be made clear to both the patient and the EAP. By the same token the patient who says "I was sent here by my boss" needs to be evaluated for motivation for treatment.

Confidentiality can be a problem with EAP patients. The patient's consent must be obtained for all communications, and the patient should be informed from the outset as to the extent to which the EAP requires information (e.g., diagnosis, expected length of stay, or prognosis). In order to address the patient's concerns, while at the same time insuring adequate communication with the EAP, the inpatient staff can clear all communications to the EAP with the patient. The patient can help complete all forms and letters that need to be sent out; telephone communications with the EAP can be held during the patient's therapy sessions; and, when appropriate, meetings with the EAP representative can be held in the patient's presence. If the hospital wishes to supplement these measures by having a nontreating member of the staff be in direct communication with the EAP representative, it should be done only with the patient's consent. Any refusal on the patient's part to furnish such consent should be adequately explored. In certain cases, refusal of consent may compromise the clinician's ability to treat the patient.

WORKING WITH THE LEGAL SYSTEM

Clinicians who are tempted toward legalistic approaches to psychiatric care are at risk to deliver poor care.[44] Every clinician must carefully examine his reaction to his patient whenever the legal, rather than the clinical, aspects of the case have taken center stage. Transference and countertransference resistances are the rule at these moments. On the other hand, the clinician who resists being mindful of the legal constraints within which inpatient therapy proceeds risks vulnerability to malpractice charges. Moreover, denial of legal realities may also be indicative of a narcissistic alliance with the patient aimed at satisfying the patient's wish for a caring, omnipotent figure. In either case, whether the clinician overidentifies with the aggressor (by trying to be a good lawyer) or overidentifies with the patient (as victim denying the medicolegal context of inpatient treatment), patient care is sure to suffer.

The Delphic injunction to "Know thyself" must join *primum non nocere* and "do the best for the patient" if clinicians are to turn the legal constraints reviewed here to clinical advantage.[45] With psychiatry and the law coming into progressively closer contact, especially in the high-risk populations treated by the inpatient psychiatrist, today's climate is one of both crisis and opportunity.

The *crisis* is that of feeling trapped by legal trends which expand clinician responsibility for tragic outcomes while diminishing the physician's authority to provide quality care. Expansion of physician responsibility is well illustrated by the ever-expanding duties to third parties created by *Tarasoff* and other such cases. A more ominous trend in the expansion of clinical responsibility is the movement toward strict liability. The following passage from a leading work on medical malpractice law exemplifies this problem: "The fact that a patient has begun treatment as the result of a suicide attempt renders liability under the concept of reasonable forseeability virtually automatic in all cases."[46]

The diminution of clinical authority in a number of areas has disturbed many clinicians. The most striking example is the trend of allowing treatment refusal by clearly psychotic patients. The inpatient clinician is then left to watch patients "rot with their rights on," as they descend into psychotic regression.[47] Similarly, the curtailment of the *parens patriae* justification for commitment has left clinicians with less authority to treat chronically suicidal and homicidal patients.

We have used the term *critogenic* injury to designate any *legally* caused harm that may ensue to the patient.[48] Since the legal profession does not have any term for such harm (though medicine has "iatrogenic" for "doctor-caused") we have borrowed from the Greek, "crites", meaning an Athenian presiding judge, to designate legally caused harm. Courts today seem to share a paradoxical pair of assumptions that (a) all inpatients are competent to refuse medications and (b) all inpatients are incompetent to assume responsibility for their own actions (e.g., self-harm or harm to others). Together these views seem to reflect the extremes of either counterdependent grandiosity or infantile dependence which can characterize the extreme positions that disturbed patients can take. If strictly adhered to, this courtroom paradox can make clinical treatment of seriously ill patients legally impossible.

The *opportunity* provided to inpatient clinicians is to begin to engage in an ethical and empirical dialogue with the legal system. Research is growing on biases (such as hindsight) when psychiatric prediction is evaluated by judges and juries.[49] Research findings will hopefully improve the quality of inpatient clinical decision making and give the legal system a more realistic view of the uncertainties inherent in clinical decision making. Perhaps the enforced contact between psychiatry and law, through today's torrent of litigation, will allow each profession to come away with a greater insight into its own presuppositions.[50-52]

Enforced contact between psychiatry and law will ultimately be beneficial to patients only if the inpatient clinician who appears in the courtroom appears as a *clinician*. He must avoid either being seduced into the role of playing "lawyer" (thereby identifying with the legal system as aggressor) or playing "hostile witness" (thereby identifying with the oppositional, adversary stance of the injured victim). Only as clinicians in the courtroom can we help the legal system to aid patients and to become mindful of the potential for injury to patients from legal proceedings that we have termed critogenic. Encouraging responses to the "malpractice crisis," such as proposals for arbitration or for creating victim compensation funds, are early signs of success.[53] Despite this note of encouragement, the inpatient clinician will only be able to treat his patient by remaining abreast of changing legal constraints and responding clinically with the best that empirical research, professional experience, and ethical theory have to offer.[50, 54-56]

ACKNOWLEDGMENTS

Dr. Harold Bursztajn is a member of the Peer Review Committee at Hampstead Hospital, Hampstead, N.H., a model of the clinical review process here advocated. We wish to thank the clinical staff and the medical director of Hampstead Hospital, R. James Farrer, M.D., for their support of the clinical dialogue which has generated many of the insights here conveyed. We also wish to thank the editor, whose painstaking efforts enriched this chapter. Without the careful work of Ms. Audrey Bleakley, the production of this manuscript would not have been possible.

REFERENCES

1. *Kaimowitz v Michigan Department of Mental Health*, Div. No. 73-19434 AW, Circuit Court of Wayne Cty. Michigan, 1973, 13 Criminal L Rep 2452.
2. Gutheil TG, Appelbaum PS: *Clinical Handbook of Psychiatry and the Law*, New York, McGraw-Hill, 1982.
3. Bursztajn H, Hamm RM: The clinical utility of utility assessment. Med Decision Making, *2:* 161–165, 1982.
4. Gutheil TG, Bursztajn H, Hamm RM, Brodsky A: Subjective data and suicide assessment in the light of recent legal developments. Part I: Malpractice prevention and the use of subjective data. Int J Law Psychiatry, *6:* 317–329, 1983.
5. Bursztajn H, Gutheil TG, Hamm RM, Brodsky A: Subjective data and suicide assessment in the light of recent legal developments. Part II: Clinical uses of legal standards in the interpretation of subjective data. Int J Law Psychiatry, *6:* 331–350, 1983.
6. American Psychiatric Association Annual Meeting: Panel: Malpractice: Problems and Solutions, Dallas, 1985.
7. Shein HM, Stone AA: Psychotherapy designed to detect and treat suicidal potential. Am J Psychiatry *125:* 1247–1251, 1969.
8. Klein JI, Glover SI: Psychiatric malpractice. Int J Law Psychiatry, *6:* 131–157, 1983.
9. Perr IN: Psychiatric malpractice issues, in Rachlin S (ed): Legal Encroachment on Psychiatric Practice, pp. 47–59. San Francisco, Jossey-Bass, 1985.
10. Gutheil TG, Bursztajn H, Brodsky A: Malpractice prevention through the sharing of uncertainty: Informed consent and the therapeutic alliance. N Engl J Med, *311:* 49–51, 1984.
11. Wulsin LR, Bursztajn H, Gutheil TG: Unexpected clinical features of the Tarasoff decision: The therapeutic alliance and the "duty to warn." Am J Psychiatry, *140:* 601–603, 1983.
12. Gelenberg A: 375,000 for tardive dyskinesia. Biol Ther Psychiatry, *3:* 41–42, 1980.
13. Appelbaum PS, Schaffner K, Meisel A: Responsibility and compensation for tardive dyskinesia. Am J Psychiatry, *142:* 806–810, 1985.
14. Davis JM, Schyre PM, Parkovic I: Clinical and legal issues in neuroleptic use. Clin Neuropharmacol, *6:* 117–128, 1983.
15. Baker B: Expect a flood of tardive dyskinesia malpractice suits. Clin Psychiatry News, *Jan:* 3, 1984.
16. Slovenko R: On the legal aspects of tardive dyskinesia. J Psychiatry Law, *7:* 295–331, 1979.
17. Tardive Dyskinesia: Report of the American Psychiatric Association Task Force on Late Neurological Effects of Antipsychotic Drugs, APA Task Force Report No. 18, Washington, D.C., American Psychiatric Association, 1979.
18. Muentz MR: Overcoming resistance to talking to patients about tardive dyskinesia. Hosp Community Psychiatry, *36:* 283–287, 1985.
19. Bursztajn H, Chanowitz B, Gutheil TG, Hamm RM: Context specific language effects in the decision to prescribe neuroleptics. Presented at the Fifth Annual Meeting of the Society for Medical Decision Making, Toronto, Canada, October 2–5, 1983.
20. *Clites v. Iowa*, Court of Appeals of Iowa, June 29, 1982.
21. *Faigenbaum v. Cohen*, reported in Clin Psychiatry News, *5:* 31, 1985.
22. *Hedin v. U.S.*, reported in Clin Psychiatry News, *5:* 31, 1985.
23. *Tarasoff v. Regents of the University of California*, 131 Cal Reptr 14 (Calif 76).
24. Appelbaum PS: The expansion of liability for patients' violent acts. Hosp Community Psychiatry, *35:* 13–14, 1984.
25. Stone AA: The Tarasoff case and some of its progeny: Suing psychotherapists to safeguard society, in *Psychiatry and Morality: Essays and Analysis*, Washington, D.C., American Psychiatric Press, 1984.
26. *Commonwealth of Massachusetts v. Cobrin*, SJC-3671, 1985.
27. In re *Kathleen M.* 493 A2D 472 (April 18, 1985, S.Ct. N.H.).
28. Halleck SH: *Law in the Practice of Psychiatry*, New York, Plenum, 1980.
29. Appelbaum PS, Mirkin, SA, Bateman, AL: Empirical assessment of competency to consent to psychiatric hospitalization. Am J Psychiatry, *138:* 1170–1176, 1985.
30. Gutheil TG, Havens LL: The therapeutic alliance: Contemporary meanings and confusions. Int Rev Psychoanal, *6:* 467–481, 1979.
31. Stone AA: Mental Health and Law: A System in Transition, U.S. Department of Health, Education, and Welfare Publication 75-176, Rockville, Md., National Institute of Mental Health, 1975.
32. Barton WE, Barton GM: *Ethics and Law in Mental Health Administration*, New York, International Universities Press, 1984.
33. *Rogers v. Commissioner of Department of Mental Health*, 390 Mass. 489 (Nov. 29, 1983).
34. *Rennie v. Klein*, 102 S. Ct. 3506 (1982).
35. APA Task Force Report No. 14: Electroconvulsive Therapy, Washington, D.C., American Psychiatric Association, 1978.
36. Soloff PH, Gutheil TG, Wexler DB: Seclusion and restraint in 1985: A review and update. Hosp Community Psychiatry, *36:* 652–657, 1985.

37. Appelbaum PS, Hamm RM: Decision to seek commitment. Arch Gen Psychiatry, *39:* 447–452, 1982.

38. Gutheil TG: Medicolegal pitfalls in the treatment of borderline patients. Am J Psychiatry, *142*(1): 9–14, 1985.

39. *Burroughs v. Board of Trustees of Alachua General Hospital,* 328 So 2d 538, Fla 1976.

40. Vaillant GE: Sociopathy as a human process. Arch Gen Psychiatry, *32:* 178–183, 1975.

41. Freud S: Some character types met with in psychoanalytic work: "The exceptions," in Strachey J (ed): *Standard Edition,* vol. 14, London, Hogarth Press, 1957.

42. Havens L: Personal communication, 1983.

43. Brill P, Herzberg J, Speller JL: Employee assistance programs: An overview and suggested roles for psychiatrists. Hosp Community Psychiatry, *36:* 727–731, 1985.

44. Gutheil TG: Legal defense as ego defense: A special form of resistance in the therapeutic process. Psychiatry Q, *51*(4): 251–256, 1979.

45. Stone AA: The new paradox of psychiatric malpractice. N Engl J Med, *31:* 1384–1387, 1984.

46. Holder RH: *Medical Malpractice Law,* New York, John Wiley & Sons, 1978.

47. Appelbaum PS, Gutheil TG: "Rotting with their rights on": Constitutional theory and clinical reality in drug refusal by psychiatric patients. Bull Am Acad Psychiatry Law, *7:* 308–317, 1979.

48. Bursztajn H: More law and less protection: "Criminogenesis", "legal iatrogenesis", and medical decision making. J Geriatr Psychiatry, *18:* 143–153, 1985.

49. Fischhoff B: Hindsight/foresight: The effect of outcome knowledge on judgment under uncertainty. J Exp Psychol (Hum Percept), *1:* 288–299, 1975.

50. Bursztajn H, Feinbloom RI, Hamm RM, Brodsky A: *Medical Choices, Medical Chances: How Patients, Families, and Physicians Can Cope with Uncertainty,* New York, Delacorte, 1981.

51. Gutheil TG, Rachlin S, Mills MJ: Differing conceptual models in psychiatry and the law, in Rachlin S (ed): *Legal Encroachment on Psychiatric Practice,* San Francisco, Jossey-Bass, 1985.

52. Schaffner KF: Causation and responsibility: Medicine, science and the law, in Spicker SF, Healey JM, Engelhardt HT (eds): *The Law-Medicine Relation: A Philosophical Exploration,* D. Reidel, 1981.

53. Brodsky A: Doctoring defensively, in *The New Republic,* p. 6. Aug 19, 1985.

54. Kahneman D, Slovic P, Tversky A (eds): *Judgment under Uncertainty: Heuristics and Biases,* New York, Cambridge University Press, 1982.

55. Modell AH: *Psychoanalysis in a New Context,* New York, International University Press, 1984.

56. Katz J: *The Silent World of Doctor and Patient,* New York, The Free Press, 1984.

chapter 18

the psychiatric medical record and issues of confidentiality

Thomas G. Gutheil, M.D.

SPECIAL CONSIDERATIONS FOR CASE RECORDS OF INPATIENTS

Many clinicians believe that inpatient psychiatry is a veritable subspecialty in its own right. This book is an expression, in effect, of this viewpoint. In an analogous manner, evolving the inpatient case record requires a grasp of certain principles unique to inpatient practice and its documentation.

The inpatient ward may be compared to an intensive care unit in general medicine. Though not always obvious or manifest, issues of life and death usually engross most patients sick enough to require admission, given the high admission threshold most contemporary facilities maintain. These ultimate issues coupled with the manifestations of florid mental illness give to the inpatient's experience a drama, intensity, and urgency rarely seen in outpatient circumstances. In these troubled times such indices invariably connote an increase in potential liability for clinicians and their institutions as well—an issue highly relevant to recordkeeping.

A second important consideration, frequently scanted in legal assessments of a given case, is that the inpatient clinician must weigh the effects of interventions on other ward patients as well as on his "own" patient or patients. The hospitalized patient is inevitably a member of a social milieu, an arrangement which contrasts with the unitary model of outpatient practice. The implications for records of a milieu orientation are reviewed in this chapter.

Finally, inpatient psychiatric treatment customarily involves multidisciplinary care delivered by different personnel whose separate contributions must be orchestrated in constructive collaboration. This poses problems for the record keeping process different from those encountered in the one patient-one therapist model characteristic of certain outpatient treatments.

Despite inevitable overlap, this discussion is divided into clinical and legal aspects of the record keeping process. Since confidentiality is a topic intimately related to recordkeeping, the third section addresses that subject. Finally the specific organization of the material in the record is outlined in the appendix to this chapter.

CLINICAL ASPECTS

Though fraught with medicolegal implications, the case record is an instrument whose primary purpose is the care of the patient. The specific functions of the record, which are reviewed here, are in the service of the clinical aims of the psychiatric record.

The Archival Function

A major function of the record is the durable storage of information about both the patient and the care delivered to him by the institution. This storage may be short-term (chart entries may be consulted minutes after they are made, e.g., in a medical emergency) or long-term (decades after a first admission a patient's readmission might require review of his chart).

The importance of writing the record in language whose meaning will endure is essential for archival reasons. Topical allusions, excessively idiosyncratic abbreviations or crypticisms, and simple illegibility are all ephemera too transient to serve archival purposes.

Case 1. A resident wrote: "LOL in betzopenia with possible 'Big S' admitted from BNH for a Charlie's special." This might be "translated" as: "Little old lady with dementia (facetiously characterized as deficiency of Betz cells) who may have schizophrenia admitted from Bad Nursing Home (i.e., a nursing home whose administration is characterized by a tendency to refuse readmission of the patient after psychiatric intervention, in contrast to a GNH) for that extensive work-up of reversible causes of dementia especially favored by the Chief Resident that year, one Dr. Charles."

The "original" is shorter, terser, more richly evocative and, no doubt, almost telepathic in its semantics for those staff on the ward during that particular year. We can, however, readily predict that the coherency of this entry will fade rapidly into obscurity with the passage of time. One must write for the ages. The breeziness of tone of the case example, moreover, poses other difficulties that are discussed later.

The Planning Function

The chart as archive, as a repository of clinical data, observations, reports, results of examinations, etc., is useful only insofar as it generates plans of operation for treatment. We generate the data base in order to identify problems in biological, psychiatric, and social areas and to suggest directions for further exploration or intervention. A statement of the presenting problems, required explorations, and planned interventions constitute the treatment plan, the operational heart of the record.

The treatment plan, like a musical score, serves to orchestrate the con-

tributions from the members of the treatment team into an harmonious, collaborative effort. In addition, the plan points to goals (preferably measurable ones) that the interventions aim to achieve. A goal orientation avoids the twin treatment pitfalls of amorphousness, wherein treatment grinds along directionless or, like Leacock's[1] protagonist, "rides madly off in all directions," and manic grandiosity, wherein treatment is aimed at "blue-skies" goals impossible of fulfillment in this life.

Case 2. A treatment plan read: "All members of the team should get this guy by the lapels, shake some sense into him and turn his life around."

A preferable plan for the case in question might have been: "Psychotherapy for hysterical seizures and medical control of diabetes by psychiatrist; vocational assessment and training in marketable skills by occupational therapist; family therapy by social worker aimed at family's acceptance of severity of his illness; increased socialization by nursing staff."

The improved version, while still brief, specifies who will do what in precise terms that allow for measurable goals. Though the goals are not explicitly spelled out in the example, they may readily be inferred because of the precision of the task definitions. A measure of goal attainment, for example, in vocational training of marketable skills would be the patient's suitable employment.

The Documentational Function

The documentational function of the record is linked to its archival and planning functions. It serves to validate the delivery of care, an issue of great clinical and forensic power, as is further elaborated on in Legal Aspects. The power of this function can best be captured in the axiom: "If it isn't written down, it didn't happen."[2] In countless treatment settings the skilled delivery of care is gainsaid through failures in attention to documentation. Good work deserves credit by careful recording. Complex and difficult decisions made on the firing line deserve the protection from liability that scrupulous documentation provides.

Case 3. A malpractice case was lost because of the failure to *note* a patient's condition while in restraints. Though good clinical practice was followed, there was no validation of the indications for, and observations during, the procedure.

It must be stressed that, as often as not, the data to be documented are significant by their absence. Significant negatives, as in *"denies* suicidal intent"; the *absence* of change, and the *absence* of concurrent medical conditions, signs of tardive dyskinesia, or an FTA response can only be conveyed through documentation.

The Justificatory Function

In these times of heightened accountability, data must serve not only to record, guide, and document but also to justify. The need for certain interventions and their clinical, legal, or fiscal (reimbursement) validity will rest firmly only on a foundation of documented information. Among the items requiring justification are examinations, interventions and, most importantly, the admission itself.

Many patients who are ranting, raving, and out of control in the emergency setting rapidly calm down on the ward. They may thus appear to the inexperienced viewer to be ready for discharge the instant they hit the unit. This familiar clinical phenomenon might cast retrospective doubt on the need for the admission unless attention is paid to recording why *no less* a step than admission would provide appropriate clinical care. Many apparently tranquil inpatients simply can not be responsibly returned to the very outside situation that fostered their decompensation without achievement of durable changes in their clinical condition or their extrahospital environment. Furthermore, third party payers may not allow reimbursement for inadequately justified admissions, resulting in crushing economic effects on patient and family.

The Utilization Function

Closely related to the justificatory function, the utilization function addresses aspects of quality control and utilization review (an amalgam of documentation and justification with planning) affecting litigation and reimbursement as well as other important variables. Utilization review (UR) is an intrahospital "checks-and-balances" mechanism by which patients are evaluated *after* admission as to the appropriateness of the decisions to admit and/or treat. The question might be phrased: "Is this patient receiving a level of care appropriate to his/her condition or might lower level (less intense) care serve equally well?" This determination frequently affects third party reimbursement. At times UR requires that a particular form be filled out addressing the question above.

The principle here is that certain services or procedures must be accounted for in terms of indications, needs, and justification, as earlier noted. Admissions, use of special investigations like CAT scans, or special interventions like electroconvulsive therapy must be justified in terms of both clinical appropriateness and expense. Professional standards review organizations (PSRO) require similar recording. PSRO's are groups of physicians (and sometimes other professionals) who engage in peer review as a form of UR. This function was formerly termed "quality assurance." Again, the issues are checks and balances concerning medical decision-making.

The Educational Function

A good case record should instruct the trainee about etiology, precipitants, interventions, and response. It should be able to serve as a profitable focus in supervisory and training meetings.

More importantly, the act of thinking through one's conceptualization of the case in order to record it is, *in itself,* a vital method of instruction in systematic clinical evaluation and treatment planning. Many a clinically confused trainee, when asked to reread the muddy prose of a chart entry, has correctly diagnosed, through introspection, the muddy clinical thinking at the core of the problem.

Case 4. A trainee noted that his chart order that markedly increased a psychotic patient's privileges followed close upon an entry that stressed the patient's profound suicidality. The trainee realized that his countertransference anger at this abusive patient had led him to minimize the patient's lethality. The order could then be corrected.

The Research Function

For obvious reasons, recorded data are the essential raw material for research. The data for research may be gathered from project-specific research instruments or from the actual record, as often occurs in longitudinal studies. For research purposes a premium is therefore placed on recording even observations that seem incidental or uninterpretable at present. Explanatory hypotheses may emerge long after the data are gathered, if they are available for retrospective review.

LEGAL ASPECTS

The mental health system has become increasingly involved with the legal and judicial systems,[3] as has occurred in almost every sphere of modern life. The implications of this involvement are especially relevant to recordkeeping. The overlap of this section with its clinical predecessor is profound, largely because of the importance assigned by the legal system to *formal* aspects of care, particularly records. The art of therapy, the role of the unconscious in human functioning, the therapeutic alliance, ambivalence, and the various empathic, experiential, and intuitive elements of psychiatric work are poorly grasped by lawyers. Their ideological heritage stresses concrete matters such as contracts, documents, and explicit testimony, all of which may relate to the psychiatric case record. This difference in conceptual models may led to misunderstanding.[3]

Case 5. An attorney agreed to refrain from serving a writ of habeas corpus (for the immediate release of a patient) because the doctor predicted that the patient's condition would probably improve enough over the weekend to permit a Monday discharge. The patient's condition, however, worsened unexpectedly over the weekend, and discharge required postponement on *clinical* grounds. At a later commitment hearing, the attorney presented these events as though the physician had promised (i.e., contracted) to discharge the patient that Monday. In conceptualizing the matter as a breach of contract, the attorney failed to grasp the significance of the change in the patient's clinical state as determining the psychiatric decision.

From this general view, we will now turn to particular legal issues relevant to inpatient recordkeeping.

Malpractice Prevention versus Fostering Good Practice

The clinician's central concern with good patient care is certainly fostered by good record keeping. In these litigious times we should not overlook the additional important role of records in the prevention of suits for negligence and other wrongs as well as in the protection of patients' rights. Because the "fostering" and "preventing" aspects of the record are so intertwined they are presented together under the legal rubric.

Inclusions and Exclusions

The "Process-Progress" Distinction[2-5]

The court subpoena, insurance companies, and other sociopolitical forces conspire to make the record less private than is desirable. The record, therefore, should be written in *all parts* in an objective, descriptive manner. The patient's verbal expression and behavior should be recorded in diplomatic language. Unconscious fantasy content, psychodynamic formulations, dream material, and technical descriptive terms or jargon likely to be misunderstood by the laity should be scrupulously eschewed. To put it another way, the record should consist of *progress notes* only. *Process notes*, verbatim accounts, and the dynamic issues just listed should be maintained separately in the clinician's private file. A question is sometimes raised about this point when the S.O.A.P. record schema is endorsed (Subjective, Objectve, Assessment, Plan), in which "subjective" is often interpreted as verbatim—i.e., a quotation in the patient's own words. Even in this model, compromising words and quotes should be avoided.

Case 6. In a digression from the main course of examination in a malpractice trial, an attorney seized upon a note mentioning the patient's "homosexually erotized relationship" to the therapist. The attorney then attempted to discredit the therapist in relation to the comment by introducing testimony to the effect that the patient had *never* been "gay." Although the attorney had misconstrued the meaning of the phrase, this apparent "contradiction" was damaging to the therapist's credibility.

In keeping with the guideline of careful choice of terminology, one might replace "homosexuality" with "positive feeling" or "identity confusion." Another example would be substituting "developmental" for "infantile" or "primitive" when the recording of these terms is unavoidable in communicating about the patient to subsequent caretakers. In all other cases such material should simply not appear in the "public" record at all.

The Professional Tone

The professionalism rightly expected of inpatient caretakers should extend to the tone of the written record. In practice this means that the following should be excluded: judgemental or moralistic terms ("the patient is really being evil to the nurses"); inappropriate preciosity ("patient is back to being her sweet widdle self"); facetiousness or sarcasm ("if this patient gets any more grandiose, we'll have to crown him Messiah and be done with it"); casual and pejorative slang ("the patient is being a real brat and a royal pain in the ass"); gratuitous interpolations ("patient plans to work in therapy at being less entitled [hah!] in the future"); and any other lapses of professional demeanor as conveyed in written form. No matter how satisfying such entries may be to write or how cute and funny to read to one's colleagues, one must recall,[2] first, that they are rarely quite so comic when, say, they are read aloud in open court and, second, that such material invariably conveys disrespect for the patient, an attitude destructive both to one's actual attitude towards and work with the patient and to the caring posture one would wish conveyed, say, at a trial for negligence toward that same patient.[3] All the clinical descriptions given in the mock examples above can be expressed quite adequately and appropriately in neutral and objective terms. One should recall that the "eyes of the future are upon you."[2]

Referring to Other Patients and Staff

A patient's interaction with specific other patients may be highly significant and relevant to his or her care, in which case it may be important to refer to patient B in patient A's chart. For example, two patients may provoke each other and fight or sexualize and thus have to be kept apart on clinical grounds. This information should be recorded to guide and inform staff on subsequent shifts in order to prevent harm.

However, if patient A later releases his/her record to an appropriate reader, that reader is not entitled to gratuitous information about patient B. For patient B's protection, therefore, only the first name and last initial of the "other" patient(s) should be used in order to conceal his identity from future readers. Current staff, however, will still be able to identify him.

When staff members must be referred to, they whould be noted by name and discipline. For example, "patient threatened Ms. Smith, R.N.," instead of "patient threatened Betty."

Judgment Calls and Thinking Out Loud for the Record

Clinical work repeatedly requires the exercise of clinical intuition, the making of judgment calls, and the taking of calculated risks. For inpatients these critical decisions often, but not always, focus around the question of when the patient is clinically ready to leave the hospital or to experience some liberalization of constraints.

In such "judgment calls" the usual austerity and restraint that should characterize writing for the record must be compromised. Instead, the clinician should "think out loud for the record."[2, 3] This phrase means that the clinician should go to greater than usual lengths to detail the factual underpinnings and incremental steps of reasoning that lead to the decision in question. Equal care should invest the *explicit* weighing of benefits and risks and advantages and costs that enter into the clinical reasoning.

The essence of judgment calls and thinking out loud relates to the critical distinction between a legitimate error in judgment, on the one hand, and negligence on the other. Careful decision-making based on careful assessment that leads to a regrettable result is not negligence. *Failure* to make such assessment and decision, or failure to *record* same, is negligent, and, given a bad result, is thus grounds for malpractice.

Case 7. A resident was considering releasing a patient in an AMA (against medical advice) discharge rather than filing for commitment. The patient was a chronically suicidal borderline male intermittently self-lethal and highly resistant to taking responsibility for himself.

In writing up the discharge note, the resident included observations of the patient's state; notations about the goals of treatment in fostering responsibility in this patient; the justifications for this approach; reports of the views of supervisors and consultants; candid acknowledgment of the risk of suicide; review of the disadvantages of hospitalization (regression, absence of an end point, failure of even the hospital to *ensure* safety); iteration of the various extra-hospital supports and safeguards (e.g., "patient was given hospital phone number and instructed to call if situation worsens"); and an outline of contingency plans.[2]

While the amount of detail may seem excessive or unnecesary, remember that one is preparing for a calculated risk that may turn out for well or ill, no matter how necessary the plan may be for the good management of the patient. If well, a slight amount of time is lost. If ill, the presence of details documenting careful assessment and exercise of judgment becomes enormously important.

Recording comments by professional colleagues is also an important step. As an informal "peer review," this documentation demonstrates that the decision on the "judgment call" has the support of at least one or more colleagues in the field, a situation similar to the "second opinion" obtained in general medicine. Professional support for an opinion powerfully refutes the accusation of negligence since the clinician demonstrated care by obtaining consultation and assessed the "community standard" of another "average reasonable practitioner."

An Approach to Forensically Significant Events

In the practice of inpatient psychiatry some events are more likely than others to be the focus of medicolegal attention. These include (nonexhaustively): admissions and discharges; assaults, falls, accidents, and injuries; ill effects from treatments, especially sensitive treatment (e.g., electroconvulsive therapy); special procedures (seclusion, restraint); escapes or failures to return from pass; threats or other evidence of dangerousness; concurrent medical conditions (illnesses, allergies); and the like.

These clinical events and their attendant decisions require recordkeeping commensurate with their potential forensic significance. At times the documentation requires "significant negatives."

Case 8. A patient was inappropriately and without clinical basis sent by a court to a hospital because of alleged dangerousness. Realizing that this issue would adumbrate the eventual discharge, the clinician, in anticipation of discharge, regularly recorded in the progress notes the *absence* of dangerous behavior, threats, etc.

The documentation of forensically significant events should also address any potential future questions. Examples include: Was normal neurological function present after a fall with head injury? Are x-rays indicated? Vital signs? Pupil checks?, and so on.

In a complementary manner, noting evidence *for* dangerousness is useful when a possible future commitment petition is envisioned.

Special Medicolegal Issues

Certain documents with specific medicolegal significance must clearly be included in the record. These include the legal status paper (voluntary or involuntary admission by court or civil commitment); consent forms for special procedures (the consent form should always be matched by a progress note in the body of the chart outlining the conversation with the patient in which the information about the procedure in question is conveyed. The note should also comment on answers given to the patient's questions, if any. The purpose of these data is to document that consent is truly "informed"[3]); certificates of guardianship and similar papers bearing on matters of competence[3]; and the like. For court-committed patients, the relevant court documents should also be included.

Specificity about the sources of data often has medicolegal significance. Direct observation of behavior and speech must be distinguished from secondary sources.

Case 9. A record entry read, in part: "4/19/80 5 p.m. I saw Mr. Jones in the day room become agitated and strike Rhonda W. across the face (note that the alleged crime for which Mr. Jones is being evaluated, as reported by the arresting officer on admission, is assault and battery on an older woman)."

Note the distinctions between *primary observations* ("I saw"), *secondary observations* ("as reported"), and the careful use of "alleged" to refer to any actual or potential criminal charges. Note also the use of *time* (as well as date) for recording specific incidents in which time course may be essential (e.g., does Rhoda W. develop neurological symptoms 2, 10, or 18 hours after the injury?).

A more extensive discussion of record keeping may be found elsewhere.[3, 4]

Confidentiality[3]

Definition

Confidentiality is the name given to a person's right not to have revealed to third parties that information shared "in confidence" with a second party.

Practical Aspects of Confidentiality

Originally an ethical principle, confidentiality now rests on a number of explicit and implicit legal bases, at the core of which lies this principle: *identifiable information about a patient cannot be shared with third parties without that patient's explicit (usually written) consent.*

Implied in this act of consenting are several considerations.

1. Consent should be given for particular data or particular kinds of data, with the amount or degree of detail specified.

2. A single consent is good for a single release of information. A second request, even from the same source, requires a second consent.

3. Even with consent, the clinician is expected to use discretion in how much or what kind of information to release, the standard being set by the "needs of the situation," narrowly construed.

4. Oral consent, while acceptable during emergencies and other conditions, is generally far less desirable than written consent for obvious documentational reasons.

Pitfalls in Confidentiality

The most common breach of confidentiality on inpatient units occurs when staff carelessly discuss patients by name in elevators, corridors, or cafeterias of the hospital. This harmful practice must be eschewed not only because it is a genuine compromise of confidentiality but also because it is a blow to the morale of other patients in addition to those being discussed. The casual insensitivity thus demonstrated conveys a lack of respect or of seriousness of purpose regarding patients in general.

To the surprise of some clincians, confidentiality extends even to families of the patient; to the patient's attorney; to the patient's former therapist; and to the clinician's professional colleagues who are not directly involved in care of that patient.

Supervisors, on the other hand, are usually considered part of the treatment team and thus are viewed as being within the "circle" of direct information, as are ward personnel directly involved with the patient's care. Thus, ward staff who keep patient-related secrets from each other are not "observing confidentiality" but acting in a manner destructive to good patient care.[6]

Clinicians often wonder about the amount of information to share with a consultant when the later gives advice on a case. It is customary to obtain the patient's permission for the consult and, hence, for the implicit sharing of information. If there is some difficulty with this—the patient is paranoid, hesitant, reluctant, and ambivalent—I usually recommend that the clinician present the patient anonymously ("The patient is a 50-year-old man") to obtain at least some consultative benefit from a second opinion without compromising confidentiality. This approach also "spares" litigation-shy consultants: their duty here is to the clinician-consultee, not the patient, so that the latter cannot sue the consultant for malpractice.

Exceptions to the Principle of Confidentiality

This topic is extensively covered elsewhere.[3] However, a brief outline will serve here to stimulate thought about this important area. Under certain circumstances information from a patient's record may be released without the patient's consent. These include:

1. Emergency needs of the patient (the "best interests" doctrine narrowly construed, e.g., patient's lawyer needing to meet with her before an imminent trial, and asking if the patient is on your ward, while the patient, through paranoia, refuses release of any information to anyone; the family of a floridly psychotic teenager needing to be queried regarding his possible PCP use). In all such incidents, the record should reflect the basis for this (justified) breach of confidentiality. In all such cases an attempt should be made to obtain consent, and the effort should be documented.

2. For incompetent patie~~...~~ of guardian (or nex~~t~~ gencies) is requi~~r~~

3. In some juris~~d~~ ~~...~~, alas for consist~~...~~ ~~...~~ers the clinician is ~~...~~ breach confidentiality ~~...~~ ry to protect third

parties from harm from a patient, e.g., in warning the putative victim of death threats even without the patient's consent.[3] The clinician's knowledge of past crimes, however, does not mandate reporting.

4. In some jurisdictions reporting requirements govern venereal disease, child abuse, and other issues. Local statutes should be checked.

5. In the interests of the alliance all breaches of confidentiality for one of these emergency reasons should be reviewed with the patient, addressing the necessity of the breach, the impact and consequences, etc. The patients' feelings and the clinical state which necessitated the breach should be reviewed, explored, and worked through to the best degree possible.

It is hoped that this review of the structure and function of the psychiatric record not only clarifies the complex medicolegal nimbus surrounding "charting" but also offers an insight into the manner in which good clinical care may be fostered by attention to careful recording of clinical data. The appendix which follows addresses some particulars of the chart itself.

REFERENCES

1. Leacock S: *Laugh with Leacock*, New York, Pocket Books, Inc., 1980.
2. Gutheil TG: Paranoia and progress notes: A guide to forensically-informed psychiatric record-keeping. Hosp Community Psychiatry, *31:* 479–482, 1980.
3. Gutheil TG, Appelbaum, PS: *Clinical Handbook of Psychiatry and the Law*, New York, McGraw-Hill, 1982.
   ~~...~~enko R: On the need for record-keeping in ~~...~~ractice of psychiatry. J Psychiatry Law, *7:* ~~1~~40, 1979.
5. ~~Ra~~~~...~~port RG: The psychiatrist on trial. J Psychiatry Law, *7:* 463–469, 1979.
6. Gutheil TG: Legal defense as ego defense: A special form of resistance to the therapeutic process. Psychiatr Q, *51:* 251–256, 1979.

Appendix

the contents of the psychiatric inpatient record

Since the majority of inpatient facilities tend to evolve their own systems of record keeping in idiosyncratic fashion, we must limit our discussion in this appendix to those general principles defining the purpose— and, hence, the content— of the sections of the record.

The Admission Note

This section heralds the transformation of an individual into an "inpatient." This is a shift of enormous sociolegal impact, rife with implications of changed status, altered rights, liabilities, duty of care, potential stigma, and the like. In keeping with the seriousness of the patient's passage over this "administrative cliff," this section should emphasize the justificatory aspect of the record. Why was admission the best (or the only, or the only feasible, or the most appropriate) approach? Why would no less a step suffice? What was the "last straw" for this patient that "broke the back" of extrahospital functioning? The answer to these questions must be clear in the note.

Ideally, hospital admission is a carefully planned and weighed prescription. In reality, it is often a precipitous event, partaking of the urgency of a life-or-death emergency room intervention. Like the emergency room work-up, the admission note should focus on critical, decisive elements. Deeper, more discursive elaboration must await the definitive write-up. Thus, after identifying data, chief complaints, and a cogent "present illness" have been recorded, a brief past history relating social circumstances and family history should be taken. Particular attention should be paid to past *medical* history, noting past and current medical conditions and their pharmacotherapy, if any; current medications, drugs, and alcohol, including O.T.C. preparations; allergies or previous adverse drug reactions; and dietary considerations. The tentative formulation and working diagnosis should guide the early interventions, expressed in goal-directed fashion ("Thorazine 50-mg test dose, then 50 t.i.d. for hallucinations). The working diagnosis and acute interventions should be recorded together with planned investigations and laboratory tests.

Often the informants, or those who accompany the patient, are extremely important to the patient, though this may not always be obvious. The admission note should record their names and *phone numbers* as well as similar data for previous mental health or medical and social contacts, if available. If this information is not obtained upon admission it is often far more difficult to track down later.

Of course, a physical examination, including careful neurological assessment, is a central part of each admission work-up.

The Status Paper

This vitally important document is, quite literally, the only indication that what is happening is medical hospitalization and not kidnapping or false imprisonment. Clinical experience reveals the surprising finding that the most dangerously vague status indicators accompany patients sent by the courts. For this reason, particular scrutiny must be given to "the papers" sent with court-ordered patients. Ambiguities should be clarified as rapidly as possible with the clerk of the court.

The Definitive Write-Up

Whether termed "case study," "anamnesis," "staffing report," "conference plan," or some similar title, this section of the record should reflect a detailed portrait of the patient at the present time. Rather than merely expanding the admission note, the write-up should describe the result of medical, neurological, and laboratory examinations; reports of detailed family, social, sexual, cultural, religious, educational, and vocational history-taking; data gathered by the various disciplines; and a more confident statement of diagnosis, clinical formulation, and the various planned modalities of treatment, with attention to the utilization perspective noted earlier in chapter 18.

In some institutions this section is maintained separate from the chart as a teaching device. When it is part and parcel of the record, of course, the cautions about diplomatic use of terminology should be kept in mind.

Team Treatment Plan

As the operational core of the chart and the veritable compass of the course of hospitalization, this section should focus on data gathering, task assignment, and goal definition. Often a problem-oriented format helps to organize this section. Regular updating should keep the plan contemporary and up to date with the evolution of the illness, the treatment, the hospital course, newly emerging data, and the pooled wisdom of supervisors, consultants, and others.

Progress Notes

These regular recordings of the developments of the hospital course should follow the principles outlined in the chapter above. Most of the considerations described apply particularly to progress notes.

Progress notes should always be dated (and for significant events, given a time indicator as well) and should always be signed by name and discipline. Additional titles sould be added when pertinent (e.g., S. Wilson, R.N., night supervisor).

Frequency of entry should be governed by the evolution of hospitalization and treatment, but a workable rule of thumb might be: semi-weekly notes for 2 weeks, weekly thereafter, and—for slow reconstitution/rehabilitation courses—monthly. *Ad hoc* entries should, of course, be made whenever significant events occur.

The Discharge Summary

In addition to marking the termination of one phase of total treatment (hospitalization) and the onset of another (after-care), this section also heralds passage over another "administrative cliff" to outpatienthood. The outpatient state often lacks many of the implicit supports and opportunities for monitoring care that would be present in the hospital. This fact places a burden on the treatment planners to address this deficit, which they must do in the discharge summary.

Many institutions, moreover, send *only* the discharge summary to other caretakers when information is requested (with patient's release, of course). Thus, of the whole record, the discharge summary is "the part that flies." This fact places two potentially contradictory burdens on its author: completeness, since all the critical data must be included, and austerity, since this document is the most "public" piece of the chart, by virtue of its transmissibility.

The discharge summary should contain identifying data; chief complaint; brief statement of the admission picture enriched by subsequent information and understanding; a summary of the hospital course specifically including forensically important events (allergic reactions, injuries, etc., as earlier noted) and their outcomes or remedies; a comparison of admission and discharge diagnoses; statements of condition (e.g., "improved") and prognosis (e.g., "guarded"); and a very detailed outline of planned after-care, preferably including specifics of the first planned outpatient or aftercare appointment.

Example of after-care plan. Perphenazine, (32 mg h.s. daily) 10 pills were given to pt.; a prescription for 2 weeks' supply given, to be filled by patient's mother. Needs to be monitored by Dr. Smith; pt. has 1st appt. with him on 5/17/85 at 2:30 p.m.; given appt. slip. Therapy per Jonesville CMHC clinic; case reviewed with Ms. Adams, M.S.W., who will follow pt. 1st appt. 5/14/85 at 10 a.m. Pt. given map to clinic.

If some aspect of dangerousness characterized the admission (suicide attempt, homicide threats) specific mention should be made of an assessment of *present* dangerousness at discharge. If discharge is occurring (as not uncommonly happens) in the context of a calculated risk, this decision should be meticulously spelled out with determinants, risks, and benefits of discharge and benefits of alternative courses of action made explicit. The care with which this is done here may prove decisive (in the event of even an adventitious post-discharge bad outcome) in differentiating a justified judgment call from negligence.

Miscellaneous

Other important parts of the record include: consent forms (witnessed) for special procedures; laboratory and consultation reports; and special forms (e.g., seclusion reports and other statutorily required documents). Most of these should be initialled or countersigned by the responsible clinician to indicate that they have been reviewed.

chapter 19

the economics of inpatient psychiatry

Joseph T. English, M.D., and Richard G. McCarrick, M.D.

INTRODUCTION

Today's psychiatrist who works in or has any contact with inpatient psychiatric units must deal not only with the patients themselves but also with complex administrative tasks, financial policy reimbursement guidelines, and government regulations. Indeed inpatient psychiatrists should develop not only a familiarity with these tasks but a competency in dealing with them that rivals their ability to handle the clinical concerns of their patients. In the future they also face the reality of tighter financial resources and increasing government regulations. Yet, the issues of economics and financing have always been important to the physicians and administrators who run inpatient psychiatric units in the United States. A brief historical review can illustrate this point and emphasize the need for psychiatrists as a group to take an active role in policy debates on the economics of health care.

HISTORICAL REVIEW OF THE FINANCING OF INPATIENT UNITS

One of the earliest examples of concern about financing of a psychiatric hospital was in Samuel Tuke's *Description of the Retreat*, published in 1813. The York Retreat was founded in 1792 by Samuel's grandfather, William Tuke, and other Quakers in York, England. This hospital served as a model for reform of care for the mentally ill in 19th century America. In Samuel Tuke's account of the origin of the hospital, he stated that:

Proposals for raising money and forming the Establishment, were prepared and laid before Friends, at the conclusion of the next Quarterly Meeting; which were generally approved. A subscription was immediately entered into; and the contributions were one hundred pounds, for a life-annuity of 5% per annum annual subscriptions £L11.0.6 for three years certain, and donations amounting to £191.3s[1]

The principles of the York Retreat were followed in 19th century America by the medical practitioners of "moral treatment." They made up the original membership of the Association of Medical Superintendents of American Institutions for the Insane, which eventually became the American Psychiatric Association, and were also the founders and major contributors to the early volumes of the *American Journal of Insanity*. They believed that the damaged brain tissue of the mentally ill could be reconstructed by re-socializing the patients. They prescribed a complete milieu of treatment, much like that of the York Retreat, and thus led to the development of large asylums.[2]

One of the earliest examples of the establishment of a mental institution based on the York Retreat model was the Bloomingdale Asylum, founded by Thomas Eddy and a group of philanthropists. In 1816 the New York State legislature agreed to give the institution $10,000 annually, and the hospital agreed to accept all patients regardless of financial position according to a sliding scale of fees (fees for the poor were levied on the town). However, despite the high goals of the medical superintendents of Bloomingdale Hospital and other asylums, economic pressures caused another picture to emerge. A period of high inflation after 1850 raised the costs of institutional construction and maintenance, and legislatures were hesitant to appropriate funds for new facilities despite increasing numbers of patients being treated. Municipalities were usually supposed to pay the asylum for treating its indigent insane, but these fees were often set before costs rose. Thus institutions were forced to cut expenses by sacrificing the "milieu," which was essential to moral treatment. Because they actually had a poor record of curing their patients the asylums began to house increasing numbers of chronic patients.[3]

Even with the deteriorating conditions of the early asylums by the middle of the 19th century, most indigent insane had to endure much worse conditions in jails, almshouses, or the community. These conditions were brought to the attention of the public and various state legislatures in a dramatic fashion by Dorothea Dix, a retired schoolteacher from Boston, Mass. In her crusading style she called for the establishment of state hospitals for the indigent insane and attracted other prominent reformers to the movement. Her first success came in her home state, in which the legislature passed a bill greatly enlarging the state hospital to receive the indigent insane. Dix then carried her fight to other states. In Rhode Island, she lobbied one of the wealthiest but most parsimonious men in the state to pledge $40,000 to build that state's first state hospital. From there she went on to every state east of the Rockies, personally carrying her message for new and better state hospitals to individual legislatures. Her tenacity and lobbying skills were great. From the state level she then proceeded to the Federal government, where she worked for a number of years for passage of a bill by both houses of Congress which granted states 12,000,000 acres of Federal lands to sell, with the proceeds of the sale to be used for bettering the condition of the indigent insane. In her arguments she called the insane the "wards of the nation." However, when this bill was passed in 1854, President Franklin Pierce

vetoed it because, in the opinion of his administration, government could not become involved in granting aid for any humanitarian cause whatsoever.[4]

Thus the model of care for the chronically mentally ill in the state hospitals was set in the 1800's, and the state hospital population continued to grow to a peak national census of 560,000 in 1955.[5] In the decade prior to 1955 the foundations were laid for the shift away from the state and to the Federal government as the primary source for funding for psychiatric care and away from the state hospital and to general hospital psychiatric units as the locus of care for mental patients. In 1946, the National Mental Health Act, establishing the National Institute of Mental Health, was passed and signed into law. Robert Felix and other psychiatrists, fresh from the administrative and clinical experiences of World War II, were instrumental in promoting the passage of this bill. Initially $7,500,000 was authorized to promote research in psychiatry, to provide for training of personnel, and to aid states in developing new programs. Through the alliance of the psychiatric profession and very influential lobbyists in Washington, Federal support of mental health research increased dramatically in the 1950's. During that decade, the National Institute of Mental Health focused its efforts of program development on community mental health: short-term inpatient care, outpatient care, partial hospitalization, emergency services, and consultation/ education. Beginning in 1948, Federal funds that states were required to match dollar for dollar were made available to state mental health programs. The guidelines specifically stated that Federal funds could not be used to train personnel or obtain equipment for state hospitals. These Federal grants to states for program development increased from $20,000 per state in 1948 to $65,000 per state in 1962.[6]

While these changes in policy and funding were being made in Washington, a revolutionary advance had been made in the care of the mentally ill with the introduction of the psychotropic drug chlorpromazine, and practitioners were learning of the successes that British psychiatrists were having with the "open-hospital" system. These events led to a small but significant decrease in state hospital populations in the late 1950's.[7]

In 1963, President Kennedy's "Message on Mental Illness and Mental Retardation" set the Federal philosophy for mental health funding for the next decade and a half. He based his message on the findings of the Joint Commission on Mental Illness and Health which had been formed in 1955. Kennedy called for the establishment of community mental health centers, which "ideally . . . could be located at an appropriate community general hospital, many of which already have psychiatric units. . . ." Under this plan the Federal government would provide from 45 to 75% of construction and staffing costs with declining support over a period of 8 years. Kennedy envisioned that services provided by these centers would be "financed in the same way as other medical and hospital costs."[8] However, even by 1975, these centers showed a heavy dependency on categorical Federal funding.

The next spur to the growth of general hospital psychiatric inpatient units was the enactment of the Medicaid and Medicare programs. Medicaid pays for medical care for the poor by providing Federal matching funds to the states and in determining reimbursement does not permit distinctions between psychiatric and other diagnoses. It is established that Medicaid provides 25% of the funding for all mental health care for everyone in the United States (70% of those expenditures were for inpatient care). Medicare provides both hospital insurance and supplemental medical insurance. The hospital insurance is available to all persons over 65, and the coverage for mental health services is less than that provided for other disorders. Coverage of inpatient services in a psychiatric hospital is limited to 190 days in a lifetime.

Private insurance plans have provided fewer benefits for psychiatric illness. Initially, when health insurance expanded during World War II, insurers included more liberal inpatient and outpatient psychiatric coverage. However, because of a broadened concept of mental illness and a widened availability of services insurers found that large claims were being made

for ambulatory psychiatric care. As a result they imposed arbitrary limits on coverage, most evident in the area of outpatient benefits. However, these limits have affected hospitalization coverage much less, and a 1975 study concluded that over 63% of the United States civilian population had some coverage for hospital psychiatric care.

As a result of the historical trends outlined, today's picture of inpatient psychiatric care is very different than it was in 1955. At that time, state hospitals were responsible for 99% of total patient episodes in psychiatry (both inpatient and outpatient), and in 1977 they accounted for 49% of the episodes. Acute general hospital psychiatric beds increased from 7,000 in 1955 to 19,000 in 1977. Yet, interestingly the funding for state and county hospitals has not changed proportionately. Expenditures for psychiatric services by state and county mental hospitals still account for 48.7% of all expenditures for psychiatric services (not including private outpatient practice). General hospitals account for 13.7%, private psychiatric hospitals 7%, VA neuropsychiatric hospitals 6.3%, community mental health centers 12%, residential treatment centers for emotionally disturbed children 4.2%, and other multi-service centers 1.8%.[10] In New York State, for example, while the census in state psychiatric centers has declined by approximately 69,000, the staff in these facilities has increased from 24,000 in 1955 to 36,000 today. The State Purposes Budget for the New York State Office of Mental Health represented 83.3% of the total state mental health budget for 1982–83 while local assistance funding for community-based care was only 16.7% of the total budget.[11]

To look at the broad picture again in 1982, health care expenditures were approximately $322,000,000,000, representing 10.5% of the gross national product. In the 1970's, the inflation rate in the medical sector was significantly above the nation's overall inflation rate. In the early 1980's economists feared that the Medicare and Social Security income maintenance programs would become bankrupt. Thus, a bipartisan political effort was made to reform past methods of fin ing health and hospital care. Psychiatry, as well as all other medical specialists, is being subjected to a dramatic increase in regulatory activity at every level. Alternate systems of providing health care services most efficiently are being encouraged, and investor-owned hospitals are increasing; the number of investor-owned hospital beds rose from 33% of all psychiatric hospital beds in 1969 to 51.6% in 1979.

Perhaps most critical to general hospital inpatient psychiatry is the advent of prospective payment systems of reimbursement of costs. One example is the DRG (Diagnosis Related Group) reimbursement for Medicare, but the future will probably bring this form of reimbursement for most types of public and private insurance.

GENERAL PRINCIPLES OF INPATIENT REIMBURSEMENT SYSTEMS

A health care delivery system that is to meet the needs of people should provide for access to the system for those in need at a convenient site. The system should include accountability which includes service accountability (quality and volume) as well as fiscal accountability. However, the best health care delivery system that could be designed with respect to access and accountability is of little value if it cannot be financed. Hospitals need financing sufficient to maintain quality and stability of service and facilities as well as to provide a high level education for future health practitioners where needed.

Although the focus of this chapter is on the economics of inpatient psychiatry, since a hospital is a single economic unit it is difficult to focus exclusively on one segment of a hospital's operation. Specific decisions made with respect to inpatient reimbursement impact in often unpredictable ways on ambulatory care activities. The degree of impact is dependent on the related ambulatory care reimbursement system. The principles of reimbursement adopted for inpatient reimbursement, with future development, could be applied to ambulatory care reimbursement and result in a better coordinated system.

COST SHIFTING VERSUS COST ANALYSIS

In the past, the phrase "cost containment" has been interpreted in different ways. The use of the term by Medicaid or Medicare representatives is generally related to containing the costs of their particular programs, despite the fact that a "cost shifting" may occur to other programs. Costs can be contained in ways having no impact on a hospital's costs, such as shifting responsibility for costs to other payers or limiting benefits. On the other hand, cost containment efforts through a "cost analysis" process are not directed to any particular program. Ideally, benefits accruing from regulatory effort should be shared appropriately by all who utilize or pay for hospital inpatient services. There should be a certain degree of regulation and control in the hospital system. Voluntary cost containment efforts on the part of hospitals have had some measure of success. However, to leave complete control in the hands of an industry is an unacceptable approach to those responsible for cost containment. The best system may be one in which the parameters of operation are established by a regulatory agency in such a way that the system methodology provides positive incentives for hospitals to continue or initiate voluntary cost containment efforts. Another basic consideration is that reimbursement systems must be responsive to changing situations, needs, inequities, programs, resources, and many other external factors. The system should have the ability for change. In turn, hospitals should examine their internal procedures and their relationship with their communities so that they may provide vital acute health care services in the most efficient manner. The burden is placed on any regulatory agency to ensure a level of financing that will permit hospitals to provide these services at appropriate levels.

One goal in developing a reimbursement mechanism is to ensure that the system include methods of establishing equitable payment from all sources. For all practical purposes equitable payment from a hospital viewpoint is the receipt of proper reimbursement for the services it provides. From a charge-paying patient's viewpoint it is to pay a reasonable amount for the services received. From the third party payer's viewpoint it is to reimburse a hospital at an amount reflecting the cost of services provided to its beneficiaries or enrollees. The viewpoints of all three participants most directly involved in the reimbursement process are thus compatible with respect to "equitable payment." Given this overall viewpoint, the question becomes how proper and reasonable payments are to be determined.

ALLOWABLE, REASONABLE, AND JUSTIFIABLE COSTS

The general principle under which a cost analysis process operates is that hospitals should receive, and be limited to, reimbursement for costs that are determined to be allowable, reasonable, and justifiable in the efficient production of necessary services. The determination of whether a cost is allowable is related exclusively to the nature of the expense, as opposed to the amount. A broad general definition of allowable costs would include all costs that are incurred in the provision of inpatient services. Certain hospital expenses, such as fund raising, are not related to patient care and are not considered in the reimbursement process. Once the total allowable costs in a hospital have been identified the focus shifts to the next step in the process, which is to determine the reasonableness and justifiability of the amount of such costs. Reasonable costs are those allowable costs that have survived the cost analysis process by being lower than or equal to the cost standards developed to identify the efficient production of service. Justifiable costs are those allowable costs which exceed the standards developed but are justified as being a necessary cost in a specific hospital because of special acceptable circumstances. The definition or identification of "necessary inpatient service" is a consideration outside the reimbursement process or methodology, which is structured to implement these care-related considerations and decisions.

PEER GROUP COMPARISONS

A significant fact that any cost containment program must deal with is the wide and unexplained variations in hospital costs. An obvious regulator response is to develop the cost analysis system around cost comparisons among similar hospitals and not reimburse costs that exceed an acceptable level developed from the comparison. Basically, this approach follows the rationale that if a hospital can provide services at a certain cost per day or per discharge, then other similar hospitals should be able to do the same within reasonable boundaries. This approach is referred to as "peer group comparisons." An alternative to peer group comparisons in the cost analysis process is to develop cost standards from sources external to the hospital industry. This would require specific cost standards for direct and indirect costs to be applied to an individual hospital's costs incurred in providing needed direct and support services in meeting the treatment requirements of its inpatients. This is at present a formidable task when one considers the very limited data sources available outside of hospitals' current operations on which such standards could be based. Reimbursement limitations on a hospital's incurred costs must be based on reliable data and explicitly considered decisions. Failure to do so would result in a successful challenge by those adversely affected. Therefore, a peer group comparison system, properly developed with consideration and acceptance of differences in hospitals' operations, cases, specialties, and community responsibilities, is probably the best technique available for cost analysis at this time. It permits flexibility in that an in-depth cost analysis for certain costs can be initiated under an "exception" concept and, it provides a clarification as to why hospital costs vary within a standard economic region.

The original criteria used to identify "like" hospitals in which cost comparisons would be meaningful were hospital size, geographic area, and whether the hospital is teaching or non-teaching and sponsor (voluntary, proprietary, public). The assumptions leading to the use of those limited criteria were that hospitals of approximately the same size in the same geographic area having the same sponsorship generally provided the same services if differentiated as teaching or nonteaching hospitals. Any determination of reasonableness and justifiability demands a standard against which an individual hospital's costs can be measured, usually a peer group cost comparison methodology. In a peer grouping system, the comparable costs, after adjustment for wage and fringe differentials, of "like" hospitals are compared, and costs exceeding a group-developed norm are not eligible for reimbursement. The key elements in a peer grouping cost comparison system are (a) the criteria used in identifying like hospitals, (b) the identification of comparable costs, (c) the uniformity in the reporting system, and (d) the methodology used in adjusting hospital costs to reflect wage and fringe benefit differentials.

For all practical purposes, a peer grouping cost comparison system results in an industry-set standard and has been used in most hospital reimbursement formula having cost containment provisions. The rationale is that hospitals with similar service demands should incur similar costs when adjusted for certain acceptable cost differentials. In the identification of comparable cost, the prime consideration should be whether a particular cost is one incurred by all hospitals and would be expected to be incurred in a comparable amount when related to a unit of measure such as a day of care or a discharge. If the costs do not meet these two criteria, then a peer group comparison including such costs loses a certain amount of validity.

THE IMPORTANCE OF CASE MIX

Hospital costs are a product of the level of services rendered, the intensity of manpower, and the technology necessary to provide that level of service. Historically, the types and numbers of services per patient or hospital stay have been used to determine the case mix of a hospital. Case mix is a term used to describe patients by specialty service and type of clinical problem. Two hospitals could admit and discharge the same number of patients and yet show a wide disparity in costs due to the case mix.

It has been difficult to establish absolute values for case mixes that would accurately reflect costs. As a result, various characteristics of hospitals have been used to arrive at an approximate value. Some of the characteristics used are bed size, accreditation status, number of specialties, patient population, and presence of teaching programs. A significant difference in interhospital costs can be explained by the differences in the case mix.

Currently there is a two-step process to determine interhospital differences in case mix. The first step is to group hospitals on the basis of teaching status and/or bed size. Then ceilings are placed on reimbursement costs based on the group average. This ceiling is some percentage above the group average. This range between the ceiling and the group average is said to allow for differences in interhospital case mixes. If a hospital's costs are above the ceiling they are only reimbursed at the ceiling. As a result some hospitals have been overpaid while others have been underpaid.

There have been recent attempts to generate a more precise case mix measure. The measure must meet four basic criteria to be applicable. First, it must be derived from reliable and readily available data. The measure must be acceptable to physicians and understood by the hospital community. Lastly, the benefits of the measure must outweigh the costs.

Diagnosis Related Groups, or DRG's, is an attempt to provide a classification scheme for patients. DRG's see hospitals as multi-product companies whose line of products are numbers and types of patients treated. DRG's are based on the characteristics of the patients and not the hospitals. The length-of-stay of the patient is assumed to directly affect the type and quantity of resources consumed.

THE PROBLEM OF UNREIMBURSED CARE

Another major problem for all nonpublic hospitals which any reimbursement system must deal with is the loss of revenue from bad debts and from the costs of providing charity care. Hospitals should be viewed as business enterprises that can exist only if revenues are sufficient to meet necessary costs. All businesses sell merchandise or provide services to persons from whom they are unable to collect payment. After an approved collection process fails to generate payment from those determined able to pay for the services rendered the loss of revenue to the hospital should be considered a cost of doing business. Such losses are financed, as in any other industry, by an adjustment in prices to all others who utilize the services offered. Some believe that it is appropriate to segregate and treat differently the costs related to charity care. Charity care costs can be financed through a "pooled fund" approach, as is done in New York State. The size of the available pool is based on those state-wide health resources that are committed to care for the poor, who are not eligible for assistance in meeting medical needs.

The bad debt/charity care issue is a national issue that has demanded attention for some time. This is particularly true in view of proposals for inpatient revenue control systems that will affect a hospital's ability to provide services to the uninsured and poor. Hospitals are required by law to provide emergency services without reliance on ability to pay. In addition hospitals do incur bad debts and probably always will to some extent, even after adoption of aggressive collection procedures. To date, hospitals have depended principally on any surplus generated from charge-paying patients to offset the bad debt and charity care costs. This surplus may disappear under a prospective payment system.

The bad debt/charity care problem may be viewed as a community problem, as opposed to a hospital specific problem. Regional bad debt/charity care pools can be established through a common regional percentage to be included in each hospital's revenue and paid into the pool by each hospital. The pooled funds would then be distributed throughout the region on the basis of need in accordance with a system for identifying need. The intent is that each regional pool have sufficient funds to cover the same degree of need determined on a state-wide basis that is to be financed through this mechanism in any given year.

SOURCES OF FINANCING FOR INPATIENT PSYCHIATRY

An analysis of the historical development of the financing of the care of psychiatric inpatients in the United States has shown that the bulk of the funding has come from public sources. On the other hand, general medical care had developed most of its support through private sources, and indigent persons were cared for by philanthropic institutions or as charity cases in general hospitals.[11] Within psychiatry the state provided much of the public funding until the 1950's, as most of the inpatients were in state hospitals. As has been noted, by 1982 health care expenditures represented 10.5% of the gross national product, and approximately $40-50,000,000,000, or 15% of the total amount, was for mental health services. General hospitals utilize 13.7% of mental health funding, and this represents a balance of Federal, state, and private funding.

THE FEDERAL GOVERNMENT

The Federal government has long been a direct source of funding for inpatient psychiatric care through the Veterans Administration hospitals, which today represent 6.3% of national expenditures on mental health. We have traced the growth of Federal expenditures in mental health through the development of the Community Mental Health Act of 1963 and the implementation of Medicaid and Medicare legislation. Inpatient psychiatric services were one of the five essential mental health services, originally defined through the Community Mental Health Act, that a community mental health center must provide. Most of the inpatient services of these centers are provided in general hospital psychiatric units which are part of the CMHC's. By 1977, the Federal government had invested $1,500,000,000 in 650 community mental health centers.

MEDICAID

The Medical Assistance program (Medicaid), which was enacted at the same time as Medicare, has provided greater coverage of mental illness than has Medicare. The Medicaid program provides Federal matching funds to the states, and the matching rate is related to each state's per capita income. The Federal share runs from 50 to 77.55%. Medicaid prohibits states from refusing benefits on the basis of diagnosis. So eligible persons with a psychiatric diagnosis may receive the same services as all other types of patients under provisions of the various state plans, the one important exception being that no Federal funds are available for the care of persons between 21 and 65 in either a psychiatric hospital or a psychiatric skilled nursing home.

As has been analyzed, the Medicaid program has been a major source of revenue for mental health services in the past 20 years. Approximately 25% of the $16,300,000,000 Medicaid paid out nationwide went to mental health services, and 70% of those benefits were for inpatient care.[9] In the 1980's, the Federal government has been investigating ways of controlling its costs in the Medicaid program. Proposals include placing a cap on Federal spending on Medicaid, elimination of the requirement to pay reasonable costs, and a general tightening of eligibility for Medicaid services. In the future Medicaid may also adopt a prospective payment system of reimbursment of costs.

MEDICARE

Medicare was initiated in 1966 by Title XVIII of the Social Security Act to provide assistance to the elderly. The Senate Special Committee on Aging had discovered that one-quarter of the population over 65 had an income at or below the poverty line and that senior citizens commonly spent 30% of their income on health care. Initially, Medicare provided medical care benefits only for those 65 and older covered by Social Security, but in 1972, the program was amended to extend benefits to those over 65 who did not meet the criteria for the regular Social Security program but who were willing to pay a premium for coverage, and in 1972 the program was extended to cover the disabled and their dependents and those suffering from chronic renal disease. Hospital insurance is provided by Part A, and supplemental medical insurance is provided by Part B of Medicare. Part A is financed through a payroll tax and trust fund and is available to all persons over 65 and some disabled persons under 65, while Part B is a voluntary enrollment program in which the insured pays a monthly premium.

Part A provides coverage of inpatient services in a psychiatric hospital up to 190 days in a lifetime. Until 1983 the Federal government reimbursed hospitals for all medical, including psychiatric, services based on the reasonable cost basis of reimbursement, a retrospective system of payment. Thus, hospitals would submit their costs of caring for a patient, and the Federal government would reimburse them. The 1972 amendments to Medicare attempted to control costs by providing authorization to establish limits on institutional payments, generally, to the lesser of cost or charges, among other provisions. However, these cost control measures were ineffective, and in April 1983, Alice Rivlin, Director of the Congressional Budget Office, stated that the Hospital Insurance Trust Fund was in danger of bankruptcy and that the increased outlays of the Supplemental Medical Insurance were adding significantly to the deficit. So, Congress passed the Social Security Amendment of 1983, which included the substitution of a hospital prospective payment system for its former method of reimbursement.

PROSPECTIVE PAYMENT

In a prospective payment system, a determination is made in advance of the hospital providing a service as to what it will be paid. If a hospital spends more than it has been allocated, it endures financial loss, while if it spends less, it achieves a financial surplus. Under the new Medicare reimbursment system, the payments to hospitals are based on "diagnostically related groups." The DRG grouping decides on the amount of the patient's bill for hospital services in advance, reflecting the cost of treating an average patient in the DRG grouping. Determination of a specific DRG is based on the principal admitting diagnosis, a secondary diagnosis, age, sex, discharge status, and surgical procedures. Thus, a hospital can project its revenue for a year based on predicting the cases it will treat. There is a powerful incentive to reduce the cost of the services it provides.

There are a number of potential difficulties with this system of reimbursement. For instance, does a variation in cost between institutions represent differences in efficiency or differences in services provided, patients served, or quality of service? Inner city and teaching hospitals deal with more seriously ill patients and have additional expenses for teaching, research, and the development of new technology. Some of these concerns have been addressed by the inclusion of patient mix factoring.

When the DRG system was proposed, even more difficulties were foreseen in psychiatry. Diagnosis is a poor predictor of resource utilization for psychiatric patients. It is also important to note that the studies which influenced the development of the DRG system included very few psychiatric patients in the data base.

POTENTIAL CLINICAL AND SYSTEMIC IMPACT OF DRG's

The basic purpose of DRG's is to shift reimbursement from a provider-determined to a payer-determined system. The economic locus of control over patients and their treatment is taken away from physicians, who inevitably must respond to the forces of the reimbursement system. The potential impact of DRG's on actual clinical practice of psychiatry has been well reviewed by Ralph A. O'Connell M.D.[13] All aspects of psychiatric practice from the initial decision of whom to admit to the increasingly crucial importance of discharge planning and medical record keeping, will be affected. There will be intense pressure for hospitals to adopt selective admissions practices and engage in skimming of those patients with uncomplicated and prognostically favorable conditions while referring away those problematic cases that will require greater utilization

of resources to those medical centers mandated by law or public policy to accept all patients. It can be anticipated that diagnostic problems will arise from the fact that the DRG's derived from the ICD-9-CM of the World Health Organization, which differs in some respects from the DSM-III of the American Psychiatric Association. Economic incentives will influence diagnosis toward the higher paying DRG's, the so-called DRG creep, a practice which will be difficult to control by the customary chart review in the absence of any reliable external method of validating psychiatric diagnosis. The geometric and arithmetic means for length-of-stay in the DRG's are low and seem to be at variance with clinical experience. The time pressure will compromise the valuable practice of observation before making a definitive diagnosis and treatment plan. There will be a further erosion in the importance of psychotherapy as a valuable tool in the inpatient treatment of certain psychiatric conditions. Economic considerations will encourage a careful search for potential medical or surgical co-morbidities in view of the possibility of the greater financial return to the hospital from such combinations. There will be an emphasis on accelerated research for biological markers in psychiatry that might be useful indications of diagnostic states or predictors of treatment outcome. Hospitals will explore the possibility of acquiring or gaining administrative control over day hospitals, nursing homes, and community residences in a concerted effort to avoid prolonged hospitalizations for treatment-resistant patients. Many of these predicted consequences are due to the fact that DRG's, as presently constituted, have no measure of such environmental factors as stressors, the availability of social or family support, alternative community treatment resources, well-established after-care programs, or the need for post-discharge placement. Within the diagnostic group itself, no account is taken of severity of the illness, history of previous response to treatment, psychopathology, ego strengths, chronicity, compliance with treatment, or legal status. This is despite the fact that many clinicians and hospital administrators consider all of these variables to be highly predictive of length-of-stay and utilization of hospital resources.

Depending on the final form which DRG's take, a number of systemic consequences for the entire field of mental health care delivery can be anticipated. Goldman et al.[14] have presented such a possible scenario. Inequities in access to treatment for economically problematic groups such as the poor, children and adolescents, and the elderly may develop. Hospitals which offer long-term rehabilitative care to patients may disappear. Even in acute care hospitals, there will be a shift in favor of inpatient units with a biomedical-organic orientation and away from those with a psychosocial-reconstructive orientation. There will be an increase in the number of transfers of patients with complicated or resistant psychiatric problems from private facilities to government-sponsored inpatient facilities. Increased readmission rates for mental disorders may diminish the savings associated with the limited payments for the index hospital stay. New mechanisms of peer review and quality assurance will need to be developed to prevent the premature discharge of patients still acutely ill. The simultaneous existence of multiple systems for establishing payment rates will undoubtedly lead to increased administrative overhead. Cost shifting will result in an implicit increase in charges to all non-medicare beneficiaries in the short run. Future limitations on funding for psychaitric residency training could exacerbate the documented shortage of psychiatrists in the United States, and economic constraints on the practice of psychiatry could further dampen the interest of medical students in the field as a career choice.

Organized psychiatry responded to the predicted difficulties of implementing DRG's in their present form by addressing these problems to the Congress and obtaining a period of exemption to study the problems of DRG reimbursement unique to psychiatry and thus to help determine the best methods to introduce a better prospective payment system for psychiatric patients.[15] A task force of the American Psychiatric Association conducted a major study which confirmed that DGR's failed to explain a number of critical variables with regard to resource utilization by psychiatric patients.[16] The APA study confirmed the inaccuracy of the Medicare DRG system for psychiatric patients. This inaccuracy is much worse than for surgical patients and somewhat worse than for medical patients. Consistent with other studies, the APA study shows there is little relationship between a psychiatric DRG payment and the resources needed for patient treatment within that DRG. This lack of accuracy implies the absence of essential predictability and raised the possibility that hospitals would modify their admission and transfer practices in order to reduce financial risk.[17,18] It is clear that in this present and future period of financial retrenchment, the leaders of psychiatry must organize, as they have done in the past, and retain an active role in public policy and financial planning, and reaffirm psychiatry's roots as a medical specialty.

COMMUNITY PSYCHIATRY

Over the past 20 years, the Federal, state, and local governments have provided financing for a variety of community programs and direct financial support for chronic psychiatric patients which has helped enable chronic psychiatric patients to remain outside of state hospitals and thus to utilize the services of general hospital psychiatric units when needed. In 1974, Supplemental Security Income was introduced in which the Federal government provides basic monthly income to eligible patients. As states have transferred some of their mental health budgets away from state hospitals and to community programs a multitude of grant programs to localities has been established. One state which was an early pioneer in these efforts was New York, and the following are some examples of program financing. Community Support Services, introduced in 1977, receives 100% funding of net costs, and its goal is to coordinate service agencies in providing comprehensive and integrated mental health services. Under Demonstration Grants local governments and voluntary nonprofit agencies provide up to 80% of the development costs for community residential facilities while Community Residence Funds provide up to 50% of funds for the acquisition or construction of community residences for the mentally disabled. Yet, despite the amount of funds available the present development of community programs and residences for the mentally disabled meets only a small fraction of the need in this segment of care.

PRIVATE INSURANCE

Private insurance to cover the costs of hospitalization and physician's fees has grown from a single plan at Baylor Hospital in 1929 to cover teachers at the University of Texas to, in 1978, over 72,000,000 people being enrolled in Blue Cross plans. Eighty-five percent of the membership today is enrolled through group plans. Although coverage for outpatient mental health services has been quite limited, the already quoted figure of 63% of the civilian population (in a 1975 analysis) has some coverage for inpatient psychiatric care. Blue Cross and Blue Shield, private insurance companies, and the Federal government are scrutinizing methods of cost containment. There has been a dramatic increase in regulatory guidelines and activity in examining requests for reimbursement, and insurance companies may also eventually shift to a prospective payment system of reimbursement.

Health insurance organizations providing coverage for the costs of psychaitric care include Blue Cross-Blue Shield Plans, insurance companies, and independent plans such as commnunity, group, and individual pre-paid practice plans; self-insured employer-employee-union plans; and programs sponsored by private groups of physicians. The amount of protection provided to health insurance beneficiaries varies substantially according to the type of service and to the provisions of particular insurance programs from complete coverage to very little. A typical pattern for a contract covering employee groups is basic benefits for supplementary major medical coverage. Supplementary benefits apply when basic coverage has been exhausted or when they pay for a greater variety of services, such as private duty nursing and prescribed drugs. A second, less common, pattern may be a plan providing comprehensive coverage without the distinction between basic and supplementary benefits. Beyond the full payment under basic benefits, major medical programs usually pay 75-80% of charges for covered services after the payment of an initial deductible by the beneficiary. For group coverage, the employer usually pays part of or all of the premium costs. Individual policies with insurance companies and Blue Cross-Blue Shield are usually held by persons without affiliations which would entitle them to group coverage, or they may be purchased to supplement other forms of health insurance protection. Benefits under individual programs are usually less extensive than those under group policies, often being limited to basic coverage of hospital care and in-hospital physician's services. Because the independent plans exist under many arrangements, there is substantial variety in the ways they provide coverage and in the extent of the psychiatric benefits offered. Some operate their own facilities and employ medical personnel. Others pay hospitals, physicians, and other providers for services rendered under contract or on a fee-for-service basis. Self-insured employer-employee union plans provide psychiatric insurance protection through group and individual practice arrangements or major medical type of coverage.

UNFAVORABLE PROVISIONS FOR PSYCHIATRY

Although the role of private health insurance in financing medical health care is expanding, discrimination with regard to coverage for psychiatric disorders continues to represent a source of frustration to providers, who are attempting to deliver clinically indicated modalities of care in various treatment settings. This discrimination can also be an economic burden for the mentally ill and their families.

There were several factors contributing to the development and perpetuation of special circumstances surrounding insurance coverage for psychiatric disorders. During the period when health insurance programs covering large populations were developing there already was an established pattern of public responsibility for the care of the mentally ill. Until recently state and local government programs made few efforts to hold patients liable for the cost of their mental health care. Therefore subscribers and insurers have had little incentive to ensure coverage for services which were already financed through government expenditure. Moreover the demand for inclusion of mental health benefits in insurance programs, both from purchasers of group coverage and from beneficiaries, has been slow to develop. Public attitudes towards mental illness in the United States have generally become more enlightened as overall educational levels have increased, as well as through informational efforts by representatives of the mental health field. However, concern about the stigma attached to mental illness and reluctance to seek treatment persists, even when financial liability is not a factor. Many persons fear that the use of psychiatric services will adversely affect their employment status. Many also feel that mental health care is something they will never need. Thus, pressure on employers and, hence, on insurers to include psychiatric benefits has been less, particularly in comparison with other types of employee benefits, such as dental coverage. Employers, for their part, have only recently begun to recognize their employees' need for mental health care and the potential long-run economics in the form of increased worker productivity which may result from utilization of mental health services.

Insurers have pointed to the need to protect themselves against excessive costs by defining the risks being insured. In regard to psychiatric disorders, stereotypes of lengthy custodial care persist. There is continuing concern about lack of adequate criteria for and professional consensus in defining and verifying the existence and extent of mental disorders; determining the necessity of treatment, the appropriate modality, and the length of care required; and measuring significant improvement or recovery. Attempts to

verify information on particular cases may be met with refusal or reluctant compliance due to the need to maintain confidentiality. Often cited as evidence of insurers' concern are the experiences of a number of insurance companies in the early 1950's which provided outpatient coverage for psychiatric conditions on the same basis as for other illnesses. Heavy utilization and high cost to the insurers resulted. In these instances it was alleged that the high utilization largely represented psychotherapeutic services provided to a small number of beneficiaries who were not disabled, were employed and earning above average incomes, and were continuing to carry out their usual activities. This experience led to sharp restrictions on benefits for all types of psychiatric care which are still evident in many insurance programs.

Current approaches to psychiatric care, with its emphasis on community-based acute treatment, pharmacotherapy, and the expanding role of the general hospital in providing short-term inpatient care, have served to move mental health services toward the mainstream of medical care, wherein they may be considered insurable on a comparable basis with other types of health services. While there have been increases in the estimate of the number of people with some benefits for mental health services under private insurance in the United States, less is known about the extent of psychiatric benefits available to policy holders and to what degree these benefits are more limited than those for other types of illness. The mental health benefits provided by different types of insurance organizations and the provisions of specific plans offered by any one insurer vary widely. Differences exist among insuring organizations and policies, not only in number of days of care, visits, or other units of service provided but also in such areas as deductible and co-insurance requirements, definition of a hospital, types of facilities and practitioners covered, and inclusion of professional consultations, as opposed to treatment visits. Of special significance for mental health care are exclusions or limitations on coverage of services in facilities operated by branches of government. Despite these variations, examination of the mental health provisions of numerous plans offered by different types of private health insurance organizations reveals some general patterns of coverage.

Blue Cross-Blue Shield plans usually provide health insurance on a cooperative basis. Blue Cross plans cover hospital care, and affiliated Blue Shield plans offer medical benefits. The plans emphasize group coverage, although individual coverage is possible with less extensive benefits. All Blue Cross plans offer some hospitalization benefits for mental conditions, though there is significant diversity among the plans in the number of days of care provided. Blue Cross coverage for mental illness has generally lagged behind that offered by insurance companies, a circumstance related to the plan's traditional contractual relationship with general hospitals. Blue Cross plans generally reimburse hospitals on the basis of contracts with "member" hospitals. Although benefits are paid for care in non-member hosptials, they usually represent a smaller proportion of the charges. Some plans have requirements which hospitals must meet to become members which result in the exclusion of some mental hospitals. For this and other reasons not all psychiatric facilities are member hospitals. At the time that Blue Cross plans were organized in the 1930's and 1940's, most general hospitals had little, if any, capability for providing psychiatric care. The situation has gradually changed as many general hospitals now admit and treat psychiatric patients. Although extension of mental health benefits has been significant in the past 20 years, coverage for psychiatric disorder is seldom on the same basis as that for other illnesses. A common benefit for general illness under major group contracts is 120–125 days of care in a general hospital. For psychiatric disorders, 30 days is a common allowance. Care in private psychiatric hospitals is covered on the same basis as mental health care in general hospitals by most plans. However, some plans exclude coverage in private psychiatric hospitals. Further, for psychiatric disorders the designated number of days of care is often the maximum that will be covered in a specified time period, often 12 months,

whereas for other types of illness the coverage usually refers to days of care per admission. Coverage of physician's services for psychiatric disorders under basic benefits is often largely limited to in-hospital care. Basic Blue-Cross-Blue Shield benefits are often extended by various types of major medical contracts, usually offered jointly by affiliated Blue Cross-Blue Shield plans. These policies generally provide additional protection against cost of services covered by basic benefits, as well as providing for coverage of a wider variety of services. These policies usually pay 75 to 80% of charges for covered services after the patient pays an initial deductible.

Although discriminatory provisions against mental disorders in relation to other illnesses are still evident, there is a trend in group coverage toward comparable benefits for psychiatric disorders for inpatient hospital care and in-hospital physician's services, both under basic and major medical types of coverage. Individual insurance policies generally provide less extensive mental health benefits than group coverage. This is due to the fact that under individually written policies, adverse selection can be a considerable problem since those individuals most likely to require care may be more likely to purchase the coverage. In the majority of cases coverage for mental disorders is probably limited to hospitalization benefits, and these are likely to cover fewer days of care than inpatient benefits provided for general illness. Independent plans, which include community, group and individual prepaid practice plans, employer-employee-union plans, and private medical clinic programs, are diverse in organization and function, as well as in the types and extent of health insurance protection provided.

Experience data for individual insurance programs reflect utilization and costs under specific benefits structures which vary in types of services covered, amounts and extent of benefits, and requirements for cost sharing by the patient. In addition to the kinds and levels of benefits available, other factors affecting utilization under insurance programs include the age, sex, cultural, and socio-economic composition of the insured population and the availability and cost of alternative service providers in different geographic areas. Furthermore, the experience data do not document total utilization and costs for mental health services for some members of the covered population. Undoubtedly there were some subscribers whose requirements for care exceed the benefits, some to whom no covered provider was available or accessible, and some who were unaware or chose not to use the benefits available to them for various reasons. In addition, mental disorders are frequently treated under a general medical diagnosis because of presenting complaints for such conditions as gastritis and chronic alcohol abuse. Therefore, efforts to summarize and interpret experience data should be viewed with these qualifications in mind. Even with these considerations, it appears that hospital care for active treatment of mental conditions can be insured under basic benefits in the same context as that for other illnesses. Utilization of hospital care for mental conditions does not seem excessive. Experience data from insurers indicate that per capita charges for inpatient psychiatric services are likely to represent only a small fraction of those for all other medical conditions. While length-of-stay for mental disorders is, on the average, greater than that for other conditions, the per diem charges are usually less. Restrictions on insurance coverage for inpatient mental health care appear to stem largely from concern about the costs of long-term custodial care. As a result of this legitimate concern misconceptions about excessive duration and cost have continued, and unwarranted discriminations against mental health services have persisted. For patients with chronic psychiatric illness, as with other chronic conditions, it is important to differentiate between long-term treatment and custodial care. Although custodial care appropriately may be excluded from insurance coverage, benefits for inpatient treatment for mental disorders should be the same as those for any illness. The determining factor should not be the chronic nature of the illness but whether active treatment is involved. There is no justification for differentiating

between the benefits available for mental health care and those available for treatment of heart disease, diabetes, or other chronic medical conditions requiring continuing or periodic care on an inpatient basis.

When benefits for mental health care are expanded and the stigma associated with receiving treatment for mental disorders diminishes, an increase in insurers' cost attributable to psychiatric care probably will result. However, with psychiatric problems no longer masked under other diagnoses and with early detection and appropriate treatment of these conditions, it is also possible that such costs will be offset by reduced expenditures for care of other illnesses.

THE ACTIVE TREATMENT CONCEPT

Most third party payers expect that certain requirements be met before services furnished in a psychiatric hospital can be reimbursed. Generally the stipulation states that payment for inpatient psychiatric hospital services is to be made only for "active treatment." It thus becomes important for economic reasons to clearly distinguish between "active treatment" and "custodial care." For service in a psychiatric hospital to be designated as "active treatment" it must meet three conditions. First, the psychiatric services must be provided under an individualized treatment or diagnostic plan developed by a physician in conjunction with staff members of appropriate other disciplines on the basis of a comprehensive evaluation of the patient's restorative needs and potentialities. Thus, an isolated service such as a single session with a psychiatrist or a routine laboratory test not furnished under a planned program of therapy or diagnosis would not constitute active treatment, even though the service was therapeutic or diagnostic in nature. The plan of treatment must be explicitly recorded in the patient's medical record.

Secondly, the psychiatric service must reasonably be expected to improve the patient's condition or must be for the purpose of diagnostic study. It is not necessary that a course of therapy have as its goal the restoration of the patient to a level which would permit discharge from the institution, although treatment must, at a minimum, be designed both to reduce or control the patient's psychotic or neurotic symptoms which necessitated hospitalization and improve the patient's level of functioning. The kinds of service which would meet this requirement would include not only psychotherapy, drug therapy, and electroconvulsive therapy but also adjunctive therapies such as occupational therapy, recreational therapy, and milieu therapy, provided the adjunctive therapeutic services are expected to result in an improvement in the patient's condition. If, however, the only activities prescribed for the patient are primarily diversional, social, or recreational in nature, it would not be regarded as treatment to improve the patient's condition and would not be reimbursable. In many large psychiatric hospitals these adjunctive services are present and are part of the life experience of every patient. In a case where milieu therapy or one of the other adjunctive therapies is involved it is particularly important that this therapy be a planned program for the particular patient and not one in which life in the hospital is designated as milieu therapy. It is also noteworthy that the mere administration of a drug or drugs does not of itself necessarily constitute active treatment. Thus the use of mild tranquilizers or sedatives solely for the purpose of relieving anxiety or insomnia would not constitute active treatment, whereas the administration of antidepressant or tranquilizing drugs which are expected to significantly alleviate a patient's psychotic or neurotic symptoms would be considered active treatment.

Third, the psychiatric services must be supervised and evaluated by a physician. Physician participation is an essential ingredient of active treatment. The services of qualified individuals other than physicians, such as social workers, occupational therapists, or group therapists, must be prescribed and directed by a physician to meet the specific psychiatric needs of the individual. In short, the physician must serve as a source of information and guidance for all members of the therapeutic team who work directly with the patient in various roles. It is the responsibility of the physician to periodically evaluate the therapeutic program and determine the extent to which treatment goals are being realized and whether changes in direction or emphasis are needed. Such evaluations should be made on the basis of periodic consultations and conferences with other therapists, review of the patient's medical record, and regularly scheduled patient interviews. The treatment furnished the patient should be documented in the medical record in such a manner and with such frequency as to provide a full picture of the therapy administered as well as an assessment of the patient's reaction to it.

In certain instances, inpatient hospital services are reimbursable when a patient receives medical or surgical care in a psychiatric hospital but does not satisfy the requirements dealing with active psychiatric treatment. Such cases arise when a physician certifies that the medical or surgical service requires a hospital level of care and hospitalization in a psychiatric institution, rather than in a general hospital, is appropriate because of some factor related to the patient's medical condition. The patient's past history of psychiatric problems or the current psychiatric condition would furnish a proper basis for the exercise of medical judgment in concluding that admission to the psychiatric hospital is medically necessary.

ACKNOWLEDGMENTS

The authors wish to acknowledge the research assistance of Lonny J. Behar, M.D., resident in psychiatry at St. Vincent's Hospital and Medical Center of New York, in the preparation of this chapter.

REFERENCES

1. Goshen C: *Documentary History of Psychiatry: A Source Book on Historical Principles,* p. 478, New York, Philosophical Library, 1967.
2. Caplan RB: *Psychiatry and the Community in Nineteenth Century America,* pp. 4 and 26, New York, London, Basic Books, Inc., 1969.
3. Rothman DJ: *The Discovery of the Asylum: Social Order and Disorder in the New Republic,* pp. 270–282, Boston, Little, Brown, 1971.
4. Deutsch A: *The Mentally Ill in America,* pp. 158–178, New York, London, Columbia University Press, 1949.

5. Talbott JA: Deinstitutionalization: Avoiding disasters of the past. *Hosp & Community Psychiatry, 30* (9): 621–624, 1979.

6. Foley HA, Sharfstein SS: *Madness and Government. Who Cares for the Mentally Ill?*, pp. 17–28, Washington, D.C., American Psychiatric Press, 1983.

7. Brill H, Patton RE: Analysis of population reduction in New York State mental hospitals during the first four years of large-scale therapy with psychotropic drugs. *Am J Psychiatry,* 116: 495–508, 1959.

8. Kennedy J: Message from the President of the United States relative to mental illness and mental retardation. *Am J Psychiatry,* 120: 729–737, 1964.

9. English JT, Kritzler ZA, Scherl DJ: Historical trends in the financing of psychiatric services. Psychiatr Ann, *14* (5): 321–331, 1984.

10. Kellerman SL: Is deinstitutionalization working for the mentally ill. Testimony presented at the Public Hearing to Examine the Effectiveness of Treatment Programs for the Mentally Ill. City of New York, Dept. of Mental Health, Mental Retardation & Alcholism Serv., 1982.

11. Scherl DJ, English JT: Current trends in financing psychiatric services: The initial response of psychiatry to prospective payment. Psychiatr. Ann, *14* (5): 332–339, 1984.

12. Information from the New York State Office of Mental Health, 1984.

13. O'Connell RA: Time-limited treatment: The DRG challenge, in Schatzberg AF (ed): *Common Treatment Problems in Depression,* Washington, D.C., American Psychiatric Press, 1985.

14. Goldman HH, et al.: Prospective payment for psychiatric hospitalization: Questions and issues. *Hosp & Community Psychiatry, 35* (5): 460–464, 1984.

15. English JE: Proposals to establish a prospective payment system under Medicare, in *Economic Fact Book for Psychiatry,* Washington, D.C., American Psychiatric Press, 1983.

16. English JT, et al.: Diagnosis-related groups and general hospital psychiatry: The APA study. Am J Psychiatry, *143:* 131–139, 1986.

17. Taube CA, Lee ES, Forthofer RN. Diagnosis-related groups for mental disorders, alcoholism and drug abuse: Evaluation and alternatives. *Hosp & Community Psychiatry, 35:* 452–455, 1984.

18. Lave FG, Jr.: *The Psychiatric DRGs: Are They Different?, Med Care,* in press, 1985.

index